Fundamentals of

Applied
Pathophysiology

FOURTH EDITION

Fundamentals of
Applied Pathophysiology

An Essential Guide for Nursing and Healthcare Students

EDITED BY

IAN PEATE OBE FRCN

Principal
School of Health Studies
Gibraltar

WILEY Blackwell

Registered Office(s)
John Wiley & Sons, Inc., 111 River Street, Hoboken, NJ 07030, USA
John Wiley & Sons Ltd, The Atrium, Southern Gate, Chichester, West Sussex, PO19 8SQ, UK

Editorial Office
9600 Garsington Road, Oxford, OX4 2DQ, UK

For details of our global editorial offices, customer services and more information about Wiley products, visit us at www.wiley.com.

Wiley also publishes its books in a variety of electronic formats and by print-on-demand. Some content that appears in standard print versions of this book may not be available in other formats.

Limit of Liability/Disclaimer of Warranty
The contents of this work are intended to further general scientific research, understanding and discussion only and are not intended and should not be relied upon as recommending or promoting scientific method, diagnosis or treatment by physicians for any particular patient. In view of ongoing research, equipment modifications, changes in governmental regulations and the constant flow of information relating to the use of medicines, equipment and devices, the reader is urged to review and evaluate the information provided in the package insert or instructions for each medicine, equipment or device for, among other things, any changes in the instructions or indication of usage and for added warnings and precautions. While the publisher and authors have used their best efforts in preparing this work, they make no representations or warranties with respect to the accuracy or completeness of the contents of this work and specifically disclaim all warranties, including without limitation any implied warranties of merchantability or fitness for a particular purpose. No warranty may be created or extended by sales representatives, written sales materials or promotional statements for this work. The fact that an organization, website or product is referred to in this work as a citation and/or potential source of further information does not mean that the publisher and authors endorse the information or services the organization, website or product may provide or recommendations it may make. This work is sold with the understanding that the publisher is not engaged in rendering professional services. The advice and strategies contained herein may not be suitable for your situation. You should consult with a specialist where appropriate. Further, readers should be aware that websites listed in this work may have changed or disappeared between when this work was written and when it is read. Neither the publisher nor authors shall be liable for any loss of profit or any other commercial damages, including but not limited to special, incidental, consequential or other damages.

Library of Congress Cataloging-in-Publication Data

Names: Peate, Ian, editor.
Title: Fundamentals of applied pathophysiology : an essential guide for
   nursing and healthcare students / edited by Ian Peate.
Description: Fourth edition. | Hoboken, NJ : Wiley-Blackwell, 2021. |
   Includes bibliographical references and index.
Identifiers: LCCN 2021003661 (print) | LCCN 2021003662 (ebook) |
   ISBN 9781119699491 (paperback) | ISBN 9781119699545 (Adobe PDF) |
   ISBN 9781119699477 (epub)
Subjects: MESH: Pathologic Processes | Nursing Care–methods |
   Physiological Phenomena
Classification: LCC RB113 (print) | LCC RB113 (ebook) | NLM QZ 140 | DDC
   616.07–dc23
LC record available at https://lccn.loc.gov/2021003661
LC ebook record available at https://lccn.loc.gov/2021003662

Cover Design: Wiley
Cover Image: © Stocktrek Images/Getty Images

Set in 10/12pt MyriadPro by SPi Global, Pondicherry, India
Printed and bound by CPI Group (UK) Ltd, Croydon, CR0 4YY

C9781119699491_280824

This text is dedicated to my late sister,
Maureen Ann Paterson (nee Peate).

Contents

Preface   *viii*
Acknowledgements   *x*
Contributors   *xi*
About the companion website   *xv*

Chapter 1 **Learning the language: Terminology**   **1**

Chapter 2 **Cell and body tissue physiology**   19

Chapter 3 **Homeostasis**   49

Chapter 4 **Cancer**   64

Chapter 5 **Inflammation, immune response and healing**   96

Chapter 6 **Shock**   130

Chapter 7 **The nervous system and associated disorders**   153

Chapter 8 **The heart and associated disorders**   185

Chapter 9 **The vascular system and associated disorders**   217

Chapter 10 **The blood and associated disorders**   252

Chapter 11 **The renal system and associated disorders**   290

Chapter 12 **The respiratory system and associated disorders**   322

Chapter 13 **The gastrointestinal system and associated disorders**   361

Chapter 14 **Nutrition and associated disorders**   398

Chapter 15 **The endocrine system and associated disorders**   428

Chapter 16 **The reproductive systems and associated disorders**   464

Chapter 17 **Pain and pain management**   500

Chapter 18 **The musculoskeletal system and associated disorders**   539

Chapter 19 **Fluid, electrolyte balance and associated disorders**   566

Chapter 20 **The skin and associated disorders**   593

Chapter 21 **The ear, nose and throat, and eyes, and associated disorders** 623

Appendix A: Reference values in venous serum (adults)   654
Index   657

Preface

The fourth edition

Being in a position to write the preface for the fourth edition of *Fundamentals of Applied Pathophysiology: An Essential Guide for Healthcare Students* is an absolute privilege. We have listened to feedback from a wide range of sources. This edition brings with it a number of changes; however, we have tried to retain the user-friendly approach that readers tell us they enjoy.

I have introduced a series of new activities, including website activities, that are intended to help you learn in an engaged way and to apply your learning when you are in the care setting, wherever this may be. This edition has been updated; the pathophysiology and important issues related to care have been reviewed. The illustrations are there to assist in understanding and appreciating the complex conditions that are being discussed. By using a fundamental approach to the subject, this can help readers acquire a key understanding of applied pathophysiology.

This edition retains its nursing and healthcare focus and considers the wider context of care provision. An essential requirement for those who offer care and support to people in contemporary care environments is an integrated, multidisciplinary approach. The healthcare student is an important participant within the multidisciplinary care team. In this book, a multidisciplinary approach is acknowledged as well as the recognition that care is delivered in dynamic environments to a diverse groups of people and communities.

This text has been written with the intention of making the subject of pathophysiology understandable and stimulating. Our bodies have astonishing capacity as they respond to illness in a number of physiological and psychological ways; we are able to compensate for the changes that occur as result of the disease process, the pathophysiological processes and the impact they can have on a person. This text can help in developing critical thinking, encouraging innovation and creativity in relation to the health and well-being of the people that you have the privilege to care for.

New features have been added, along with two new chapters: *Learning the Language* and *Homeostasis*. These two chapters are provided earlier on in the text so as to help prepare the reader for some of the more complex discussions to follow. Each chapter concludes with questions that aim to trigger reflection and encourage further thought. In the snapshots (case studies), pseudonyms are used to maintain confidentiality. Nurses and those who offer care owe a duty of confidentiality to all those they care for (Nursing and Midwifery Council, 2018).

Where appropriate, we have included boxed information that will help you when you are providing care. Red flags are incorporated that contain significant information alerting you to be cautious in your approach, and orange flags alert the reader to psychological considerations and also information regarding the management of medicines as related to the chapter.

The snapshots have been developed further and usually include data concerning the patient's vital signs and blood analysis. This can help relate important concepts to care, offering more insight into the patient's condition and therefore needs. Some of the snapshots include a NEWS2 score (national early warning score) where applicable (Royal College of Physicians, 2017).

Many of the values cited are a range, and blood pressure in respect of the NEWS2 score is noted as systolic. Local policy and procedure should be adhered to when using NEWS2.

Although an elevated blood pressure is an important risk factor for cardiovascular disease, it is low or falling systolic blood pressure that is most significant in the context of assessing acute illness severity. We have adopted the Royal College of Physician's (2017) stance on this parameter related to a range of systolic blood pressure.

Each chapter provides questions that are there to test your pre- and post-knowledge. There are a range of self text multiple choice questions at the end of each chapter. Selected chapters provide a list of further resources that the reader may wish to access in order to increase and advance learning.

Pathophysiology considers the cellular and organ changes that occur when disease is present, as well as the effects these changes have on the ability to function. When something interrupts normal physiological functioning, such as illness, this then becomes a pathophysiological issue. It must always be remembered that normal health is not and can never be exactly the same in any two people, and as such the term *normal* has to be treated with caution. An understanding of pathophysiology 'normal' and 'abnormal' can assist the student help the patient in a competent, compassionate safe and effective manner.

This text is a foundation text that can help the reader grow personally and professionally with regards to the provision of care, and is primarily intended for nursing students who come into contact with those who may have a number of physical healthcare problems, in the hospital and community setting. The text focuses on the adult person. Illness and disease are discussed explicitly, highlighting the fact that people do become ill and they do experience disease.

You need not read the text from cover to cover, you are encouraged to dip in and out of it. The aim is to entice and encourage you, whet the appetite, so you may read further, and in so doing we hope to instil a sense of curiosity in you. The first six chapters set the scene, and you may want to think about reading these first and then move on to a more specific area of interest.

We have enjoyed putting this new edition together, and we truly hope that you enjoy reading it and applying it to practice situations.

Ian Peate
Gibraltar
March 2021

References

Nursing and Midwifery Council (2018). *The Code. Professional Standards of Practice and Behaviour for Nurses, Midwives and Nursing Associates* https://www.nmc.org.uk/globalassets/sitedocuments/nmc-publications/nmc-code.pdf last accessed June 2020.

Royal College of Physicians (2017). *National Early Warning Score (NEWS) 2 standardising the assessment of acute illness severity in the NHS* https://www.rcplondon.ac.uk/projects/outputs/national-early-warning-score-news-2 last accessed January 2021.

Acknowledgements

Thank you to all of my colleagues, who have been so supportive in providing their expertise and time contributing to this new edition of this well-established text. I am grateful to you all for your commitment, particularly during the COVID-19 pandemic. I would like to also thank those who contributed to chapters in the previous edition.

I would like to thank my partner, Jussi Lahtinen, for his support and encouragement and my dear friend Mrs Frances Cohen.

Thank you to all of my colleagues, who have been so supportive in providing their expertise and time contributing to this new edition of this well-established text.

Contributors

Jim Blanchflower, BSc Pharmacology, PGCE, MSc (Health Practice)
Senior Lecturer, School of Nursing and Midwifery, University of Salford, Manchester, UK

Jim Blanchflower is lecturer in physiology, pharmacology and pathophysiology in the School of Nursing and Midwifery at Salford University.

He has been involved in educating healthcare professionals for over 25 years. This includes advanced practitioners, nurses, midwives, pharmacists and physiotherapists.

He has several publications in the area of non-medical prescribing, and has presented at conferences for non-medical prescribing, sepsis and antibiotic resistance.

He also works with strength athletes, particularly powerlifters, helping them to upgrade their performance by improving training practices and nutrition. He is the president of the North-West Powerlifting Federation.

Carl Clare, RN DipN, BSc (Hons), MSc (Lond), PGDE (Lond)
Programme Lead MSc Nursing, Senior Lecturer, Department of Adult Nursing and Primary Care, School of Health and Social Work, University of Hertfordshire, Hatfield, Hertfordshire, UK

Carl began his nursing career in 1990 as a Nursing Auxiliary. He later undertook three years of student nurse training at Selly Oak Hospital (Birmingham), moving to The Royal Devon and Exeter Hospitals, then Northwick Park Hospital, and finally The Royal Brompton and Harefield NHS Trust as a Resuscitation Officer and Honorary Teaching Fellow of Imperial College (London). Since 2006, he has worked at the University of Hertfordshire as a Senior Lecturer in Adult Nursing. His key areas of interest are long-term illness, physiology, sociology and cardiac care. Carl has previously published work in cardiac care, resuscitation and pathophysiology.

Louise Henstock, BSc (Hons) Physiology, BSc (Hons) Physiotherapy, MSc Sports & Exercise Management, SFHEA, PGCAP, HCPC, MSCP
Lecturer & Admissions Tutor, School of Health and Society, University of Salford, Greater Manchester, UK; Visiting Lecturer Cambridge University, Cambridge, UK

Louise began her career at St. James's University Hospital, Leeds, before becoming a senior musculoskeletal physiotherapist working at Leeds General Infirmary. She has worked as a physiotherapy lecturer since 2003, initially at York St. John University, gaining her master's degree in Sports and Exercise Management and a Postgraduate Certificate in Academic Practice. She moved to the University of Salford in 2010, where she is currently employed as a physiotherapy lecturer and admissions tutor. Her key areas of interest are musculoskeletal physiotherapy and physiology. In 2017, Louise was awarded Best Teacher in the Health School & Best Overall Teacher at Salford University, and was also the winner of a VC Distinguished Teaching Award in 2014. In 2017, Louise became a Senior Fellow of the Higher Education Academy. Louise has also guest-lectured at the University of Cambridge.

Barry Hill MSc, Advanced Practice, PGC Academic Practice, BSc (Hons) Intensive Care Nursing, DipHE Adult Nursing, O.A. Dip Counselling Skills, Registered Nurse (RN), Registered Teacher (NMC RNT/TCH); Senior Fellow (SFHEA), Programme Leader (Senior Lecturer) Adult Nursing, Northumbria University, Clinical Editor *British Journal of Nursing*
Director of Employability, Department of Nursing, Midwifery and Health,
Programme Leader, BSc (Hons) Adult Nursing, Northumbria University, Newcastle upon Tyne, UK

Barry Hill leads and teaches on a range of undergraduate and postgraduate healthcare-related programmes. Clinically, Barry worked at Imperial College NHS Trust across all three adult intensive care units including neuro, trauma, cardiac and general critical care, whilst undertaking a clinical master's degree in advanced practice. Prior to joining Higher Education, Barry was Matron for Plastics Orthopaedics ENT and Major Trauma division, managing and leading the ENT, Airway, Head and Neck and Plastics, including breast surgery.

Barry has been awarded a GEM Award (Going the Extra Mile) in 2019, Northumbria University; 2019 Finalist – 'Educator of the Year 2019' Student Nursing Times Awards; 2018 Student Led Teachers Award (SLTA) Winner of the 'Best Lecturer Award 2018' Northumbria University; and 2009 'Outstanding Service Care & Research Awards OSCAR' (Clinical Education), Imperial College. Barry is Clinical Series Editor for *British Journal of Nursing* (*BJN*) and on the editorial board. Barry has published books, book chapters, and academic journal articles. He is currently studying a Doctor of Philosophy (PhD) at Northumbria University in his third year.

Noleen P. Jones, EN, RN, DipN, Dip Management, BSc, FHEA
Principal Lecturer (Ag), School of Health Studies, Gibraltar

Noleen began her nursing career as a Nursing Auxiliary in 1987 before training to be an Enrolled Nurse, eventually qualifying as a Staff Nurse in 1992. She worked in Critical Care as a newly qualified Registered Nurse until 2013, where she held the posts of Senior Sister and Lead Nurse for Education and Training before she moved into practice development for a year. It was during this time that Noleen's links to the School of Health Studies strengthened. Noleen became a Lecturer with the School of Health Studies in Gibraltar in 2014. Her key interests are cardiac care, respiratory care and teaching practice skills.

Claire Leader, PGCAP, MA, BSc (Hons), RN, RM, HFEA
Senior Lecturer (Adult Nursing), Nursing, Midwifery & Health, Northumbria University, Newcastle upon Tyne, UK

Claire began her nursing career in 1998 after graduating from York University. Between 1998 and 2003, Claire worked as an Emergency Nurse in the UK as well as overseas before commencing her Midwifery education and obtaining a

first class honours degree at the University of Huddersfield. Claire practised as a midwife in large tertiary referral centres in Sheffield and Newcastle upon Tyne before taking on the role of Research Nurse & Midwife in 2009. During this time Claire worked closely with Principal Investigators in the development and delivery of research sponsored by the National Institute of Health Research (NIHR) in a number of specialties whilst also studying part time for the Masters in Sociology and Social Research, for which she received a distinction. In 2018, Claire moved to her current post at Northumbria University, teaching on programmes of education within the department of Nursing, Midwifery and Health as well as developing research as part of collaborations and through her own PhD on workforce well-being.

Louise McErlean, RGN, BSc (Hons), MA (Herts)
Lecturer, Department of Nursing, School of Health and Social Work, Ulster University, Northern Ireland, UK

Louise is a lecturer in Nursing at Ulster University. Louise commenced her nursing career in Glasgow in 1986, specialising in Intensive Care Nursing. Louise has worked in Glasgow, Belfast, London and Hertfordshire. Louise moved to Higher Education in 2005 and has taught on anatomy and physiology, pathophysiology and skills modules within adult nursing. Her interests include physiology, clinical skills, simulation and nurse education.

Janet G. Migliozzi, DMS, RGN, BSc (Hons), MSc (London), PGDEd, PGCMed.Sim, FHEA
Senior Lecturer, Department of Nursing, Health and Wellbeing, School of Health and Social Work, University of Hertfordshire, Hatfield, Hertfordshire, UK

Janet completed her initial training in London and commenced her career in 1988. She has worked at a variety of hospitals across London, predominantly in vascular, orthopaedic and high-dependency surgery before specialising in infection prevention and control and communicable disease. Janet has worked in higher education since 1999 and is involved in teaching across a range of healthcare professions programmes both at an undergraduate and postgraduate level. She is also involved in the research supervision of students undertaking advanced clinical practice pathways. Her key interests include clinical microbiology, particularly in relation to healthcare-associated infections, global communicable disease and public health. Patient safety at the local and global levels is also an area of interest. Janet has published in journals and books in areas including immunology, minimising risk in relation to healthcare-associated infection and pathophysiology.

Valerie Nangle, MPhil, FHEA, RGN
Assistant Professor, Coventry University (London), Spitalfields, London, UK

Prior to becoming a nurse educator teaching students on undergraduate nursing courses, she worked in coronary care and high-dependency units in London before specialising and practising for 20 years as a cardiac rehabilitation and secondary prevention nurse specialist.

Valerie's academic clinical research interests are concerned mainly with migrant health and inequalities in health focusing on the health of refugees and asylum seekers. Her academic research areas of interest include nursing students with dyslexia and disabilities experiences within clinical practice areas. She continues to practice clinically, and volunteers with a migrant health clinic and as a cardiac nurse consultant with the Irish diaspora in the UK, focusing on primary prevention of coronary heart disease and hypertension.

Ian Peate, OBE, FRCN
Visiting Professor St George's University of London and Kingston University, London, Visiting Professor Northumbria University, Visiting Senior Clinical Fellow University of Hertfordshire, Head of School, School of Health Studies, Gibraltar

Ian began his nursing a career at Central Middlesex Hospital, becoming an Enrolled Nurse practicing in an intensive care unit. He later undertook three years of student nurse training at Central Middlesex and Northwick Park Hospitals, becoming a Staff Nurse and then a Charge Nurse. He has worked in nurse education since 1989. His key areas of interest are nursing practice and theory. Ian has published widely. He is the editor-in-chief of the British Journal of

Nursing. He was awarded an OBE in the Queen's 90th Birthday Honours List for his services to Nursing and Nurse Education and was bestowed a Fellowship from the Royal College of Nursing in 2017.

Hazel Ridgers, RN (Adult), PGCAP, MA, FHEA
Freelance Lecturer and Researcher in Nursing and Health, London, UK

Hazel trained as a Nurse with King's College, London, and took up her first staff Nurse post in older people's care at Guys and St Thomas' hospital in 2006. She developed an interest in the health and well-being of older people living with HIV, and undertook sexual health and HIV specialisation courses early in her nursing career. She has worked in HIV and sexual health as a nurse, research nurse and clinical teacher. Hazel began her career in nursing education in 2010 working in both clinical practice and higher education settings with a focus on clinical skills, simulation and sexual health. Hazel was the lead for a Nursing Associate programme and is currently a freelance lecturer and researcher in Nursing and Public Health.

Melanie Stephens, PhD
Senior Lecturer in Adult Nursing and Head of Interprofessional Education, School of Health and Society, University of Salford, Manchester, UK

Melanie is a health service researcher and member of the Ageing and Dementia Hub with specific research interests in pressure redistributing properties of seating, postural management, tissue viability and interprofessional working. She has undertaken research in order to provide an evidence base for products used in the 24-hour management of pressure ulcers and postural care. She co-led an amendment to the UK Tissue Viability Guidelines for Seating 2017 with service users. She is experienced in using qualitative and mixed methods of enquiry, working with practitioners and commerce to develop research for the use in the clinical environment. Prior to becoming a nurse educator, Melanie worked as a Tissue Viability Nurse Specialist. She has also held nursing posts in Intensive Care, Burns and Plastics Surgery, Gynaecology Oncology, Endocrinology and Care of older adult ward.

Anthony Wheeldon, MSc (Lond), PGDE, BSc (Hons), DipHE, Registered Nurse (RN)
Associate Subject Group Lead for Adult Nursing, Department of Adult Nursing and Primary Care, School of Health and Social Work, University of Hertfordshire, Hatfield, Hertfordshire, UK

Anthony began his nursing career at Barnet College of Nursing and Midwifery in 1992. After qualification, he worked as a staff nurse and senior staff nurse in the Respiratory Directorate at the Royal Brompton and Harefield NHS Trust in London. In 2000, he started teaching on post-registration cardio-respiratory courses before moving into full-time nurse education at Thames Valley University in 2002. Anthony has a wide range of interests including the promotion of inclusivity, success and attainment in nurse education, as well as cardio-respiratory care, anatomy and physiology, respiratory assessment, and the application of bioscience in nursing practice. Since 2006, Anthony has worked at the University of Hertfordshire, where he teaches on pre- and post-registration nursing courses. He is currently an Associate Subject Group Lead for Adult Nursing.

About the companion website

This book is accompanied by a companion website:

www.wiley.com/go/fundamentalsofappliedpathophysiology/student4e

The student website includes:

- Interactive multiple choice questions
- Interactive true/false exercises
- Searchable glossary
- Further reading and resources

The instructor website includes:

www.wiley.com/go/fundamentalsofappliedpathophysiology/instructor4e

- Image Bank
- PowerPoint slides

Chapter 1

Learning the language: Terminology

Ian Peate

Principal, School of Health Studies, Gibraltar

Contents

Introduction 2
Anatomy and physiology 2
Terminology 8
Pathophysiology... 13
The determinants of health 14
Using a nursing/medical dictionary:
   hints and tips... 15

Searching for definitions on the
   Internet and hand-held devices...............16
Conclusion 16
Multiple choice questions.............................17
Further resources..18
References..18

Key words

- Terminology
- Anatomy
- Physiology
- Pathophysiology
- Latin
- Greek
- Prefix
- Suffix
- Word roots
- Forms

Fundamentals of Applied Pathophysiology: An Essential Guide for Nursing and Healthcare Students, Fourth Edition. Edited by Ian Peate.
© 2021 John Wiley & Sons Ltd. Published 2021 by John Wiley & Sons Ltd.
Student companion website: www.wiley.com/go/fundamentalsofappliedpathophysiology/student4e
Instructor companion website: www.wiley.com/go/fundamentalsofappliedpathophysiology/instructor4e

- What do you understand by the term *prefix*?
- What do you understand by the term *suffix*?
- How is the root word altered by a prefix or a suffix?
- List the anatomical planes.

Learning outcomes

On completion of this chapter the reader will be able to:

- Discuss the terms *anatomy*, *physiology* and pathophysiology

- Further understand prefixes and suffixes used in anatomy, physiology and pathophysiology

- Understand directional terms

- Describe the anatomical planes, anatomical regions of the body and the body cavities

Don't forget to visit the companion website for this book (www.wiley.com/go/fundamentalsofappliedpathophysiology/student4e) **where you can find self-assessment tests to check your progress, as well as lots of activities to practise your learning.**

Introduction

The terms used in science, especially in nursing and medicine, are saturated with Latin and Greek terminology. Latin names are used for every part of the body, and Greek terms are common since the Greeks are said to be the founders of modern medicine. All healthcare professionals use pathophysiology as they work with the people whom they offer care to and offer treatment for those who are experiencing some type of health condition.

Anatomy and physiology

Anatomy is concerned with the study of the structure and location of body parts, and physiology is the study of the function body parts; these two terms are interlinked. Knowing where the body parts are located can help you understand how they function. McGuiness (2010) explains that thinking of the numerous functions of the heart and the four chambers along with the valves (this is the anatomy) and visualising these various structures can help in comprehending how blood flows through the heart and how the heart beats (this is related to its function and therefore its physiology).

Anatomy

The body map

Learning anatomical terminology is like learning a new language and can help you talk confidently about the body; the anatomical directional terms and body planes present a universally recognised anatomical language. When undertaking the study of anatomy and physiology, it is essential that you have a key or directional terminology in order to give you an accurate description as you or others refer to the precise location of a body part or structure.

All parts of the body are described in relation to other body parts, and a standardised body position known as the anatomical position is used in anatomical terminology. An anatomical position is established from an imaginary line that runs down the centre or mid-line of the body. When in this position, the body is erect and faces forward with the arms to the side, the palms face forward with the thumbs to the side and the feet are slightly apart with the toes pointing forward.

The standard body 'map' or anatomical position (just like a map) is that of the body standing upright (orientated with north at the top), with the feet at shoulder width and parallel, toes forward (see Figure 1.1); humans are bilaterally symmetrical. This position is used to describe the body parts and positions of patients irrespective of whether they are lying down, lying on their side or facing down.

As well as understanding the anatomy and the physiology (the structure and function), understanding directional terms and the positions of the various structures is also necessary. Table 1.1 lists common anatomical descriptive terms that you will need to become acquainted with.

Figure 1.2 depicts anatomical positions.

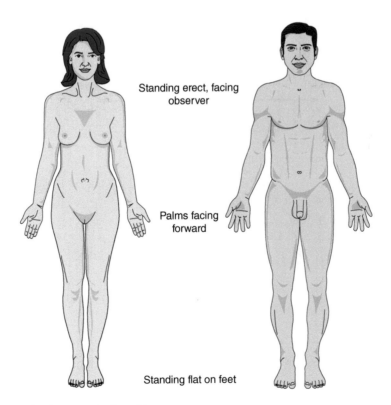

Standing erect, facing observer

Palms facing forward

Standing flat on feet

Figure 1.1   Standard anatomical position.

Table 1.1 Anatomical descriptive terms.

Anatomical term	Relationship to the body
Anterior	Front surface of the body or structure
Posterior	Back surface of the body or structure
Deep	Further from the surface
Superficial	Close to the surface
Internal	Nearer the inside
External	Nearer the outside
Lateral	Away from the mid-line
Median	Mid-line of the body
Medial	In the direction of the mid-line
Superior	Located above or towards the upper part
Inferior	Located below or towards the lower part
Proximal	Nearest to the point of reference
Distal	Furthest away from the point of reference
Prone	Lying face down in a horizontal position
Supine	Lying face up in a horizontal position

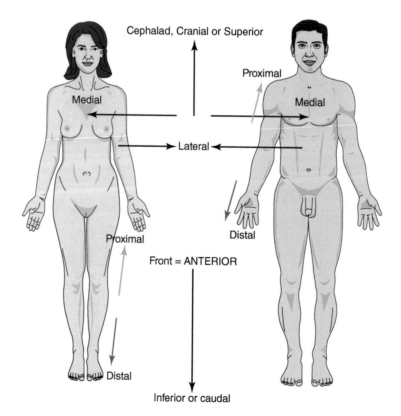

Figure 1.2 Directional anatomical positions.

Anatomical planes of the body

A plane is an imaginary two-dimensional surface that passes through the body. There are three planes that are generally referred to in anatomy and healthcare (see Figure 1.3):

- Sagittal
- Frontal
- Transverse

The sagittal plane, the vertical plane, is the plane that divides the body or an organ vertically into the right and left sides. If this vertical plane runs directly down the middle of the body, it is known as the midsagittal, or median, plane. If it divides the body into unequal right and left sides, then it is called a parasagittal plane.

The frontal plane is the plane dividing the body or an organ into an anterior portion and a posterior portion. The frontal plane is often referred to as a coronal plane (the word *corona* is Latin for 'crown').

The transverse plane divides the body or organ horizontally into the upper (superior) and lower (inferior) portions.

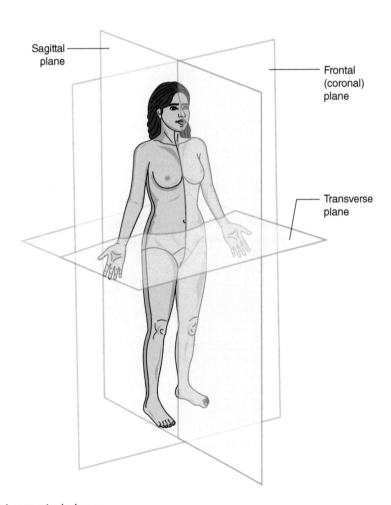

Sagittal plane

Frontal (coronal) plane

Transverse plane

Figure 1.3   Anatomical planes.

Anatomical regions of the body

The body is divided up into regions, like a map, and the anatomical regions of the body refer to a particular area/region of the body, which helps to compartmentalise the body. The body is divided into the following:

- Head and neck
- Trunk (thorax and abdomen)
- Upper limbs (arms)
- Lower limbs (legs).

Tables 1.2, 1.3, 1.4, and 1.5 present the correct terminology for each region.

Body cavities

Body cavities are spaces within the body that contain the internal organs. The cavity can be filled with air or with organs. Minor body cavities include the oral cavity (mouth), the nasal

Table 1.2 Anatomical regions of the head and neck.

Anatomical term	Area of body related to
Cephalic	Head
Cervical	Neck
Cranial	Skull
Frontal	Forehead
Occipital	Back of head
Ophthalmic	Eyes
Oral	Mouth
Nasal	Nose

Table 1.3 Anatomical regions of the trunk (thorax and abdomen).

Anatomical term	Area of body related to
Axillary	Armpit
Costal	Ribs
Mammary	Breast
Pectoral	Chest
Vertebral	Backbone
Abdominal	Abdomen
Gluteal	Buttocks
Inguinal	Groin
Lumbar	Lower back
Pelvic	Pelvis/lower part of abdomen
Umbilical	Navel
Perineal	Between anus and external genitalia
Pubic	Pubis

Table 1.4　Anatomical regions of the upper limbs.

Anatomical term	Area of body related to
Brachial	Upper arm
Carpal	Wrist
Cubital	Elbow
Forearm	Lower arm
Palmar	Palm
Digital	Fingers (also relates to toes)

Table 1.5　Anatomical regions of the lower limbs (legs).

Anatomical term	Area of body related to
Femoral	Thigh
Patellar	Front of knee
Pedal	Foot
Plantar	Sole of foot
Popliteal	Hollow behind knee
Digital	Toes (also relates to fingers)

cavity, the orbital cavity (eye), middle ear cavity and the synovial cavities (these are spaces within the synovial joints).

There are two main cavities in the body:

1. The dorsal cavity is located in the posterior region of the body.
2. The ventral body cavity occupies the anterior region of the trunk.

The dorsal cavity is subdivided into two cavities:

1. Cranial cavity: Encloses the brain and is protected by the cranium (skull)
2. Vertebral/spinal cavity: Contains the spinal cord and is protected by the vertebrae

The ventral cavity is subdivided into the following:

1. The thoracic cavity: It is surrounded by the ribs and muscles, the intercostal muscles. The thoracic cavity contains the lungs, heart, trachea, oesophagus and thymus. It is separated from the abdominal cavity by the diaphragm.
   The abdominopelvic cavity:
   a. The abdominal cavity: Contains the stomach, spleen, liver, gallbladder, pancreas, small intestine and most of the large intestine. The abdominal cavity is protected by the muscles of the abdominal wall and partly by the diaphragm and ribcage
   b. The abdominopelvic cavity: Contains the urinary bladder, some of the reproductive organs and the rectum
   The pelvic cavity is protected by the bones of the pelvis.
   Figure 1.4 depicts the body cavities.

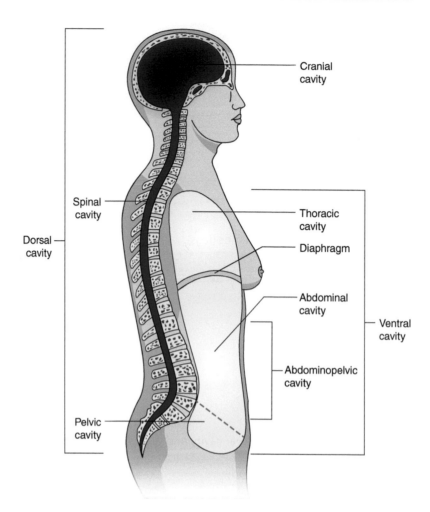

Figure 1.4   The cavities of the body.

Physiology

Human physiology concerns itself with the study of the body's function. Anatomy and physiology therefore are the study of the structure and the function of the human body, respectively.

The human body is organised in a most precise way whereby atoms combine in appropriate ways forming molecules in the chemical organisation of the body. The molecules combine to form cells and cells organise themselves collectively as functioning masses that are known as tissues and then organs and systems. Chapter 2 of this text describes cells and the organisation of tissues within the body

Terminology

Already in this chapter you may have come across some complex terms. It is important to learn the language (the terminology) that is used in the provision of healthcare; this is an important part of safe and effective care. Whilst it is not a pre-course requirement to be proficient in Latin or Greek in order to learn anatomical terminology to become a nurse or healthcare practitioner, it is essential that you understand and are able to use the terminology.

There are three basic parts associated with medical terms; see Table 1.6.

The word *root* is the core of the word and provides the basic meaning to the subject of the word; the prefixes and the suffixes modify the word. In the word *hepatitis*, for example, the word root is *hepa*, which means liver. When the suffix 'itis' ('itis' means inflammation) is added, then this changes the word root, and it becomes *hepatitis* – inflammation of the liver.

Word roots act as the foundation for most medical terms and often (but not always) describe the part of the body that is involved (see Figure 1.5).

Table 1.6   Basic components.

Component	Description
Word root	This is usually found in the middle of the word and is its central meaning
Prefix	The prefix comes at the beginning of the word and usually identifies some subdivision or part of the central meaning
Suffix	This comes at the end of the word and modifies the central meaning as to what or who is interacting with it or what is happening to it

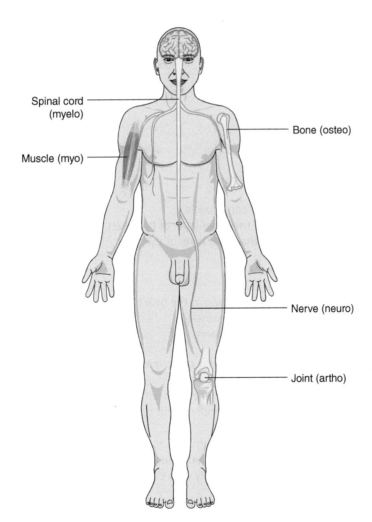

Figure 1.5   Word roots are the foundation of most medical terms and describe the part of the body involved.

The prefix is added to the beginning of the word root and also changes the meaning of the word. If the root word is *nutrition* and the prefix 'mal' is added (this means bad), then *malnutrition* means bad or poor nutrition.

Look at this example:

Hypothermia

The word root is 'therm' (heat)

'Hypo' means low (this is the prefix)
Hypothermia = low heat

Take a look at this word:
myocarditis
Now let us break this up:

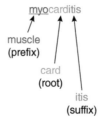

myocarditis

muscle
(prefix)

card
(root)

itis
(suffix)

myo	card	itis	Inflammation of heart muscle
Muscle	Heart	Inflammation	

The prefix can change the word:

Myocarditis = inflammation of heart muscle
Endocarditis = inflammation of the inner layer of the heart
Pericarditis = inflammation of the outer layer of the heart

The suffix can also alter the word:

Cardiologist = a practitioner specialising in the heart
Cardiomyopathy = damage to heart muscle
Cardiomegaly = enlargement of the heart

In these examples, the prefix and suffix can change the meaning of the word but, the root *cardio* stays the same.

There are many frequently used prefixes and suffixes, and you will already know some of them. See Table 1.7 for a list of some prefixes and suffixes that are used in a number of medical terms.

As is the case when learning any language, it can take time to learn all the words, and indeed, the learning may be lifelong. When you are in practice, you will be able to reinforce your learning, using your new vocabulary with confidence. Take your time, seek clarification if needed and be patient with yourself.

Knowing the various anatomical terms can make it easier to understand the various pathophysiological concepts that can help you provide care that is patient centred, safe and effective.

Table 1.7 Some prefixes, suffixes, their meaning and examples.

Prefix/suffix	Meaning	Example
a/an	No, not, without, lack of	Anoxia (without oxygen), anuria (without urine), asepsis (without sepsis), asymptomatic (without symptoms)
ab	Away from	Abduction (to move away from the mid-line), abnormal (away from normal)
ad	Towards	Adduction (to move towards the mid-line), adrenal (towards the kidney), addiction (drawn towards or a strong dependence on a drug or substance)
aemia	Of blood	Leukaemia (cancer of blood cells), anaemia (lack of red blood cells)
algia	Pain	Cephalgia (headache), mastalgia (breast pain), myalgia (muscle pain)
ante	Before/in front of	Antepartum (before birth), anterior (to the front of the body), anteprandial (before meals)
arthro	Joint	Arthroscope (an instrument used to look into a joint), arthritis (joint inflammation), arthrotomy (incision of a joint)
baro	Pressure/weight	Isobaric (having equal measure of pressure), bariatrics (the field of medicine that offers treatment to people who are overweight), baroreceptor (a sensor reacting to pressure changes)
brady	Slow/delayed	Bradycardia (slow heart rate), bradykinesia (slowness in movement), bradylalia (abnormally slow speech)
cyto	Cell	Leucocyte (white blood cell), erythrocyte (red cell), cytology (study and function of cells)
derm	Skin	Dermatitis (inflammation of the skin), dermatome (a surgical instrument used for cutting slices of the skin), dermatology (the study of skin)
dys	Difficulty/impaired	Dysphasia (difficulty swallowing), dyspepsia (disordered digestion), dysuria (difficulty in urination)
ectomy	To cut out	Appendicectomy (removal of the appendix), mastectomy (removal of the breast), prostatectomy (removal of the prostate)
endo	Inner	Endocardium (lining of the heart), endocarditis (inflammation of the heart), endotracheal (within the trachea)
erythro	Red	Erythrocyte (red blood cell), erythropaenia (reduction in the number of red blood cells), erythema (reddening of the skin)
haem	Blood	Haematogenesis (the formation of blood), haematology (the study of blood), haemarthrosis (bleeding within the joint)
hydro	Water	Hydrophobia (abnormal dread of water), hydrocephalus (accumulation of fluid within the cranium)
hyper	Above/beyond/excessive	Hypertension (high blood pressure), hyperflexion (movement of a muscle beyond its normal limit), hyperglycaemia (high blood glucose)
hypo	Below/under/deficient	Hypotension (low blood pressure), hypothermia (low temperature), hypoglycaemia (low blood glucose)
intra	Within	Intravenous (within the veins), intraocular (within the eye), intracerebral (within the brain)
ism	Condition/disease	Hirsutism (heavy/abnormal growth of hair), hyperthyroidism (overactivity of the thyroid gland)
itis	Inflammation	Appendicitis (inflammation of the appendix), mastitis (inflammation of the breast), myocarditis (inflammation of heart muscle)
macro	Large	Macroscopic (large enough to be seen with the naked eye), macrocytic (an abnormally large cell), macroglossia (an abnormally large tongue)

(Continued)

Table 1.7 (*Continued*)

Prefix/suffix	Meaning	Example
mega/megaly	Enlarged	Cardiomegaly (enlarged heart), splenomegaly (enlarged spleen), hepatomegaly (enlarged liver)
micro	Small	Microscopic (so small can only be seen with a microscope), microcephaly (small brain), microsomia (small body)
myo	Muscle	Myocardium (heart muscle), myocyte (muscle cell), myometrium (uterine muscle)
neo	New	Neonate (new born), neoplasm (new growth [tumour]),
nephro	Kidney	Nephritis (inflammation of the kidneys), nephrostomy (an incision made into the kidney)
neuro	Nerve	Neuroma (a tumour growing from a nerve), neuralgia (pain felt along the length of a nerve), neuritis (inflammation of a nerve)
ology	Study of	Dermatology (study of the skin), neurology (study of the nervous system), cardiology (study of the heart)
oma	Tumour (swelling)	Melanoma (a cancer of melanocytes), carcinoma (a type of cancer), retinoblastoma (tumour of the eye)
ophth	Eye	Ophthalmology (study of the eye), ophthalmoscope (an instrument used to examine the inside of the eye), ophthalmotomy (an incision made into the eye)
osteo	Bone	Osteomyelitis (bone infection), osteosarcoma (bone cancer), osteoarthritis (inflammation of the joints)
ostomy	To make an opening (a mouth)	Colostomy (an opening into the colon), jejunostomy (an opening into the jejunum)
otomy	To cut into	Tracheotomy (cutting into the trachea), craniotomy (a hole made into the skull), thoracotomy (cutting into the chest)
oto	Ear	Otology (study of the ear), otosclerosis (abnormal bone growth inside the ear)
para	Beside/alongside	Parathyroid (adjacent to the thyroid), paraumbilical (alongside the umbilicus)
patho	Disease	Neuropathy (disease of the nervous system), nephropathy (disease of the kidney), retinopathy (disease of the retina)
penia	Deficiency	Leucopoenia (deficiency of white cells), thrombocytopenia (deficiency of thrombocytes)
peri	Around	Pericardium, (the serous membrane around the heart) periosteum, (a covering enveloping the bones), peritoneum (the serous membrane lining the walls of the abdominal and pelvic cavities)
plasm	Substance	Plasma (liquid part of blood and lymphatic fluid), cytoplasm (substance of a cell lying outside of the nucleus)
plasty	Repair	Arthroplasty (surgical repair or replacement of a joint), myoplasty (muscle surgical repair of a muscle)
pneumo	Breathing/air	Pneumonia (a type of chest infection), pneumothorax (a collapsed lung), pneumograph (a device used for recording respiratory movement)
poly	Many/much	Polycystic (many cysts), polyuria (much urine), polyarthritis (arthritis affecting more than four joints)
rhino	Nose	Rhinitis (inflammation of the mucous membrane of the nose), rhinoplasty (surgical repair of the nose)
rrhoea	Discharge	Diarrhoea (frequently discharged faeces), rhinorrhoea (excessive discharge of mucus from the nose), galactorrhoea (excessive production of breast milk)

(*Continued*)

Table 1.7 (*Continued*)

Prefix/suffix	Meaning	Example
sclero	Toughen/hard	Sclera (hard/tough layer of the eyeballs), scleroderma (hardening and contraction of the skin and connective tissue), sclerosis (abnormal hardening of body tissue)
sub	Under	Sublingual (underneath the tongue), subarachnoid (underneath the arachnoid [layer of the brain]), submucosa (tissue below mucus membrane)
tachy	Fast/rapid	Tachycardia (fast heart rate), tachypnoea (fast respiratory rate),
toxo	Poison	Cytotoxic (having a destructive action on cells), toxaemia (blood poisoning resulting from the presence of toxins), ototoxic (being toxic to the ear)
uria	Urine	Haematuria (presence of blood in the urine), nocturia (passing urine at night), pyuria (pus in the urine)
vaso	Vessel	Vasoconstriction (narrowing the vessel), vasodilation (widening of the vessel), vasospasm (sudden contraction of a vessel)

Pathophysiology

Pathophysiology brings together a blend of pathology and physiology that considers the connection between disordered physiology and disease or illness. Pathology defines the illness itself, and physiology examines how these injuries or diseases change natural biological processes. The study of pathophysiology requires the use of clinical reasoning that is then used to make a diagnosis and prescribe treatment to address the effects of disease. Learning how pathology, physiology and anatomy interconnect can ensure that care provided is appropriate, safe and effective.

A number of terms and definitions are used that are related to pathophysiology (see Table 1.8).

Table 1.8 Terms and definitions related to pathophysiology.

Term	Definition
Pathology	Study of structural alterations in cells, tissues and organs that helps to identify the cause of disease
Pathogenesis	Pattern of tissue changes that are associated with the development of disease
Aetiology	Study of the cause(s) of disease and/or injury
Idiopathic	These are diseases with no identifiable cause
Iatrogenic	Diseases and/or injury that occur as a result of medical (or nursing) intervention
Clinical manifestations	Also known as signs and symptoms
Nosocomial	Diseases that are acquired as a consequence of being in a hospital environment
Diagnosis	The naming or identification of a disease
Prognosis	Expected outcome of a disease
Acute disease	Sudden appearance of signs and symptoms that last a short time
Chronic disease	Develops more slowly, lasting a long time or a lifetime
Remissions	Periods when clinical manifestations disappear or diminish significantly
Exacerbations	Periods when clinical manifestations become worse or more severe
Sequelae	Any abnormal conditions that follow on and are the result of a disease, treatment or injury

Pathophysiology, according to Singh *et al*. (2017), is the study of the changes of normal mechanical, physical, and biochemical functions, caused by a disease or resulting from an abnormal syndrome. The chapters in this text address these key pathophysiological concepts. Medical terminology is used to express and describe the various pathophysiological concepts.

Pathophysiology is a key component of nursing practice, enabling the healthcare practitioner to take on a number of important responsibilities, such as understanding and ordering diagnostic tests, caring for and treating people with acute and chronic illnesses, managing medications and managing general health and well-being as well as disease prevention for patients and their families. Nurses and other healthcare practitioners who can recognise the pathophysiological signs and symptoms of the conditions of those whom they offer care to will be able to provide a higher quality of safer and effective care. Asking questions such as 'why is the person experiencing this?' helps one understand what is going on in a person's body at the cellular level, helping you decide how to help them.

Pathophysiology is used to understand the progression of disease so as to identify the disease and implement treatment options for patients. Information gathered is used to identify the next course of the disease so that the most suitable course of action can be provided to the patient with the appropriate care they need. The medical procedures and medications that are administered to patients will depend very much on the nature of the disease. The main objectives when understanding pathophysiology is to assist you to:

- Use critical thinking to understand the pathophysiological principles for care provision.
- Analyse and explain the effects of disease processes at a systemic and cellular level.
- Discuss the many variables that may be at play affecting the healing of the organ and tissue systems.
- Analyse the environmental risks of the progression and development of particular diseases.
- Explain how compensatory mechanisms can be used to make a response to physiological alterations.
- Compare and contrast the effects of culture, ethics and genetics and how these can have an impact on disease progression, treatment and health promotion as well as disease prevention.
- Evaluate and review diagnostic tests and determine if the evaluation and review have any relationship to the signs and symptoms that the patient is experiencing

The determinants of health

Whilst it is important to understand the pathophysiological changes that a patient may be experiencing, the healthcare provider must also appreciate the socio-economic and cultural factors that can impact patient outcomes. These 'non-medical' factors are as important as whether the most appropriate test or diagnostic tool is being used or treatment prescribed. It is important to understand the molecular and genetic determinants of disease; however, the non-biological factors have potential influence interactions with patients and their families.

There are many factors that come together to impact the health of individuals and communities. Regardless of whether people are healthy or not, health is determined by a person's circumstances and environment. To a large extent, factors such as where we live, the state of our environment, genetics, our income and education level, and our relationships with friends and family all have significant impacts on health. However, the more commonly considered factors, for example, access and use of healthcare services, may have less of an impact. The social determinants of health are outlined in Figure 1.6. The determinants of health include political, social, economic, environmental and cultural factors which shape the conditions in which we are born, grow, live, work and age. Creating a healthy population requires greater action on these factors, not simply on treating ill-health.

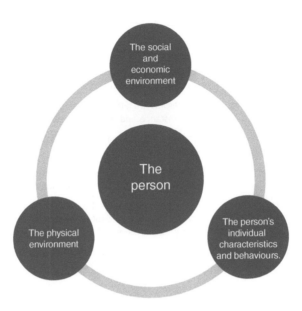

Figure 1.6   The determinants of health *Source:* World Health Organization, 2020.

Using a nursing/medical dictionary: hints and tips

Learning to use a nursing or medical dictionary and other resources (be these electronic or hard copy) to help find the definition of a term is an important aspect of understanding the correct use of the numerous medical terms. When starting to work with an unfamiliar resource (print or otherwise), spend some time reviewing its user guide. The time spent at this stage can help later when you are looking up unfamiliar terms.

Accuracy in spelling medical terms is extremely important, Changing just one or two letters has the potential to completely change the meaning of a word, and the consequences of this can be grave. Some frequently used terms and word parts are confusing because they look and sound alike; however, their meanings are very different (see Table 1.9). Beware, you may encounter alternative spellings used in England, Australia, Canada and the United States of America.

If you know how to spell the word

- With the first letter of the word, start in the appropriate section of the dictionary. Look at the top of the page for clues (there may be catch words there). The top left word is the first term on the page, and the top right word is the last term on that page.
- Now, search alphabetically for words that begin with the first and second letters of the word you are searching for. Continue looking through each letter until you have found the term that you are looking for.
- When you think you have found it, be sure to check the spelling, letter by letter, working from left to right. Terms with similar spellings have very different meanings (for example, prostrate and prostate).
- When the term has been located, carefully check all of the definitions.

If you do not know how to spell the word

Listen carefully to the term and then write it down. If you cannot find the word on the basis of your spelling, begin to look for alternative spellings based on the beginning sound; for

Table 1.9 Confusing terminology.

Term/word	Means	Comments
arteri/o	Artery	*Endarterial* means pertaining to the interior or lining of an artery ('end-' means within, *arteri* means artery, and '-al' means pertaining to).
ather/o	Plaque or fatty substance	An atheroma is a fatty deposit within the wall of an artery (*ather* means fatty substance, and '-oma' means tumour).
arthr/o	Joint	*Arthralgia* means pain in a joint or joints (*arthr* means joint, and '-algia' means pain).
-ectomy	Surgical removal	An appendicectomy is the surgical removal of the appendix (*append* means appendix, and '-ectomy' means surgical removal).
-ostomy	Surgical creation of an artificial opening to the body surface	A colostomy is the surgical creation of an artificial excretory opening between the colon and the body surface (*col* means colon, and '-ostomy' means the surgical creation of an artificial opening).
-otomy	Cutting or a surgical incision	A colotomy is a surgical incision into the colon (*col* means colon, and '-otomy' means a surgical incision).

Source: Stansfield *et al.,* 2015.

example, F can sound like F but, the word may begin with PH (such as pharynx, phlegm), K can sound like K, but the word may begin with CH (cholera, for example) or C (crepitus). Psychologist begins with P, but it sounds as though it should begin with an S.

Look under categories

Medical dictionaries may use categories such as diseases and syndromes so as to group disorders with these terms in their titles:

- Venereal disease would be found under Disease, venereal.
- Fetal alcohol syndrome would be found under Syndrome, fetal alcohol.

Multiple-word terms

When searching for a term that includes more than one word, begin the search with the last term. If you do not find it there, then move forward to the next word. Congestive heart failure, for example, is sometimes listed under heart failure, congestive.

Searching for definitions on the Internet and hand-held devices

Internet search engines are helpful resources in locating definitions and details about medical conditions and terms. It is important, however, that you use websites such as the National Institute for Health and Care Excellence (NICE) or Scottish Intercollegiate Guidelines Network (SIGN), which are known to be reputable information sources.

Beware of suggested search terms. If you do not spell a term correctly, a website might take a guess at what it is that you are searching for. Be sure to double-check that the term you are defining is the term intended.

Conclusion

Medical terminology can sometimes seem very intimidating and complicated, as many terms used in nursing and medicine are derived from Latin and Greek terminologies. In order to understand the terminology used, it is essential when learning to break it down into its parts so that you can see how it all fits together – like the carriages of a train. In translating medical terms, it is important to understand the word root (the foundation of the term), which can have a prefix and suffix attached to it.

In order to communicate safely with other healthcare professionals, it is imperative that the language being used is consistent, so as to reduce any risk of confusion. Learning the language requires practice.

It is vital to understand the pathophysiological changes that a patient may be experiencing so as to provide the most appropriate care intervention. It is equally important to have an understanding of the impact of socio-economic and cultural factors that can impact on patient outcomes, the 'non-medical' factors.

Activities

Here are some activities and exercises to help test your learning. For the answers to these exercises, as well as further self-testing activities, visit our website at **www.wiley.com/go/fundamentalsofappliedpathophysiology/student4e**

Multiple choice questions

1. A vagotomy is:
   (a) The surgical removal of the vagina
   (b) A surgical procedure that cuts one or more branches of the vagus nerve
   (c) A medical procedure that causes menopause
   (d) A specific test to determine type of deafness
2. Lymphadenopathy refers to:
   (a) Radical remove of all lymph glands
   (b) Removal of lymph glands in the axilla
   (c) Any disorder of the lymph nodes or lymph vessels
   (d) Infection of the lymph nodes
3. True or false: Haemostasis is the same as homeostasis
4. What is the difference between the word prostate and prostrate?
5. The term affect means
   (a) Loss of memory
   (b) Lack of feelings
   (c) The feeling experienced in connection with an emotion
   (d) None of the above
6. The dorsal cavity is located in the:
   (a) Lower aspect of the brain
   (b) Anterior region of the trunk
   (c) Posterior region of the body
   (d) None of the above
7. The term cubital relates to:
   (a) the foot
   (b) the head
   (c) the abdomen
   (d) the elbow

8. The abdominal cavity contains:
   (a) the stomach, spleen, liver, gall bladder, pancreas, small intestine and most of the large intestine
   (b) the stomach, spleen, liver, urinary bladder, pancreas, small intestine and most of the large intestine
   (c) the stomach, spleen, liver, gall bladder, pancreas, ovaries, small intestine and most of the large intestine
   (d) the stomach, spleen, liver, gall bladder, pancreas, testes, small intestine and most of the large intestine

9. The abdominopelvic cavity contains:
   (a) the gall bladder, some of the reproductive organs and the rectum
   (b) the urinary bladder, the stomach, some of the reproductive organs and the rectum
   (c) the urinary bladder, some of the reproductive organs and the rectum
   (d) the urinary bladder, spleen, some of the reproductive organs and the rectum

10. True or false:
    The pelvic cavity is protected by the vertebrae.

11. Chronic disease is said to:
    (a) Develop more slowly and lasts for a long time
    (b) Is incurable
    (c) Appears suddenly and lasts a short time
    (d) is only associated with the older person

12. The term hepatomegaly refers to:
    (a) an enlarged brain
    (b) enlarged spleen
    (c) an enlarged kidney
    (d) an enlarged liver

13. An arthroplasty is:
    (a) surgical repair of an artery
    (b) surgical repair or replacement of a joint
    (c) another term for a coronary artery bypass
    (d) surgical intervention used to relieve arterial obstruction

14. True or false:
    The frontal plane is the plane dividing the body or an organ into an anterior portion and a posterior portion.

15. True or false
    The prefix come at the beginning of the word.

Further resources

National Health Services (2018). *Abbreviations Commonly Found in Medical Records*. https://www.nhs.uk/using-the-nhs/nhs-services/the-nhs-app/abbreviations/ last accessed February 2020.
National Institute for Health and Care Excellence (NICE) www.nice.org.uk.
Scottish Intercollegiate Guidelines Network (SIGN) www.sign.ac.uk.

References

McGuiness, H. (2010). *Anatomy and Physiology: Therapy Basics*, 4th edn. London: Hodder Education.
Singh, I., Weston, A., Kundur, A. and Dobie, G. (2017). *Haematology Case Studies with Blood Cell Morphology and Pathophysiology*. London: Academic Press Elsevier.
Stansfield, P., Hui, Y.H. and Cross, N. (2015). *Essential Medical Terminology*, 4th edn. Chicago: Jones and Bartlett.
World Health Organization (2020). *Health Impact Assessment*. https://www.who.int/hia/evidence/doh/en/ last accessed February 2020.

Chapter 2

Cell and body tissue physiology

Anthony Wheeldon

*Senior Lecturer, Department of Adult Nursing and Primary Care,
School of Health and Social Work, University of Hertfordshire, Hatfield, Hertfordshire, UK*

Contents

Introduction 20
Anatomy of the cell 21
The cell membrane..22
Cytoplasm 27
Role of cytoplasm...27
Nucleus 27
Mitosis and meiosis 28

The organelles 32
Types of cells 35
Tissue repair 42
Conclusion 43
Multiple choice questions..............................44
Glossary of terms...45
References...48

Key words

- Plasma membrane
- Organelles
- Connective tissue
- Passive transport
- Nucleus
- Cell cycle
- Muscle tissue
- Active transport
- Cytoplasm
- Epithelial tissue
- Nervous tissue
- Bulk transport

Fundamentals of Applied Pathophysiology: An Essential Guide for Nursing and Healthcare Students, Fourth Edition. Edited by Ian Peate.
© 2021 John Wiley & Sons Ltd. Published 2021 by John Wiley & Sons Ltd.
Student companion website: www.wiley.com/go/fundamentalsofappliedpathophysiology/student4e
Instructor companion website: www.wiley.com/go/fundamentalsofappliedpathophysiology/instructor4e

Test your knowledge

- What are the three main parts of a human cell?
- Describe the structure and function of a human cell.
- Describe the phases of a cell cycle.
- Make a list of the major cellular organelles.
- Name the four tissue types, and explain the differences between them.

Learning outcomes

On completion of this chapter, the reader will be able to:

- Outline the structure and function of a human cell.

- List and describe the functions of the organelles.

- Explain the phases of a cell cycle.

- Explain the cellular transport system.

- Describe the structure and function of epithelial tissue, connective tissue, muscle tissue and nervous tissue.

- Explain the process of tissue repair (inflammation).

Don't forget to visit the companion website for this book
(www.wiley.com/go/fundamentalsofappliedpathophysiology/student4e)
where you can find self-assessment tests to check your progress, as well as lots of activities to practise your learning.

Introduction

To understand the human body and how it works (and also how it fails to work properly), it is important to understand the anatomy and physiology of the cell. Living organisms show wide diversity as regards their size, shape, colour, behaviour and habitat. In spite of this, however, there are many similarities between organisms, and this fundamental similarity is known as the 'cell theory'. This theory states that all living organisms are composed of one or more cells and the products of cells. Despite the fact that the cells belong to different organisms, and cells within the same organism may have different functions, there are many similarities between them. For example, there are similarities in their chemical composition, their chemical and biochemical behaviour and in their detailed structure.

All cells have many characteristics, but these characteristics can differ from cell to cell, such as the following:

- Cells are able to carry out certain specific functions, i.e. they are active.
- Cells need to consume food to live and to carry out their functions. Although they do not have mouths, they are still able to 'catch' and digest their food and use it for growth and

reproduction. The correct term for this is *endocytosis* – they surround and engulf organisms such as bacteria and digest them.

- Cells can grow and repair.

- Similarly, cells can reproduce themselves. They do this by a process known as simple fission. This means that they reproduce themselves by dividing into two, and then each new cell grows to its full size before it divides by simple fission, and so on. In other words, cells replicate themselves.
- Like humans, cells can become irritable if something upsets or stimulates them.
- The nutrition that cells take in is also used for the storage and release of energy (just like humans), thus enabling them to grow and repair themselves.
- Similarly, just as humans do not utilise all the food they eat – some of it cannot be used and so is excreted – cells excrete what they do not need or cannot use.
- Just as all humans will eventually die, so will cells. Some have a short life, whilst others survive many years – but eventually they will die.

So, cells are not all that different from humans in many respects. They do what humans do – albeit in different ways.

Anatomy of the cell

Each cell has a structure that is almost as complex as the human body (Figure 2.1). For example, each cell contains as many molecules as the body has cells. There is no such thing as a typical cell. However, each cell is surrounded by a membrane and contains protoplasm. This protoplasm consists of a nucleus, which is kept separate from the rest of the cell by a nuclear membrane (although the nuclear membrane disappears during the process of cell division), and an

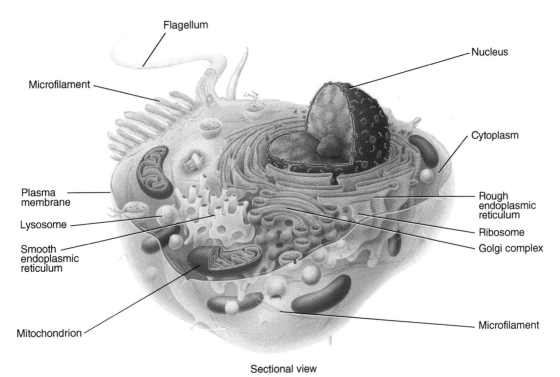

Sectional view

Figure 2.1   Simplified structure of a cell.

opaque substance called cytoplasm (Watson, 2005). The cells themselves consist of water, proteins, lipids, carbohydrates and various ions such as potassium (K$^+$) and magnesium (Mg^{2+}). Within the cytoplasm, there are also many complex protein structures called organelles.

Cells vary in size from 2 to 20 µm. For example, a lymphocyte (a type of blood cell) is about 8–10 µm in diameter.

All the cells in the body, apart from those on the surface of the body, are surrounded by a fluid that is known as extracellular fluid (i.e. fluid outside of the cell).

The cell membrane

The cell membrane can vary from 7.5 to 10 nm in thickness. It acts just like a 'skin' that protects the cell from the outside environment. In addition, it regulates the movement of water, nutrients and waste products into and out of the cell.

The cell membrane is made up of a double layer (bilayer) of phospholipid (fatty) molecules with protein molecules interspersed between them (Figure 2.2). A phospholipid molecule consists of a polar 'head' which is hydrophilic (water loving) and 'tails' which are hydrophobic (water hating). The hydrophilic 'heads' are attracted to water and are found on the inner and outer surfaces of the cell (water is the main component of both extracellular and intracellular environments), whilst the hydrophobic 'tails' are found in the middle of the cell membrane where they can avoid water. These phospholipid molecules are arranged as a bilayer with the heads facing outwards. This means that the bilayer is self-sealing. It is the central part of the plasma membrane, consisting of the hydrophobic 'tails', that makes the cell membrane impermeable to water-soluble molecules, and so prevents the passage of these molecules into and out of the cell (Marieb and Keller, 2017). However, if the membrane consisted of just these phospholipid molecules, then cells would not be able to function – within the cell membrane, there are also plasma membrane proteins (PMPs), which can be either integral or peripheral.

Some of the integral PMPs are embedded amongst the tails of the phospholipid molecules, whilst others penetrate the membrane completely (Figure 2.2). Subunits of some of these integral proteins can form channels which allow for the transportation of materials into and out of the cell. Other subunits are able to bind to carbohydrates to form receptor sites. These receptor sites are important, as will be discussed in Chapter 5 titled 'Inflammation, Immune Response and Healing'.

Peripheral PMPs bind loosely to the surface of the cell membrane and so can be easily separated from it. Some of them function as enzymes to catalyse cellular reactions, whilst others are receptors for hormones and other chemicals, or function as binding sites for attachment to other structures (Marieb and Keller, 2017).

Functions

- Endocytosis and exocytosis – the transport of fluids and other matter into and out of the cell.
- Endocytosis is the intake of extracellular fluid and particulate material (small particles) ranging in size from macromolecules to whole cells (e.g. the bacteria engulfed and destroyed by macrophage cells).
- Exocytosis is the bulk transport of material out of the cells.

There are three types of endocytosis:

1. Phagocytosis – involves the ingestion of large particles, even whole microbial cells.
2. Pinocytosis – involves the ingestion of small particles and fluids.
3. Receptor-mediated endocytosis – involves large particles, notably proteins, but also has the important feature of being highly selective.

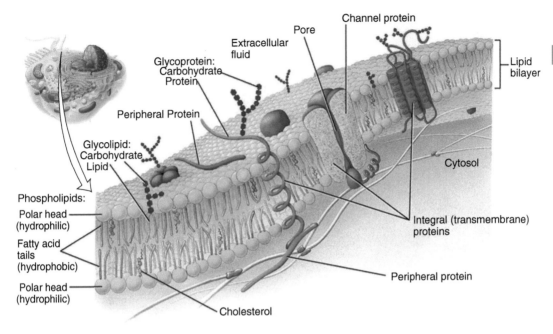

Figure 2.2   The cell membrane.

Endocytosis involves part of the cell membrane being drawn into the cell along with the particles or fluid to be ingested (Figure 2.3). This membrane is then pinched off to form a membrane-bound vesicle within the cell, whilst at the same time the cell membrane as a whole reseals itself. Inside the cell, the fate of this vesicle depends upon the type of endocytosis involved as well as the material it contains. In some cases, the endocytic vesicle ultimately fuses with an organelle called a lysosome, after which the ingested material can be processed. Endocytosis is also the means by which many simple organisms obtain their nutrients.

Transport across the cell membrane

One of the key properties of the cell membrane with regards to transport is its selective permeability. This refers to its ability to let certain materials pass through, whilst preventing others from doing so. This selective permeability is based on the hydrophobicity (water hatred) of its component molecules. Because the phospholipid tails in the centre of the bilayer are composed entirely of hydrophobic fatty acid chains (lipids are fats), it is very difficult for water-soluble (hydrophilic) molecules to penetrate to the membrane interior. The result is a very effective permeability barrier.

However, this barrier can be penetrated, but only by way of specific transport systems. These control what goes into and out of the cell, or what crosses from one subcellular compartment to another. Cell membranes control metabolism by restricting the flow of glucose and other water-soluble metabolites in and out of cells and between subcellular compartments. This is known as compartmentation. The cells store energy in the form of transmembrane ion gradients by allowing high concentrations of particular ions to accumulate on one side of the membrane.

Ions pass from inside to outside of the cell (or the other way round) so that there are more supplies of these ions just outside the cell or inside it, and the membrane controls

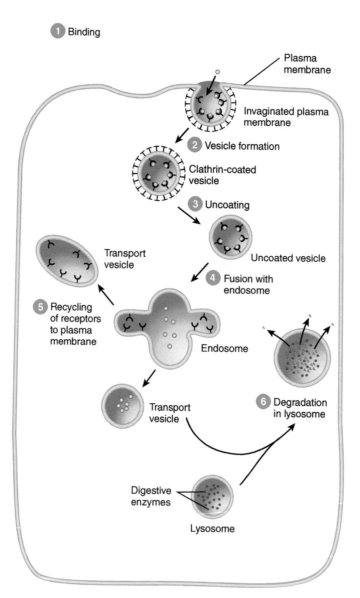

Figure 2.3   Endocytosis.

the speed/rate at which these ions pass through the membrane. The controlled release of such ion gradients can be used to:

- Extract nutrients from surrounding fluids
- Pass electrical messages (known as nerve excitability)
- Control cell volume and stop cells bursting from excess fluid.

To return to the cell membrane itself, there are four factors that decide the degree of permeability of a membrane:

1. Size of molecules – large molecules cannot pass through the integral membrane proteins, but small ones such as water and amino acids can.

2. Solubility in lipids (fats) – substances that easily dissolve in lipids can pass through the membrane more easily than non–lipid-soluble substances. Lipid-soluble substances include oxygen, carbon dioxide and steroid hormones.

3. If an ion has an electrical charge opposite to that of the membrane, then it is attracted to the membrane and can more easily pass through it.

4. Carrier integral proteins can carry substances across the membrane, regardless of their size, ability to dissolve in lipids or membrane electrical charge.

There are two ways in which substances can move across the membrane: passive or active. Passive processes are:

- Diffusion
- Facilitated diffusion
- Osmosis
- Filtration.

Active processes are:

- Active transport pumps
- Endocytosis
- Exocytosis.

A passive process is one in which the substances move on their own down a concentration gradient from an area of higher to one of lower concentration. The cell does not expend any energy on the process. Think of it as rolling down a hill from an area of high altitude to one of lower altitude. Little energy is expended in just rolling down a hill.

Diffusion is the most common form of passive transport, in which a substance of higher concentration moves to an area where there is a lower concentration of that substance (Colbert et al., 2019). This difference between the areas of high concentration and of low concentration is known as a concentration gradient. This process of diffusion is essential for respiration. It is through diffusion that oxygen is transported from the lungs to the blood, and carbon dioxide makes the opposite journey from the blood to the lungs (Colbert et al., 2019).

Facilitated diffusion is similar to diffusion, but with one exception. For this process to take place, there needs to be a substance that helps – a facilitator. Glucose is moved using this process. Although glucose can move part of the way through the membrane on its own, it needs something else (a carrier/transport protein) to give it that extra push to get it completely through the membrane (Colbert et al., 2019; McCance et al., 2018).

Osmosis is the process in which water travels through a selectively permeable membrane so that concentrations of a substance that is soluble in water (known as a solute) are the same on both sides of that membrane. This is known as osmotic pressure (Figures 2.4 and 2.5). The higher the concentration of the solute on one side of the membrane, the higher the osmotic pressure available for the movement of the water (Colbert et al., 2019).

Filtration is similar to osmosis, except that pressure is applied in order to 'push' water and solutes across that membrane. The heart is a major supplier of the force that can lead to one type of filtration (renal filtration) as it pushes blood into the kidneys, where filtration of the blood can take place (Colbert et al., 2019).

An active process is one in which substances move against a concentration gradient from an area of lower to one of higher concentration. To do this, the cell must expend energy; this is released by splitting adenosine triphosphate (ATP) into adenosine diphosphate (ADP) and phosphate. ATP is a compound of a base, a sugar and three phosphate groups (triphosphate).

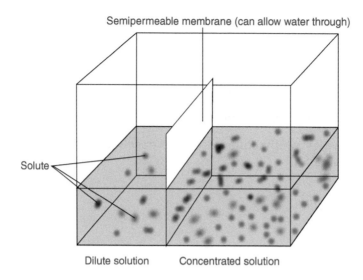

Figure 2.4   Osmosis.

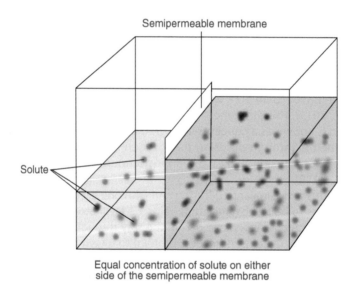

Figure 2.5   Osmosis and movement of solute.

These phosphate groups are held together by high-energy bonds, which when broken release a high level of energy. Once one of these phosphate bonds has been broken and a phosphate group has been released, that compound now has only two phosphate groups (diphosphate). The released phosphate group in turn joins up with another ADP group, thus forming another molecule of ATP (with energy stored in the phosphate bonds), and the whole process continues to recur.

The energy is required because the cell is attempting to move a substance to an area that already has a high concentration of that substance. Think again of a hill. When walking up a hill, a lot of energy is expended. Obviously, the higher the concentration already present, the more the energy required to move further molecules of the particular substance into that area – the steeper the hill, the more energy is used. For example, cells contain a lot of potassium (K^+); therefore, energy is required to transport more potassium through the membrane and into the cell.

Now, we turn to what is inside the cell membrane, starting with the cytoplasm.

Cytoplasm

Cytoplasm is a ground substance (also known as a matrix) in which various cellular components are found. 'Cyto' means cell, so any word that has 'cyto' in it has to do with cells.

Cytoplasm, itself, is a thick, semitransparent, elastic fluid containing suspended particles and the cytoskeleton. The cytoskeleton provides support and imparts shape to the cell. In addition, it is involved in the movement of structures in the cytoplasm because some cells can change shape, e.g. phagocytic cells.

Role of cytoplasm

- Chemically, cytoplasm is 75–90% water plus solid compounds – mainly carbohydrates, lipids and inorganic substances, and it is the substance in which chemical reactions occur.
- The cytoplasm receives raw materials from the external environment (such as from digested food) and converts them into usable energy by decomposition reactions.
- As well as the breakdown of raw materials to make energy, the cytoplasm is also the site where new substances are synthesised (produced) for the use of the cell.
- It is the place where various chemicals are packaged for transport to other parts of the cell, or to other cells in the body.
- It is in the cytoplasm that various chemicals facilitate the excretion of waste materials.

Nucleus

When considering the nucleus, a simple analogy is to think of it as the brain of the cell. Prokaryotic cells do not have a nucleus, but eukaryotic cells do. Eukaryotic cells are found in animals and plants, whilst prokaryotic cells are very typical of bacteria. In many ways, prokaryotic cells are less complex and often smaller than eukaryotes.

However, not all human cells possess a nucleus. An example of a cell without a nucleus is the red blood cell. Chapter 10 describes the concave shape of the mature red blood cells. This is because the lack of a nucleus means the red blood cell 'collapses in' on itself. Also, just to make it more confusing, some cells can have more than one nucleus, e.g. some muscle fibre cells (see Figure 2.12).

Some facts about the nucleus are as follows:

- The nucleus is the largest structure in the cell.
- It is surrounded by a nuclear membrane. This nuclear membrane has two layers and, like the cell membrane, is selectively permeable.
- The protoplasm within the nucleus is not called cytoplasm – it is called nucleoplasm.
- The nucleus assumes a great responsibility for both mitosis and meiosis (see later).
- Inside the nucleus is found the genetic material, consisting principally of deoxyribonucleic acid (DNA). When a cell is not reproducing, the genetic material is a threadlike mass called chromatin.
- Before cell division, the chromatin shortens and coils into rod-shaped bodies called chromosomes.
- The basic structural unit of a chromosome is a nucleosome – composed of DNA and protein.

- DNA has two main functions:
  1. It provides the genetic blueprint which ensures that the next generation of cells is identical to existing ones.
  2. It provides the plans for the synthesis of protein by the cell.
- All this information is stored in genes.
- Inside the nucleus are little spherical bodies called nucleoli, and these are responsible for the production of ribosomes from ribosomal ribonucleic acid (rRNA).
- In humans, there are 23 pairs of chromosomes in each cell with a nucleus, with the exception of the spermatozoa and ova (sperm and eggs).
- Sperm and ova only have 23 single chromosomes (i.e. one of each).
- The chromosomes are the same for males and females except for one pair – the X and Y chromosomes. It is these chromosomes that determine whether a baby is going to be male or female.

Mitosis and meiosis

These are the processes by which the cell reproduces itself. Most human cells reproduce asexually by mitosis, but the spermatozoa and ova reproduce by meiosis. Whereas the cells reproducing by mitosis finish up as exact copies of the parent cells with a pair of each of the 23 chromosomes, the cells reproducing by meiosis just finish up with one each of the 23 chromosomes.

Mitosis

In order for the body to grow, and also for the replacement of body cells that die, cells must be able to reproduce themselves, and in order for genetic information not to be lost, they must be able to reproduce themselves accurately. They do this by cloning themselves. In some organisms, this can occur by simple fission, where the nucleus in a single cell becomes elongated and then divides to form two nuclei in the same cell, each new nucleus carrying identical genetic information. The cytoplasm then divides in the middle between the two nuclei, and so two identical daughter cells result, each with its own nucleus and other essential organelles.

In humans, cell reproduction is a complex process called mitosis, in which the number of chromosomes in the daughter cells has to be the same as in the original parent cell. Mitosis can be divided into four stages:

1. Prophase
2. Metaphase
3. Anaphase
4. Telophase.
   - Before and after it has divided, the cell enters a stage known as interphase – this was thought to be a resting period for the cell, but the cell is actually very busy during this period because it has to get ready for replication.
   - Extra organelles are manufactured by the replication of existing organelles.
   - Also, the cell builds up a store of energy which is required for the process of division.

Prophase

The first stage after interphase is prophase:

- During prophase (Figure 2.6), the chromosomes become shorter, fatter and more easily visible, and each chromosome now consists of two chromatids, each containing the same genetic information (i.e. the DNA has replicated itself during interphase).
- The nucleolus and nuclear membrane disappear, leaving the chromosomes in the cytoplasm.

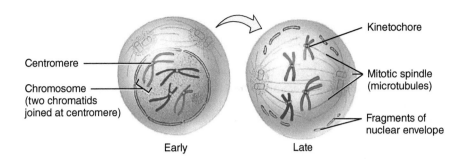

Figure 2.6   Prophase.

Metaphase

During metaphase (Figure 2.7), the 46 chromosomes (two of each of the 23 chromosomes), each consisting of two chromatids, become attached to the spindle fibres.

Anaphase

- During anaphase (Figure 2.8), the chromatids in each chromosome are separated.
- One chromatid from each chromosome then moves towards each pole of the spindle.

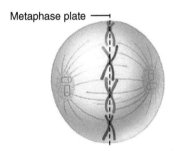

Figure 2.7   Metaphase.

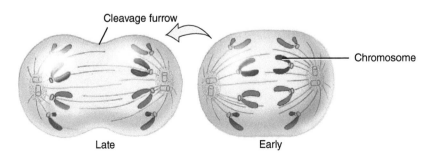

Figure 2.8   Anaphase.

Telophase

- There are now 46 chromatids at each pole, and these will form the chromosomes of the daughter cells.
- The cell membrane constricts in the centre of the cell, dividing it into two cells.
- The nuclear spindle disappears, and a nuclear membrane forms around the chromosomes in each of the daughter cells (Figure 2.9).
- The chromosomes become long and threadlike again, and are very difficult to see.

Cell division is now complete, and the daughter cells themselves enter the interphase stage in order to prepare for their replication and division.

Cell cycle

Looking now at the cell cycle (Figure 2.10) and supposing that one full cycle represents 24 hours, then the actual process of replication (mitosis) would only last for about 1 hour out of those 24 hours. The rest of the time, the cell is undertaking the replication of its DNA. It also

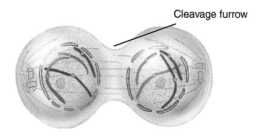

Figure 2.9   Telophase.

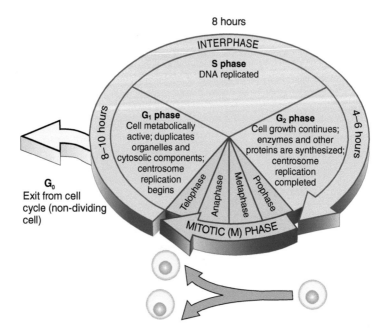

Figure 2.10   Cell cycle.

has to produce two of everything that is in the cell. In addition, it has to go through the process of obtaining and digesting nutrients so that it has the raw materials for this duplication, as well as the energy required in order to carry out various functions of the cell.

Meiosis

During the reproduction of humans, the egg is penetrated by a sperm, which then releases its DNA to combine with the DNA of the egg, so that the resulting embryo has two copies of each of the 23 chromosomes in nucleated cells. If the sperm and eggs had two copies of each chromosome (like other cells), the resulting fusion and developing embryo would have four copies of each chromosome. This means that the next generation would have four copies of each chromosome. The generation after that would have eight copies, and so on. This is obviously not practical, so the sperm and eggs undergo a process known as meiosis to ensure that the resulting embryo will only carry two copies of each chromosome in each cell with a nucleus.

For descriptive purposes, meiosis can be divided into eight stages (not the four of mitosis). However, they have the same names, but are known as either I or II (Table 2.1). As with mitosis, these phases are continuous with one another. However, there are differences as well as similarities between mitosis and meiosis.

First meiotic stage

Prophase I

This is similar to prophase in mitosis.

- However, instead of being scattered randomly, the chromosomes are arranged in 23 pairs. For example, the two chromosome number ones will pair up, as will the two chromosome number twos.
- Within each pair of chromosomes, genetic material may be exchanged between the two chromosomes.
- It is these exchanges that are partly responsible for the differences between children of the same parents.
- This process is called 'gene cross-over'.

Metaphase I

As in mitosis, the chromosomes become arranged on the spindles at the equator. However, they remain in pairs.

Anaphase I

One chromosome from each pair moves to each pole, so that there are now 23 chromosomes at each end of the spindle.

Table 2.1   Stages of meiosis.

First meiotic stage	Second meiotic stage
Prophase I	Prophase II
Metaphase I	Metaphase II
Anaphase I	Anaphase II
Telophase I	Telophase II

Telophase I

The cell membrane now divides the cell into two halves, as in mitosis. Each daughter cell now has half the number of chromosomes that each parent cell had.

Second meiotic stage

- The cells produced by the first meiotic division now divide again.
- Prophase II, metaphase II, anaphase II and telophase II are all similar to their equivalent stage in mitosis, with the exception that the DNA has not been replicated before prophase II, so there are only 23 single chromosomes in each of the granddaughter cells.

Fusion of the gametes

- When the gametes, each with 23 chromosomes, fuse together, a cell known as a zygote with 23 paired chromosomes (i.e. 46 in all) is formed.
- One chromosome in each pair comes from the mother and one from the father.
- The zygotic cell then divides (by mitosis) many times to form the embryo.

The organelles

All cells contain many organelles (little organs).

Endoplasmic reticulum

It is believed that the endoplasmic reticulum (ER; Figure 2.11) is formed from the nuclear membrane.

The ER consists of membranes that form a series of channels (called cisternae) that divide the cytoplasm into compartments. The cisternae are concerned with the transport of materials, primarily proteins. The alteration or addition of proteins for export from the cell can occur within the cisternae. They also contain a number of enzymes of importance in cell metabolism, such as digestive enzymes, enzymes involved in the synthesis of steroids and enzymes responsible for a variety of reactions leading to the removal of toxic substances

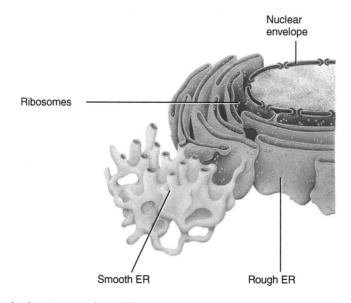

Figure 2.11   Endoplasmic reticulum (ER).

from the cell (McCance *et al.*, 2018). The ER present in liver cells has a role in drug detoxification.

There are two types of cisternae:

1. Granular (rough) ER – associated with ribosomes
2. Agranular (smooth) ER – free of ribosomes.

Granular ER is particularly well developed in cells that actively synthesise (produce) and export proteins. Agranular ER is found in steroid hormone-secreting cells, such as the cells of the adrenal cortex or the testes. Ribosomes include tiny particles of RNA on which the synthesis of proteins needed by the cell takes place, and they are formed in the nucleoli.

Golgi apparatus

The Golgi apparatus is a collection of membranous tubes and elongated sacs – actually, flattened cisternae stacked together. It plays a part in concentrating and packaging some of the substances that are made in the cell, e.g. lysosomal enzymes. The complex also plays a part in the assembly of substances for secretion outside of the cell. Secretory cells (such as those found in the mucous membrane) have many Golgi stacks, whereas non-secretory cells have few Golgi stacks per cell.

Proteins for export from the cell are synthesised on the ribosomes, and then travel through the ER to the Golgi vesicles (a vesicle is a fluid-filled sac). Vesicles leaving the Golgi fuse with the cell membrane by the process of exocytosis. The contents of the vesicles are then exported out of the cell. In addition, the Golgi is itself involved in the formation of glycoproteins.

Lysosomes

Lysosomes are organelles bound to the membrane and contain a variety of enzymes. Lysosomes have a number of functions:

- Digestion of material taken up by endocytosis, e.g. pathogenic organisms.
- Breakdown of cell components; e.g. during embryological development, the fingers and toes are webbed – the cells between the toes and fingers are removed by the lysosomal enzymes. After a baby's birth, the uterus, which weighs around 2 kg at full term, is invaded by phagocytic cells that are rich in lysosomes – these reduce the uterus to its non-pregnant weight of about 50 g within about 9 days.
- In normal cells, some of the synthesised proteins may be faulty – lysozymes are responsible for their removal.
- Contribute to hormone production, e.g. thyroxine – a hormone affecting a wide range of physiological activities, including the metabolic rate.

It is important that lysosomes do not rupture and release their contents inside living cells; otherwise the lysosomal enzymes would start to digest the cell. In certain degenerative diseases, such as rheumatoid arthritis, enzymes released by the breakdown of lysosomes from macrophages may be a significant factor by attacking living cells and tissues.

Peroxisomes

Peroxisomes are organelles similar in structure to lysosomes, but are much smaller. They are particularly abundant in liver cells. They contain several enzymes that are toxic to body cells. The role of peroxisomes in cells appears to be one of detoxification of harmful substances, such as alcohol and formaldehyde. More importantly, they neutralise dangerous free radicals. Free radicals are highly reactive chemicals that contain electrons that have not been paired off, and so are 'free' to disrupt the structure of molecules (Marieb and Hoehn, 2019).

Mitochondria (single = mitochondrion)

Mitochondria (often known as the powerhouses of the cell) consist of three membranes. The inner membrane has many folds that increase the surface area available for chemical reactions to occur. This process is collectively known as internal respiration. The mitochondrial matrix (the space surrounded by the inner membrane) contains enzymes of the tricarboxylic acid (TCA) cycle, as well as enzymes involved in fatty acid oxidation. The inner membrane is of the same thickness as the outer membrane and is responsible for oxidative phosphorylation. The mitochondria themselves are often found concentrated in regions of the cell associated with intense metabolic activity.

By using ATP, the mitochondria are able to generate the energy needed by the cell for it to function by converting the chemical energy contained in molecules of food. The production of ATP requires the breakdown of food molecules, and it occurs in several stages, each requiring the appropriate enzyme. An enzyme is a protein that can initiate and speed up a chemical reaction (it acts as a catalyst). The enzymes in the mitochondria are stored in the membranes in the required order so that the reactions occur in the correct sequence. This is very important, as it would be disastrous if the chemical reactions occurred out of sequence.

Mitochondria are self-replicating – just like the cells. DNA that is incorporated into the mitochondrial structure controls the replication process.

Cytoskeleton

The cytoskeleton is a lattice-like collection of fibres and fine tubes in the cytoplasm, and it is involved in the cell's maintenance and alteration of its shape as required.

There are three components of the cytoskeleton:

1. Microfilaments
2. Microtubules
3. Intermediate filaments.

Microfilaments

Microfilaments are rod-like structures, 6 nm in diameter, consisting of a protein called actin. In muscle, both actin (thick) and myosin – another protein (thin) – are involved in the contraction of muscle fibres. In non-muscle cells, microfilaments help to provide support and shape to the cell, and also assist in the movement of cells as well as movement within the cells.

Microtubules

Microtubules are relatively straight, slender, cylindrical structures that range in diameter from 18 to 30 nm. They consist of a protein called tubulin. Microtubules, like microfilaments, help to provide shape and support for cells. They also provide conducting channels through which various substances can move through the cytoplasm, and assist in the movement of pseudopodia.

Intermediate filaments

Intermediate filaments range in diameter from 8 to 12 nm and also help to determine the shape of the cell. Examples of intermediate filaments are neurofilaments found in the nerve.

Centrioles, cilia and flagella

Centrioles

Centrioles are found in most animal cells and are cylindrical structures. They are composed of nine sets of microtubules arranged in a circular pattern. They are involved in cell reproduction.

Cilia and flagella

Cilia and flagella extend from the surface of some cells and can bend, thus causing movement. In humans, cilia generally have the function of moving fluid or particulates over the surface of cells. Ciliated cells of the respiratory tract move mucus that has trapped foreign particles over the surface of respiratory tissues. A flagellum is usually a much larger structure than a cilium and is often used like a tail to propel the cell forward. The only example of a cell in the human body with a flagellum is the sperm, where the flagellum acts as a tail and propels the sperm towards the ova.

Types of cells

Figure 2.12 illustrates some of the cells that make up certain tissues.

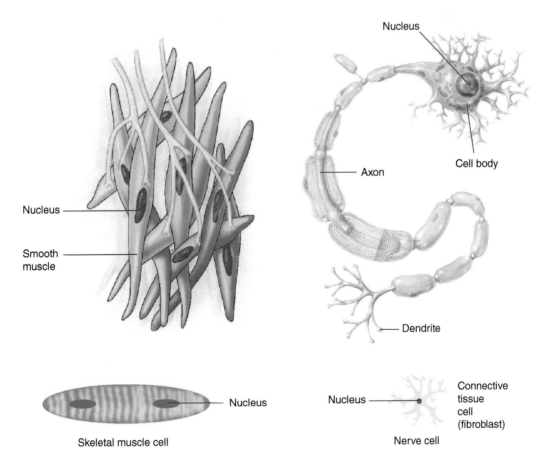

Figure 2.12   Types of cells.

Tissues

A human begins as a single cell – the fertilised egg. As soon as fertilisation takes place, the egg divides continuously. However, these cells do not divide endlessly and haphazardly. They divide and grow together in such a way that they become specialised, e.g. muscle cells, skin cells, cells of the lens of the eye and blood cells (Marieb and Keller, 2017). Cells group together to become tissues. Tissues are basically groups of cells that are similar in structure and generally perform the same functions (McCance *et al.*, 2018). There are four primary types of tissues:

1. Epithelial
2. Connective
3. Muscle
4. Nervous.

Most organs of the body contain all four types of tissue. All four have distinct functions that help to maintain homeostasis. For instance:

1. Epithelial tissue is concerned with 'covering'.
2. Connective tissue is concerned with 'support'.
3. Muscle tissue is concerned with 'movement'.
4. Nervous tissue is concerned with 'control' (Wheeldon, 2016).

Specialised cells form themselves into tissue in one of two ways. The first way is by mitosis. Cells formed as a result of mitosis are clones of the original cell. Therefore, if one cell with a specialised function undergoes mitosis, and subsequent generations of daughter cells continue to undergo mitosis, then the resulting hundreds of cells will all be of the same type and have the same function – they will become tissue. For example, epithelial cell sheets (such as skin) are formed as a result of mitosis (McCance *et al.*, 2018).

The second way involves the migration of specialised cells to the site of tissue formation and then assembling there. This is particularly seen during the development of the embryo when, for example, cells migrate to sites in the embryo where they differentiate and assemble into a variety of tissues (McCance *et al.*, 2018). This movement of cells is known as chemotaxis. Chemotaxis is discussed in detail in Chapter 5, but put simply, it is the 'movement along a chemical gradient caused by chemical attraction' (McCance *et al.*, 2018).

Epithelial tissue

Epithelial tissue lines and covers areas of the body, as well as forming the glandular tissue of the body. So, the exterior of the body is covered by one type of epithelial tissue (the skin), whilst another type of epithelial tissue lines some digestive system organs, such as the stomach and the small intestines, and the kidneys. In effect, epithelial tissue covers most of the internal and external surfaces of the body.

Epithelial tissue is classified into two ways:

1. By the number of cell layers:
   * Simple – where the epithelium is formed from a single layer of cells (Figure 2.13).
   * Stratified – where the epithelium has two or more layers of cells (Figure 2.14).
2. Shape:
   * Squamous
   * Cuboidal
   * Columnar.

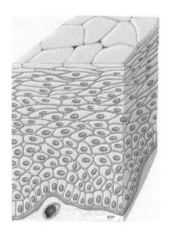

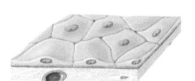
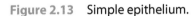

Figure 2.13   Simple epithelium.   **Figure 2.14**   Stratified epithelium.

Simple epithelial tissues are most concerned with absorption, secretion and filtration, but because they are usually very thin, they are not involved in protection.

Simple squamous epithelium rests on a basement membrane (basal layer). The basement membranes provide a layer of cells that supports and separates epithelial tissue from the underlying connective tissue. Squamous epithelial cells fit very closely together to form a thin sheet of tissue. It is this type of epithelial tissue that is found in the alveoli of the lungs and the walls of capillaries. Rapid diffusion or filtration can take place through this very thin tissue. Oxygen and carbon dioxide exchange takes place through the epithelial tissue lining the alveoli of the lungs, whilst nutrients and gases can pass through the epithelial tissue from the cells into and out of the capillaries. In addition, simple squamous epithelial cells form serous membranes that line certain body cavities and organs (Wheeldon, 2016).

Simple cuboidal epithelial tissue consists of one layer of cells resting on a basement membrane. However, because cuboidal epithelial cells are thicker than squamous epithelial cells, they are found in different places of the body and perform different functions. This epithelial tissue is found in glands, such as the salivary glands and the pancreas, as well as forming the walls of kidney tubules and covering the surface of the ovaries (Marieb and Keller, 2017).

Simple columnar epithelium (Figure 2.15), whilst being composed of a single layer of cells, is made up of a single layer of quite tall cells that, like the other two types, fit closely together. This epithelial tissue lines the entire length of the digestive tract from the stomach to the anus and contains goblet cells. Goblet cells produce mucus, and those simple columnar epithelial tissues that line all the body cavities that are open to the body exterior are known as mucous membranes (Marieb and Keller, 2017).

Stratified epithelial tissue, unlike the simple epithelial tissue, consists of two or more cell layers. Because these stratified epithelial tissues have more than one layer of cells, they are stronger and more robust than the simple epithelia. This means that a primary function of stratified epithelia is protection.

Stratified squamous epithelial tissue (Figure 2.14) is the most common stratified epithelium in the human body, and it consists of several layers of cells (Marieb and Keller, 2017). Although this epithelial tissue is called squamous epithelium, in actual fact, it is not made up entirely of squamous cells. It is the cells at the free edge of the epithelial tissue that are composed of squamous cells, whilst those cells that are close to the basement membrane are composed of either cuboidal or columnar cells. Squamous epithelium is found in places that are most at risk of everyday damage, including the oesophagus, the mouth and the outer layer of the skin (Marieb and Keller, 2017).

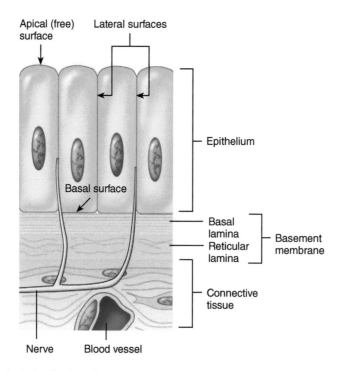

Figure 2.15   Epithelial cells classified according to shape.

Stratified cuboidal epithelial tissue has only two cell layers and is fairly rare in the human body, only being found in the ducts of large glands. The same can be said of the stratified columnar epithelial tissue.

There is a fourth type of epithelial tissue, known as transitional epithelium. This is a highly modified stratified squamous epithelium, and it forms the lining of just a few organs/ structures – all of which form part of the urinary system – the urinary bladder, the ureters and part of the urethra. This type of tissue has been modified to cope with the considerable stretching that these organs undergo. So, when one of these organs or structures is not stretched, the tissue has many layers with the superficial (those in the top layer) cells being rounded and looking like domes. However, when distended with urine, the epithelium becomes thinner, the surface cells flatten and they become just like squamous cells. These transitional cells are able to slide past one another and change their shape, allowing the wall of the ureter to stretch as a greater volume of urine flows through. Similarly, it allows for more urine to be stored in the bladder (Marieb and Keller, 2017).

Glandular epithelium

Glandular epithelial tissue is found within glands. According to Marieb and Keller (2017), a gland consists of several cells that make and secrete a particular product.

Two major types of glands develop from epithelial sheets:

1. Exocrine glands
2. Endocrine glands.

Exocrine glands have ducts leading from them, and their secretions empty through these ducts to the surface of the epithelium. Examples of exocrine glands include the sweat glands, the liver and the pancreas.

Endocrine glands, on the other hand, do not possess ducts. Instead, their secretions diffuse directly into the blood vessels that are found within the glands. All endocrine glands secrete hormones. These glands include the thyroid, the adrenal glands and the pituitary gland.

Connective tissue

Connective tissue is found everywhere in the body, and it connects body parts to one another. It is the most abundant and widely distributed of all four primary tissue types. It varies considerably in structure and has four main functions:

1. Protection
2. Support
3. Binding together other tissues (Marieb and Keller, 2017)
4. Acting as storage sites for excess nutrients (McCance *et al.*, 2018).

However, the most common structure and function of connective tissue is to act as the framework on which the epithelial cells gather in order to form the organs of the body (McCance *et al.*, 2018).

There are several common characteristics of connective tissue. One is that there are few cells in the tissue, but surrounding these few cells there is a great deal of what is known as the extracellular matrix. This extracellular matrix is composed of ground substance and fibres, and it varies in consistency from fluid to a semisolid gel. The fibres are made up of fibroblasts – one of the connective tissue cells – and are of three types:

1. Collagen (white) fibres
2. Elastic (yellow) fibres
3. Reticular fibres.

Collagen fibres have great strength, whilst elastic fibres can stretch and then recoil. The reticular fibres form the internal 'skeleton' of soft organs such as the spleen.

The ground substance is composed largely of water plus some adhesion proteins and large polysaccharide molecules, and it is these adhesion proteins that serve as a glue that attaches the connective tissue cells to the fibres. The change of consistency within the ground substance from fluid to a semisolid gel depends upon the number of polysaccharide molecules that are present. An increase in polysaccharide molecules causes the matrix to move from being a fluid to being a semisolid gel. The ground substance can store large amounts of water, so it serves as a water reservoir for the body (Marieb and Hoehn, 2019).

Connective tissue forms a 'packing' tissue around organs of the body (very much like the packing that can surround a delicate object in a parcel in transit) and so protects them. It is able to bear weight and to withstand stretching and various traumas, such as abrasions. There is a wide variation in types of connective tissue; e.g. fat tissue is composed mainly of cells and a soft matrix. Bone and cartilage have very few cells but do contain large amounts of hard matrix, and that is what makes them so strong (Marieb and Keller, 2017).

There are also variations in the blood supply to the tissue. Although most connective tissues have a good blood supply, there are some types, e.g. tendons and ligaments, which have a poor blood supply, whilst cartilage has no blood supply. That is the reason why these structures heal very slowly when they are injured – often a broken bone will heal much quicker than a damaged tendon or ligament (Marieb and Keller, 2017).

Bone

Bone is the most rigid of the connective tissues, and it is composed of bone cells surrounded by a very hard matrix containing calcium and large numbers of collagen fibres. Because of their hardness, bones provide protection, support and muscle attachment (Marieb and Keller, 2017).

Cartilage

Cartilage, which is not as hard, but is more flexible than bone, is found in only a few places in the body, e.g. hyaline cartilage, which supports the structures of the larynx. It attaches the ribs to the sternum and covers the ends of the bones where they form joints (Marieb and Hoehn, 2019). Other types of cartilage include fibrocartilage, which, because it can be compressed, forms the discs between the vertebrae of the spinal column, and elastic cartilage where some degree of elasticity is required, e.g. in the external ear.

Dense connective tissue

Dense connective tissue forms strong, stringy structures such as tendons (which attach skeletal muscles to bones) and the more elastic ligaments (that connect bones to other bones at joints). Dense connective tissue also makes up the lower layers of the skin (known as the dermis). These tissues have collagen fibres as the main matrix element, with many fibroblasts found between the collagen fibres (Marieb and Keller, 2017). These fibroblasts are the cells that are involved in the manufacture of the fibres.

Loose connective tissue

Loose connective tissue is softer and contains more cells, but fewer fibres, than other types of connective tissue (with the exception of blood). There are four types of loose connective tissue:

1. Areolar tissue
2. Adipose tissue
3. Reticular tissue
4. Blood.

Areolar tissue

Areolar tissue is the most widely distributed connective tissue type in the body. It is a soft tissue that cushions and protects the body organs that it surrounds. It helps to hold the internal organs together. It has a fluid matrix that contains all types of fibres which form a loose network, so giving it its softness and pliability. It provides a reservoir of water and salts for the surrounding tissues. All body cells obtain their nutrients from this tissue fluid and also release their waste into it. It is also in this area that, following injury, swelling can occur (known as oedema) because the areolar tissue soaks up the excess fluid just like a sponge does, causing it to become puffy (Marieb and Hoehn, 2019).

Adipose tissue

Adipose tissue is commonly known as 'fat' and is actually areolar tissue in which there is a preponderance of fat cells. It forms the subcutaneous tissue which lies beneath the skin where it insulates the body and can protect it from the extremes of both heat and cold (Marieb and Hoehn, 2019). In addition, adipose tissue protects some organs, such as the kidneys and eyeballs.

Reticular connective tissue

Reticular connective tissue consists of a delicate network of reticular fibres that are associated with reticular cells (similar to fibroblasts). It forms an internal framework to support many free blood cells – mainly the lymphocytes – in the lymphoid organs, such as the lymph nodes, spleen and bone marrow (Marieb and Hoehn, 2019).

Blood

'Blood, or vascular tissue, is considered a connective tissue because it consists of blood cells, surrounded by a non-living, fluid matrix call blood plasma' (Marieb and Hoehn, 2019). Blood is concerned with the transport of nutrients, waste material, respiratory gases (such as oxygen and carbon dioxide), as well as many other substances throughout the body.

Muscle tissue

There are three types of muscle tissue, and these are responsible for helping the body to move, or to move substances within the body:

1. Skeletal muscle
2. Cardiac muscle
3. Smooth muscle.

Skeletal muscle

Skeletal muscle is attached to bones and is involved in the movement of the skeleton. These muscles can be controlled voluntarily and form the 'bulk' of the body (the flesh). The cells of skeletal muscle are long, cylindrical and have several nuclei. In addition, they appear striated (have stripes). They work by contracting and relaxing, with pairs working antagonistically; i.e. one muscle contracts, and the opposite muscle relaxes. So, for example, if the muscles in the front of the arm contract and the ones at the back of the arm relax, then the arm bends.

Cardiac muscle

Cardiac muscle is only found in the heart, and it pumps blood around the body. It does this by contracting and relaxing, just like skeletal muscle, and it appears striated. However, unlike skeletal muscles, it works in an involuntary way – the activity cannot be consciously controlled. The cells of cardiac muscle do not have a nucleus.

Smooth muscle

Also known as visceral muscle, smooth muscle (see Figure 2.12) is found in the walls of hollow organs, e.g. the stomach, bladder, uterus and blood vessels (hence 'visceral' because these organs are also known as 'viscera'). Smooth muscle has no striations, and like cardiac muscle it works in an involuntary way. Smooth muscle causes movement in the hollow organs; i.e. as it contracts, the cavity of an organ becomes smaller (constricted), and when it relaxes the organ becomes larger (dilated). This allows substances to be propelled through the organ in the right direction, e.g. faeces in the intestines. Because smooth muscle contracts and relaxes slowly, it forms a wavelike motion (known as peristalsis) that pushes, in the case of the intestines, the faeces through the intestines (Figure 2.16).

Nervous tissue

Nervous tissue is concerned with control and communication within the body by means of electrical signals. The main type of cell that is found in nervous tissue is the neuron (see

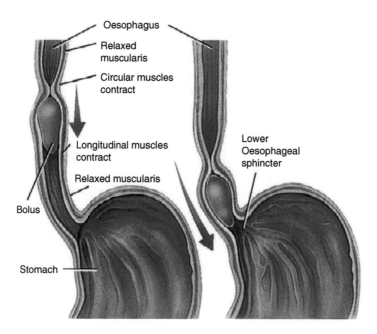

Figure 2.16   Peristalsis.

Figure 2.12). All neurons receive and conduct electrochemical impulses around the body. The structure of neurons is very different from that of other cells. The cytoplasm is found within long processes or extensions – some in the leg being more than a metre long. These neurons receive and transmit electrical impulses very rapidly from one to the other across synapses (junctions). It is at the synapses that the electrical impulse can pass from neuron to neuron, or from a neuron to a muscle cell. The total number of neurons is fixed at birth, and cannot be replaced if they are damaged (McCance *et al.*, 2018).

In addition to the neurons, nervous tissue includes cells known as neuroglia-supporting cells. These supporting cells insulate, support and protect the delicate neurons. The neurons and supporting cells make up the structures of the nervous system:

- The brain
- The spinal cord
- The nerves.

Tissue repair

The many tissues of the body are always at risk of injury or disease. Inflammation is the body's immediate reaction to tissue injury or damage, because when tissue injury or damage does occur, this stimulates the body's inflammatory and immune responses to spring into action so that the healing process can begin almost immediately.

There are four major signs and symptoms of an inflammatory response (Nairn and Helbert, 2007):

1. Pain
2. Swelling
3. Heat
4. Redness.

There may also be nausea, sweating, a raised pulse, a lowered blood pressure and even a loss of consciousness. These symptoms are the body's response to the pain and to shock.

Inflammation is usually initiated by damage to a cell. Following this damage, three simultaneous processes occur:

1. Mast cell degranulation – mast cells are tissue cells which contain granules in their cytoplasm. These granules are similar to, but smaller than, the granules found in basophils in the blood. These granules contain, amongst other substances, histamine which, during the process of degranulation, is released into the tissues. It causes some inflammatory symptoms and works with the two other processes listed here to provide the full range of inflammatory symptoms.
2. The activation of four plasma protein systems – these systems are the complement, clotting and kinin systems, and immunoglobulins (antibodies). The complement system activates and assists inflammatory and immune processes. It also plays a major role in the destruction of bacteria. The clotting system traps bacteria that have entered the wound and also interacts with platelets to stop any bleeding. The kinin system helps to control vascular permeability, whilst immunoglobulins help in the destruction of bacteria.
3. The phagocytic cells move to the area of damage in order to phagocytose bacteria or any other non-self debris in the wound.

A typical inflammatory response to injured tissue consists of the following:

- Arterioles near the injury site constrict briefly, followed by vasodilation which increases blood flow to the site of the injury (redness and heat).
- Dilation of the arterioles at the site increases the pressure in the circulation, which increases the movement of plasma proteins and blood cells into the tissues in the area, so causing oedema (swelling).
- The nerve endings in the area are stimulated, partly by pressure (pain).
- The clotting and kinin systems, along with platelets, move into the area and block any tissue tears by commencing the clotting process.
- Phagocytes and lymphocytes move into the area and start to destroy any infectious organisms found there and remove pus.
- These blood cells remain in the area until tissue regeneration (repair) takes place – known as resolution.

Thus, inflammation can be summed up as the presence of:

- Vasodilation – redness/heat
- Vascular permeability – oedema
- Cellular infiltration – pus
- Thrombosis – clots
- Stimulation of nerve endings – pain.

Conclusion

This chapter has looked at the building blocks of the human body, namely the cells. Cells are extremely complicated parts of the body, but it is important to understand them and their functions in order to understand how the human body itself functions. Cells form tissues, which then form all the structures, systems and organs of the body. Therefore, it is necessary to also understand tissues. The remainder of this book will look at the various systems, structures and organs of the body – how they function as well as what can go wrong with them.

Activities

Here are some activities and exercises to help test your learning. For the answers to these exercises, as well as further self-testing activities, visit our website at **www.wiley.com/go/fundamentalsofappliedpathophysiology/student4e**

Multiple choice questions

1. Which of the following statements is incorrect?
   (a) Cells contain an opaque substance called cytoplasm.
   (b) All cells are the same shape and size.
   (c) Water, proteins, lipids, carbohydrates and ions are found within cells.
   (d) The nucleus is separated from the rest of the cell by a nuclear membrane.
2. Which of the following statements is true?
   (a) The cell membrane consists of a bilayer of phospholipid molecules, interspersed with protein molecules
   (b) Phospholipid heads are hydrophobic (water hating)
   (c) Phospholipid tails are found on the outer surface of the cell, where they attract water
   (d) Phospholipid molecules are arranged as a single layer with the heads facing inwards
3. What is phagocytosis?
   (a) The bulk transport of material out of the cells
   (b) Ingestion of small particles and fluids
   (c) The transport of fluids from cell to cell by facilitated diffusion
   (d) The ingestion of large particles
4. Which of the following is a passive process?
   (a) Endocytosis
   (b) Active transport pumps
   (c) Osmosis
   (d) Exocytosis
5. Which of the following statements about cytoplasm is true?
   (a) Cytoplasm converts raw materials from the external environment into usable materials
   (b) Cytoplasm is the site where new substances are synthesis, ready for use by the cell
   (c) In cytoplasm, various chemicals are packaged for transport to other parts of the cell or to other cells in the body
   (d) All of the above
6. Which of the following statements is correct?
   (a) The nucleus is the smallest structure of the cell
   (b) The protoplasm in the nucleus is called cytoplasm
   (c) Before cell division, the nucleosomes shorten and coil into rod-shaped bodies called chromatins
   (d) The basic structural unit of a chromosome is a nucleosome, which is composed of DNA and protein
7. Which of the following organelles is responsible for the digestion of material taken up by endocytosis?
   (a) Golgi apparatus
   (b) Mitochondria
   (c) Lysosomes
   (d) Endoplasmic reticulum

8. Which of the following best describes the function of mitochondria?
   (a) The detoxification of harmful substances
   (b) The generation of energy
   (c) The packaging of the substances made in the cell
   (d) Transport of proteins

9. Which of the following structures enables cells to propel themselves?
   (a) Flagella
   (b) Cilia
   (c) Centrioles
   (d) All of the above

10. What is the most abundant tissue in the human body?
    (a) Muscle
    (b) Epithelial
    (c) Connective
    (d) Nervous

11. Which of the following statements is true?
    (a) Nervous tissue is concerned with 'movement'
    (b) Epithelial tissue is concerned with 'covering'
    (c) Muscle tissue is concerned with 'control'
    (d) Connective tissue is concerned with 'protection'

12. Which of the following best describes the structure of simple cuboidal epithelium?
    (a) Multiple layers of thin cells
    (b) Single layer of column-shaped cells
    (c) Multiple layers of cuboid-shaped cells
    (d) Single layer of cuboid-shaped cells

13. Which of the following is an example of loose connective tissue?
    (a) Blood
    (b) Cartilage
    (c) Ligaments
    (d) Bone

14. Which of the following statements on muscle tissue is true?
    (a) Skeletal muscle is involuntary
    (b) Cardiac muscle is non-striated
    (c) Smooth muscle is involuntary
    (d) Smooth muscle is striated

15. Which of the following are signs of inflammation?
    (a) Pain
    (b) Swelling
    (c) Heat
    (d) All of the above

Glossary of terms

Active transport   The process in which substances move against a concentration gradient from an area of low concentration to one of higher concentration. It requires the release and use of energy.

Active transport pump   Also known as a sodium pump, this is situated in the plasma membrane and uses the energy produced by the ATP reaction to pump sodium ions (Na^+) out of the cell and potassium ions (K^+) into it.

Adenosine diphosphate (ADP)   Found inside cells, it helps to produce ATP during reactions which produce cellular energy and is itself formed from ATP at a later stage. It is this continual synthesis and breaking down of ADP and ATP that produces the energy.

Adenosine triphosphate (ATP)   A compound of an adenosine molecule with three attached phosphoric acid molecules. Essential for the production of cellular energy.

Amino acid   The building block of proteins. The type of protein that is produced depends upon the number and types of amino acids that are used to construct it.

Carbohydrate   An organic compound that is composed of carbon, hydrogen and oxygen. Sugars (including glucose) and starch are carbohydrates. They are very important as an energy store.

Carrier/transport protein   A small molecule that helps in the movement of ions across a cell membrane.

Catalyst   A substance that speeds up a reversible chemical reaction. Enzymes are catalysts.

Chemical reaction   A process in which molecules are formed, changed or broken down.

Chromatid   One of the two strands of chromatin. Two identical chromatids form a chromosome after nuclear reproduction.

Chromatin   The material which forms chromosomes. It consists of DNA and proteins.

Chromosomes   Tightly coiled chromatin. This is the form in which the genetic material of all cells is organised.

Concentration gradient   The gradient that demonstrates the difference between an area of high concentration and one of low concentration of a substance.

Cytoplasm   Collective name for all the contents of the cell, including the plasma membrane, but not including the nucleus.

Deoxyribonucleic acid (DNA)   Found in the nucleus, it contains all the genetic information of an organism.

Diffusion   The passive movement of molecules or ions from a region of high concentration to one of low concentration until a state of equilibrium is achieved.

Endocytosis   The general name for the various processes by which cells ingest foodstuffs and infectious microorganisms.

Enzyme   A protein that speeds up chemical reactions.

Eukaryotic cell   A cell that normally includes, or has included, chromosomal material within one or more nuclei.

Exocytosis   The system of transporting material out of cells.

Extracellular fluid   The fluid outside of the cell that bathes the body's cells.

Extracellular matrix   Found in connective tissue, this is non-living material that is made up of ground substance and fibres. It separates the living cells found in this tissue.

Facilitated diffusion   Similar to diffusion, this requires the help of another substance – a carrier protein – for the process to take place (i.e. a facilitator).

Fibre   Any long, thin structures. The body contains many of them, including nerve fibres and muscle fibres.

Fibroblast   The most common connective tissue cell and found only in the tendons. It is responsible for the production and secretion of extracellular matrix materials.

Gene   The smallest physical and biological unit of heredity that encodes for a molecular cell product.

Genetic material   Mainly DNA (deoxyribonucleic acid) that contains genetic information.

Glucose   Also known as dextrose, it is the principal sugar found in the blood. It is essential for life. An absence can lead to diabetes, coma and even death.

Glycoprotein   A protein linked to carbohydrates.

Goblet cell   A mucus-secreting cell found in epithelial tissue.

Ground substance   The part of the extracellular matrix (found in connective tissue) that is composed mainly of water, with some adhesion proteins and large polysaccharide molecules.

Hormone   A chemical messenger that is linked to the endocrine system, and that exerts physiological control over the function of cells or organs other than those that created it.

Inorganic substance   A compound that does not contain carbon (e.g. water).

Internal respiration   The use of oxygen by cells in the enzymatic release of energy from organic compounds. This is known as aerobic respiration. Anaerobic respiration does not require oxygen, but does require a substance such as nitrate or iron to do the same job as oxygen (accept electrons during the chemical reaction). Only human cells with mitochondria can undertake aerobic respiration.

Ion   An atom or group of atoms that carries either a positive or a negative electrical charge.

Lipid   An energy-rich organic compound that is soluble in organic substances such as alcohol and benzene.

Lysosome   An organelle within the cell that is an important part of the cell's digestive system because it secretes lysozyme and other similar enzymes, which are very important in the phagocytosis of microorganisms.

Lysozyme   A bacteria-destroying enzyme found in lysosomes, sweat, tears, saliva and other bodily secretions.

Meiosis   The process by which the gametes (spermatozoa and ova) are reproduced.

Membrane   The outer covering of a cell and of a nucleus within a cell.

Metabolism   The collective name for all the physical and chemical processes occurring within a cell/living organism, but often referring only to reactions involving enzymes.

Metabolite   A substance involved in the process of metabolism – either to cause it, assist it or occurring as a result of the process.

Mitosis   The process by which cells (other than the gametes) are reproduced by simple division of the nucleus and the cell itself.

Neuroglia-supporting cell   A cell found in nervous tissue; its role is to support the delicate neurons by insulating, supporting and protecting them.

Nuclear membrane   The outer shell of the nucleus within the cell.

Nucleolus   A small spherical body found in the cell nucleus that is involved in the production of ribosomes.

Nucleoplasm   The protoplasm found within the nucleus.

Nucleosome   The basic structural unit of a chromosome.

Organelle   A structural and functional part of a cell that acts like human organs to fulfil all the needs of the cell so that it can grow, reproduce and carry out its functions.

Osmosis   The passive movement of water through a selectively permeable membrane from an area of high concentration of a chemical to an area of low concentration.

Osmotic pressure   The pressure that must be exerted on a solution to prevent the passage of water into it across a semipermeable membrane from a region of higher concentration of solute to a region of lower concentration of solute.

Oxidative phosphorylation   The process by which energy released during aerobic respiration and is linked to the production of adenosine triphosphate (ATP).

Passive transport   The process by which substances move on their own down a concentration gradient from an area of high concentration to one of lower concentration. No cellular energy is required for this process.

Phagocytosis The method by which cells ingest large particles, including whole microorganisms.

Pinocytosis The method by which cells ingest small particles and fluids.

Prokaryotic cell The opposite of a eukaryote cell; their DNA/RNA is not contained within a discrete nucleus. They are generally very small bacteria, for example.

Protoplasm The collective name for everything within the cell, including the cytoplasm, nucleus and the organelles, as well as the plasma membrane.

Ribosomal ribonucleic acid (rRNA) A highly selective method by which the cell is able to ingest large particles (particularly proteins).

Receptor site Also known as the membrane receptor molecule. This is a protein on the membrane of cells that is able to receive certain other proteins that match them (e.g. hormones and antibodies).

Receptor-mediated endocytosis Involved in the translation of the genetic material encoded in DNA into proteins. It works in conjunction with ribosomes and messenger RNA (mRNA) and transfer RNA (tRNA).

Ribosome An organelle found in cytoplasm that plays a major role in the synthesis of proteins from RNA.

Selective permeability The ability of the cell membrane to allow only certain substances to pass into or out of the cell.

Simple fission The asexual reproduction of cells by means of division of the nucleus and the cell body.

Solute A substance that is dissolved in a solution.

Transmembrane ion gradient The gradient in the concentration of ions on either side of a plasma membrane. It is involved in the production of cellular energy.

Tricarboxylic acid cycle Also known as the Krebs cycle. This is an aerobic pathway that occurs in the mitochondria and is necessary for the production of energy there.

Vesicle A spherical space within the cell cytoplasm that is involved in the storage and transfer of substances for the cell.

References

Colbert, B.J., Ankney, J. and Lee, K.T. (2019). *Anatomy and Physiology for Health Professionals: An Interactive Journey*, 4th edn. Boston: Pearson.

Marieb, E.N. and Keller, E.N. (2017). *Essentials of Human Anatomy and Physiology*, 12th edn. Harlow: Pearson.

Marieb, E.N. and Hoehn, K.N. (2019). *Human Anatomy and Physiology*, 11th edn. Boston: Pearson.

McCance, K.L., Huether, S.E., Brashers, V.L. and Rote, N.S. (2018). *Pathophysiology: The Biologic Basis for Disease in Adults and Children*, 8th edn. St Louis: Elsevier.

Nairn, R. and Helbert, M. (2007). *Immunology for Medical Students*, 2nd edn. St Louis: Mosby.

Watson, R. (2005). Cell structure and function, growth and development. In: Montague, S.E., Watson, R. and Herbert, R.A. (eds.), *Physiology for Nursing Practice*, 3rd edn. Edinburgh: Elsevier, pp. 49–69.

Wheeldon, A. (2016). Tissue. In: Peate, I. and Nair, M. (eds.), *Fundamentals of Anatomy and Physiology for Student Nurses*. Chichester, UK: Wiley-Blackwell.

Chapter 3

Homeostasis

Ian Peate

Principal, School of Health Studies, Gibraltar

Contents

Introduction 50
Cell stability 51
Stable psychological conditions...................52
Homeostatic processes 52
Set points 53

Vital signs and homeostasis 57
Conclusion 61
Multiple choice questions...............................61
References..63

Key words

- Regulation
- Internal and external environments
- Feedback systems
- Hormones
- Pituitary gland
- Hypothalamus
- Nervous system
- Electrolytes
- Homeostatic disorders
- Recognising and reporting

Test your prior knowledge

- Why is homeostasis important?
- What are receptors and effectors and what do they do?
- What is the coordination centre?
- Which system has longer-lasting effects, nervous system or hormonal system?
- How should concerns regarding a patient's condition be escalated to senior staff?

Fundamentals of Applied Pathophysiology: An Essential Guide for Nursing and Healthcare Students, Fourth Edition. Edited by Ian Peate.
© 2021 John Wiley & Sons Ltd. Published 2021 by John Wiley & Sons Ltd.
Student companion website: www.wiley.com/go/fundamentalsofappliedpathophysiology/student4e
Instructor companion website: www.wiley.com/go/fundamentalsofappliedpathophysiology/instructor4e

Aim

This chapter aims to help you to develop and apply your understanding of homeostatic mechanisms within the body to enable you to offer high-quality, safe and effective informed care.

Learning outcomes

On completion of this chapter, the reader will be able to:

- Discuss and define homeostasis.

- Provide examples of chemical and nervous system responses involving homeostasis.

- Understand the 'three-part feedback system'.

- Describe the impact of disordered homeostasis on a person's health and well-being.

- Describe how any changes in a patient's condition should be escalated to senior staff.

Don't forget to visit the companion website for this book
(www.wiley.com/go/fundamentalsofappliedpathophysiology/student4e)
where you can find self-assessment tests to check your progress, as well as lots of activities to practise your learning.

Introduction

This chapter introduces the reader to the concept of homeostasis. Homeostasis is the key to life, and vital signs, for example, are a measure of homeostasis. Being healthy for many people means being independent of clinical intervention and to be able to undertake the activities of living. In order to do this, the body needs to engage with homeostasis. Understanding the theoretical underpinning of homeostasis for health is essential for safe and effective care, for accurate clinical decision-making and for restoration of patients to health.

The word *homeostasis* is derived from the Greek words for 'similar' and 'standing still'; the term refers to any process that living things employ to actively maintain stable conditions that are necessary for survival. In 1930 the term was used by Walter Cannon, a doctor. In his text, *The Wisdom of the Body*, he describes how the body maintains constant levels of temperature and other vital conditions, for example, the water, salt, sugar, protein, fat, calcium and oxygen contents of the blood.

In health, the body does all the work that is required to maintain itself by a wide range of living processes, including the excretion of waste products and the inhalation of oxygen so as to release energy from sugar. It also uses the process of homeostasis to maintain itself in balance, it makes just the right number of cells to replace those cells that have worn out and it produces just the right amount of hormones to signal a reaction that is needed to make things happen. Maintaining homeostasis requires the body to continuously monitor its internal conditions. From body temperature to blood pressure to the levels of certain nutrients, each physiological condition has a particular set point. When disruption of homeostasis is mild and temporary, the cells of the body can quickly restore balance in the internal environment. However, if disruption is sustained and extreme, then homeostasis may fail (Tortora and Derrickson 2017).

Nurses often care for people whose ability to maintain homeostasis will be impaired. When this occurs, it becomes essential that the nurse can detect subtle changes indicating altered homeostasis, initiate the most appropriate response and escalate concerns to other healthcare staff and to commence care that is evidence-based. It is also important to be able to clearly communicate the changes to the patient, their family or carers and be able to explain any treatments that are provided or that are being considered.

Cell stability

The life of a cell is dependent on the composition and stability of the physical chemical characteristics of the surrounding external environment. Chapter 2 of this text discusses cell stability in more detail. The cell, an open system, provides the substrates that the cell needs for living; changes in the physical and chemical conditions beyond a narrow range will lead to the cell's death. All living things are composed of cells; some are single celled (unicellular) and some are multicellular. In multicellular organisms, as in the human being, the medium that surrounds the cell (represented by the extracellular fluid and known as the internal environment) is continuously monitored by a number of control systems in the body.

The external environment is changing constantly, and those external changes can be measured, such as the outside temperature, water levels, air pressure, oxygen levels and nitrogen levels. The internal environment (the environment beneath the skin) is affected by these changes; however, for life to be maintained, the internal environment needs to be stable.

All cells in the body are made of chemicals, and they will only survive in very specific conditions. Changes in heat and energy will put the cells at risk. Proteins and enzymes, which permit bodily reactions to occur, will be in danger when these changes occur. The chemistry will become dysfunctional and so would we. Our metabolism would cease unless the body reacts so as to regain its balance (homeostasis).

Cells and proteins are very sensitive to changes in variables in the internal and external environments. Cells have to be kept at certain temperatures, they require a specific pH (this is a measure of hydrogen ion concentration related to the acid-base balance), there must be osmotic balance (the balance between water and solutes) and energy levels (glucose and oxygen) amongst other requirements. They all have to be tightly controlled and kept within a non-lethal range; homeostatic mechanisms provide this control. Organisms can reproduce, they are individual living things, responding to stimuli, growing and maintaining homeostasis. The trillions of cells in the body are also required to communicate, to let each other know what is happening. All this occurs as part of the internal environment via enzymes and the nervous system. The cells use hundreds of different signal molecules, and if there is any alteration in cellular communication, disease onset and progression will be effected (McCance, 2019).

The cells of the human body function within a narrow range of parameters, and there are numerous mechanisms that operate to enable this balance to be maintained. Many chapters of this text address the imbalance due to illness (pathophysiological changes). If there is disruption at the cellular level, this disturbs normal homeostatic control. Disruption of homeostasis arises because of internal and external stimuli and psychological stressors.

If the conditions of the internal environment are favourable, then each cell keeps itself alive and thereby makes its functional contribution to the tissue of which it is a part. In a similar way, tissues contribute to organs, which, in turn, are part of systems (see Figure 3.1). A homeostatic cycle can be constructed in which the systems of the body work

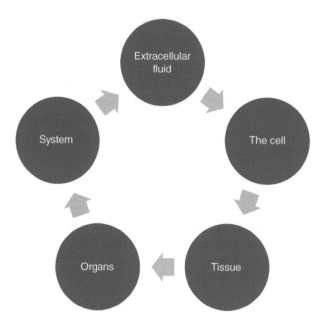

Figure 3.1   Homeostatic cycle.

interdependently, making their functional contributions to the adequate maintenance of extracellular fluid. This suggests that the function of all systems of the body is to maintain a tight control over the variables of the internal environment, providing living conditions for each cell to functionally contribute to the body as a whole. The maintenance of a stable condition of the internal environment is known as homeostasis. If an intense change in the external environment overcomes the ability of the control systems to function, or if a control system causes homeostatic failure, there is a real possibility of illness or even death.

Stable psychological conditions

In the social sciences, homeostasis refers to how a person under challenging stresses and motivations maintain a stable psychological condition. When high trait anxiety and a critical mass of psychosocial stressors come together, this can overwhelm the individual and the normal homeostasis of anxiety. This can tip someone into a state of excessive and persistent anxiety in which normally harmless situations seem threatening.

A society maintains its stability homeostatically despite competing political, economic and cultural factors. The law of supply and demand is an example, whereby the interaction of supply and demand maintains market prices at a reasonably stable level.

Homeostatic processes

There are three components required for homeostasis:

1. A receptor (detecting stimuli – recognising and responding to stimuli)
2. A control centre (receives and processes information from receptors around the body)
3. An effector (an organ, tissue or cell that produces a response).

Each of these components is required to perform specific tasks permitting regulation of the internal environment.

Receptors and effectors

Usually, monitoring of the body occurs automatically through body systems such as the nervous and endocrine systems (see Chapters 7 and 15, respectively, in this text). The body has a number of detectors known as receptors that receive information concerning changes in its internal environment. There are receptors that detect changes in chemicals (chemoreceptors), blood pressure (baroreceptors), temperature (thermoreceptors), touch or heat that is so extreme that they cause pain (nociceptors). Each of the receptors is tuned to a particular frequency, called its modality, and detects one specific variable. The receptors monitor the level of the parameter being regulated.

When a receptor receives information concerning a change of state in the variable that it has been designed to monitor, it sends signals to the brain for central coordination (the control centre), so that all of the information is gathered in one place.

A response message is then sent out to produce an appropriate behaviour or response. This response could be electrical (sent via the nervous system) or chemical (sent through the endocrine system), and it stimulates a change, or an effect, to return the internal conditions to an optimum state. Effectors, for example, include glands (causing hormone release) and muscles (causing muscle contractions), altering the parameter in whichever direction is needed. This change has been brought about by organs or cells that are known as 'effectors', and this is because they effect a response (see Figure 3.2). Receptors restore optimum levels, for example:

- Core body temperature
- Blood glucose levels
- Electrolyte and water concentrations
- pH of body fluids
- Blood and tissues oxygen and carbon dioxide levels
- Blood pressure.

Set points

As the internal and external environments of the body are continually changing, adjustments have to be made constantly to stay at or near a specific value; this is the set point.

Whilst it accepted that there are normal fluctuations from the set point, the body's systems will usually attempt to revert to this point. If the body becomes too warm, for example, alterations are made to cool the individual. If blood glucose levels increase after a meal, then adjustments are made to lower those levels. When adjustments to the set point are needed, the feedback loop works to maintain the new setting. There are two types of feedback: negative and positive.

Negative feedback

Nearly all physiological variables are controlled by negative feedback mechanisms. When a response reverses the original stimuli, then the system is operating by negative feedback.

In Figure 3.3, the regulation of blood pressure is considered. Watson (2018) provides an example of negative feedback and the maintenance of homeostasis in the regulation of blood pressure. When the heart beats faster or harder, the blood pressure increases. If a stimulus causes the blood pressure to rise, the baroreceptors (these are pressure-sensitive nerve cells) located in walls of particular blood vessels send impulses to the brain (the control centre) having sensed higher pressure. The brain responds by sending out impulses to the heart and blood vessels (the effectors). Usually, as a result the heart rate responds and decreases, and blood vessels dilate, with the blood pressure responding by returning to normal. Blood pressure is discussed further in Chapter 9 of this text.

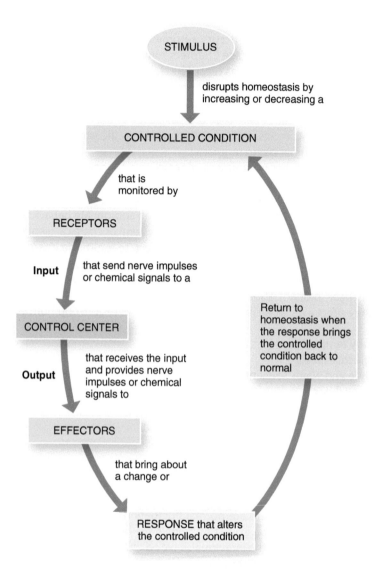

Figure 3.2   Regulation through feedback, a feedback system (*Source:* Tortora and Derrickson (2017). Reproduced with permission of John Wiley and Sons, Inc.).

There are many more examples of negative feedback mechanisms that occur in the body. Thermoregulation, control of blood glucose and osmoregulation are but three examples.

Positive feedback mechanisms

The use of positive feedback mechanisms is less common in the control of physiological variables. When a response improves the original stimuli, then the system is operating by positive feedback. Figure 3.4 uses the positive feedback control of labour contractions during birth of a baby as an example of homeostatic regulation by a positive feedback mechanism.

When labour commences, the cervix and uterus stretch (the stimulus), stretch-sensitive nerve cells located in the cervix (the receptors) will transmit nerve impulses (the input) to

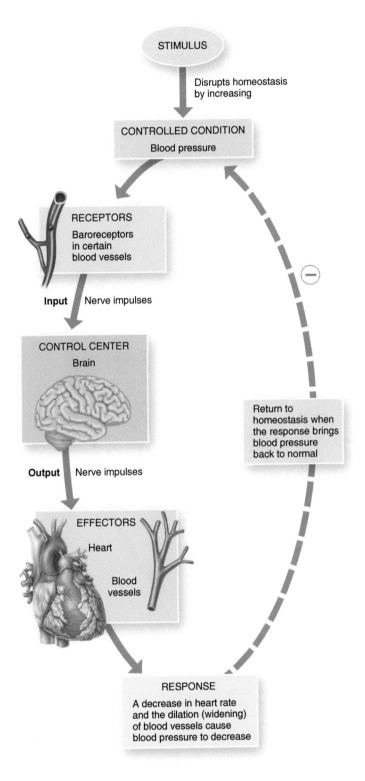

Figure 3.3 Homeostatic regulation of blood pressure by a negative feedback system. The broken return arrow with a negative sign that is surrounded by a circle represents negative feedback (*Source:* Tortora and Derrickson (2017). Reproduced with permission of John Wiley and Sons, Inc.).

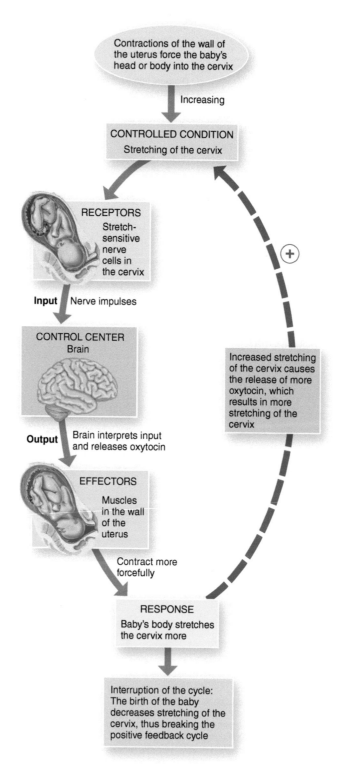

Figure 3.4 Positive feedback control of labour contractions during the birth of a baby. The broken return arrow with a positive sign that is surrounded by a circle represents positive feedback (*Source:* Tortora and Derrickson (2017). Reproduced with permission of John Wiley and Sons, Inc.).

the brain (this is the control centre). The brain responds, causing the pituitary gland to release the hormone oxytocin (the output), which then stimulates the walls of the uterus (the effector) to powerfully contract (the response) and to contract at a faster rate. When the fetus moves as a result of the contractions, this will also result in further stretching of the cervix and more oxytocin is released, resulting in even more forceful contractions. This cycle continues until the baby is born, the birth ends and the stretching of the cervix ceases, the release of oxytocin ends as well as the positive feedback mechanism.

A further example of a positive feedback mechanism is blood clotting. Once a vessel is damaged, a cascade of reactions occurs, platelets begin to adhere to the injured site and chemicals are released, attracting more platelets so as to prevent blood loss. The platelets will continue to amass, releasing chemicals until a blood clot has been formed. Chapter 10 considers blood and blood-related disorders.

Chapters in this text all draw on the principles of homeostasis and homeostatic imbalances; see Table 3.1. Each individual body system works in conjunction with other body systems, and they all interrelate with each other to ensure that an organism functions normally. It may appear that the body systems are seemingly unrelated; they are, however, very much connected. Working together, these systems maintain internal stability and balance (homeostasis). Disease in one body system can disrupt homeostasis and cause problems in other body systems. Disease pertains to impairment of normal body function, a disruption in homeostasis, a state of dis–ease (a lack of ease).

Vital signs and homeostasis

Vital signs measure homeostasis, and as such they are central to helping restore the patient's health (Cedar, 2017). Vital signs, such as the respiratory rate, depth and rhythm, oxygen saturation, pulse rate, rhythm and volume, blood pressure, temperature and a change in behaviour are regarded as an essential part of monitoring patients, whether in hospital or in other care settings/environments. When changes in vital signs occur, this indicates that there is homeostatic imbalance. Changes in vital signs prior to clinical deterioration are well documented, and early detection of preventable outcomes is key to timely intervention.

When nurses continually assess (measure) vital signs to determine whether the health of the patient is improving or deteriorating, they are using objective measures of homeostasis. The results of assessment of vital signs can help the nurse and others to implement clinical interventions with the aim of restoring homeostasis.

Vital signs serve as a communication tool regarding patient status – their physiological status. The physical deterioration of patients within acute mental health settings must also be observed, recorded and actively managed. It is essential that the assessment of vital signs, the documentation and their reporting are undertaken according to local policy and procedure and aligned to professional requirements (Nursing and Midwifery Council, 2018).

When there is an aberration in vital signs and the parameters have changed, this must be reported through appropriate channels. The nurse adheres to established ways of working and best practice.

When undertaking assessment, the nurse observes, for example, for pyrexia, tachycardia, tachypnoea, low oxygen saturations, hypotension, pallor, anorexia, tiredness and widening peripheral-core temperature gap (Brady, 2019). The frequency of these observations will depend on the person's condition and the likelihood of deterioration. Recordings are noted on an observation chart so as to determine trends and to highlight any deterioration and to prompt action. NEWS2 is the national early warning score and is being increasingly used in a number of care areas. It is based on an aggregate scoring system whereby a score is allocated to physiological measurements, already recorded in routine practice (Royal College of

Table 3.1   Systems and homeostasis.

Systems	Relationships
The cell	In Chapter 2, cell and tissue physiology are addressed. The cell is an open system providing the substrates that the cell requires for living. Changes in physical and chemical conditions beyond a narrow range will lead to the cell's death, and homeostatic imbalance occurs (disease) (Chapter 4 considers cancer).
Inflammation, immune response and healing	Inflammation and the immune response can be considered defence systems or defence responses (Chapter 5). The process of healing can only occur when homeostasis has occurred. The lymphatic system is functionally part of the immune system.
Shock	An organism responds with a number of reactions during each stage of shock as it attempts to maintain cellular homeostasis (Chapter 6). The relationship between homeostasis and stress responses is stark in shock. Stress responses have cell-autonomous and cell-extrinsic components, which contribute to tissue-level adaptation to stress conditions. There is disequilibrium/disruption.
The nervous system	The nervous system (Chapter 7) is the major control system of homeostasis; it monitors, responds and regulates. Maintaining a steady state requires the nervous system to control body function. Prompt regulation of bodily activities occurs through rapid nerve impulses that are transported through the central and peripheral nervous systems. The central nervous system comprises the brain and spinal cord; the peripheral nervous system comprises all of the nervous system that is outside of the central nervous system.
The heart	The heart is required to pump out blood through blood vessels, systematically (around the body). The blood contains the requisites for cell function. The heart is discussed in Chapter 8. Chapter 9 considers the vessels in the vascular system. Chapter 10 discusses erythrocytes that transport oxygen; lymphocytes that have a role to play in immunity and thrombocytes that are responsible for controlling bleeding.
The renal system	The renal system (Chapter 11) is another key system in the maintenance of homeostasis. It is a regulatory system. The chemical composition of body fluids and elimination of waste (toxic) products are key responsibilities of the renal system. In order to maintain homeostasis, the internal environment has to remain relatively stable, often within narrow margins. The kidneys regulate the water concentration in the blood and excrete toxic waste. When they fail to work properly, dialysis treatment or a transplant may be required. Fluid, electrolyte and acid-base balance are controlled by the action of the kidneys and other systems that work in close proximity (Chapter 19 considers fluid and electrolyte balance).
The respiratory system	This remarkable body system has the capacity to maintain a consistent internal environment. The respiratory system (Chapter 12), enables O_2 to reach body cells and to eliminate CO_2. Respiratory homeostasis is concerned with the regulation of blood gas composition that is compatible with maintaining cellular homeostasis.
The digestive system	The body requires a constant supply of nutrients from digested food, essential for body functions and the maintenance of health; this is the work of the digestive system (Chapter 13). The gastrointestinal tract and accessory organs enable food to enter the body and be used for body function. The digestive system contributes to homeostasis by transferring nutrients from the external environment to the internal environment.

(Continued)

Table 3.1 (*Continued*)

Systems	Relationships
The endocrine system	The endocrine system is a regulatory system and plays an important role in homeostasis as hormones, secreted into the bloodstream, regulate the activity of body cells. Regulation of bodily activity occurs due to the action of various endocrine glands that regulate metabolism, and therefore the activity levels of a number of organs of the body, through the secretion of chemical messengers (hormones) that are transported in body fluids to target cells.
The reproductive systems	The reproductive systems do not contribute to the maintenance of a constant internal environment that is essential for the survival of cells. The reproductive systems (Chapter 16) enable continuation of the species; they are responsible for gametogenesis. The reproductive systems aid in the homeostasis of an organism, the sex hormones affect organs and if there is homeostatic imbalance this has the potential to cause disease. The ability to reproduce and to perpetuate the species is dependent on a complex relationship between the reproductive organs and the hypothalamus, the anterior pituitary gland as well as the target cells of the sex hormones.
Pain and pain management	Pain creates a state of imbalance (physically and psychologically), and the aim is to address the disequilibrium, returning the organism to internal stability. The various components of pain (discussed in Chapter 17) are directly associated with the homeostatic and adaptive nature of pain. Pain is a threat to homeostatic function; this usually motivates individuals to engage in a range of behaviours, the common denominator being survival.
The musculoskeletal system	The musculoskeletal system (Chapter 18) contributes to the maintenance of homeostasis in a number of ways, including thermoregulation, muscle homeostasis and growth. The skeleton provides protection, support and movement. Bone marrow has a major role in the formation of blood cells (Chapter 10). It also helps maintain the level of calcium in the blood, and the skeletal system acts as a reservoir for minerals.
Fluid and electrolyte balance	Chapter 19 describes the importance of fluid and electrolytes, highlighting how essential they are in homeostasis and for the body to function. Electrolytes help regulate myocardial and neurological function, fluid balance, oxygen delivery, acid-base balance and other biological processes. All other body systems will require fluid and electrolytes to be in balance.
The skin	Skin (Chapter 20) has multiple roles in homeostasis, including protection, temperature regulation, sensory perception, biochemical synthesis and absorption. In addition, the skin contributes to the adaptive immune system. The sensory receptors located in the skin send information to the central nervous system, where action is initiated. The skin plays an important role in vitamin D production.
The senses	The senses help the body react to stimuli by responding to changes in pressure, temperature, perception, and so forth, alerting the body to danger. The body responds and reacts to protect itself from danger or maintain homeostatic balance. The senses (Chapter 21) contribute to homeostasis, helping to measure external factors, detecting changes in the external environment of the body and relaying their findings. The sensory system transports information to the central nervous system from special and general organs where information is interpreted and homeostasis is maintained.

Table 3.2 The SBAR communication tool.

Component	Example
Situation	I am (name), (X) nurse on ward (X)
	I am calling about (patient X)
	I am calling because I am concerned that … (e.g. BP is low/high, pulse is XX, temperature is XX, NEWS2 is XX)
Background	Patient (X) was admitted on (XX date) with … (e.g. myocardial infarction/chest infection)
	They have had (X operation/procedure/investigation)
	Patient (X)'s condition has changed in the last (XX minutes)
	Their last set of vital signs were (XX)
	Patient (X)'s normal condition is … (e.g. alert/drowsy/confused, pain free)
Assessment	I think the problem is (XXX) and I have … (e.g. given O_2/analgesia, stopped the infusion) OR
	I am not sure what the problem is but patient (X) is deteriorating
	OR
	I don't know what's wrong, but I am very worried
Recommendation	I need you to …
	Come to see the patient in the next (XX minutes) AND
	Is there anything I need to do in the meantime? (e.g. stop the fluid/repeat vital signs)
At the end of the interaction, ask the receiver to repeat key information to ensure understanding.	

Source: NHS Improvement (ND), 2020.

Physicians, 2017). There are six physiological parameters that form the basis of the scoring system:

1. Respiration rate
2. Oxygen saturation
3. Systolic blood pressure
4. Pulse rate
5. Level of consciousness or new confusion
6. Temperature

Concerns, deviations and any deterioration must be proactively escalated. The use of communication tools such as SBAR (NHS Improvement 2020) can help ensure that information to be transferred is transmitted accurately between individuals:

- Situation
- Background
- Assessment
- Recommendation

The SBAR Communication tool is detailed in Table 3.2.

Whilst tools such as the SBAR can aid in communication and the use of an early warning score such as NEWS2 can help identify the deteriorating patient, it is the nurse's interpretation and synthesis of data that are key to safe and effective care provision.

Conclusion

Homeostasis is the preservation of relatively stable conditions in the body's internal environment; this comes about as a result of interactions between all of the body's regulatory processes. During an episode of illness, the pathophysiology of homeostasis is a complex process, and the body tries to manage its return to stability. This chapter has explored some of the events that can disrupt homeostasis. It has also highlighted the importance of recording and interpreting the patient's vital signs and observations followed by analysis of the underlying pathophysiology. It has been emphasised that the prompt escalation of any concerns is an integral part of the healthcare professional's duties.

The overall goal of homeostasis is to maintain equilibrium around the set point. Whilst there are normal fluctuations from the set point, the systems of the body will usually attempt to correct these. When a change in the internal or external environment (a stimulus) is detected by a receptor, the system responds and attempts to adjust the anomalous parameter towards the set point. If, for example, the body becomes too warm, adjustments are made to cool the person. If the blood's glucose rises after a meal, adjustments are made to lower the blood glucose level by moving the nutrient into tissues, or to store it for later use.

When a patient's vital signs are assessed, the nurse is undertaking an objective measure of homeostasis. When there is ill health or disease, homeostasis is challenged, and vital signs indicate this as they fall outside of their normal range. Undertaking accurate measurement of vital signs is essential in diagnosis, clinical decision-making and treatment. The nurse must record and report any abnormality so as to intervene rapidly when appropriate.

Activities

Here are some activities and exercises to help test your learning. For the answers to these exercises, as well as further self-testing activities, visit our website at **www.wiley.com/go/fundamentalsofappliedpathophysiology/student4e**

Multiple choice questions

1. Homeostasis is best described as:
   (a) Maintaining a near-constant internal environment
   (b) Maintaining a near-constant external environment
   (c) The ability to produce blood cells
   (d) Keeping the body in a fixed and unaltered state
2. Where in the body is the temperature monitored and controlled?
   (a) The baroreceptors
   (b) The skin
   (c) The cauda equina
   (d) The hypothalamus
3. The term *thermogenesis* means:
   (a) Temperature regulation
   (b) Shivering
   (c) Sweating
   (d) Heat production

4. The following are examples of effectors:
   (a) Glands and muscles
   (b) Glands and neurones
   (c) Neurones and synapses
   (d) Synapses and glands
5. Name two sense organs that are sensitive to chemicals:
   (a) Nose and lungs
   (b) Skin and kidneys
   (c) Mouth and nose
   (d) Nose and kidneys
6. In thermoregulation, what type of feedback is involved?
   (a) Positive
   (b) Negative
   (c) Neutral
   (d) Positive and negative
7. Cells can function:
   (a) Only in a narrow range of temperatures and pH
   (b) In a wide range of temperatures
   (c) In diverse range of pH
   (d) Only when the pH is acidic
8. The respiratory system helps to maintain homeostasis by:
   (a) Regulating oxygen levels
   (b) By causing the contraction of muscles
   (c) Releasing histamine
   (d) Evoking thermogenesis
9. A receptor:
   (a) Is only located on the surface of the skin
   (b) Detects stimuli
   (c) Always causes energy release
   (d) Will not function in disease
10. When a response improves the original stimuli, the system is:
    (a) Operating by neutral feedback.
    (b) Operating by dynamic feedback
    (c) Operating by positive feedback
    (d) Failing
11. The main stimulus for increasing intake of fluids is:
    (a) Decreased urinary output
    (b) Headache
    (c) Thirst
    (d) A coated tongue
12. In most cases, a disruption in homeostasis:
    (a) Causes the cells of the body to respond quickly
    (b) Is mild and balance is restored
    (c) Is usually temporary
    (d) All of the above
13. The systems that most often provide corrective measures are:
    (a) The reproductive systems
    (b) The renal and reproductive systems
    (c) The nervous and endocrine systems
    (d) The gastrointestinal and endocrine systems

14. Which is correct concerning the homeostatic responses?
    (a) Nerve impulses typically cause rapid change
    (b) Nerve impulses typically result in a slower response
    (c) Hormones typically cause rapid change
    (d) Nerve impulses are redundant

15. The endocrine system secretes messenger molecules that are called:
    (a) Neurones
    (b) Peptides
    (c) Hormones
    (d) Gametes

References

Brady, M. (2019). Homeostasis. In: Gormley-Fleming, E. and Peate, I. (eds), *Fundamentals of Children's Applied Pathophysiology. An Essential Guide for Nursing and Healthcare Students*. Oxford: Wiley, Chapter 4, 67–81.

Cedar, S.H. (2017). Homoeostasis and vital signs: Their role in health and its restoration. *Nursing Times* [online], 113(8): 32–35.

McCance, K. (2019). Cellular biology. In McCance, K.L. *et al.* (eds), *Pathophysiology. The Biologic Basis for Disease in Adult and Children*, 8th edn. St Louis: Elsevier, Chapter 1, pp. 2–45.

NHS Improvement (ND) (2020). *SBAR Communication Tool – Situation, Background, Assessment, Recommendation* https://improvement.nhs.uk/documents/2162/sbar-communication-tool.pdf *last accessed* March 2020.

Nursing and Midwifery Council (2018). *The Code. Professional Standards of Practice and Behaviour for Nurses, Midwives and Nursing Associates* https://www.nmc.org.uk/globalassets/sitedocuments/nmc-publications/nmc-code.pdf *last accessed* March 2020.

Royal College of Physicians (2017). *National Early Warning Score (NEWS) 2. Standardising the Assessment of Acute Illness Severity in the NHS. Executive Summary and Recommendation* https://www.rcplondon.ac.uk/projects/outputs/national-early-warning-score-news-2 *last accessed* March 2020.

Tortora, G.J. and Derrickson, B.H. (2017). *Tortora's Principles of Anatomy and Physiology*. New Jersey: Wiley.

Watson, R. (2018). *Anatomy and Physiology for Nurses*, 14th edn. Edinburgh: Elsevier.

Chapter 4

Cancer

Carl Clare

Senior Lecturer, Department of Adult Nursing and Primary Care, School of Health and Social Work, University of Hertfordshire, Hatfield, Hertfordshire, UK

Contents

Introduction	65
Biology of cancer	66
Causes of cancer	69
Staging of cancers	73
Signs and symptoms of cancer	74
Treatment of cancer	75
Prevention of cancer	77
Examples of cancers	79
Conclusion	88
Multiple choice questions	89
Conditions	90
Further resources	91
Glossary of terms	92
References	94

Key words

- Cancer
- Tumour
- Oncogene
- Chemotherapy
- Carcinogen
- Malignant
- Radiotherapy
- Immunotherapy
- Carcinoma
- Neoplasm
- Cytotoxic

Fundamentals of Applied Pathophysiology: An Essential Guide for Nursing and Healthcare Students, Fourth Edition. Edited by Ian Peate.
© 2021 John Wiley & Sons Ltd. Published 2021 by John Wiley & Sons Ltd.
Student companion website: www.wiley.com/go/fundamentalsofappliedpathophysiology/student4e
Instructor companion website: www.wiley.com/go/fundamentalsofappliedpathophysiology/instructor4e

Test your prior knowledge

- What is the difference between a malignant tumour and a benign tumour?
- Name three methods of treating cancer.
- What can cause lung cancer?
- What is the aim of palliative treatment?

Learning outcomes

On completion of this chapter, the reader will be able to:

- Discuss the process of carcinogenesis and explain the difference between benign and malignant tumours.

- List and explain the ways in which the body tries to prevent cancers from growing.

- Describe the role of genes and environmental factors in the development of cancers.

- Understand the staging of cancers and describe some of the more common cancers.

- Describe the signs and symptoms of cancer and explain what causes them.

- List and discuss the many ways in which cancers can be treated.

 Don't forget to visit the companion website for this book (www.wiley.com/go/fundamentalsofappliedpathophysiology/student4e) **where you can find self-assessment tests to check your progress, as well as lots of activities to practise your learning.**

Introduction

According to Cancer Research UK (2019a), approximately 166 544 people died of cancer in the UK in 2017, most of whom were over 65 years of age.

Cancer is a disease of abnormal cell growth, cell division and cell differentiation. The disease 'cancer' actually consists of a group of diseases, all of which are underpinned by (and caused by) uncontrolled abnormal cell growth. Cancers are always life-threatening but not always fatal. There are many causes of cancers, just as there are many types of cancers.

According to McCance (2018a), the cells of multicellular organisms are not concerned just with the individual cell, but rather with the survival of the entire multicellular organism. These cells can be thought of as specialised members of a society – a cellular society. This means that all cells work for the good of the organism. Because of this, the processes of cell division, proliferation and differentiation are normally regulated so that they are in balance – particularly a balance between the rate of cell birth and the rate of cell death (see Chapter 2).

However, as in any society, there are always some abnormal cells that disobey all social control mechanisms; in this case, the social control mechanisms of cell division, proliferation and differentiation. These are the cells that will proliferate to form tumours in the body, and indeed, as McCance (2018a) points out, virtually every cell in the body has the potential to become a tumour if it mutates.

Carcinogenesis is a multistep mechanism and is caused by an accumulation of cellular and chemical errors, particularly concerning the deoxyribonucleic acid (DNA) of a cell. Altered DNA bases – known as mutations – are the cause of any changes that lead to cells becoming cancers, and several mutations within the DNA are required for carcinogenesis to happen. Carcinogenesis always begins with a single cell whose DNA has been damaged for some reason. This cell starts to grow in an abnormal and uncontrolled way. Following the process of division and reproduction, as discussed in Chapter 2, each new daughter cell, because it has inherited its parent's DNA, also grows in an uncontrolled way. Normally, a cell is programmed to stop growing when it reaches its correct size, but because of the DNA abnormality (mutation), it continues past this point and grows ever larger.

The body does have mechanisms to deal with cells that are abnormal, which means that these cells that carry a genetic mutation causing uncontrolled growth should either commit suicide (apoptosis) or should be killed by the body's own defences (see Chapter 2). In order to become a cancer, these abnormal cells have to multiply literally billions of times. It takes a long time for a single cell to develop billions of daughter cells, and this is why cancers are generally considered to be diseases of old age. Unfortunately, there are exceptions to this, and some cancers develop in children (some even in babies). Examples are some cancers of the eye – retinoblastoma, and of the blood – certain leukaemias. However, the idea that cancer is generally a disease linked with old age still holds true, and there is a high incidence of cancer occurring after the age of 40 years.

Cancer can occur in almost any cell, but the most common cancers are to be found in the:

- Breast
- Prostate gland
- Lung
- Bowel
- Skin.

Over the past few years, there have been some changes in the incidence rates of the various cancers. For example, the incidence of stomach and colon cancer has reduced, whilst the incidence of skin and kidney cancers has increased (Smittenaar *et al.*, 2016).

Despite all the advances in diagnosis, care and treatment of cancer, the overall rate of cancer deaths has increased. Rates of cancer related to the Human Papilloma Virus (HPV), specifically oral, anal, and cervical, are showing a significant increase in incidence. However, at present the effect of the HPV vaccination programme introduced in the UK in 2008 are yet to show an effect (Smittenaar *et al.*, 2016).

Biology of cancer

For whatever reason, the DNA of a cell becomes altered, causing the cell to grow uncontrollably. This is known as the initiation period. What happens after the cell starts to grow uncontrollably determines whether or not cancer will occur.

Apoptosis (or cell suicide) is a process that is continually occurring within the body. This is because altered and damaged cells are constantly being produced in the body. To understand why this should be so, one only needs to look at the process by which DNA and cells are replicated. This process is an extremely rapid one (as it needs to keep pace with the needs of the body in terms of replacing altered and damaged cells). For example, skin cells are constantly being replaced because of damage caused by being worn away and dislodged every time the skin comes into contact with any surface. Because of the speed at which this very complicated process of DNA replication occurs, it can be no surprise when mistakes occur. There are several mechanisms by which cellular apoptosis can be induced (Figure 4.1); e.g. internal cell stresses can lead to apoptosis via the cell's own mitochondria.

Another mechanism that the body possesses to try and prevent the development of damaged cells is their destruction by the body's own immune system. One of the many functions of the immune system is called immune surveillance, and this does just what it says. Certain white blood cells of the immune system (including cytotoxic T lymphocytes) move through the body looking for any abnormal or 'alien' cells (e.g. bacteria and viruses). Each cell carries receptors on its outer membrane, and some of these receptors are specific identification (ID) receptors that identify them as belonging to that particular body. If these cytotoxic T lymphocytes come across a cell that does not carry these particular ID receptors for that body, then they will kill it. Either there is activation of death receptors on the cell wall or there is activation of apoptosis using an enzyme known as granzyme.

Although cancerous cells will belong to the same body as the cytotoxic T lymphocytes, because of their alteration, due to the altered DNA, the ID receptors on these cancerous cells may have slight alterations in their formation. Luckily, even though there is only a slight alteration to the ID receptors carried by cancerous cells, they are still different enough for the T cells to recognise them as not being 'correct' cells, and to destroy them. However, unfortunately, some of the cells (known as precancerous cells) are able to develop strategies to hide their dif-

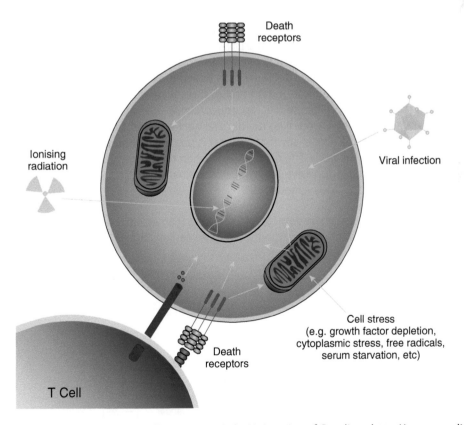

Figure 4.1 Apoptosis. *Source:* Cell Migration Lab, University of Reading, http://www.reading.ac.uk/cellmigration/apoptosis.htm.

ferences from the immune system, and so escape being destroyed by the T cells. Once the precancerous cells have achieved this evasion of the body's immune system, they can then proceed to divide and replicate in order to cause cancers, because all their daughter cells will also have this ability to evade the T lymphocytes (Gorczynski and Stanley, 2006; Vickers, 2005).

Once the precancerous cell has developed a strategy for avoiding both apoptosis and the T lymphocytes, it can then proceed to clone itself, and the cancer starts to develop. To transform a single precancerous cell into a cancer requires more than just a straightforward cloning of this cell, because, in addition to the cell cloning itself, new blood vessels need to form (known as angiogenesis). These new blood vessels need to develop because all cells require a good blood supply so that oxygen and nutrients can reach them and keep them alive (as well as allowing for the removal of carbon dioxide and other toxins). In order for these new blood vessels to develop, the cancerous cell needs to produce angiogenic growth factors. The other thing to consider is that the cancerous cells need extra blood flow (more than a normal cell) because they are growing so rapidly and to such a great size that they require extra oxygen and nutrients for the growth to continue and for the extra metabolism that is required by the cancerous cell.

There are several models that demonstrate the development of cancers, and the two most relevant ones are the following:

- Molecular biology model – Figure 4.2 illustrates the process of the development of cancer from the cellular perspective. A normal cell can become precancerous as a result of DNA changes (1) during reproduction/cloning. The precancerous cell can then become a cancer as a result of further alteration in its DNA (2) during cloning, and the final DNA change (3) can cause the cancerous cell to become metastatic and to spread throughout the body. Thus, it can be seen that the DNA needs to continue to mutate for a normal cell to reach the metastatic stage – it is not just a single mutation.
- Clinical model – in this model (Figure 4.3), which looks at the actual clinical disease as opposed to the biochemical underpinning, the cancer commences with a normal cell, which starts to overproliferate (i.e. reproduce/clone excessively), so that although these cells are 'normal', they are dividing rapidly. The next stage occurs when there are sufficient cancerous cells to be able to say that a cancer is present, although it is still only situated in one place within the body. The third stage is when the cancerous cells start to invade the surrounding tissue (aggressive behaviour), and finally the cancer spreads to other, often remote, parts of the body – metastasis.

Often, once a cancer can be detected, it is already at an advanced stage and thus the prognosis is poorer than if it had been diagnosed at an earlier stage.

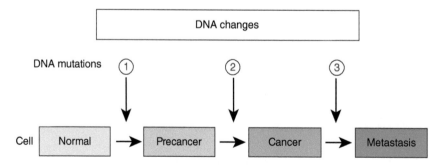

Figure 4.2   Molecular biology model (*Source*: King, 2000).

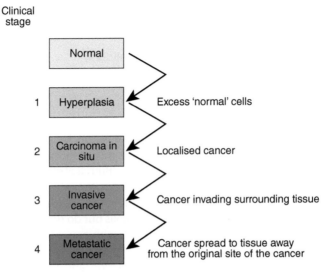

Figure 4.3   Clinical model (*Source:* King, 2000).

Causes of cancer

The main causes of cancer appear to be linked to interactions between genes and the environment.

Genes

The role of genes in the development of cancer is very important, and there are three types of genes that are involved:

1. Proto-oncogenes
2. Oncogenes
3. Tumour suppressor genes.

Proto-oncogenes possess the genetic codes for the proteins that are needed for normal cell division and growth, whilst oncogenes are proto-oncogenes that have mutated and so have become cancer-causing genes that increase the rate at which cells divide and proliferate. One of the problems with proto-oncogenes is that many of them have fragile sites that can easily break once they are exposed to carcinogens. Once this occurs, then the proto-oncogenes are converted into oncogenes. Unfortunately, since oncogenes have been discovered in only 15–20% of cancers found in humans, there has to be something else which causes cancerous cells to develop, and tumour suppressor genes, e.g. *p*53, provide the answer. Tumour suppressor genes work to suppress or even prevent cancer by repairing any damaged cell DNA, as well as slowing down or even stopping cell division.

These tumour suppressor genes also help to inactivate carcinogens as well as improving the ability of the immune system to destroy cancer cells (Cosgrove *et al.*, 2016). When these mutated cancer-causing cells occur in germline cells (i.e. sperm and ova), then the cancer-causing genes can be inherited from one generation to the next, and so produce families in which there is a predisposition for certain cancers, such as breast cancer (Robson *et al.*, 2015). Therefore, it is now known that certain forms of cancer oncogenes can be inherited within some families. However, if the oncogene is only to be found in somatic cells, then it would not be inherited by future generations. Examples of inherited cancers, for which a specific oncogene has been isolated, include the following:

- Retinoblastoma – cancer of the eye (found in children)
- Wilms' tumour – cancer of the kidney (also found in children)
- Familial breast cancer.

Environmental factors

The link between cancer genes and environmental factors is one of increasing interest. The frequency of the cancer-causing mutations and the seriousness of their effects can be altered by a large number of environmental factors (Burrell et al., 2013). Chemicals that cause mutations in cells can cause cancers, and so it is appropriate to describe these particular chemicals as carcinogens. In addition, there are other environmental agents that may enhance the development of genetically altered cells but do not cause new mutations. So, it would seem that it is often the interplay of genes with environmental factors that leads to carcinogenesis, and they cannot be viewed in isolation (Carbone et al., 2018)

Environmental factors, such as chemicals, radiation and viruses, can cause cancer by increasing the frequency with which cells mutate. Environmental agents that cause cancer are known as carcinogens, and most carcinogens are mutagens (they increase the frequency of mutations). What is apparent is that most of the agents that are known to cause cancer (carcinogenesis) also cause genetic changes (mutagenesis), whilst factors that cause genetic change also cause cancer.

Many environmental agents are known to be carcinogenic, including:

- Radiation
- Alcohol
- Chemicals
- Some foods
- Air pollution
- Smoking
- Viruses.

At the same time, however, most human cancers appear to arise spontaneously, and develop without any known prior exposure to a carcinogenic agent, but this may be because the carcinogenic agents have not yet been identified.

Radiation

- Ultraviolet radiation – ultraviolet (UV) sunlight (or solar radiation) causes basal cell carcinoma and squamous cell carcinoma (see Chapter 20). These are two common cancers that are found in people who havev pale skin with a light complexion. This type of radiation causes mutations in two tumour suppressor genes. In addition, the very malignant pigmented moles known as melanomas are linked to the amount of exposure to UV light.
- Ionising radiation – the list of carcinomas caused by ionising radiation is extremely long, and includes:
  - Acute leukaemias in adults and children
  - Thyroid cancer
  - Breast cancer
  - Lung cancer
  - Stomach cancer
  - Cancer of the colon

- Oesophageal cancer
- Urinary tract cancer
- Multiple myeloma.

Ionising radiation is thought to inhibit cell division. This is of particular importance where the cells only live for a short time, which leads to rapid cell division, e.g.:

- Lymphocytes
- Cells of lymphoid tissue
- Bone marrow cells
- Intestinal epithelial cells.

The developing foetus is especially at risk, even at such low doses that may not cause any problems to adults. This is because during pregnancy, foetal organ development occurs very early and at an extremely rapid rate; therefore, even small doses of radiation can completely alter the integrity of the cells and hence normal development. This is why pregnant women – especially in the early stage of pregnancy – should not have X-rays taken (unless there is no alternative and their condition is life-threatening).

Smoking

It has been known for a long time that cigarette smoking is carcinogenic, and that it remains one of the most important causes of cancer. A hundred years ago, lung cancer was a rare disease, but as the incidence of cigarette smoking increased, so the incidence of lung cancer rose to epidemic proportions. Smoking not only leads to lung cancer, it also increases the incidence of cancer of the bladder, pancreas, kidney, larynx, oral cavity and oesophagus. The reason for this is that there are 70 carcinogens in tobacco smoke that can cause tumours.

Diet

Many toxic, mutagenic and carcinogenic chemicals can be found in the human diet. Sources of toxic carcinogenic substances within our diet include various compounds that are produced during the cooking of fat or protein. In addition, there are naturally occurring carcinogens that are associated with plant food substances, e.g. alkaloids and by-products of moulds/fungi.

Alcohol

Alcohol is linked with increased rates of incidence of oral cancer and cancer of the pharynx, larynx, oesophagus and liver – particularly if taken with large quantities of tobacco in the form of cigarettes, cigars and in pipes. Alcohol interacts with smoke, and this increases the risk of malignant tumours. Although the rationale for this has not been proved, it is thought that it possibly acts as a solvent for the carcinogenic smoke products. Alcohol consumption has also been linked to breast cancer and colorectal cancer.

Sexual and reproductive behaviour

The possible mechanism for the carcinogenesis of cervical and other cancers of the sexual organs is a viral infection transmitted between sexual partners. According to Lowy and Schiller (2012), the age of first sexual intercourse allied to the number of sexual partners (or the number of sexual partners of a partner) are the major factors leading to the risk of the development of cervical cancer.

Certain types of the human papillomavirus (HPV) are known to be a cause of cervical cancer. HPV has also been identified with many other cancers of the anogenital region, such as cancers of the penis, vulva and anus (Lowy and Schiller, 2012).

Environmental pollution

Because of the huge quantities of air that humans inhale every day (about 20 000 L), even small amounts of carcinogens and other pollutants in the atmosphere can cause problems. There is particular concern with the industrial emissions of pollutants, such as arsenic, benzene, chloroform and vinyl chloride, and there is an increasing focus on fine particulate matter (Vineis and Fecht, 2018). Consequently, it is recognised that living close to certain industries and in areas of significant traffic congestion are risk factors for developing certain cancers, although, again, other factors have to be taken into account – especially lifestyle factors (such as drinking and smoking, as discussed earlier). According to Si (2018), indoor pollution is generally considered to be a greater risk than outdoor pollution, partly because of second-hand or environmental tobacco smoke, but also due to the amount of time we spend indoors compared to outdoors.

Along with smoke, another indoor air pollutant of significance is radon gas – this is a natural radioactive gas that is present in certain soils (e.g. granite). It can become trapped in houses and produce carcinogenic radioactive decay products (Eggertson, 2015).

Occupation

Exposures to carcinogenic substances as a result of one's occupation have been recognised for a long time as a cause of cancer. In Victorian times, for example, there was a high incidence of testicular cancer amongst boy chimney sweeps.

Asbestos accounts for the largest number of occupational cancers in recent years, although the situation is improving as the risks of asbestos have become common knowledge. What is particularly of concern is that a combination of asbestos exposure and cigarette smoking can lead to a significant increase in the risk of lung cancer (Vineis and Wild, 2014). In actual fact, a large percentage of cancers of the upper respiratory tract, lung, bladder and peritoneum can be linked causally to various occupational factors.

Hormones

The relationship between hormones and human cancer has been widely studied. Hormones, such as steroids, can be immunosuppressive. However, much of the current research on hormones and cancer focuses on the sex steroids, which include:

- Oestrogen
- Progesterone
- Testosterone.

According to McCance (2018b), most evidence to date supports the role of hormones as promoters of carcinogenesis in target tissues rather than as primary carcinogens. However, oestrogen is now being seen as a cause of cancer, but its exact mechanism is unknown.

Oral contraceptives

A large cohort study of 1.8 million women followed over an average of 10.9 years has shown a small increase in the incidence of breast cancer in women taking contemporary oral contraceptives (Mørch et al., 2017). This risk increases with the length of time the contraceptives are taken and persists for up to 5 years in those who have used oral contraceptives for longer periods. Other studies (Kabat et al., 2010) have identified subgroups of women using oral contraceptives who have an increased risk of breast cancer. These subgroups include the following:

- Women who have used oral contraceptives for many years prior to the age of 25 years
- Those who used them before 1971

- Extended use before the first full-term pregnancy
- Use at the age of 45 years or older
- History of biopsy-confirmed benign breast disorders
- Nulliparous, premenopausal women, with an early menarche
- Women with only one child
- Family history of breast cancer.

In contrast, complete/incomplete pregnancies and the use of oral contraceptives reduce the risk of ovarian cancer (Huber *et al.*, 2020). This is because ovarian cancer appears to develop from the epithelial cells on the ovarian surface, and the main stimulus for division of these cells is ovulation itself. What happens is that after each ovulation, epithelial cells then replicate in order to ensure that the exposed surface of the ovary (following ovulation and release of the egg) is covered. So, those factors that help to prevent ovulation also help to protect against ovarian cancers. The risk of endometrial cancer is reduced by 55% in women who have taken oral contraceptives for 5 years, as opposed to those who have not used oral contraceptives. In addition, it is also thought that oral contraceptive usage may reduce colo-rectal cancers (Long *et al.*, 2010).

Male hormones

The male sex hormone (i.e. testosterone) actually stimulates the growth of target tissues for cancers, such as the prostate – hence the risk of benign or malignant prostate tumours.

Viruses

A group of viruses known as oncogenic viruses can cause cancers:

- Papovaviruses
- Adenoviruses
- Herpesviruses
- Hepadenoviruses.

Burkitt lymphoma and nasopharyngeal carcinoma are caused by the Epstein-Barr virus (EBV), whilst HPV is found in cervical cancer (Mui *et al.*, 2017).

Staging of cancers

Following the diagnosis of a cancer, the patient will be told the stage that the cancer has reached. The stage of a cancer at the time of diagnosis can give an indication of the likely prognosis for the patient. The staging system is linked to the spread of the cancer (metastasis). The common sites for the metastatic spread of cancer include the brain, the lungs, the bones and the liver (Figure 4.4).

There are four general cancer stages – although most types of cancer also have specific staging criteria (NHS, 2018):

- Stage 1 – The cancer is small, and there is no spread of the cancer from the original site of the cancer.
- Stage 2 – The cancer has grown, but has not spread.
- Stage 3 – The cancer is larger and has spread to local tissues or lymph nodes.
- Stage 4 – The cancer has spread to at least one other organ in the body.

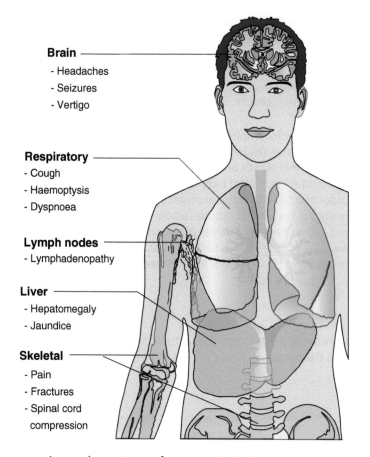

Brain
- Headaches
- Seizures
- Vertigo

Respiratory
- Cough
- Haemoptysis
- Dyspnoea

Lymph nodes
- Lymphadenopathy

Liver
- Hepatomegaly
- Jaundice

Skeletal
- Pain
- Fractures
- Spinal cord
  compression

Figure 4.4   Common sites and symptoms of cancer metastasis.

Cancers that have started to spread have a much poorer prognosis than cancers that are still confined to their original site. Stage 1 cancers have a much better chance of responding to treatment, whilst stage 4 cancers are very often terminal. Consequently, the earlier a patient is diagnosed, the better the chances of overcoming cancer.

Signs and symptoms of cancer

Cancers can present in many ways depending upon the type of cancer and where it is situated, e.g. the brain, kidney, blood or breast, but there are some common factors to most of them:

- General run down condition (general malaise, anorexia/loss of appetite, loss of weight)
- Marked change in bowel or bladder habits
- Nausea or vomiting for no apparent reason
- Bloody discharge of any kind; failure to stop bleeding in the usual time
- Presence of swelling, lump or mass anywhere in the body
- Any change in the size or appearance of moles or birthmarks
- Unexplained stumbling
- Unexplained pain (or persistent crying of an infant or child).

The problem that the healthcare provider has in diagnosing cancer is that these signs and symptoms can be related to many other medical conditions. This is why there is sometimes a delay in diagnosing cancer until the cancer has developed and may have started to metastasise.

Treatment of cancer

Whilst there are different treatments for different cancers, there are certain principles and types of treatment that are generally accepted as standard. There are six types of treatment that are mainly used at the moment – depending upon the individual cancer and patient:

- Drug therapy
- Radiation therapy
- Immunotherapy
- Surgical removal
- Hormone therapy
- Photodynamic therapy.

The first, very important, point to make is that the earlier the cancer is diagnosed and treatment begins, the better will be the prognosis. If the cancer is still localised (i.e. it has not spread to other parts of the body) at the time of diagnosis, then the plan would be the removal of the primary cancer by surgery, accompanied by drug therapy and/or radiation therapy. Unfortunately, not all cancers are amenable to surgery, e.g. the blood cancers such as leukaemias and lymphomas.

If the cancer is detected late, or if surgery does not remove all of the primary cancer and metastasis occurs, then other forms of treatment are necessary – mainly drug therapy and radiotherapy. In this scenario, it is often not possible to cure the cancer and the treatment is based on preventing the growth of the cancer, or at least slowing it down.

Drug therapy

The other name for drug therapy is chemotherapy, and there are two different types of chemotherapy that are used in the treatment of cancer:

- Cytotoxic chemotherapy
- Cytostatic chemotherapy.

The difference between the two types of chemotherapy is that cytotoxic chemotherapy has the potential to cure a patient, whereas cytostatic drugs are not able to get rid of the cancer but can prevent it growing too large.

Red flag

Cytotoxic drugs

Cytotoxic drugs are harmful to normal tissue and potentially harmful to staff if not dealt with properly. Students should not handle cytotoxic drugs without supervision from an appropriately trained member of staff. The administration of cytotoxic drugs should include the use of appropriate personal protective equipment (PPE).

Local policy should be followed for dealing with the urine, faeces, blood and vomit of a patient receiving cytotoxic drugs. This will include the use of PPE when handling bodily fluids and waste for several days after the administration of the drug.

Side effects

Unfortunately, because all these drugs affect normal cells as well as cancerous cells, treatment using these drugs can cause many severe side effects (Perry *et al.*, 2012). These side effects can include the following:

- Secondary cancers, including leukaemia – these can occur because the normal blood cells, including the white blood cells which form a major part of the immune system (see Chapter 5), are particularly sensitive to many of these drugs, and a reduction in white blood cells can lead to further tumours arising because of a lack of immune surveillance.
- Infections – a reduction in white blood cells can leave the body open to serious infections, including septicaemia, because the immune system has been compromised.
- Sterility – the germ cells in the ovaries and testes are also very sensitive to these chemotherapeutic drugs, and young people in particular can become sterile as a result of the treatment.
- Hair loss – this occurs because the cells of the hair follicles are rapidly dividing (as can be seen from the speed at which hair grows), and as some chemotherapeutic drugs target rapidly dividing cells because cancerous cells are themselves rapidly dividing cells, normal rapidly dividing cells are also destroyed.
- Nausea and vomiting – these are frequent side effects of chemotherapy because the drugs can activate the centres in the brainstem that can cause vomiting.
- Skin damage – these occur in the same way that hair loss occurs, because skin cells have to rapidly replicate to replace the skin cells that are damaged with normal wear and tear.

Radiation therapy

Ionising radiation damages cell DNA. Once the DNA of a cell is damaged, one of three results can occur:

- The death of the cancerous cell
- The cell becomes so severely damaged that any changes in its environment will cause it to die
- The cell becomes damaged but can eventually repair itself.

Radiation therapy attempts to kill the cancer cell, but as with chemotherapy, normal cells can also be killed by the radiation.

Immunotherapy

Current attempts at using immunotherapy to cure tumours are based on the idea that the immune system can eradicate existing tumours by means of immune surveillance, and thus the modification of immune system cells may be a pathway to cancer therapy (Farkona *et al.*, 2018). Immunotherapy is still not standard therapy in clinical practice, but recent advances show promising results in areas such as prostate therapy (Schweizer and Drake, 2014).

Surgical removal

Surgical therapy is used when the cancer has not yet spread. In addition, it is generally agreed that if there is any chance that local lymph nodes may be involved but there is no evidence that the disease has spread, then the lymph nodes should also be removed.

As with chemotherapy, there are two types of surgery – surgery to cure the disease and palliative surgery. Palliative surgery, which means alleviating the symptoms without curing the cancer, has two purposes:

- To prevent symptoms that would have occurred without the surgery
- To relieve symptoms that are already present.

Hormonal therapy

Hormonal therapy has been used for some years now. Although how this works is not really known, it is thought to work by blocking receptors on the cancerous cells; it prevents a cell from receiving normal growth stimulation signals.

Examples of hormones being used in cancer therapy include:

- Corticosteroids – used in leukaemias, malignant lymphomas, Hodgkin's disease and breast cancer
- Androgens – used in breast cancer
- Oestrogens – used in breast cancer and prostate cancer.

Red flag

Steroids

The use of steroids in the treatment of cancer carries the same potential risk of the patient developing diabetes as it does in any other situation. Therefore, regular checks should be made of the patient's blood sugar.

Photodynamic therapy

Light on its own does not damage cells, whether they are malignant cells or normal cells. However, when light combines with oxygen, it can have a serious effect on photosensitive chemicals such as porphyrins (an example of a porphyrin is haemoglobin, which binds and transports oxygen in the body). It is now possible to produce a drug consisting of a modified porphyrin and to give it systemically; then the target cancer can be eliminated by using a special light that is focused on the cancer and not the surrounding tissues. This can cause the death of the malignant cells of the cancer. Photodynamic therapy has now been successfully used to treat:

- Cancers of the bladder
- Head and neck cancers
- Cancer of the oesophagus
- Skin cancers
- Non-small cell lung cancer.

Gene therapy

Gene therapy is still experimental, but there is ongoing work that is looking at using the fact that genetics plays an important part in the causes of cancer. The eventual hope is that it will be possible to replace the affected genes with normal ones.

Prevention of cancer

Although the treatment of cancers has improved dramatically over the last 20 years or so, it is still better to try and prevent cancers occurring in the first place. As was discussed earlier, there are many environmental and lifestyle factors that play a part in causing the development of cancers. These include smoking, diet, alcohol, occupation, sexual behaviour and UV radiation. By reducing or even removing these factors, it is possible, to a large extent, to prevent many cancers occurring, although, because of the genetic factors previously mentioned, cancers will never go away.

Increasing fruit and vegetable intake has the potential to reduce the risk of getting several cancers, including bowel cancer, breast cancer, cancer of the mouth, larynx and nasopharynx, and even lung cancer. In addition, bowel cancer and breast cancer, amongst others, can be prevented by reducing smoking as well as the intake of alcohol. A reduction in meat and alcohol intake, along with an increase in eating more fruits and vegetables, can reduce bowel cancer by as much as 70%. A diet that includes increased amounts of fruit and vegetables and reduced amounts of fat and alcohol can reduce breast cancer by as much as 40% if started before puberty (15% if started after puberty), whilst a diet high in fruit and vegetables can prevent an estimated 25% of lung cancers – in both smokers and non-smokers. So, it can be seen that diet is one environmental factor that can be used to reduce the incidence of many cancers.

For many years now, the link between smoking and lung cancer has been well known and well documented, although there are still many arguments about the role of passive smoking in causing lung cancer.

Taking sensible precautions in strong sunshine can prevent a lot of skin cancers, particularly the very malignant melanomas.

In addition to considering environmental factors as a means of preventing cancer, there are also certain drugs that can help to reduce cancers. For example, tamoxifen has been found to prevent breast cancers, particularly in women from families who carry a genetic defect that causes breast cancer. The major risk factor for breast cancer is excessive oestrogen production, and tamoxifen is an anti-oestrogen drug, which is why it helps to prevent breast cancer. However, in a major trial in the United States, it was found that women who took tamoxifen had twice as many endometrial cancers than the control group, in addition to a higher-than-expected incidence of problems such as pulmonary embolus and deep vein thrombosis. However, because the risk probability of developing breast cancer for some women in families who carry the breast cancer gene defects is as high as 80%, many of them believe that the risk of developing these other problems is outweighed by the risk of developing breast cancer if tamoxifen is not taken (Cuzick et al., 2015).

The fifth most common cause of cancer deaths in women is ovarian cancer, and oral contraceptive pills have been found to be effective against endometrial and ovarian cancer. In fact, it is so effective against ovarian cancer that oral contraceptive pills have now halved the risk of developing it.

Another drug that appears to prevent a particular type of cancer, colon cancer, is aspirin. Colon cancer is the third most important cause of cancer-related deaths in both men and women. It is not only aspirin that is effective, but also non-steroidal anti-inflammatory drugs that are taken for arthritis and similar diseases.

Finally, it is necessary to look at the potential role of vaccines in preventing various cancers. There have been many approaches that have been used to develop vaccines for use in the treatment of cancer. At present, prophylactic approaches to cancer focus on the use of vaccines that will induce immunity to viruses that are known to be associated with the development of a tumour, in the same way that any vaccination induces immunity to the causative organism, e.g. measles, mumps or rubella. An example of a vaccine in use to give immunity to a cancer is the HPV vaccine. HPV vaccines prevent the development of cervical carcinoma because HPV is a known cause of cervical cancer (Giuliano et al., 2015).

Medicines management

HPV vaccines

The HPV vaccine has been shown to be effective in preventing precancerous changes and is recommended for women between 15 and 26 years of age. Latest research shows that the HPV vaccine is safe in pregnancy and is not associated with an increased rate of miscarriage (Arbyn *et al.*, 2018).

Another possible vaccine against a virus that causes cancer would be a vaccine against hepatitis B, and such a vaccine would reduce the incidence of liver cancer. As we are able to identify other cancers that are caused by viruses, this prophylactic measure of vaccination against those particular viruses could help to prevent these cancers and save many lives.

In contrast to the use of vaccines against viruses that cause cancer, most other tumour vaccine approaches are designed to enhance or to initiate effective tumour immunity in patients who already have cancer.

Snapshot   HPV vaccine

Stephanie is a 13-year-old girl currently attending a local school. In line with government recommendations, the school nurse is offering the HPV vaccine to all girls and boys in year 8. Whilst a letter has been sent out to the parents of all children, Stephanie has returned her form without parental consent but has consented to the vaccine herself. The school nurse is aware of the guidance on consent (https://www.nhs.uk/conditions/vaccinations/how-is-hpv-vaccine-cervarix-gardasil-given/) and considers Stephanie to be of an age that she can consent to the vaccine without parental approval. The nurse discusses the risks and benefits of the vaccine with Stephanie and also discusses the reason that she has not acquired parental consent. Stephanie explains that her father is opposed to her receiving the vaccine as he feels that it encourages sexual activity in the young. When the HPV vaccine was first introduced, there was a concern that parents would be upset by the vaccine being offered and schools would receive multiple phone calls from concerned parents; however, this does not seem to have happened and, in general, parents are very positive about the vaccine (Hilton *et al.*, 2011). Research into sexual activity following the HPV vaccine has shown no difference in age of onset of sexual activity, condom use or risky behaviours (Marchand *et al.*, 2013), and it is suggested that this should be included in discussions and information leaflets for parents.

Examples of cancers
Acute lymphoblastic leukaemia

Snapshot   Acute lymphoblastic leukaemia

Sarah Vaughan is a 34-year-old accountant who is married with no children. She has recently been diagnosed with acute lymphoblastic leukaemia (ALL) following a history of recurrent fevers, easily bruised skin and a general feeling of lethargy and weakness. Diagnosis was confirmed by blood tests and a bone marrow biopsy, which Mrs Vaughan found rather unpleasant. Mrs Vaughan has been advised that she will undergo treatment in three stages, including total body irradiation after which she will have to avoid going out in the sun for several months.

The results from a full blood count for Sarah show a typical pattern for ALL: there is anaemia, a low white cell count (though this can be normal or high as well), a low level of neutrophils (neutropenia) and a low platelet count (thrombocytopenia).

Vital signs

On admission to ward, the following vital signs were noted and recorded:

Vital sign	Observation	Normal
Temperature:	38.2°C	36.0–37.9°C range
Pulse:	80 beats per minute	60–100 beats per minute
Respiration:	20 breaths per minute	12–20 breaths per minute
Blood pressure:	115/68 mmHg	100–139 mmHg (systolic) range
O₂ saturation:	98%	94–98 %

A full blood count and urea and electrolytes were performed.

Test	Result	Guideline normal values
White blood cells (WBC)	14×10^9/L	4 to 11×10^9/L
Neutrophils	0.8×10^9/L	2.0 to 7.5×10^9/L
Lymphocytes	1.4×10^9/L	1.3 to 4.0×10^9/L
Red blood cells (RBC)	5.3×10^{12}/L 3.4 $\times 10^{12}$/L	4.5 to 6.5×10^{12}/L
Haemoglobin (Hb)	80 g/L	130–180 g/L
Platelets	100×10^9/L	150 to 440×10^9/L
C reactive protein	6.2 mg/L	<5 mg/L
Urea	8 mmol/L	2 to 6.6 mmol/L
Potassium	5.1 mmol/L	3.4–5.6 mmol/L
Sodium	138 mmol/L	135–147 mmol/L

Take some time to reflect on this case and then consider the following:

1. Mrs Vaughan is slightly unusual in presenting with ALL. Which adult patient groups are most likely to develop ALL?
2. What are the three stages of treatment for ALL?
3. What is total body irradiation, why is it carried out and why will Mrs Vaughan need to avoid direct sunlight afterwards?
4. Mrs Vaughan is of child-bearing age. What should she be told about her fertility now and in future?

NEWS 2

Sarah Vaughan

Physiological parameter	3	2	1	0	1	2	3
Respiration rate				20			
Oxygen saturation %				98			
Supplemental oxygen				No			
Temperature °C					38.2		
Systolic BP mmHg				115			
Heart rate				80			
Level of consciousness				A			
Score	0	0	0	0	1	0	0
Total	1						

Clinical investigation

Bone marrow biopsy

Bone marrow biopsy is the removal of bone marrow for the purposes of investigating its structure. There are two main sites that bone marrow is sampled from, the hip being the most common site; but the breast bone can also be used.

Bone marrow biopsy is done under local anaesthetic, and sometimes the patient may receive a sedative prior to the procedure.

Once the site has been cleaned and local anaesthetic infiltrated into the skin, the clinician inserts a large bore needle through the skin and the cortex of the bone into the marrow. The insertion of the needle can be painful, but this does not last long.

The large size of the needle is necessary to ensure that an intact 'core' of bone marrow is removed from the patient. The whole procedure lasts approximately 15–20 minutes.

After the procedure, the patient will have a sore area at the site of the needle insertion for a few days, which can be treated with over-the-counter analgesia. The patient should also be warned to observe the wound for 24 hours for any signs of bleeding or infection (see Figure 4.5).

Once a sample has been taken, it is sent to the pathology department, and the cells will be examined under a microscope. The pathologist may also 'stain' the cells to help identify certain structures. Results are generally available one to three weeks later.

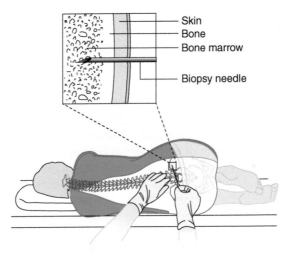

Figure 4.5   Bone marrow biopsy.

ALL is a primary disorder of the bone marrow in which the normal marrow cells are replaced by immature or undifferentiated blast cells. When the quantity of normal marrow is depleted to below the level necessary to maintain peripheral blood cells within normal ranges, then the following occur:

- Anaemia
- Neutropenia
- Thrombocytopenia.

Red flag

Neutropenia

Patients with neutropenia are susceptible to infection which can become severe very quickly. It is important that if a patient develops any of the following symptoms, they should contact their doctor:

- A temperature of 38 °C or higher
- Chills or sweating
- Headaches
- Facial flushing
- Sore throat or mouth
- Mouth ulcers
- Swollen glands
- Lack of energy
- Flu-like symptoms.

The exact cause of ALL is unknown, but the following are suspected of being involved in the development of this disease:

- Environmental causes
- Infectious agents (especially viruses)
- Genetic factors
- Chromosomal abnormalities.

ALL is the most common malignancy in children, with over 400 new cases diagnosed in children under the age of 15 years each year in the UK, with the incidence being higher amongst Caucasian children. ALL is classified according to the cell type involved.

ALL results from the growth of an abnormal type of leucocyte in the bone marrow, the spleen and the lymph nodes. These abnormal cells have little cytoplasm and a round nucleus – they resemble lymphoblasts. With ALL, the normal bone marrow cells may be displaced or replaced. The changes that occur in blood and bone marrow result from an accumulation of leukaemic cells and a deficiency of normal cells:

- Red cell precursors and megakaryocytes from which platelets are formed are decreased, leading to anaemia, bleeding and bruising.
- Normal white cells are decreased, which makes the patient liable to pick up infections.
- The leukaemic cells may infiltrate into the lymph nodes, spleen and liver, thus causing a diffuse adenopathy and hepatosplenomegaly.
- The increase in the size and amount of marrow and/or this infiltration of leukaemic cells causes bone and joint pain.
- Invasion of the central nervous system (CNS) by leukaemic cells can lead to headaches, vomiting, cranial nerve palsies, convulsions and coma.
- Weight loss, muscle wasting and fatigue occur when the body cells are deprived of nutrients because of the immense metabolic needs of the proliferating leukaemic cells.

Therefore, the signs and symptoms of ALL are:

- An increase in lethargy and general malaise
- Persistent fever of unknown cause

- Recurrent infection
- Prolonged bleeding (e.g. after dentistry)
- Bruising easily
- Pallor
- Enlarged lymph nodes
- Pain, particularly abdominal, bone and joint
- CNS involvement leading to headache and vomiting.

Treatment and prognosis

The treatment for ALL includes:

- Supportive therapy, including:
  - Control of infections, anaemia, bleeding, etc.
- Specific therapy, including:
  - Cytotoxic chemotherapy – e.g. dexamethasone, vincristine, imatinib, asparaginase, methotrexate
  - Radiation therapy
  - Bone marrow transplantation (BMT) to replace the damaged marrow with noncancerous marrow.

The prognosis of ALL is good these days – almost 90% of children (Inaba *et al.*, 2013) and nearly 50% of adults survive more than 5 years. However, later relapses can still occur after long remissions.

Lung cancer

Case study   Mental health

Geoffrey Simpson is a 76-year-old gentleman with a history of a non-productive cough and occasional chest pain. Recently he has noticed he is becoming increasingly short of breath and he reports blood in his handkerchief when he coughs and he states he has been losing weight but puts it down to his loss of appetite. Following referral to hospital, a CT scan and bronchoscopy, Mr Simpson was diagnosed with stage 4 non-small cell lung cancer and bony metastases. The treatment plan is for chemotherapy to treat the primary tumour and bisphosphonate drugs and radiotherapy for the bony metastases. Mr Simpson retired from the shipbuilding industry 12 years ago and states he has never been a smoker, eats healthily enough and drinks only moderate amounts of alcohol. Today he has presented to his GP with significant lethargy and 'feeling down'. The GP notes the following vital signs, all of which are normal for Mr Simpson. Following a consultation, the GP diagnoses depression and prescribes 50 mg sertraline once a day.

Vital sign	Observation	Normal
Temperature	36.2°C	36.0–37.9°C range
Pulse	80 beats per minute	60–100 beats per minute
Respiration	25 breaths per minute	12–20 breaths per minute
Blood pressure	150/81 mmHg	100–139 mmHg (systolic) range
O_2 saturation	93%	94–98 %

Take some time to reflect on this case, and then consider the following:

1. What is the difference between small cell lung cancer and non-small cell lung cancer?
2. Looking at Mr Simpson's NEWS2 score, should the GP be escalating Mr Simpson's care to the ED?
3. Why does Mr Simpson's treatment plan include bisphosphonate drugs and radiotherapy for the bone metastases?
4. What is the incidence of depression in patients with a diagnosis of cancer?

NEWS 2

Geoffrey simpson

Physiological parameter	3	2	1	0	1	2	3
Respiration rate							25
Oxygen saturation %			95				
Supplemental oxygen				No			
Temperature °C				36.2			
Systolic BP mmHg				115			
Heart rate				80			
Level of consciousness				A			
Score	0	0	1	0	0	0	3
Total	4						

Clinical investigation

Bone scan
Bony metastases can be detected by a bone scan (radioactive scintigraphy). A radioactive tracer is injected into the bloodstream (the dose of radiation is less than a normal X-ray) via a cannula. Over a period of hours, the radioactive isotope will be taken up by the bones. Whilst they wait, the patient will be asked to drink plenty of water to flush out any isotope not taken up by the bones. The areas where the isotope is found to be abnormally present or absent can be seen by performing a specialised scan, and these areas are suggestive of bony cancers. Often a computerised tomography (CT) scan will be undertaken as a standard follow-up procedure, especially in complex areas such as the spine.

Medicines management

Take note of any special instructions when administering bisphosphonate medication.
Many bisphosphonates should be taken on an empty stomach and at least half an hour before eating (some drugs require 2 hours). Some bisphosphonates require the patient to remain upright for half an hour because they carry a risk of oesophageal perforation. There have been concerns that long-term bisphosphonate use may increase the risk of oesophageal cancer; however, the evidence for this is limited, and one recent meta-analysis suggests the risk is very small (Ye and Zhou, 2016).

Orange flag

Depression

Depression is a common finding in patients with cancer, with an incidence of 20% compared to 5% in the population in general (Pitman *et al.*, 2018). The incidence of depression in older patients with cancers has also been found to increase with age (Goldzweig *et al.*, 2018), with the incidence rising to 88% in those over 86 years of age with a diagnosis of cancer. It is recognised that clinical depression is under-diagnosed in patients with cancer and is associated with an increased level of distress and a reduced quality of life. Clinicians should be aware that anti-depressant drugs can exacerbate some cancer symptoms and also interact with chemotherapy. Sertraline and citalopram seem to be the first-choice drugs as they have fewer interactions and are generally well tolerated (Pitman *et al.*, 2018).

Lung cancer is the most common cause of death from cancer in men and the second most common cause of death from cancer in women, and in 2018, it was calculated that it is responsible for 1.8 million deaths each year throughout the world.

The causes of lung cancer are the following:

- The greatest cause is long-term exposure to inhaled carcinogens, particularly tobacco smoke.
- People who do not smoke tobacco may still get lung cancer, due to a combination of genetic factors and exposure to passive smoking.
- Radon gas may also play a part in the development of lung cancer, as may air pollution.

Signs and symptoms of lung cancer are (Kasper *et al.*, 2015):

- Dyspnoea (difficulty in breathing)
- Haemoptysis (coughing up blood)
- Chronic cough and wheezing
- Chest or abdominal pain
- Cachexia, fatigue and loss of appetite
- Dysphonia (hoarse voice)
- Difficulty in swallowing.

Unfortunately, for many patients, by the time that they seek medical attention because the symptoms have become so apparent, the cancer has already metastasised.

Treatment of lung cancer depends upon the particular type of lung cancer and how far it has metastasised, but common treatments include:

- Surgery
- Chemotherapy, e.g. cisplatin and vinorelbine
- Radiation therapy.

The 5-year survival rate for all types of lung cancer is very low, although again the earlier it is diagnosed and treated, the better the long-term prognosis (Hirsch *et al.*, 2017). Consequently, this makes the prevention of this particular cancer a real priority.

Breast cancer

Throughout the world, breast cancer is the fifth most common cause of death from cancer (after lung cancer, stomach cancer, liver cancer and colon cancer), whilst among women throughout the world, breast cancer is the most common cancer (Bray *et al.*, 2018). The incidence of breast cancer has increased significantly since the 1970s, and this is partly explained by modern lifestyles in the Western world. Breast cancer is not purely a cancer of women, because males can also have breast cancer, although this is less common than it is in females (Ottini *et al.*, 2010). The reason for this phenomenon is that the breast is composed of exactly the same tissues in both males and females. The lifetime risk for getting breast cancer is 1 in 11 for women and 1 in 1000 for men (King and Robins, 2006). The 5-year survival rates for breast cancer in England is as high as 98% for stage one cancer, but only 26% once the cancer has reached stage 4 (ONS, 2019).

There are different sorts of breast cancer (although these can overlap), including (Figure 4.6):

- Ductal carcinoma (where the milk ducts become cancerous)
- Lobular carcinoma (cancer of the lobules attached to the ducts)
- Inflammatory breast carcinoma (diffuse cancer of the breast).

The causes of breast cancer have been mentioned earlier, particularly with regard to hereditary breast cancer. In addition, the younger a woman is when her first child is born, the lower the risk of her developing breast cancer (Tamimi, 2017).

Signs and symptoms of breast cancer can include (Figure 4.7):

- Painless/painful lump in the breast
- A lump under the arm or above the collar bone (enlarged lymph nodes)
- Nipple discharge/bleeding from the nipple
- Oedema of the arms
- Nipple retraction
- Prominently visible veins in the breast
- Pitting of the skin of the breast (known as 'peau d'orange' because it resembles the skin of an orange).

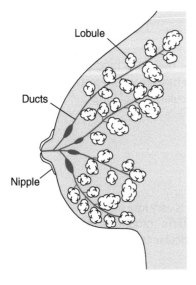

Figure 4.6 Diagram of breast showing lobules and ducts.

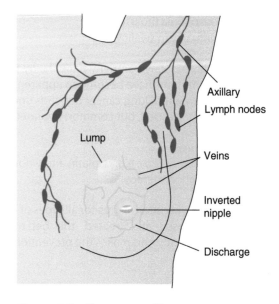

Figure 4.7 Symptoms of breast cancer.

The ideal treatment for breast cancer is surgery – the main treatment when the tumour is localised and has not metastasised, followed by:

- Chemotherapy – before, after or instead of surgery where patients are unsuitable for surgery
- Hormonal therapy (e.g. tamoxifen) – once chemotherapy has been completed
- Immunotherapy – e.g. trastuzumab (Herceptin®; a monoclonal antibody that slows the growth of breast cancer cells)
- Radiation therapy – to eliminate any microscopic cancer cells that may remain near the site of the primary tumour following surgery.

Surgery can range from a simple lumpectomy (just involving the cancerous lump itself) to a radical mastectomy – removal of the whole breast tissue and neighbouring lymph nodes (Marieb and Hoehn, 2010).

Orange flag

Breast reconstruction surgery

The rate of take-up of breast reconstruction surgery post mastectomy in the UK is approximately 10%. Whilst there is considered to be significant psychological benefit to reconstructive surgery, some studies have shown that there appears to be no significant long-term or short-term psychological difference between women who opt for reconstruction than those who do not (Owens *et al.*, 1988) though other studies have shown self-image is affected (Sisco *et al.*, 2015). However, it should be noted that there are differences between those who do not opt for reconstruction and those who do, with those who opt for reconstruction tending to be younger, married and of a higher socio-economic class (Rowland *et al.*, 1995). Breast reconstruction can take two forms, autologous (flap) reconstruction using the patient's own tissue, and implant-based reconstruction. A study by Ng *et al.* (2016) suggests that women who undergo autologous reconstruction have greater satisfaction than those undergoing implant reconstruction. Reviewing the literature, the clear outcome is that though breast reconstruction surgery seems to be a simple choice with clear psychological benefits, the research in the area suggests it is a very complex decision. Each woman should be treated as an individual, and assumptions based on simplistic views of what women would want in this situation should not be allowed to influence information giving and decision-making for the individual woman.

Snapshot   Breast cancer

Evelyn is a 38-year-old lady with learning disabilities who has been diagnosed with stage 3 breast cancer. Evelyn was unaware of the need for self-examination, and unfortunately the breast cancer was not diagnosed until it had progressed, and the lymph nodes were involved. The diagnosis was only made when Evelyn reported significant pain in her left breast and was examined by the GP. It is known that women with learning disabilities have the same risk of breast cancer as women without but are diagnosed later in the course of the disease due to a lack of awareness of self-examination and screening programmes (Walsh *et al.*, 2019). Since diagnosis Evelyn's pain relief has been slowly increased, but the pain remains uncontrolled. It is known that pain in people with learning disabilities is under-recognised and under-treated due to a series of factors such as communication difficulties, atypical pain experience and behavioural factors (Millard and Knegt, 2019). Evelyn lives in sheltered accommodation with care staff aiding her with medication compliance. Unfortunately, the carers are not confident with the *pro re nata* (prn) use of opiate drugs, and thus breakthrough pain is not being treated with the 'top-up' opiates that are available. Meanwhile, medical staff are unwilling to increase the routine opiate dose for Evelyn due to the risks of opiate medications. It was decided that Evelyn should be moved onto fentanyl transdermal patches. Fentanyl is considered to be a reliable drug for non-oral administration of pain relief. The administration of a drug via transdermal patch is recognised as a valuable route as it avoids the peaks and troughs of oral administration, ensuring a consistent pain-relieving effect and reducing the chance of overdose.

Medicines management

Opiates have a well-recognised side-effect profile including respiratory depression and lethargy. Many patients remain wary of taking opiates due to the fear of overdose or addiction. However, research has shown that fentanyl patches have no greater risk of addiction than oral opiates, and overdose is uncommon without deliberate misuse. Fentanyl patches are associated with lower side effects of constipation, urinary retention, and nausea and are thus better tolerated (Cachia and Ahmedzai, 2011).

Conclusion

Cancer is always an emotional subject because of the historically very high mortality rate associated with it. Over the past few years, great strides have been made in the prevention and treatment of many cancers, but it still remains a tremendous challenge to researchers and clinical staff. Greater knowledge of the biochemical, economic, social and psychological aspects of these diseases has led to a greater understanding of them and, in some parts of the world, an ability to defeat, or at least ameliorate, many of them. However, it is certainly true that the incidences of many of them are increasing (even though they can be better treated). This is related to the facts that many are diseases linked with old age, because they take so long to develop, and people in many countries are living much longer. In the past, they would have died from other causes before the cancers caused problems. So, there have been many triumphs in the treatment and prevention of cancers, but there is no room for complacency.

Activities

Here are some activities and exercises to help test your learning. For the answers to these exercises, as well as further self-testing activities, visit our website at **www.wiley.com/go/fundamentalsofappliedpathophysiology/student4e**

Multiple choice questions

1. The 'programmed suicide' of the cell is known as:
   (a) Apoptosis
   (b) Mitosis
   (c) Meiosis
   (d) Amitosis

2. Which of the following cancers has increased in incidence?
   (a) Stomach
   (b) Colon
   (c) Kidney
   (d) Brain

3. The type of blood cell that is known as a hunter/killer cell for abnormal cells are called:
   (a) H lymphocytes
   (b) K lymphocytes
   (c) P lymphocytes
   (d) T lymphocytes

4. The creation of new blood vessels to support tumour growth is known as:
   (a) Neogenesis
   (b) Newgenesis
   (c) Angiogenesis
   (d) Vascular genesis

5. Wilms' tumour is a cancer of:
   (a) The lung
   (b) The breast
   (c) The eye
   (d) The kidney

6. What sort of radiation causes melanoma?
   (a) Ionising
   (b) Ultraviolet
   (c) Electromagnetic
   (d) Particle

7. Why is ionising radiation particularly dangerous to the developing foetus?
   (a) The foetus receives blood cells from the mother
   (b) Ionising radiation causes heat
   (c) Foetal cell division occurs very quickly
   (d) Foetuses are susceptible to nuclear radiation

8. How many carcinogens are there in tobacco smoke?
   (a) 20
   (b) 30
   (c) 50
   (d) 70

9. Human papillomavirus (HPV) is associated with cancers of:
   (a) The anus
   (b) The penis
   (c) The vulva
   (d) All of the above

10. What naturally occurring gas is known to be associated with cancer risk?
    (a) Randon
    (b) Random
    (c) Radon
    (d) Radson

11. Photodynamic therapy is the use of what to treat cancer?
    (a) Lasers
    (b) Light
    (c) X-rays
    (d) Freezing liquid

12. Increasing the intake of fruit and vegetables can help to reduce the incidence of which cancers?
    (a) Bowel
    (b) Breast
    (c) Mouth
    (d) All of the above

13. Neutropenia should be suspected if the patient develops:
    (a) A sore throat
    (b) A urine infection
    (c) A swollen limb
    (d) A low temperature

14. The incidence of depression in cancer patients is approximately:
    (a) 5%
    (b) 10%
    (c) 15%
    (d) 20%

15. With a localised breast tumour, the best treatment is:
    (a) Chemotherapy
    (b) Radiotherapy
    (c) Hormone therapy
    (d) Surgery

Conditions

The following is a list of types of cancer. Take some time and write notes about each of the conditions. You may make the notes taken from textbooks or other resources (e.g. people you work with in a clinical area), or you may make the notes based on people you have cared for. If you are making notes about people you have cared for, you must ensure that you adhere to the rules of confidentiality.

Pancreatic cancer	
Acute myeloid leukaemia	

Thyroid cancer	
Prostate cancer	
Cervical cancer	

Further resources

BMC Cancer

http://www.biomedcentral.com/bmccancer

This is an open access (i.e. free) cancer journal. Here you will find peer-reviewed articles on topics ranging from cell biology to the treatment of cancer.

British Cancer Journal

http://www.nature.com/bjc/index.html

This is a multidisciplinary cancer journal. Articles from each issue are available free of charge immediately upon publication, and all content is free to access for 12 months after publication.

Cancer Research UK

http://www.cancerresearchuk.org/

This is the website of one of the leading cancer research charities in the UK. Here you will find a very useful and extensive information section and patient stories.

Cancer Symptoms

https://www.cancer.gov/publications/pdq/information-summaries/adult-treatment

An alphabetical list of adult cancer treatment summaries for patients and professionals.

Inside Cancer

http://www.insidecancer.org/

This website provides multimedia presentations about cancer, including animated slide shows on the biology of cancer, causes and prevention, and interviews with researchers in the field. This is a good place to start your study.

Glossary of terms

Adenopathy   Enlargement of lymph nodes.

Alkaloid   Naturally occurring chemical that is basic (i.e. not acidic).

Allele   A gene on one of a pair of chromosomes that codes for the same physical or other feature as its corresponding one on the other chromosome.

Anaemia   Blood lacking in iron. Often used to mean a deficiency in red blood cells.

Angiogenesis   Growth of new blood vessels.

Angiogenic growth factor   Substance within the body that is involved in the development of new blood vessels.

Anorexia   Loss of appetite/weight.

Antibiotic   Drug used to kill bacteria.

Antibody   Protein in the blood that binds specifically to a particular foreign substance (its antigen). It is a major part of the immune system.

Antigen   A foreign substance (e.g. an infecting micro-organism) that can be recognised by the immune system and generates an antibody response.

Apoptosis   Programmed cell death. It is a form of cell death in which the cell activates an internal death programme; it is a form of cell suicide.

Basal cell carcinoma   A cancer involving the surface epithelium of the skin.

Benign   Causes no problem. In cancer, it means a growth that is not malignant.

Blast cell   An immature cell.

Cachexia   This is a syndrome that includes anorexia, weight loss, anaemia, marked weakness, and altered protein, lipid and carbohydrate metabolism. This most severe form of malnutrition is often associated with the later stages of cancer.

Cancer   Unregulated growth of cells and tissue that are invasive and able to metastasise.

Carcinogen   Something capable of causing cancer.

Cell differentiation   The process by which cells take on different roles.

Cell division   The reproduction of cells to produce two identical daughter cells. Also known as binary fission.

Colorectal cancer   A cancer that involves the colon and the rectum.

Cytoplasm   The collective name for all the contents of the cell, including the plasma membrane, with the exception of the nucleus.

Cytotoxicity   Lethal to cells.

Cytotoxic T lymphocyte   A specialised white blood cell that is capable of destroying other cells of the body that are damaged or have become infected.

Daughter cell   The resultant cell following cell division.

Dysphonia   Hoarse voice.

Dyspnoea   Difficulty in breathing.

General malaise   Generally lethargic, with loss of appetite and loss of weight.

Germline cell   A sperm or egg that possesses genes that can be passed on to offspring.

Gray   The unit that defines the amount of energy released from radiation. It is usually abbreviated to Gy, and it replaces the older unit of radiation energy, the 'rad', which was equivalent to 0.01 Gy.

Haemoglobin   A protein consisting of globin and four haem groups that is found within erythrocytes (red blood cells). Responsible for the transport of oxygen.

Haemoptysis   Coughing up of blood.

Hepatosplenomegaly   Enlarged liver and spleen.

Lymph node   Part of the lymphatic system, it contains many white cells to destroy bacteria that are trapped within the lymph node.

Lymphoblast   An immature lymphocyte (a white blood cell).

Malignant   Invasive, has a tendency to grow and may spread to other parts of the body.

Megakaryocyte   A large bone marrow cell that gives rise to platelets.

Melanoma   A cancerous outgrowth of melanocytes (pigmented cells of the skin).

Menarche   The time when the first menstruation occurs.

Metastasise   The spread of cancerous cells to other parts of the body – often distant to the site of the original cancer.

Mutagen   Something that can affect genes and cause changes (mutations).

Mutation   A change in one or several bases in DNA.

Neoplasm   A new growth of tissue. It may or may not be malignant.

Nucleotide sequence   The sequence of the bases of DNA that make up genes.

Nulliparous   Never having given birth to a viable infant.

Oncogene   A gene that contains proteins that contribute to carcinogenesis.

Oncogenic virus   A virus that causes cancers.

Ovulation   The release of eggs from the ovary.

Palliative   Easing the situation – making it better, but not a cure.

Porphyrins   An important group of several protein pigments involved in various processes – bound to the iron in haemoglobin.

Precancerous cell   A cell that is at the stage before it becomes cancerous.

Precursor   Something that will eventually turn into something else (e.g. a red cell precursor will eventually become a red cell).

Premenopausal   The period before the end of menstruation (i.e. the menopausal period).

Primary cancer   The tumour that first appears; the site of this first cancer.

Prognosis   A prediction about how a person's disease will progress.

Prophylactic   Preventative.

Proto-oncogene   A gene that, due to mutation, can become an oncogene.

Radiation therapy   The use of ultraviolet or ionising radiation to treat cancer.

Solute   A substance that is dissolved in liquid (solvent).

Solvent   The liquid in which solutes are dissolved.

Somatic cell   A cell that possesses genes that are not passed on to offspring (i.e. cells of the body other than the sperm and ova).

Spleen   An organ in the abdomen that removes and destroys old, damaged or fragile red blood cells. Also, it has an important role to play in immunity.

Squamous cell carcinoma   A cancer involving squamous cells, usually of epithelial tissue.

Terminal cancer   Cancer that cannot be cured and leads to death.

Thrombocytopaenia   A deficiency in thrombocytes (platelets).

Toxic   A substance that is poisonous or damaging to something else.

Tumour   Lump in or on the body caused by the abnormal growth of cells. It can be either malignant or benign.

Tumour suppressor gene   A gene whose function is to suppress the growth and development of tumours.

Vaccine   A substance that can be given to a host in order to provoke an immune response and therefore confer immunity on the host without making the host severely ill (e.g. polio vaccine).

Vector   An organism that houses parasites and transmits them from one host to another. A prime example is the mosquito that transfers the malaria parasite to humans. Also, a means of carrying a substance so that it can be transferred somewhere else. Viruses are often used as vectors to transfer genes to where they are required in gene therapy.

References

Arbyn, M., Xu, L., Simoens, C. and Martin-Hirsch, P.P. (2018). Prophylactic vaccination against human papillomaviruses to prevent cervical cancer and its precursors. *Cochrane Database of Systematic Reviews*, (5).

Burrell, R.A., McGranahan, N., Bartek, J. and Swanton, C. (2013). The causes and consequences of genetic heterogeneity in cancer evolution. *Nature*. 501(7467): 338–345.

Bray, F., Ferlay, J., Soerjomataram, I., Siegel, R.L., Torre, L.A. and Jemal, A. (2018). Global cancer statistics 2018: GLOBOCAN estimates of incidence and mortality worldwide for 36 cancers in 185 countries. *CA: A Cancer Journal for Clinicians*, 68(6): 394–424.

Cachia, E. and Ahmedzai, S. H. (2011). Transdermal opioids for cancer pain. *Current Opinion in Supportive and Palliative Care*, 5(1): 15–19.

Cancer Research UK (2019a). *Cancer Mortality for All Cancers Combined*. [online] accessed 08/06/20 from https://www.cancerresearchuk.org/health-professional/cancer-statistics/mortality/all-cancers-combined#ref-

Carbone, M., Amelio, I., Affar, E.B., Brugarolas, J., Cannon-Albright, L.A., Cantley, L.C. and Gandara, D. (2018). Consensus report of the 8 and 9th Weinman Symposia on Gene x Environment Interaction in carcinogenesis: Novel opportunities for precision medicine. *Cell Death & Differentiation*, 25(11): 1885–1904.

Cosgrove, D., Park, B. H. and Vogelstein, B. (2016). Tumor suppressor genes. *Holland-Frei Cancer Medicine*, 1–20.

Cuzick, J., Sestak, I., Cawthorn, S., Hamed, H., Holli, K. *et al.* and IBIS-I Investigators (2015). Tamoxifen for prevention of breast cancer: extended long-term follow-up of the IBIS-I breast cancer prevention trial. *The Lancet Oncology*, 16(1): 67–75.

Eggertson, L. (2015). More needed to reduce radon-related cancer. *CMAJ: Canadian Medical Association Journal*. 187(7): 485.

Farkona, S., Diamandis, E. P. and Blasutig, I. M. (2016). Cancer immunotherapy: The beginning of the end of cancer?. *BMC Medicine*, 14(1): 73.

Giuliano, A.R., Kreimer, A.R. and de Sanjose, S. (2015). The beginning of the end: Vaccine prevention of HPV-driven cancers. *Journal of the National Cancer Institute*. 107(6): djv128.

Goldzweig, G., Baider, L., Rottenberg, Y., Andritsch, E. and Jacobs, J. M. (2018). Is age a risk factor for depression among the oldest old with cancer?. *Journal of Geriatric Oncology*, 9(5): 476–481.

Gorczynski, R.M. and Stanley, J. (2006). *Problem-Based Immunology*. Philadelphia: Saunders Elsevier.

Hilton, S., Hunt, K., Bedford, H. and Petticrew, M. (2011). School nurses' experiences of delivering the UK HPV vaccination programme in its first year. *BMC Infectious Diseases*, 11(1): 226.

Hirsch, F.R., Scagliotti, G.V., Mulshine, J.L., Kwon, R., Curran, W.J., Jr., Wu, Y. L. and Paz-Ares, L. (2017). Lung cancer: current therapies and new targeted treatments. *The Lancet*, 389(10066): 299–311.

Huber, D., Seitz, S., Kast, K., Emons, G. and Ortmann, O. (2020). Use of oral contraceptives in BRCA mutation carriers and risk for ovarian and breast cancer: A systematic review. *Archives of Gynecology and Obstetrics*, 301: 875–884.

Inaba, H., Greaves, M. and Mullighan, C.G. (2013). Acute lymphoblastic leukaemia. *The Lancet*, 381(9881): 1943–1955.

Kabat, G.C., Jones, J.G., Olson, N. *et al.* (2010). Risk factors for breast cancer in women biopsied for benign breast disease: A nested case-control study. *Cancer Epidemiology*, 31(1): 34–39.

Kasper, D.L., Fauci, A.S., Hauser, S.L., Longo, D.L., Jameson, J.L. and Loscalzo, J. (2015). *Harrison's Principles of Internal Medicine*, 19th edn. New York: McGraw-Hill.

King, R.J.B. (2000). *Cancer Biology*, 2nd edn. Harlow: Pearson/Prentice Hall.

King, R.J.B. and Robins, M.W. (2006). *Cancer Biology*, 3rd edn. Harlow: Pearson/Prentice Hall.

Long, M.D., Martin, C.F., Galanko, J.A. and Sandler, R.S. (2010). Hormone replacement therapy, oral contraceptive use and distal large bowel cancer: A population-based case-control study. *American Journal of Gastroenterology*, 105(8): 1843–1850.

Lowy, D.R. and Schiller, J.T. (2012). Reducing HPV-associated cancer globally. *Cancer Prevention Research*, 5(1): 18–23.

Marchand, E., Glenn, B.A. and Bastani, R. (2013). HPV vaccination and sexual behavior in a community college sample. *Journal of Community Health*, 38(6): 1010–1014.

Marieb, E.N. (2010). *Essentials of Human Anatomy and Physiology*, 10th edn. San Francisco: Pearson/Benjamin Cummings.

McCance, K.L. (2018a) Cellular biology. In: McCance, K.L., Huether, S.E., Brashers, V.L. and Rote, N.S. (eds), *Pathophysiology: The Biologic Basis for Disease in Adults and Children*, 8th edn. Missouri: Mosby Elsevier.

McCance, K.L. (2018b) Cancer epidemiology. In: McCance, K.L., Huether, S.E., Brashers, V.L. and Rote, N.S. (eds), *Pathophysiology: The Biologic Basis for Disease in Adults and Children*, 8th edn. Missouri: Mosby Elsevier.

Millard, S. K. and de Knegt, N. C. (2019). Cancer pain in people with intellectual disabilities: Systematic review and survey of health care professionals. *Journal of Pain and Symptom Management*. 58(6): 1081–1099.

Mørch, L. S., Skovlund, C. W., Hannaford, P. C., Iversen, L., Fielding, S. and Lidegaard, Ø. (2017). Contemporary hormonal contraception and the risk of breast cancer. *New England Journal of Medicine*, 377(23): 2228–2239.

Mui, U. N., Haley, C. T. and Tyring, S. K. (2017). Viral oncology: Molecular biology and pathogenesis. *Journal of Clinical Medicine*, 6(12): 111.

National Health Service (NHS) (2018). *What Do Cancer Stages and Grades Mean? [online]* accessed 08/06/20 from https://www.nhs.uk/common-health-questions/operations-tests-and-procedures/what-do-cancer-stages-and-grades-mean/

Ng, S. K., Hare, R. M., Kuang, R. J., Smith, K. M., Brown, B. J. and Hunter-Smith, D. J. (2016). Breast reconstruction post mastectomy: Patient satisfaction and decision making. *Annals of Plastic Surgery*, 76(6): 640–644.

Office for National Statistics (ONS) (2019). *Cancer Survival in England – Adults Diagnosed. 2013-2017* [online] accessed 08/06/20 from https://www.ons.gov.uk/peoplepopulationandcommunity/healthandsocialcare/conditionsanddiseases/datasets/cancersurvivalratescancersurvivalinengland adultsdiagnosed

Ottini, L., Palli, D., Rizzo, S., Federico, M., Bazan, V. and Russo, A. (2010). Male breast cancer. *Critical Reviews in Oncology/Haematology*. 73(2): 141–155.

Owens, R.G., Ashcroft, J.J., Slade, P.D. and Leinster, S.J. (1988). *Psychological effects of the offer of breast reconstruction following mastectomy. Psychosocial Oncology*. Oxford: Pergamon.

Perry, M.C., Doll, D.C. and Freter, C.E. (2012). *Perry's The Chemotherapy Source Book*. Philadelphia: Lippincott Williams & Wilkins.

Pitman, A., Suleman, S., Hyde, N. and Hodgkiss, A. (2018). Depression and anxiety in patients with cancer. *BMJ*, 361: k1415.

Robson, M.E., Bradbury, A.R., Arun, B., Domchek, S.M., Ford, J.M. *et al.* (2015). American Society of Clinical Oncology Policy Statement Update: Genetic and genomic testing for cancer susceptibility. *Journal of Clinical Oncology*, 33(31): 3660–3667.

Rowland, J.H., Dioso, J., Holland, J.C., Chaglassian, T. and Kinne, D. (1995). Breast reconstruction after mastectomy: who seeks it, who refuses?. *Plastic and Reconstructive Surgery*, 95(5): 812–822.

Schweizer, M.T. and Drake, C.G. (2014). Immunotherapy for prostate cancer: Recent developments and future challenges. *Cancer and Metastasis Reviews*, 33(2–3): 641–655.

Si, H. (2018). Indoor air pollution, lung cancer and solutions. *Cancer Cell Research*, 19: 464–470

Sisco, M., Johnson, D.B., Wang, C., Rasinski, K., Rundell, V.L. and Yao, K.A. (2015). The quality-of-life benefits of breast reconstruction do not diminish with age. *Journal of Surgical Oncology*, 111(6): 663–668.

Smittenaar, C. R., Petersen, K. A., Stewart, K. and Moitt, N. (2016). Cancer incidence and mortality projections in the UK until 2035. *British Journal of Cancer,* 115(9): 1147–1155.

Tamimi, R.M. (2017). *Epidemiology of Breast Cancer*. In *Pathology and Epidemiology of Cancer*. Springer: Cham, pp. 151–172.

Vickers, P.S. (2005). Acquired defences. In: Montague, S.E., Watson, R. and Herbert, R.A. (eds), *Physiology for Nursing Practice*, 3rd edn. Edinburgh: Elsevier.

Vineis, P. and Wild, C.P. (2014). Global cancer patterns: Causes and prevention. *The Lancet.* 83(9916): 549–557.

Vineis, P. and Fecht, D. (2018). Environment, cancer and inequalities—The urgent need for prevention. *European Journal of Cancer*, 103, 317–326.

Walsh, S., O'Mahony, M., Lehane, E., Farrell, D., Taggart, L., Kelly, L. and Martin, A. M. (2019). Cancer and breast cancer awareness interventions in an intellectual disability context: A review of the literature. *Journal of Intellectual Disabilities*, 1744629519850999.

Ye, W. W. and Zhou, Y. (2016). Oral bisphosphonates and risk of esophageal cancer: a meta-analysis. *International Journal of Clinical and Experimental Medicine*, 9(9): 17050–17059.

Chapter 5

Inflammation, immune response and healing

Janet G. Migliozzi

Senior Lecturer, Department of Nursing, Health and Wellbeing, School of Health and Social Work, University of Hertfordshire, Hatfield, Hertfordshire, UK

Contents

Introduction 97
Infectious microorganisms 98
Spread of infection 98
Types of infectious microorganisms............ 103
The immune system 111
Inflammatory response....................................118
Conclusion 121

Test your knowledge..121
Multiple choice questions...............................122
Conditions...123
Further resources...124
Glossary of terms...125
References..128

Key words

- Virus
- Infectious
- Immune system response
- Microorganism
- Pathogen
- Bacterium
- Reservoir of infection
- Lymphocytes
- Vaccination
- Phagocytes
- Inflammatory response
- Prions

Fundamentals of Applied Pathophysiology: An Essential Guide for Nursing and Healthcare Students, Fourth Edition. Edited by Ian Peate.
© 2021 John Wiley & Sons Ltd. Published 2021 by John Wiley & Sons Ltd.
Student companion website: www.wiley.com/go/fundamentalsofappliedpathophysiology/student4e
Instructor companion website: www.wiley.com/go/fundamentalsofappliedpathophysiology/instructor4e

Test your prior knowledge

- List the ways in which bacteria are transmitted.
- How does a virus cause disease?
- What is a prion?
- Describe the roles of tears within the immune system.
- What are the physical signs of inflammation?

Learning outcomes

On completion of this section, the reader will be able to:

- List and describe the various types of infectious microorganisms that affect humans.

- Discuss how infectious diseases are transmitted to humans.

- Outline the components of the immune system and their functions.

- Explain the process of inflammation and its role in tissue repair.

Don't forget to visit the companion website for this book (www.wiley.com/go/fundamentalsofappliedpathophysiology/student4e) **where you can find self-assessment tests to check your progress, as well as lots of activities to practise your learning.**

Introduction

From the moment that someone is born and for the rest of their life, they are constantly in danger. Some of the dangers come from inside the body and are known as genetic defects, whilst others come from external sources. Two of the dangers that beset everyone throughout life are infectious diseases and injuries. Fortunately, the human body has inbuilt mechanisms to protect it from these dangers, namely the immune system and wound healing.

Infectious diseases occur as a result of invasion of the body by microorganisms which cause damage to the tissues of the body. Every infectious disease is characterised by an interaction between the responses of both the infected human host and the infecting organism. Microorganisms are everywhere – they colonise humans, animals, food, water and soil, and infectious diseases are acquired by humans following contact with an exogenous pathogen present within a reservoir of infection.

The immune system, which is actually an intricate system of cells, enzymes and proteins, is the system that has evolved within humans (and other animals) to protect against these infectious pathogenic microorganisms. In particular, white blood cells are essential to the functioning of the immune system, and this chapter will explain about these and the other elements of the body that constitute the immune system.

This chapter will commence by looking at the microorganisms that can cause disease and then will look at how the immune system fights these microorganisms and how it helps to heal injuries.

Infectious microorganisms

Microorganisms are microscopic cells that either live in the environment, on the skin, or inside bodies. They can cause infectious diseases, and can do this as long as two conditions are met:

1. They are allowed to grow and reproduce in the right conditions for that microorganism
2. They are in the right location for their growth and reproduction.

These conditions are important because different microorganisms have differing and sometimes exacting needs for their growth and reproduction. If environmental conditions are not right, they will not flourish. However, once the conditions are right for them, microorganisms multiply at an astonishing rate within the host tissues, causing destruction or degeneration so that the host becomes unwell and cannot function properly.

It is not actually the presence of microorganisms that is the problem; rather, it is the fact that during their growth and reproduction (as well as part of the protection against the immune system), they produce waste products known as toxins, and it is these that cause the problems. However, not all of these microorganisms pose problems for humans. In fact, humans need bacteria to help to break down food and digest it. These bacteria are known as commensal bacteria.

Unfortunately, even commensal microorganisms can become pathogenic if they find themselves in the wrong place. For example, microorganisms that live in the colon and are beneficial there may invade the urinary bladder, where they become pathogenic microorganisms because they are now in the wrong place. A good example of one of these is *Escherichia coli* (*E. coli*), which normally lives in the gut. However, if it migrates to the bladder, then it causes cystitis. When infections are caused in this way, they are known as endogenous infections ('endogenous' means 'from within' – in this case the body). All other infections are known as exogenous infections – they come from outside of the body.

Spread of infection

The causative organisms of infectious disease in humans can be transmitted from the reservoir of infection by 1 of 10 ways:

1. Droplet spread
2. Air currents (airborne transmission)
3. Aerosol
4. Water
5. Direct contact
6. Soil
7. Inoculation
8. Fæcal-oral route
9. Vector
10. Contaminated intermediates.

Droplet spread

Microbial organisms are spread in mucous droplet nuclei that travel only short distances – less than 1 metre from the reservoir to the host. This spread can come from coughing and sneezing (as discussed below), but also by talking or laughing. In one sneeze, 20 000 droplets may be produced and expelled from the person who is the reservoir. Droplet transmission should not be confused with airborne transmission – although there are many similarities. Disease-causing organisms that do not spread more than 1 metre from the host reservoir are not regarded as airborne, because they are not carried on currents of air, but just rely upon the force of the expulsion to travel the short distance to a new host. Examples of disease spread by droplet transmission include:

- Influenza
- Pneumonia
- Pertussis (whooping cough).

Air currents (airborne transmission)

Airborne transmission refers to the spread of agents of infection by droplet nuclei in dust. These droplets may spread by more than 1 metre from the reservoir to the host.

A good example of droplet transmission is what happens during sneezing and coughing. When someone coughs or sneezes, they expel a fine spray into the air around them. That spray is made up of many, many droplets of mucus that could contain infectious microorganisms. These droplets of mucus and bacteria/viruses are small, and light enough, to remain airborne for a long time. Consequently, anyone coming into contact is likely to breathe in the mucus/ bacteria/virus droplets, and so become infected in turn. Infectious microorganisms that can be spread in this way include:

- Measles
- Tuberculosis (TB)
- Staphylococcal and streptococcal infections
- Certain fungal diseases – spread by the spores – such as histoplasmosis.

Aerosol transmission

Both domestic and industrial water supplies are sources of aerosol transmission. It has a similar action to that which occurs with droplet transmission, except the reservoir is water, rather than another human. If someone with asthma requires salbutamol via an aerosol – that works quickly because the drug carried in the tiny droplets of water is able to work on the lining of the respiratory tract immediately. The same thing happens with aerosol transmission of infectious organisms.

Examples of diseases that are spread by this method include:

- Legionnaire's disease
- Tuberculosis (TB).
- Coronavirus – This is one of the major pathogens that primarily targets the respiratory system causing pneumonia-type illness. Previous outbreaks of coronaviruses include the severe acute respiratory syndrome (SARS) and the Middle East respiratory syndrome (MERS). More recently, following a worldwide outbreak of respiratory illness (COVID-19), a global pandemic caused by a new seventh member of this group of viruses, SARS-COV2, was declared in 2020 (Rothan *et al.*, 2020).

Waterborne transmission

In waterborne transmission, pathogens are usually spread by water that has been contaminated with untreated, or poorly treated, sewage. The pathogenic organisms enter the host either by contact with the mucosa, or by contact with broken skin. Examples of infections spread through water include:

- Leptospirosis – often picked up from rat urine whilst swimming in a river
- Schistosomiasis (commonly known as bilharzia) – caused by a fluke (similar to a worm) which is a parasite found in freshwater snails that inhabit the edges of major waterways, such as the River Nile (Percival *et al.*, 2014).

Direct contact

Contact transmission is the spread of an infectious organism by direct, or indirect, contact. Direct contact transmission is also known as 'person-to-person transmission'. This is the direct transmission of an infectious organism by physical contact between its present host and a susceptible recipient host. The most common forms of direct contact transmission are:

- Touching
- Kissing
- Sexual intercourse.

There are many diseases that can be transmitted by direct contact, and these include:

- Viral respiratory tract diseases (e.g. the common cold, influenza)
- Staphylococcal infections (e.g. septicaemia)
- Hepatitis A
- Measles
- Scarlet fever
- Sexually transmitted infections (e.g. syphilis, gonorrhoea, genital herpes)
- Infectious mononucleosis (glandular fever)
- HIV (human immunodeficiency virus), which causes AIDS (acquired immunodeficiency syndrome).

Potential pathogens can also be transmitted by direct contact from animals (or animal products) to humans, e.g. rabies, anthrax.

Indirect contact transmission occurs when the infectious microorganism is transmitted from its present reservoir to a potential susceptible host by means of a non-living object.

Soil

Soil has already been mentioned as a potential reservoir for infectious microorganisms. The route of entry from the soil into the body is usually by a skin lesion. Infection can occur:

- When playing sport on a contaminated playing field
- Whilst gardening on soil that has been contaminated by the use of animal manure
- Whilst farming on land that has been fertilised with animal manure
- Any fall on contaminated ground in which the skin becomes broken.

Examples of infectious diseases that can occur from soil include:

- Tetanus
- Gas gangrene.

Inoculation

Inoculation can be accidental, for example by being bitten or scratched. Examples of infections caused this way include:

- Cat scratch disease
- Rabies.

Inoculation can occur following an injection, as can occur with healthcare professionals not taking proper precautions, or by someone injecting themselves with drugs. Examples of infections caused this way include:

- HIV
- Hepatitis B.

Fæcal-oral route

This transmission of infectious microorganisms can occur in several ways, including:

- Hand-to-mouth – This is seen particularly in young children, who may explore the anal area, and then put their hands in their mouths.
- Sewage-contaminated food or water – This occurs, particularly if fresh vegetables, salads and fruit are not properly washed before being eaten. It is a particular problem in certain countries, where human sewage is used to fertilise fields in which salads are grown.
- Certain sexual practices, in which there is oro-anal stimulation ('rimming').

Examples of infectious diseases, transmitted via this route, include:

- Gastroenteritis
- Enteric fevers.

Vector transmission

Vector transmission is commonly held to be inoculation by the bite of a sucking arthropod (such as a 'tick') which is also a host, but there are other types of vector transmission. Vectors are animals that carry pathogens from one host to another. Arthropods are the most important group of disease vectors.

Contaminated intermediates

This is caused by indirect contact transmission, and it occurs when the infectious microorganism is transmitted from its initial reservoir to a potential susceptible host by means of a non-living object. These non-living objects, or inanimate intermediates, are called fomites. Examples of fomites include:

- Clothes, bedding and towels
- Tissues and handkerchiefs
- Drinking cups and eating utensils
- Toys.

Other fomites can transmit infections, such as:

- Chicken pox
- Staphylococci and streptococci infections
- Tetanus.

(Tortora *et al.*, 2018)

Snapshot   Infected wound

Mr Brian Hendrich, a 66-year-old retired town planner was discharged from hospital 8 days ago following a large bowel resection for diverticular disease. He had been attending his GP practice for wound dressing changes as his wound was not healing well and had started to become painful, inflamed and had begun to discharge purulent fluid. He has been admitted to a surgical ward for exploration and possible debridement of the infected wound. Swabs taken from the wound reveal that it is growing Methicillin-Resistant *Staphylococcus aureus* (MRSA).

Vital signs

On admission to the ward, the following vital signs were noted and recorded:

Vital sign	Observation	Normal
Temperature:	38.6°C	36.0–37.9°C range
Pulse:	98 beats per minute	60–100 beats per minute
Respiration:	22 breaths per minute	12–20 breaths per minute
Blood pressure:	158/94 mmHg	100–139 mmHg (systolic) range
O_2 saturation:	98%	94–98%

A full blood count and urea and electrolytes was performed.

Test	Result	Guideline normal values
White blood cells (WBC)	27×10^9/L	4 to 11×10^9/L
Neutrophils	13.3×10^9/L	2.0 to 7.5×10^9/L
Lymphocytes	2.8×10^9/L	1.3 to 4.0×10^9/L
Red blood cells (RBC)	5.4×10^{12}/L	4.5 to 6.5×10^{12}/L
Haemoglobin (Hb)	156 g/L	130–180 g/L
Platelets	224×10^9/L	150 to 440×10^9/L
C-reactive protein	9 mg/L	<5 mg/L
Urea	5.4 mmol/L	2–6.6 mmol/L
Potassium	4.2 mmol/L	3.4–5.6 mmol/L
Sodium	138 mmol/L	135–147 mmol/L

Take some time to reflect on the following questions:

1. What is MRSA and what are its common causes?
2. What measures need to be taken whilst Mr Hendrich is in hospital to prevent cross-infection to other patients?
3. Outline the treatment protocol that Mr Hendrich will require to treat his MRSA infection.

Clinical investigation

Microscopy, Culture and Sensitivity (M, C & S)

The Microscopy, Culture and Sensitivity test of a sample is a common request made to the microbiology laboratory. The aim of the test is to identify the microorganism initially by looking at the sample under the microscope (Microscopy) and then growing a sample from the original culture to aid further identification (Culture) and provide an indication of which antimicrobial the organism responds to or is 'sensitive' to (Sensitivity) in order to guide the clinical diagnosis and management of the patient's condition, which may include the prescribing of appropriate antimicrobial therapy.

Red flag

Specimen collection

MRSA represents one of the most important threats to safe health care and its detection and eradication is essential to ensure its control. Obtaining swabs is part of an effective programme for early detection and eradication of MRSA, both in hospital and the community. Practitioners should know which type of microorganism they are testing for, as this will determine the type of swab to be used (HPA, 2014). In addition, the Royal College of Nursing states that practitioners must be competent in specimen collection and ensure that they have the right knowledge and skills to obtain and correctly process samples for specimen collection (RCN, 2020).

Types of infectious microorganisms

There are many different types of microorganism that can infect humans (Table 5.1), and each of them requires different environmental conditions in which to survive and to grow and reproduce, as well as different modes of transfer to humans. Some of them are more well known to humans than others, and perhaps the three most well-known microorganisms are:

- Bacteria
- Viruses
- Fungi.

Bacteria

Bacteria come in a great many sizes and shapes, and their diameter ranges from 0.2 to 2.0 µm (micrometre), whilst their length ranges from 2 to 8 µm.

Table 5.1   Other types of infectious microorganisms.

Protozoa
Rickettsiae
Chlamydiae
Helminths
Slow viruses (prions)

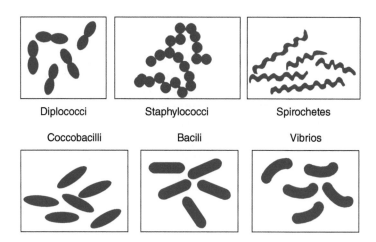

| Diplococci | Staphylococci | Spirochetes |
| Coccobacilli | Bacili | Vibrios |

Figure 5.1   Shapes of bacteria.

Bacteria have three basic shapes (Figure 5.1):

1. Spherical (known as a coccus), e.g. streptococcus, staphylococcus
2. Rod-shaped (known as a bacillus), e.g. diplobacillus, streptobacillus
3. Spiral (known as a spiral), e.g. vibrio, spirochetes.

Cocci

Cocci are usually round, but they can also be oval, elongated or even flattened on one side. When cocci divide to reproduce, the cells can remain attached to one another. Cocci that remain in pairs after dividing are called diplococci. Cocci that divide and remain attached in chain-type patterns are called streptococci. Cocci that divide and form grape-like clusters are known as staphylococci (see Figure 5.1).

Bacilli

Most bacilli appear as single rods. However, some that appear in pairs after they have divided are called diplobacilli. Those that occur in chains are known as streptobacilli, whilst those bacilli that have a more oval shape are called coccobacilli (see Figure 5.1).

Spiral

Spiral bacteria have one or more twists – they are never straight. Bacteria that look like curved rods are called vibrios. Spirella have a helical shape. Spirals that are helical and flexible are known as spirochetes (see Figure 5.1).

Bacterial reproduction

Bacteria reproduce simply by means of simple fission, also known as binary fission (Figure 5.2). Initially, in reproduction, DNA divides into two and then a transverse wall or septum divides the cytoplasm of the cell, which eventually divides into two, so that there are two daughter cells from each cell, which are clones of the parent cell (see Chapter 2).

Viruses

Viruses are obligate intracellular parasites, and they vary from 20 to 200 nm (nanometre) in size; for example, the polio virus is 30 nm in size, whilst the vaccinia virus (the cause of chicken pox) is 400 nm in size – as big as a small bacterium.

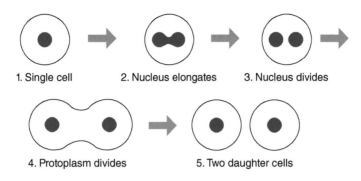

Figure 5.2   Bacterial reproduction – simple fission.

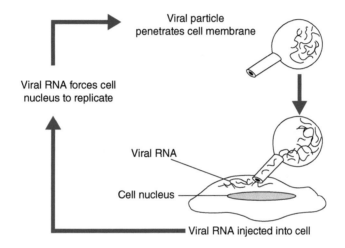

Figure 5.3   Viral replication.

Viruses have varied shapes and chemical composition, but unlike bacteria (or human body cells), they do not contain RNA and DNA – but only contain either RNA or DNA.

Infection of host cells

Figure 5.3 illustrates the stages involved in viral replication.

First, the virus has to be transmitted, and the commonest ways in which a virus is transmitted are:

- Via inhaled droplets (e.g. rhinovirus – causes the common cold)
- In food and/or water (e.g. hepatitis A – causes hepatitis)
- By direct transfer from other infected hosts (e.g. HIV – causes AIDS)
- From the bites of arthropods (such as mosquitoes) that are acting as *vectors* (e.g. yellow fever).

Unconventional slow viruses: Prions

Prions are virus-like structures that are associated with long incubation periods of months and years before disease is evident. The slow virus agent is a mutant form of a host protein know as a prion which can transmit the disease. The long incubation period, which can last as long as 30 years, means that the study of these organisms is difficult. In humans, these agents cause damage to the central nervous system, leading to acute spongiform encephalopathy, which refers to the changes in the structure and appearance of brain tissue (Murray *et al.*, 2020). Examples of slow virus disease in humans include Creutzfeldt-Jakob Disease (CJD) and Variant CJD (vCJD). CJD is transmitted predominantly by injection and transplantation of contaminated tissue, e.g. corneas, contact with contaminated instruments, e.g. brain electrodes, treatment with human growth factor, blood transfusion and food (Murray *et al.*, 2020). The initial diagnosis of the disease is made on clinical grounds, as it is not possible to directly detect prions in tissues through microscopy or serology, and no treatment exists for CJD.

Red flag

Decontamination of medical instruments in cases of known or suspected prion disease

The prion is resistant to common methods of decontamination for medical instruments. Therefore, instruments used on patients undergoing high-risk surgical procedures, e.g. involving structures such as the brain, spinal cord, cranial nerves (in particular the optic nerve) and the pituitary gland, who have an increased risk of CJD/vCJD, require additional/alternative decontamination procedures. Single-use disposable surgical instruments and equipment should be used where possible, and subsequently destroyed by incineration or sent to the instrument store.

Effective tracking of reusable instruments should be in place, so that instruments can be related to use on a particular patient.

Fungi

Fungi are characteristically multicellular organisms with a thick cell wall. They may grow as threadlike filaments known as hyphae, although there are many other forms of growth that occur with fungi. Of these other forms of fungi, the more familiar to us are the single-celled yeasts, and of course the mushrooms.

Fungi are free-living organisms, and are common causes of local infections on skin and hair. However, a number of fungi are also associated with significant disease, and many of these are acquired from the external environment. Pathogenic species invade tissues and digest material externally by releasing enzymes. They also take up nutrients directly from host tissues – as do all good parasites. The various forms of fungi can be seen in Figure 5.4.

Protozoa

Protozoa are single-celled microorganisms that range in size from 2 μm (micrometre) to 100 μm. Many species of protozoa are free-living (i.e. they can exist outside of a cell). Some protozoa are important parasites of humans. Infections are most prevalent in tropical and subtropical regions, but they can also occur in temperate regions.

Although protozoa can cause disease directly (e.g. by the rupture of red cells in malaria), usually the pathology of a protozoal infection is caused by the immunological response of the infected host. Most protozoal infections are actually not life-threatening, unless the infected host has a compromised immune system. The very obvious exception to the previous statement concerns malaria, which kills more than 1.5 million people every year (most of whom are young children, with an immature immune system).

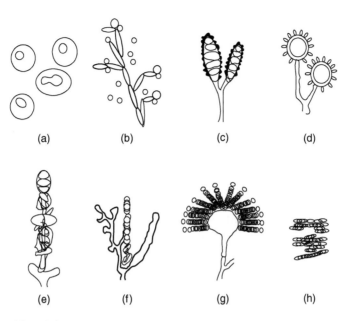

Figure 5.4   Typical fungi shapes.

Medicines management

Antifungal therapy

Colonization of the mouth can occur in up to a third of the population. Oral candidiasis is uncommon in people other than infants, denture wearers and the elderly. In otherwise healthy people, candidiasis may be the first presentation of an undiagnosed risk factor. The use of antibiotic or steroid therapy increases the risk of oral candidiasis as they interfere with the mouth's normal flora and allow candidiasis (oral thrush) to develop.

For localized or mild oral candidal infection, topical treatments such as nystatin oral suspension or miconazole oral gel are usually prescribed for 7 days.

For extensive or severe candidiasis, oral fluconazole 50 mg a day may be prescribed for 7 days and may be increased for a further week if the infection has not fully resolved.

Patients, in particular those who wear dentures, should be advised of the importance of good dental hygiene and to give up smoking if applicable.

Patients using an inhaled corticosteroid are also at risk of oral candidiasis, and advice on the prevention of oral candidal infection should be given.

Recurrent episodes of oral candidal infection in patients with diabetes may require a review of their diabetic control and ongoing management.

(NICE, 2017).

Rickettsiae, Chlamydiae and Mycoplasmas

Rickettsiae

Rickettsiae belong to a group of pathogens that, whilst physically/anatomically belonging to bacteria, also have certain similarities with viruses. They are gram-negative rod-shaped bacteria or coccobacilli. Perhaps the best-known disease that they cause is typhus. They are maintained in animal reservoirs, and they are transmitted by the bites of ticks, fleas, mites and lice.

Chlamydiae

Chlamydiae are very small bacteria that are also obligate intracellular parasites.

The majority of chlamydial infections are genital and acquired during sexual intercourse. Asymptomatic infection is common, especially in women; however, in men it is usually symptomatic. Chlamydiae enter the host through minute abrasions in the mucosal surface, where they bind to specific receptors on the host cells and enter the cells by 'parasite-induced' endocytosis.

Mycoplasmas

Mycoplasmas are also tiny bacteria (actually smaller than large viruses), which differ from normal bacteria in that they lack cell walls, and consequently are not rigid structures. They can produce filaments that resemble fungi. Because of their small size and the fact that they lack rigid cell walls and therefore have a degree of plasticity, they were originally considered to be viruses. In fact, according to Tortora *et al.* (2018: 324), mycoplasmas may represent the smallest cell type that are capable of a cell-free existence and are able to replicate.

There are several species of Mycoplasma, and in humans some species may cause atypical pneumonia, pelvic inflammatory disease, pyelonephritis and puerperal fever. *Mycoplasma pneumoniae* is transmitted from person to person by the airborne route, whilst *Mycoplasma hominis* and *Mycoplasma genitalium* are transmitted by sexual contact (Goering *et al.*, 2018; Tortora *et al.*, 2018).

Helminths

'Helminths' is the correct term for all sorts of parasitic worms that infect the body.

As far as human bodies are concerned, there are three main groups of parasitic worms that cause disease:

1. Tapeworms
2. Flukes
3. Roundworms.

Tapeworms and flukes are also known as flatworms, because they have flattened bodies. They also have muscular suckers and/or hooks to enable them to attach themselves to the host. Roundworms, on the other hand, have long cylindrical bodies, and they generally lack any specialised attachment organs.

Helminth infestations are commonest in warmer countries, although in terms of intestinal species of helminth, they may also occur in temperate regions.

Transmission

Infestation by helminths can occur after:

- Swallowing eggs or larvae via the faecal-oral route
- Swallowing larvae in the tissues of another host (e.g. beef, pork, fish)
- Active penetration of the skin by larval stages
- The bite of an infected blood-sucking insect vector.

Many helminths live in the intestines, whilst others live in the deep tissues, but almost any part of the body can be infested by these parasitic helminths. Flukes and nematodes actively feed on the host tissues or on the contents of the intestines. Tapeworms, on the other hand, have no digestive system and therefore have to absorb pre-digestive nutrients from the host.

Snapshot   Systemic lupus erythematous

Agnes Muretembi, a 24-year-old lady, has been admitted to a medical ward complaining of joint and loin pain, generalised weakness and hair loss. Agnes lives at home with her 2-year-old child and her husband. She is noted to have a butterfly-type rash on her face. Following further investigation, a provisional diagnosis of systemic lupus erythematous (SLE) has been made.

Vital signs

On admission to the medical ward, the following vital signs were noted and recorded:

Vital sign	Observation	Normal
Temperature:	37.2°C	36.0–37.9°C range
Pulse:	90 beats per minute	60–100 beats per minute
Respiration:	16 breaths per minute	12–20 breaths per minute
Blood pressure:	110/65 mmHg	100–139 mmHg (systolic) range
O_2 saturation:	97%	94–98%

A full blood count and urea and electrolytes was performed.

Test	Result	Guideline normal values
White blood cells (WBC)	2.1×10^9/L	4 to 11×10^9/L
Neutrophils	2.0×10^9/L	2.0 to 7.5×10^9/L
Lymphocytes	7.9×10^9/L	1.3 to 4.0×10^9/L
Red blood cells (RBC)	2.4×10^{12}/L	4.5 to 6.5×10^{12}/L
Haemoglobin (Hb)	78 g/L	130–180 g/L
Platelets	98×10^9/L	150 to 440×10^9/L
C-reactive protein	38 mg/L	<5 mg/L
Urea	14.2 mmol/L	2–6.6 mmol/L
Potassium	7.9 mmol/L	3.4–5.6 mmol/L
Sodium	127 mmol/L	135–147 mmol/L

Take some time to consider the following:

1. What is SLE?
2. Plan the care that Agnes will require
3. What ongoing health advice will Agnes require?

NEWS2

Agnes Muretembi

Physiological parameter	3	2	1	0	1	2	3
Respiration rate				16			
Oxygen saturation %				97			
Supplemental oxygen				No			
Temperature °C				37.2			
Systolic BP mmHg				100			
Heart rate				90			
Level of consciousness				A			
Score	0	0	0	0	0	0	0
Total	0						

Medicines management

Immunosuppressants and anti-rheumatoid drugs

Immunosuppressant drugs are commonly used to prevent rejection in transplanted tissues and organs. However, they are also widely used to treat autoimmune conditions, in which the body's own immune system begins to attack itself, damages organs and causes disease, e.g. rheumatoid arthritis, systemic lupus erythematosus, psoriasis and Crohn's disease (Neal, 2020). Patients taking immunosuppressive drugs must be educated to ensure that they take their medication exactly as prescribed every day. Regular blood tests are used to monitor the effectiveness of the drugs and the need for adjustments. When immunosuppressant drugs weaken the immune system, the body becomes less resistant to infection and any infections that develop will be more difficult to treat because of this. These drugs also increase the likelihood of uncontrolled bleeding due to injury or infection. Patients taking immunosuppressant drugs should be careful to avoid catching an infection and should be informed of the following:

- Frequent hand washing
- Avoiding sports in which injuries occur
- Extra care when using sharp objects such as knives or razors
- Avoiding close contact with people who have infections or colds

Patients should be educated to seek medical advice immediately when the following symptoms occur:

- Fever or chills
- Pain in the lower back, on the sides
- Pain or difficulty urinating
- Unusual bruising or bleeding
- Urine that is blood-stained
- Stools that are bloody or black.

Immunosuppressant drugs can cause adverse reactions and birth defects, and health professionals should be aware of the following conditions before immunosuppressant drugs are prescribed: allergies, pregnancy, lactation, shingles or chickenpox, kidney or liver disease, and intestinal problems.

Whilst the most significant side effect of immunosuppressant drugs is an increased risk of infection, these groups of drugs can also put patients at a higher risk of developing cancer, as immunosuppression removes the immune system's protective mechanisms against cancer. Immunosuppressant drugs can interact with many other medications. This can cause dangerous effects in which the immunosuppressants may lose or even increase their effect. Health professionals should ensure that they are aware of any prescription or over-the-counter medications their patients are taking whilst on immunosuppressant therapy

The immune system

Immunology is the study of the immune system and its effects on the body and on invading microorganisms. However, the immune system does more than just protect the body from invasion by microorganisms, and it is linked to many different organs and cells of the body. The immune system is an intricate system of cells, enzymes and proteins, which together protect the body by making it resistant (i.e. immune to infection by microorganisms such as bacteria, viruses, fungi, as well as to larger organisms such as worms).

Organs, cells, and proteins of the immune system

The lymphatic system consists of the following:

- Tonsils and adenoids
- Thymus gland
- Lymph nodes
- Spleen
- Appendix
- Patches of lymphoid tissue in the intestinal tract.

The circulatory system consists of the following:

- Bone marrow
- Lymphocytes (white blood cells)
- Phagocytic cells (white blood cells)
- Dendritic cells
- Thrombocytes (platelets)
- Complement proteins.

The lymphatic system

The lymphatic system is similar to the blood system and consists of a specialised system of lymph vessels (similar to blood vessels) and specialised lymph nodes and tissue. Unlike the circulatory system, the lymphatic system does not have a heart to pump the lymph around. Instead, the lymph (which fills the lymph vessels) is pushed around the body by a combination of contractions of the smooth muscular walls of the lymph vessels, as well as the flexing and relaxing of striated muscle in the body due to the movement of the individual.

The peripheral lymphatic system consists of lymphatic vessels, lymphatic capillaries and encapsulated organs. These organs include the following:

- Spleen
- Tonsils
- Lymph nodes.

The lymph vessels and capillaries form an extensive network throughout the body (Figure 5.5) and connect the organs of the body to the lymphoid organs, such as the spleen, and the lymph nodes. Lymph originates from plasma that leaks from the blood capillaries, and it drains into the lymphoid organs from nearby organs of the body. The lymph nodes act like fishing nets that trap harmful toxins and infectious organisms from the blood, and allow the very high concentrations of immune cells (in this case lymphocytes) to destroy them.

The lymphatic capillaries join together to form larger lymphatic vessels, and throughout the lymphatic system are to be found lymph glands – like railway stations on a railway

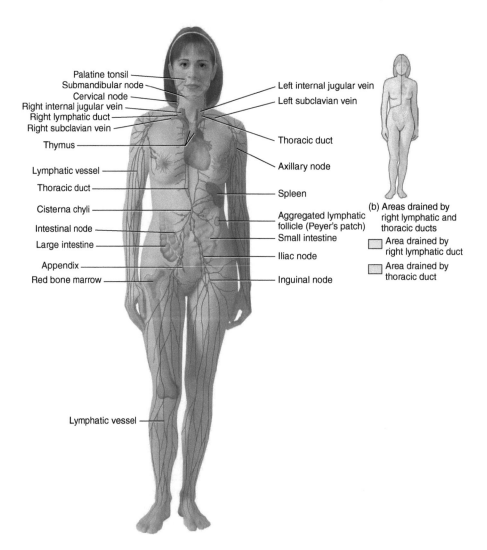

Figure 5.5   The lymphatic system.

network. All the lymph eventually arrives at two large lymph glands, called the thoracic duct and the right lymphatic duct. These two lymph ducts then empty into the great veins of the neck, and this restores fluid and proteins to the venous circulation.

Lymphoid tissue

Lymphoid tissue consists of lymph glands (lymph nodes – Figure 5.6), which are the size and shape of a broad bean, and lymphoid tissue which is found in specific organs such as the spleen, bone marrow, lung and liver.

A lymph node is made up of a meshwork of cells, and the lymph containing any antigens from infected tissues and antigen-bearing cells passes through this meshwork. Within the lymph gland, lymphocytes and phagocytes are found in large numbers, so that they can destroy invading microorganisms that have been trapped in the lymph node.

Other lymphoid organs

The spleen collects antigens from the blood for presentation to phagocytes and lymphocytes. The spleen also collects, and disposes of, dead red blood cells.

Types of immunity

There are two types of immune defence systems:

1. Non-specific (or innate) immunity
2. Specific (or acquired) immunity.

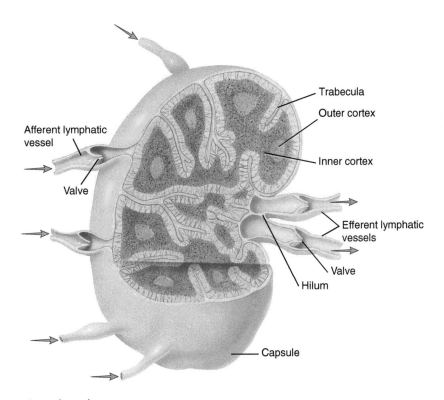

Figure 5.6 Lymph node.

Non-specific immunity

Non-specific immunity is the immunity with which we are born; hence, its more common name, 'innate immunity'.

The innate immune system can be divided into four different components, although there is some overlapping of functions:

1. Physical barriers
2. Mechanical barriers
3. Chemical barriers
4. Blood cells.

Physical barriers

Physical barriers include skin and mucosal membranes.

The skin acts as a physical barrier to prevent infectious organisms and other material, such as dirt, from getting into the more delicate and undefended organs within our body. However, skin is not only a physical barrier, but is also a chemical barrier in that sweat produced from the skin is bactericidal. Unfortunately, skin as a physical barrier does have weaknesses, namely the various orifices that connect the internal body to the outside, including the mouth, nose, urethral opening and anus.

Thus, there needs to be some other type of protection, and the body has that in the form of mucosal membranes, which coat all the passageways between the internal organs and the outside world. Mucosal membranes contain secretions that are also bactericidal as well as secreting large amounts of antibodies (antibodies will be discussed in the section on acquired immunity).

Mechanical barriers

Actions involving cilia, coughing, sneezing and tears are included in this section, as are mechanical barriers.

Cilia are the tiny hairs that are found in the nose. They are constantly moving like coral under the sea, and they move mucus containing dirt and microorganisms away from the inside of the body where they can cause problems to the outside of the body.

Sneezing and coughing work by pushing any microorganisms or irritants out of the body and into the atmosphere. With each sneeze or cough, millions of viruses are expelled into the atmosphere, and this means that there are fewer viruses in the body to cause even worse problems. This is very effective for the person who is coughing and sneezing, but unfortunately it means that there are all these viruses in tiny droplets suspended in the air, just waiting for someone else to come along and breathe them in, and in turn becoming infected with these viruses.

Tears are also a mechanical barrier. They wash any dirt particles or microorganisms away from the eyes. Tears are also a chemical barrier because they contain a bactericidal enzyme known as lysozyme.

Chemical barriers

Some of the components that are involved as chemical barriers have already been mentioned above.

Chemical barriers include the following :

• Tears
• Breast milk

- Sweat
- Saliva
- Acidic secretions, including stomach acid
- Semen.

Most of these secretions contain either bactericidal enzymes such as lysozyme, or antibodies. In addition, bacteria have great difficulty in surviving acidic secretions and are often killed if the environment is too acidic.

Blood cells

As well as the defences mentioned above, the innate system includes certain blood cells, namely leucocytes (white cells) and thrombocytes (platelets).

The actual white cells involved in the innate immune system are known as:

- Neutrophils
- Monocytes and tissue macrophages
- Eosinophils
- Basophils
- Mast cells.

Several different types of cells are involved in the innate immune system.

Orange

Psychological impact of source and protective isolation

The isolation of a patient is normally required for one of two reasons:

1. To protect others from the patient – known as **source isolation**. This is normally required when a patient is suffering from an infectious condition that is either highly contagious or highly resistant to treatment.
2. To protect the patient from others – known as **protective isolation**. This is normally required when the patient has an impaired immune system, is vulnerable to infection and is unable to protect themselves from others.

Cohort isolation of several patients with the same infection/symptoms in a shared area may sometimes be required if there are not enough facilities to isolate each patient individually. However, the decision to isolate a patient is not one that should be taken lightly, as caring experiences and patient–staff relationships are dramatically altered by the uniqueness of imposed physical, social and emotional barriers. Isolation involves serious impacts on patient health, welfare and liberty (Gammon and Hunt, 2018).

Phagocytic cells

Phagocytic cells include:

- Mononuclear phagocytes (these are the monocytes and macrophages)
- Polymorphonuclear phagocytes (neutrophils)
- Eosinophils.

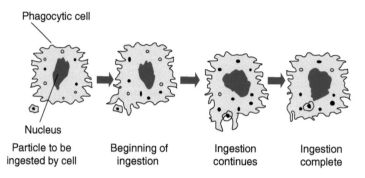

Phagocytic cell

Nucleus

| Particle to be ingested by cell | Beginning of ingestion | Ingestion continues | Ingestion complete |

Figure 5.7   Phagocytosis.

A phagocyte is a cell that ingests microorganisms, such as bacteria, as well as other foreign matter, such as dirt in a wound and wood splinters, as well as any of the body's cells that are recognised by the immune system as being 'foreign', or 'non-self' cells through a process called phagocytosis (see Figure 5.7). The neutrophils and eosinophils contain enzymes which are released when the phagocyte ingests a microorganism. These enzymes help to break down the ingested microorganism, so that the cell can utilise what it wants for its own needs and expel the rest as waste matter.

Mediator cells

A second group of cells of the innate immune system (the basophils and mast cells) are more accurately described as the helper cells of the immune system. They do not actually destroy the invading microorganisms by phagocytosis, but they help the phagocytes to do so. These mediator cells work by releasing various chemicals that have several actions. For example, some of these chemicals improve the inflammatory response to infection and injury, whilst others help the phagocytic cells reach the microorganisms. Although not usually thought of as being part of the immune system, platelets are included because they help to block off and close any cuts and breaks in the skin, and so prevent invading microorganisms from getting inside the body.

Specific immunity

It is specific immunity that gives the body immunity to specific pathogenic microorganisms, and it consists of lymphocytes (white blood cells) that target specific invading microorganisms. This allows for a much more concentrated attack on pathogenic microorganisms that have broken through the body's initial defences.

Clinical investigation

Quantitative immunoglobulin tests (IgA, IgD, IgE, IgG, IgM)

This test measures the amount of antibodies or immunoglobulins in the blood and is usually undertaken when there is suspicion of immunodeficiency. Immunoglobulins are protein molecules that are produced by plasma cells in response to bacterial invasion. The antibody binds to the specific protein (antigen) present on the bacterial surface that induced its production by the plasma cell using a lock and key analogy; i.e. the structure of the antibody matches that of the antigen. The functions of the antibodies are summarized here:

IgA – Provides localized protection from bacterial and viruses; found in saliva, sweat, tears, nasal secretions and breast milk.

IgD – Activates B cells and are located on their surface

IgE – Initiates the inflammatory response by activating mast cells and the release of histamine. Can lead to allergic reactions if present in excess. Found on the surfaces of mast cells and basophils.

IgG – Plays a role in phagocytosis and neutralizes bacterial toxins. Prevents the attachment of some viruses to body cells and activates the complement system.

IgM – Activates the complement system and causes clumping of bacteria. Plays a major role in the early phase of the immune response

Immune problems

The immune system underpins just about all of health, and so if anything goes wrong with it, then there can be serious problems for the body. The things that can go wrong include:

- Immunodeficiencies – the immune system not working properly
- Autoimmune diseases – the immune system in a person is working too well and attacking cells of the person's own body.

There are two types of immunodeficiency – primary and secondary. Primary immuno-deficiency occurs as a result of genetic mutations, whilst secondary immunodeficiency has an external cause, such as infection (HIV) or chemicals. Both types of immunodefi-ciency can range from very mild to life-threatening, and the treatment consists of sup-portive care – antibiotics and other similar drugs, as well as improvement of nutrition and general well-being. In addition, some immunodeficiencies may be helped by the injec-tion of immunoglobulins (antibodies) to replace the patient's own. With secondary immunodeficiencies, it may be possible to remove the cause of the immunodeficiency. For example, if the immunodeficiency is caused by a drug (such as is given in chemo-therapy for cancer – see Chapter 4), once the drug has been discontinued, the immuno-deficiency resolves.

Autoimmunity is often caused by an overreaction of the immune system to an antigen which can lead to the immune system attacking the body's own cells. Examples of autoim-mune diseases include:

- Diabetes (the immune system attacks the cells in the pancreas that secrete insulin).
- Rheumatoid arthritis (the cells of joints, such as fingers and knees, are attacked by the immune system).
- There is a third type of disease caused by a malfunctioning immune system, and that is an allergy. An allergy is a heightened immune response to an allergen (something that causes an allergy, such as peanuts, dust or pollen). As with immunodeficiencies, allergies can range from very mild to life-threatening.

See also Chapter 15 of this text on the endocrine system and associated disorders.

Snapshot   Type 1 diabetes mellitus

Sophie, a 9-year-old child, has presented to the paediatric emergency department with a history of abdominal pain. Sophie had spent the day at school, but has seemed to have worsened since coming home and has vomited on two occasions. Sophie's mother reports that there is no history of fever, diarrhoea, rash, pain elsewhere or dysuria and that no other family member is unwell with gastrointestinal conditions. Simple painkillers had made little difference to Sophie's discomfort. Sophie was diagnosed with autism spectrum disorder (AST) at the age of 3 and has difficulty with small spaces, communication and socialising with her peers. Sophie is normally fit and well, has no other significant past medical history, is not currently taking any medication and has no known allergies. On examination she is apyrexial, her abdomen is soft with no specific tenderness and her bowel sounds are normal. Sophie's mother reports that Sophie has been unusually thirsty over the past few days, has been getting up in the night to pass urine and appears to have lost weight (this is confirmed once Sophie has been weighed). A provisional diagnosis of type 1 diabetes mellitus is made, and Sophie is admitted to the paediatric ward for ongoing treatment.

Sophie's observations are as follows:

Heart rate: 88 beats per minute
Respiratory rate: 20 breaths per minute
Blood pressure: 110/65mm/Hg
Temperature: 36.4°C

Investigations

Urinalysis: glucose ++++, ketones none
Glucometer: blood glucose level 25.3 mmol/L,
C-peptide level: 0.3 ng/mL
Weight: 26 kg

Take some time to consider the following:

1. What is type 1 diabetes mellitus?
2. What care will Sophie require?
3. What ongoing health advice and support will Sophie and her family require?

Inflammatory response

Inflammation is the body's immediate reaction to tissue injury or damage. This damage can be caused by:

- Physical trauma
- Intense heat
- Irritating chemicals
- Infection by viruses, fungi or bacteria.

The inflammatory process (Figure 5.8) involves the movement of white cells, complement and other plasma proteins into a site of infection or injury (Delves *et al.*, 2019).

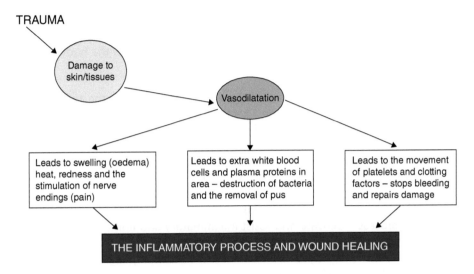

TRAUMA

Damage to skin/tissues

Vasodilatation

Leads to swelling (oedema) heat, redness and the stimulation of nerve endings (pain)

Leads to extra white blood cells and plasma proteins in area – destruction of bacteria and the removal of pus

Leads to the movement of platelets and clotting factors – stops bleeding and repairs damage

THE INFLAMMATORY PROCESS AND WOUND HEALING

Figure 5.8   The inflammatory process.

There are fundamental signs and symptoms of any tissue or bony injury, and these include at the site of the injury the following four classic signs of inflammation:

1. Swelling
2. Pain
3. Heat
4. Redness.

There may also be:

- Nausea
- Sweating
- Raised pulse
- Lowered BP.

These last few symptoms and signs are the body's response to the pain and to shock, but in terms of immunology, the first four signs and symptoms are important.

Although inflammation does cause pain and other problems, it actually has beneficial properties and effects, namely:

- The prevention of the spread to nearby tissues of infectious microorganisms and other damaging agents
- The disposal of killed pathogens and cell debris
- Preparation for repair of the damage.

(Marieb and Hoehn, 2018)

Clinical investigation

Blood tests to detect inflammation

Erythrocyte sedimentation rate (ESR) and C-reactive protein (CRP) are proteins found within the blood which circulate in the presence of inflammation and can therefore be tested for as markers of inflammation in the body.

According to Playfair and Chain (2012), inflammation can be defined clinically as the presence of redness, warmth, swelling and pain.

Inflammation is usually initiated by injury to cells and tissues of the body, and following this injury/damage, three processes occur at the same time:

1. Mast cell degranulation – the release from the mast cells into the tissues of granules containing serotonin and histamine. These work with the other two processes below to provide the complete inflammatory signs and symptoms.
2. The activation of four plasma protein systems:
   a. Complement (helps to orchestrate the inflammatory response)
   b. Clotting (stops bleeding and repairs damage)
   c. Kinin (involved in vascular permeability)
   d. Immunoglobulins (destroys bacteria), all of which work together to support the inflammatory process – activate and assist inflammatory and immune processes, and also play a major role in the destruction of bacteria.
3. The movement of phagocytic cells to the area in order to phagocytose bacteria or any other non-self debris in the wound.

Summary of inflammation

The timetable of a typical inflammatory response to tissue injury is as follows:

- Arterioles near the injury site constrict briefly.
- This vasoconstriction is followed by vasodilation, which increases blood flow to the site of the injury (redness and heat).
- Dilation of the arterioles at the injury site increases the pressure in the circulation.
- This increases the exudation of both plasma proteins and blood cells into the tissues in the area.
- This exudation then causes oedema (swelling).
- The nerve endings in the area are stimulated, partly by pressure (pain).
- The clotting and kinin systems, along with platelets move into the area and block any tissue damage by initiating the clotting process (clot formation).
- White blood cells – phagocytes and lymphocytes move into the area and start to destroy any infectious organisms in the vicinity of the trauma.
- These phagocytes and protein cells, along with the substances they produce, act at the site of the trauma in order to kill any bacteria or other microorganisms in the vicinity, but just as importantly they will remove the debris which results from the coming together of the microorganisms/other non-self matter and the forces of the immune system; this includes exudates and dead cells, also known more commonly as pus (cellular infiltration).
- These systems/blood cells/tissue cells will remain in the area until tissue regeneration (repair) takes place. This is known as resolution.

Thus, inflammation can be summed up as the presence of:

- Vasodilation – redness/heat
- Vascular permeability – oedema
- Stimulation of nerve endings – pain
- Thrombosis – clots
- Cellular infiltration – pus.

(Traske *et al.*, 2014)

Conclusion

This chapter began by looking at infectious diseases. An infection is the result of invasion of the body by microorganisms which cause damage to its tissues. Infectious diseases are characterised by the interaction of the responses of both the infected human host and the infecting organism.

Microorganisms are everywhere – they colonise humans, animals, food, water and soil. Infectious diseases are acquired by humans following contact with an exogenous pathogen present within a reservoir of infection. Such reservoirs include:

- Active human carriers of the disease
- Human carriers of the causative organism
- Animal cases of disease or carriers of the organism
- The inanimate environment.

More than 70 bacteria, viruses, fungi and parasites have been identified as pathogenic infecting organisms that are capable of causing serious diseases in humans (Goering *et al.*, 2018). Vaccines are available against some of these, and work continues to find vaccines for almost all the bacteria, viruses and parasites.

Vaccines tend to mimic and enhance the body's own defences against invading microorganisms – the immune system. The immune system is an extraordinary system, with the continued cooperation of all its components with each other being necessary for continued good health and for our protection against infecting microorganisms.

Test your knowledge

1. What are the differences between a pathogenic microorganism and a commensal microorganism?
   How are the following infectious diseases transmitted?
   a. Rabies
   b. HIV
   c. Enteric fevers
   d. Tuberculosis
   e. Influenza
   f. Tetanus
2. Discuss the effectiveness of physical, chemical and mechanical barriers to infection and what they consist of.
3. What are the organs of the lymphatic system?
4. Briefly discuss the signs and symptoms of an inflammatory response and explain what causes them.

Activities

Here are some activities and exercises to help test your learning. For the answers to these exercises, as well as further self-testing activities, visit our website at
www.wiley.com/go/fundamentalsofappliedpathophysiology/student4e

Multiple choice questions

1. Which antibody class is abundant in body secretions?
   (a) IgD
   (b) IgA
   (c) IgE
   (d) IgM
   (e) IgG

2. Antibodies released by plasma cells are involved in
   (a) Hypersensitivity reactions
   (b) Autoimmune disorders
   (c) Humoral immunity
   (d) All of the above

3. Which of the following is a part of the second line of defence against microorganisms?
   (a) Phagocytes
   (b) Cilia
   (c) Keratin
   (d) Stomach acid

4. Non-specific defence mechanisms are also called
   (a) Acquired
   (b) Adaptive
   (c) Secondary
   (d) Innate

5. The two types of lymphocytes are:
   (a) B-cells and the T-cells
   (b) Platelets and the T-cells
   (c) Platelets and erythrocytes
   (d) T-cells and erythrocytes

6. Another name for acquired immunity is?
   (a) Explicit immunity
   (b) Specific immunity
   (c) Adaptive immunity
   (d) Non-specific immunity

7. Chemical barriers to infection include:
   (a) Tears, breast milk, sweat, saliva, stomach acid
   (b) Tears, stomach acid, urine, hair
   (c) Urine, breast milk, stomach acid, sweat, faeces
   (d) Saliva, stomach acid, hair, breast milk, sweat

8. B-cells that produce and release large amounts of antibody are called:
   (a) Plasma cells
   (b) Neutrophils
   (c) Killer cells
   (d) Basophils

9. Naturally acquired active immunity would be MOST likely acquired through which of the following processes?
   (a) Infection followed by recovery from a disease-causing organism
   (b) Vaccination
   (c) Breast milk
   (d) A natural birth

10. Phagocytes belong to this type of defence mechanism
    (a) Acquired
    (b) Secondary
    (c) Innate
    (d) Adaptive

11. Which of the following in NOT considered to be a classic sign of inflammation?
    (a) Heat
    (b) Redness
    (c) Pain at the injury site
    (d) Swollen lymph glands

12. The causative organisms of infectious disease in humans can be transmitted from the reservoir of infection by:
    (a) Droplet spread
    (b) Inoculation
    (c) Vector
    (d) All of the above

13. Inappropriate and unregulated insulin release from the pancreatic beta cells is called:
    (a) Diabetes mellitus
    (b) Diabetes insipidus
    (c) Cushing's disease
    (d) Hyperinsulinaemia

14. Acute inflammation can be initiated by:
    (a) Mast cell activation
    (b) Influx of neutrophils
    (c) Lysozyme
    (d) An increase in vascular permeability

15. What is the term used to describe white blood cells migrating towards bacteria?
    (a) Phototaxis
    (b) Chemotaxis
    (c) Phagocytosis
    (d) Zeiosis

Conditions

The following is a list of conditions that are associated with inflammation, the immune response and healing. Take some time and write notes about each of the conditions. You may make the notes taken from textbooks or other resources (e.g. people you work with in a clinical area), or you may make the notes as a result of people you have cared for. If you are making notes about people you have cared for, you must ensure that you adhere to the rules of confidentiality.

Keloid	
Anaphylactic shock	

Systemic lupus erythematous	
Human immunodeficiency virus	
Hepatitis	

Further resources

Allergy UK

https://www.allergyuk.org

Allergy UK is a leading national patient charity for people living with all types of allergy. The charity works with the government, professional bodies and healthcare professionals to provide a dedicated helpline and factsheets for those people with allergic disease.

AVERT

http://www.avert.org

This website is a charitable organisation that supports and builds partnerships with local organisations who are working to directly avert the spread of HIV and AIDS. Students will find it useful as it provides a wide range of information to educate people about HIV/AIDS across the world.

CELLS alive!

http://www.cellsalive.com/index.html

Another useful website for students looking for visual images of human cells. CELLS *alive!* represents 30 years of capturing film and computer-enhanced images of living cells and organisms for education and medical research. The majority of the site is free of cost and registration for anyone with Internet access. Contains a stock video library of a range of subjects, both live recording and computer animation.

National Resource for Infection Control (NRIC)

http://www.nric.org.uk

This website is a useful resource for students who wish to increase their knowledge in relation to healthcare-associated infection and its prevention. NRIC is an online project developed by healthcare professionals, aimed at being a single-access point to existing resources within infection control for both Infection Control practitioners and all other healthcare staff.

The Biology Project

http://www.biology.arizona.edu/immunology/tutorials/immunology/main.html

This online interactive resource for learning biology contains a good resource for immunology.

The Department of Health (DH)

https://www.gov.uk/government/organisations/department-of-health

The Department of Health (DH) exists to improve the health and well-being of people in England and the website provides policy, guidance and publications for NHS and social care professionals. There are a number of useful resources relating to HIV/AIDS for students wishing to understand more about this area.

HIV Tutorial (University of Utah)

http://library.med.utah.edu/WebPath/TUTORIAL/AIDS/HIV.html

A short tutorial on human immunodeficiency virus (HIV) from the University of Utah's WebPath service that students will find useful, The tutorial covers prevention of infection, mechanism of infection, HIV structure and function, HIV-2, establishment and dynamics of HIV infection, immunodeficiency, genetic variability of HIV, transmission of HIV, primary HIV infection, onset of AIDS, persistent generalised lymphadenopathy (PGL), AIDS-related complex (ARC), and clinical AIDS.

Primary Immunodeficiency UK (PID UK)

http://www.piduk.org

Primary Immunodeficiency UK (PID UK) is an organization and registered charity supporting individuals and families affected by a primary immunodeficiency in the UK.

Public Health England (PHE)

https://www.gov.uk/government/organisations/public-health-england

Public Health England works with national and local government, industry, and the NHS, to protect and improve the nation's health and support healthier choices. PHE is addressing inequalities by focusing on removing barriers to good health and the website contains a number of useful resources relating to a wide range of health concerns.

Glossary of terms

Acquired immunity   Immunity that develops during the lifetime of an individual after coming into contact with different infectious organisms.

Active immunity   Immunity that occurs after exposure to an antigen.

Allergen   Environmental substance that elicits an immediate hypersensitivity reaction.

Allergy   Type 1 hypersensitivity reaction mediated by IgE.

Antibodies   See immunoglobulins.

Antigen   Something that causes an antibody response, e.g. an infecting microorganism.

Apoptosis   Death of a cell.

Asymptomatic   An infection in which the infected person shows no symptoms of infection (see symptomatic).

Autoimmunity   An overreaction of the immune system to an antigen which can lead to the immune system attacking the body's own cells.

Bacteria (single = bacterium)   Single-cell microorganisms that can infect the body, but also may work with the body to the mutual benefit of both (symbiosis). *E. coli* is an example of a bacterium that can be both beneficial to the body and dangerous to it, depending upon the type of *E. coli* and where it is found within the body.

Bactericidal   Deadly to bacteria – kills them.

B-cell lymphocytes   White blood cells that produce antibodies from plasma cells that are derived from these cells. Part of the humoral immunity.

Bone marrow   Site of production of blood cells.

Cell-mediated immunity   Acquired immunity that is provided by T cell lymphocytes.

Commensal   A microorganism that does not cause any problems to a human and may even be beneficial (c.f. *E. coli*). The opposite of a pathogen.

Complement   A series of enzymatic proteins that work together to aid the immune system by being involved in the processes of opsonisation, chemotaxis and the death of bacterial cells.

Contaminated intermediate   Something that is itself contaminated and can contaminate something else. It acts as a 'go-between' for the infectious organism and the targeted potential host.

Coronavirus   Large single-stranded RNA virus with club-shaped spikes reminiscent of a corona or halo that can cause a variety of illnesses in animal and causes common colds and respiratory infections in humans.

Coronavirus disease 2019 (COVID-19)   An infectious disease that causes severe acute respiratory syndrome coronavirus 2 (SARS-CoV-2). Common symptoms include fever, cough, fatigue, shortness of breath and loss of smell and taste.

C-reactive protein (CRP)   Plasma protein that increases production during inflammation. Can be used as an inflammatory marker.

Creutzfeldt-Jakob Disease   A rare, degenerative and fatal disease affecting the brain and nervous system caused by the build-up of abnormal infectious protein in the brain.

Cystitis   Inflammation of the urinary bladder – usually as a result of colonisation by an infectious microorganism.

Cytokines   Chemical messenger molecules that affect the behaviour of cells including those of the immune system.

Degranulation   The release of granules into the tissues from certain cells, particularly mast cells, eosinophils and basophils, which contain them. These granules contain, amongst other substances, serotonin and histamine, and these substances cause some of the signs and symptoms of inflammation.

Dilate   To widen – see vascular permeability.

Endocytosis   The general name for the various processes by which cells ingest foodstuffs and infectious microorganisms.

Endogenous   From inside of the body – in the case of infections, the infecting microorganism is already present in the body before becoming infectious.

Enteric fevers   Another name for typhoid or paratyphoid fever.

Enzymes   Molecules that speed up chemical reactions.

Epitopes   Receptors on the cell membrane that allow the antigen and antibody to combine with each other

Exogenous   From outside of the body, i.e. an infectious organism that comes from outside of the body.

Fluke   A type of flattened worm (similar to helminths) that can infest humans and cause schistosomiasis or liver fluke infestation.

Fungi   Microorganisms that combine to form larger structures that can be seen by the naked eye. Include yeasts as well as fibrous forms.

Gut helminths   See **helminths**.

Helminths   Also known as intestinal worms. These worms exist as parasites in the human intestines, although other types of helminth can live in the blood, lymph system, or the liver (some are even known to live in the eye).

Herd immunity   A natural population of people (the herd) who are immune to a particular infection. This can be achieved by the population having natural immunity to the infectious organism, or it may be induced by means of vaccination. This means that anyone within that population who may not be immune to the infection will still have only a low chance of becoming infected, because there is so little of the infecting organism in existence within that population.

Histamine   See serotonin.

Histoplasmosis   A respiratory infection caused by inhaling the spores of the fungus *Histoplasma capsulatum* (found in soil contaminated with bird or bat droppings).

Humoral immunity   Acquired immunity that is provided by antibodies secreted from plasma cells produced by B-cell lymphocytes.

Hyphae   Tubular filament-like threads that make up certain fungi.

Immunodeficiencies   Deficiencies in the structure or functioning of the immune system – they can be either secondary (with an external cause) or primary (usually with a genetic cause).

Immunoglobulins   Another name for antibodies. Antibodies are opsonins that are manufac tured by the B-cell lymphocytes and help the phagocytic cells to destroy invading microorganisms.

Inflammation   The body's immediate response to tissue damage or injury.

Innate immunity   The immunity that is present from birth.

Kinin System   Kinins are proteins which play a role in inflammation. The primary kinin is bradykinin, which causes dilation of vessels, acts with prostaglandins to induce pain, increases vascular permeability and may increase leucocyte chemotaxis.

Legionnaire's disease   A form of pneumonia caused by the bacterium *Legionella pneumophila*. It breeds in warm, moist conditions, such as central heating water, and is transmitted via water droplets, such as occur when taking a shower.

Leptospirosis   A disease that often affects the liver and kidneys and is caused by a bacterium found in the urine of rats. Also known as Weil's disease.

Leukocytosis   Increased production of white blood cells.

Macrophage   Develops from monocytes and is involved in phagocytosis within the tissues.

Microorganism   Any living self-contained organism that can only be seen when under a microscope, e.g. bacteria and viruses.

Mucosal membranes   The membranes containing mucus that cover all the passageways leading into or out of the body, e.g. the mouth, nose, bronchi, urethra.

Natural killer cells   Lymphocyte that is part of the innate immune system and destroys abnor-mal cells.

Neutropaenia   Decreased production of neutrophils.

Neutrophil   White blood cell that is involved in phagocytosis.

Obligate intracellular parasites   Microorganisms that are obligated to reproduce inside cells.

Oedema   The abnormal collection of fluid in the tissues. It may be localised (following an injury = swelling) or it may be generalised (as in heart failure).

Opsonisation   Process where bacteria and cells are modified to enhance phagocytosis.

Parasite   An organism living on or in another organism and obtaining nourishment at the expense of the organism that is not parasitic.

Passive immunisation   Rather than stimulate the person's own immune system to produce antibodies, the actual antibodies are given to the patient. See also **active immunisation**.

Pathogen   A microorganism that causes problems – is 'infectious'.

Pelvic inflammatory disease   An inflammation of internal female reproductive organs.

Phagocytosis   The method by which some cells ingest large particles, including whole microorganisms.

Prion   An infectious agent composed entirely of protein primarily located on the surface of central nervous system cells.

Prostaglandins   Prostaglandins are produced by the mast cells. They cause increased vascular permeability, neutrophil chemotaxis, and can induce pain.

Protozoa   The simplest and most primitive type of microorganism, although bigger than a bacterium. Examples of protozoa include those that cause malaria and sleeping sickness (see **trypanosomiasis**).

Puerperal fever   Also known as puerperal sepsis – this is an infection of the female genital tract. It occurs within 10 days of childbirth, a miscarriage, or an abortion.

Pus   A thick green or creamy-coloured fluid found at the site of a bacterial infections. It consists of millions of dead white blood cells of the immune system as well as dead bacteria.

Pyelonephritis   Inflammation of the kidney – usually as a result of bacterial infection.

Reservoir of infection   The place where infectious microorganisms reside before infecting people, e.g. human or animal carriers of the disease, or certain environments. For a disease to perpetuate itself, there must be a continual source of the organisms that cause that disease.

Salbutamol   A bronchodilator drug used in the treatment of asthma – it widens the bronchial tubes to allow asthmatics to breathe more easily.

Schistosomiasis   A tropical disease caused by a fluke (schistosoma) and is contacted by bathing in a river infested by such schistosomes.

Serotonin   Serotonin is a substance that is released from platelets in response to injury, trauma or infection. Along with other substances, such as histamine, it causes temporary, rapid constriction of the smooth muscles of large blood vessel walls and dilation of the small veins (venules). This results in increased blood flow and increased vascular permeability.

Submandibular area   The area just below the jaw (or lower mandible).

Symptomatic   The infected person shows the signs and symptoms of the infection, such as a raised temperature and respirations (see **asymptomatic**).

T cell lymphocyte   White blood cells involved in cell-mediated immunity as part of acquired immunity.

Thymus gland   Organ where lymphocytes migrate to mature into T cell lymphocytes.

Trypanosomiasis   A tropical disease caused by protozoa (Trypanosoma) that is spread by the tsetse fly, which bites humans (and cattle) and causes this disease known as sleeping sickness because of the obvious symptoms.

Vascular permeability   The widening/dilating of blood vessels to allow fluid and other matter to pass through easily.

Vectors   An organism that houses parasites and transmits them from one host to another. A prime example of a vector is the mosquito, which transfers the malaria parasite to humans.

Viruses   A group of very tiny microorganisms that are parasitic in that they can only multiply and survive within a cell that they have infected.

References

Delves, P.J., Seamus, J.M., Burton, D.R. and Roitt, I.M. (2019). *Roitt's Essential Immunology*, 13th edn. England: Wiley-Blackwell.

Goering, R.V., Zuckerman, M., Roitt, I. and Chiodini, P.L. (2018). *Mims' Medical Microbiology*, 6th edn. Edinburgh: Elsevier Mosby.

Health Protection Agency (HPA) (2014). *UK Standards for Microbiological Investigations: Investigation of Specimens for Screening for MRSA*. London: HPA. Available at: www.hpa.org.uk/webc/hpawebfile/hpaweb_c/1317132861509

Marieb, E.N. and Hoehn, K.N. (2018). *Human Anatomy and Physiology*, 11th edn. San Francisco: Pearson Benjamin Cummings.

Murray, P.R., Rosenthal, K.S. and Pfaller, M.A. (2020). *Medical Microbiology*, 9th edn. St Louis: Elsevier Health Sciences.

Neal, M.J. (2020). *Medical Pharmacology at a Glance*, 9th edn. England: Wiley-Blackwell.

National Institute for Health and Care Excellence (NICE) (2017). *Clinical Knowledge Summaries Candida-Oral*. Available at: www.http://cks.nice.org.uk/candida-oral#!scenario:1 Accessed April 2020.

Percival, S.L., Yates, M.V., Williams, D., Chalmers, R. and Gray, N. (2014). *Microbiology of Waterborne Diseases: Microbiological Aspects and Risks*, 2nd edn. London: Elsevier.

Playfair, J.H.L. and Chain, B.M. (2012). *Immunology at a Glance,* 10th edn. England: Wiley-Blackwell.

Rothan, H.A., Siddappa, N. and Byrareddy, N. (2020). The epidemiology and pathogenesis of coronavirus disease (COVID-19) outbreak. *Journal of Autoimmunity*, 109(2020): 102433

Royal College of Nursing (RCN) (2020). *Essential Practice for Infection Prevention and Control Practice: Guidance for Nursing Staff.* London: Royal College of Nursing.

Tortora, G.J., Funke, B.R. and Case, C.L. (2018). *Microbiology: An Introduction*, 13th edn. San Francisco: Pearson Benjamin Cumming.

Traske, B.C., Rote, N.S. and Huether, S.E. (2014). Innate immunity: Inflammation. In: McCance, K.L. and Huether, S.E. (2018), *Pathophysiology: The Biologic Basis for Disease in Adults and Children*, 8th edn. St Louis: Mosby.

Chapter 6

Shock

Janet G. Migliozzi

Senior Lecturer, Department of Nursing, Health and Wellbeing, School of Health and Social Work, University of Hertfordshire, Hatfield, Hertfordshire, UK

Contents

Introduction	131	Multiple choice questions	147
Types of shock	131	Conditions	149
Pathophysiology of shock	140	Further resources	150
Stages of shock	141	Glossary of terms	151
Conclusion	147	References	152
Test your knowledge	147		

Key words

- Anaphylactic shock
- Anaerobic metabolism
- Cardiac output
- Distributive shock
- Homeostasis
- Hypovolaemic shock
- Hypoperfusion
- Neurogenic shock
- Obstructive shock
- Peripheral vasodilation
- Septic shock
- Toxic shock syndrome

Fundamentals of Applied Pathophysiology: An Essential Guide for Nursing and Healthcare Students, Fourth Edition. Edited by Ian Peate.
© 2021 John Wiley & Sons Ltd. Published 2021 by John Wiley & Sons Ltd.
Student companion website: www.wiley.com/go/fundamentalsofappliedpathophysiology/student4e
Instructor companion website: www.wiley.com/go/fundamentalsofappliedpathophysiology/instructor4e

Test your prior knowledge

- What does the cardiovascular system consist of?
- What is homeostasis?
- How is blood pressure maintained at a constant level?
- What are the four main categories of shock?
- What does epinephrine do?

Learning outcomes

On completion of this section, the reader will be able to:

- Describe the different types of shock and their causative factors.

- Describe the clinical presentation of different types of shock.

- Describe the pathophysiology and stages of shock.

- Understand the care of the patient in shock.

Don't forget to visit the companion website for this book
(www.wiley.com/go/fundamentalsofappliedpathophysiology/student4e)
**where you can find self-assessment tests to check your progress, as well as
lots of activities to practise your learning.**

Introduction

The cardiovascular system consists of the heart, blood and a vascular network composed of arteries, veins, arterioles, venules and capillaries that work together to maintain tissue survival by ensuring that an adequate and constant supply of oxygen and nutrients reaches the cells and that metabolic waste products are removed.

Under normal circumstances, homeostasis is maintained by the four essential circulatory components, e.g. blood/interstitial fluid volume, blood flow, vascular resistance and the ability of the heart to contract (myocardial contractility). When one of these circulatory components fails, the others compensate. However, if compensatory mechanisms fail or if more than one of the circulatory components is affected, the cardiovascular system will fail to function, resulting in a state of circulatory shock (Sole *et al.*, 2016).

Types of shock

Any condition that leads to a reduction in cardiac output can lead to circulatory shock; consequently, the effects of shock are not limited to one organ system and can be considered to be a general systemic reaction. However, shock is typically classified by its causative factors and includes the following.

Snapshot   Carcinoma of the stomach

Mr Raj Kumar is an 84-year-old man with carcinoma of the stomach who returned to the ward an hour ago following surgery for a total gastrectomy. He has a Robinson's drain *in situ* which is draining small amounts of blood-stained fluid, a urinary catheter on hourly measurements of urine output and an intravenous infusion of Normal Saline in progress. He is currently on half-hourly observations of his vital signs and has been stable since his return from the theatre.

Forty-five minutes later, Mrs Kumar asks you to check on her husband as she is worried about him. On examination his pulse is rapid, weak and thready, and he is breathless and hypotensive. His wound is oozing slightly, the Robinson's drain is now full of blood-stained fluid and there is approximately 5 mL of dark-coloured urine in the urometer.

Take some time to reflect on the following questions:

1. What type of shock is Mr Kumar likely to be experiencing?
2. Discuss the signs and symptoms that Mr Kumar is experiencing.
3. Discuss the role of fluid therapy in managing Mr Kumar's condition.
4. Outline the immediate care that Mr Kumar will require to prevent deterioration.

Vital signs

The following vital signs were noted and recorded:

Vital sign	Observation	Normal
Temperature	36.5°C	36.0–37.9°C range
Pulse	125 beats per minute	60–100 beats per minute
Respiration	28 breaths per minute	12–20 breaths per minute
Blood pressure	88/55 mmHg	100–139 mmHg (systolic) range
O_2 saturation	92%	94–98% Or 88–92% in chronic resp. conditions

A full blood count and urea and electrolytes was performed.

Test	Result	Guideline normal values
White blood cells (WBC)	4.6×10^9/L	4 to 11×10^9/L
Neutrophils	4.2×10^9/L	2.0 to 7.5×10^9/L
Lymphocytes	2.5×10^9/L	1.3 to 4.0×10^9/L
Red blood cells (RBC)	3.7×10^{12}/L	4.5 to 6.5×10^{12}/L
Haemoglobin (Hb)	96 g/L	130–180 g/L
Platelets	154×10^9/L	150 to 440×10^9/L
C-reactive protein	3.5 mg/L	<5 mg/L
Urea	4.4 mmol/L	2–6.6 mmol/L
Potassium	3.9 mmol/L	3.4–5.6 mmol/L
Sodium	135 mmol/L	135–147 mmol/L

NEWS 2

Raj Kumar

Physiological parameter	3	2	1	0	1	2	3
Respiration rate	28						
Oxygen saturation %		92					
Supplemental oxygen				No			
Temperature °C				36.5°C			
Systolic BP mmHg	88						
Heart rate		125					
Level of consciousness	V						
Score	9	4	0	0	0	0	0
Total	13						

Red flag

Infection risks associated with peripheral IV cannulae

One in three UK patients have a peripheral intravenous cannula (PVC) *in situ* at any time, and PVC-related thrombophlebitis and infection are common complications of a PVC.

There are four possible pathways leading to a PVC infection. The insertion of a PVC provides a potential portal of entry for bacteria to cross from an unsterile external environment to the normally sterile blood. This can occur at insertion of the device from the puncture site that provides a means for microbes from the patient's skin or healthcare worker's hands to travel along the cannula into the bloodstream. The catheter hub, which can become contaminated by healthcare workers' or patients' skin flora during connection of fluids, medicine administration or during extraction of blood, also provides a common means of contamination and should be managed with an adequate aseptic non-touch technique. The third route is for the device to be contaminated directly by bacteria circulating in the bloodstream. That is, the patient has an existing bloodstream infection, and microbes are able to attach to the catheter as they pass by the device. A contaminated infusate, which may occur at the manufacturing stage (intrinsic) or during manipulation by healthcare workers (extrinsic), provides the final means of contamination, and a recent study confirms that infusates other than water, including heparin, have great potential to form crystals in the intraluminal surface of PVCs, which can induce bacterial attachment and colonisation (Nishikawa *et al.*, 2010). However, most PVC infections are preventable with proper adherence to hand hygiene, the implementation of education strategies, the use of sterile semipermeable dressings and correct location of insertion site for the device, all of which dramatically reduce the incidence of PVC-related infections.

Hypovolaemic shock

Hypovolaemic shock due to haemorrhage is the most common cause of this type of shock (Norris, 2019) and occurs as a result of fluid loss, which includes both blood loss, plasma loss and/or loss of interstitial fluid. Blood can be lost from a bleeding organ or wound; however, the circulating volume can also be reduced as a result of plasma loss, e.g. from extensive burns or damaged tissues or excessive loss of fluids from either renal impairment or inadequate fluid intake, e.g. dehydration. This loss of fluid leads to a reduction in circulatory fluid in the blood vessels, leading to insufficient quantities of blood returning to the heart. This poor venous return results in a decrease in cardiac output and subsequent decrease in blood pressure, which leads to a decrease in tissue perfusion, resulting in impaired cellular metabolism and shock. Figure 6.1 outlines the physiological events leading to hypovolaemic shock.

Cardiogenic and obstructive shock

Cardiogenic shock occurs when the heart 'fails' as a pump, resulting in abnormal cardiac functioning. Obstructive shock occurs when a mechanical or physical obstruction impedes the flow of blood, e.g. a pulmonary embolism or tension pneumothorax.

Distributive shock

The next three types of shock (anaphylactic, septic and neurogenic) are collectively known as distributive shock (see Figure 6.2) in which (irrespective of the causative factors) widespread vasodilatation and decreased peripheral vascular resistance are a common feature (Kanaparthi and Pinsky, 2011). This type of shock differs from hypovolaemic shock in that the circulating blood volume remains normal (Martini, 2017). However, cardiac output and blood pressure become impaired due to the blood vessels losing their vasomotor tone, which leads to an increase in their diameter (vasodilatation). This leads to a decrease in

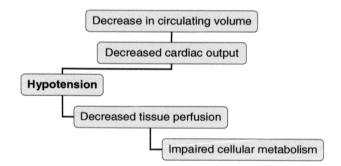

Figure 6.1   Hypovolaemic shock.

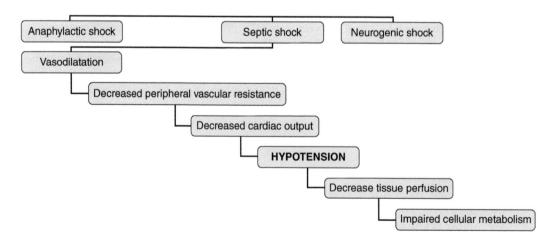

Figure 6.2   Distributive shock.

peripheral vascular resistance, resulting in the blood collecting or 'pooling' in the large veins, causing circulating blood volume to be abnormally distributed. As a result, blood pressure in the systemic circulation falls to such a low point that venous return decreases to the point that cardiac output becomes inadequate to perfuse the tissues adequately, and shock ensues (see Figure 6.2).

Snapshot Anaphylaxis

Mr David Carter, a 29-year-old old builder, was working with others on a new construction at a local district general hospital. Mr Carter had been tearing down some old guttering when he encountered a wasp's nest, and was stung several times by a large number of swarming wasps. Immediately after this, he commented to his colleagues that, in addition to the pain of the stings, he had begun to feel generally unwell, weak, lightheaded and nauseous. His work colleagues have brought him into the hospital's emergency department. On arrival, Mr Carter reports that he has begun to feel worse and is complaining of increased weakness and nausea, a tightness across his chest and some difficulty breathing. He also has several raised hives on his face and arms.

Vital signs

On admission to the emergency department, the following vital signs were noted and recorded:

Vital sign	Observation	Normal
Temperature	37.2°C	36.0–37.9°C range
Pulse	110 beats per minute	60–100 beats per minute
Respiration	28 breaths per minute	12–20 breaths per minute
Blood pressure	110/78 mmHg	100–139 mmHg (systolic) range
O_2 saturation	94%	94–98% Or 88–92% in chronic resp. conditions

A full blood count and urea and electrolytes was performed.

Test	Result	Guideline normal values
White blood cells (WBC)	6.1×10^9/L	4 to 11×10^9/L
Neutrophils	4.8×10^9/L	2.0 to 7.5×10^9/L
Lymphocytes	3.2×10^9/L	1.3 to 4.0×10^9/L
Red blood cells (RBC)	5.4×10^{12}/L	4.5 to 6.5×10^{12}/L
Haemoglobin (Hb)	141 g/L	130–180 g/L
Platelets	309×10^9/L	150 to 440×10^9/L
C-reactive protein	4.8 mg/L	<5 mg/L
Urea	4.3 mmol/L	2–6.6 mmol/L
Potassium	4.1 mmol/L	3.4–5.6 mmol/L
Sodium	138 mmol/L	135–147 mmol/L

Take some time to reflect on the following questions:

1. What type of shock is Mr Carter likely to be experiencing?
2. Discuss the signs and symptoms that Mr Carter is experiencing.
3. Discuss the role of epinephrine in Mr Carter's care.
4. What health promotion advice would you give Mr Carter for the future?

Clinical investigation

Allergy blood testing – the tryptase test

The body releases tryptase, not only as part of the body's normal response to injury but also as part of an allergic response.

Mast cells contain tryptase in both immature and mature stages, and the ratio between the two can be indicative of anaphylaxis if less than 10.

The tryptase test is advocated by NICE (2011) following any suspected case of anaphylaxis, as it can help confirm the diagnosis. With anaphylaxis, tryptase concentrations typically peak about 1 to 2 hours after symptoms begin. If a sample is drawn too early or too late, results may be normal. If a histamine test is also performed, it can be compared to the tryptase levels. Histamine concentrations peak within several minutes of the onset of anaphylaxis and fall within about an hour. If the timing of sample collection was appropriate and neither the histamine or tryptase concentrations were elevated, it is unlikely that a person had anaphylaxis, but it cannot be ruled out.

Anaphylactic shock

This form of shock (also known as anaphylaxis) occurs following a widespread allergic or hypersensitivity reaction to the presence of an allergen or antigen that can lead to severe circulatory collapse within seconds (Resuscitation Council UK, 2012). A diagnosis of anaphylaxis is likely when all the following are met:

- Acute onset of symptoms/illness
- Life-threatening airway and/or breathing and/or circulation problems
- Usually there are skin changes, e.g. rash, itching, redness.

(Resuscitation Council, 2012)

In addition, some common causes of anaphylaxis are summarised in Table 6.1.

Anaphylactic reactions can be either immunoglobulin E (IgE)-mediated or non-IgE-mediated and occur as a result of repeated exposure to an antigen or allergen (to which the individual has previously produced an antibody response), which results in an allergic response (Lewis *et al.*, 2014). The subsequent release of histamine causes massive vasodilatation of blood vessels, increases vascular permeability (which results in loss of intravascular fluid volume) and constricts respiratory smooth muscle (Lewis *et al.*, 2014). Figure 6.3 summarises this response.

Signs and symptoms of anaphylactic shock can include the following:

- Sense of impending doom, anxiety and restlessness
- Altered levels of consciousness

Table 6.1 Common causes of anaphylaxis (Turner *et al.*, 2015).

Antibiotics (penicillins and cephalosporins)
Anaesthetic agents and muscle relaxants
Aspirin and non-steroidal anti-inflammatory drugs, e.g. ibuprofen
Immunuisations
Blood products and plasma expanders
Intravenous radiocontrast media
Latex
Food allergies, e.g. shellfish, eggs, nuts and dairy products
Insect stings

137

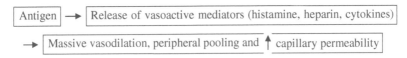

Figure 6.3 Stages involved in an anaphylactic reaction.

- Severe air hunger
- Bronchospasm and dyspnoea
- Stridor caused by laryngeal oedema
- Urticaria (hives)
- Pruritus (itching)
- Rhinitis and conjunctivitis
- Abdominal pain, vomiting and diarrhoea
- Oedema of the lips, eyes, hands, neck and throat.

Medications management

Adverse drug reactions
Analysis of patient safety incidents reported to the National Reporting and Learning System between 2005 and 2013 identified 18 079 incidents involving drug allergy. These included 6 deaths, 19 'severe harms', 4980 'other harms' and 13 071 'near-misses'. The majority of these incidents involved a drug that was prescribed, dispensed oar administered to a patient with a previously known allergy to that drug or drug class (NICE, 2014).

Snapshot   Sepsis

Ms Josephine Darko-Boateng is a 67-year-old lady who has had recurrent urinary tract infections over the last 10 years with the last episode causing pyelonephritis and severe back pain. Recent investigations could not find a specific cause for this, and she was to be reviewed in urology clinic in 6 weeks' time.

Two days ago, Josephine started to feel flu-like but had no respiratory symptoms. She took paracetamol 1 gram and went to bed. After 24 hours she felt worse. She rang her GP, who suggested it may be flu and to rest and take painkillers. The following evening, Josephine felt shaky and cold; she began to shiver and could not keep warm. She rang her friend Joan, who persuaded her to go to hospital. On arrival to the local emergency department, Josephine is confused and lethargic, and the following were observed:

Blood pressure 100/54mm/Hg	Blood sugar 6.2 mmol
Pulse 112 beats /minute	AVPU: Voice
Temp 39.2°C	Weight 76 kg height 172 cm
Oxygen saturation 94% on air	White cell count 16× 10⁹/L
Respiratory rate 26 beats/minute	

Orange flag

White coat syndrome (also called white coat hypertension) is a phenomenon in which people exhibit a blood pressure level above the normal range, in a clinical setting, although in other settings they do not exhibit it.

Urinary dipstick was undertaken, and a sample was sent for cultures. She was found to have protein, blood and nitrates in her urine, and she complained of difficulty in passing urine in the last 3 hours.

Josephine was identified as having sepsis secondary to a urinary tract infection and was commenced on Trimethoprim. Paracetamol was given for pain control, and Enoxaparin 40 mg subcutaneous given for prophylaxis against deep vein thrombosis. Blood cultures were undertaken, and she was put on fluid replacement to support her blood pressure. Oxygen at 4 litres was started.

Take some time to consider the following;

1. The signs and symptoms Ms Darko-Boateng is experiencing
2. The findings from the urinary dipstick
3. The pharmacological action of Trimethoprim

Septic shock

Septic shock is the most common type of distributive shock (Smeltzer and Bare, 2013) and occurs as a result of widespread infection. This form of shock is most commonly associated with the release of gram-negative and gram-positive bacteria into the bloodstream – a condition known as bacteraemia, in which the pathogen's release of toxins into the bloodstream results in massive vasodilatation and hypotension.

Sepsis is the systemic response to infection and includes evidence of a widespread inflammatory response. Early recognition of sepsis is imperative and includes looking for sources of infection, measuring physiological signs and symptoms to identify potential organ dysfunction. Identification for high-risk criteria known as the sepsis 'red flags' (Daniels and Nutbeam, 2018) is outlined in Table 6.2 below – a suspicion of infection and any one red flag requires immediate action. The critical point is that sepsis is not simply the presence of infection (even where this is a severe infection or infection in the blood), but rather an

Table 6.2 Sepsis red flags.

Sepsis red flags
Systolic BP ≤90 mmHG (or drop of 40 mmHg)
Temperature >38°C or <36°C
Heart rate >130 beats/min
Respiratory rate >25 breaths/min
Needs oxygen to keep saturation level >92%
Not passed urine in past 18 hours/less than 30 mL/hour if catheterised
Non-blanching rash, mottled, ashen, cyanotic
Lactate >2 mmol/L
Responds only to voice or pain/unresponsive
Recent chemotherapy

Source: Daniels and Nutbeam, 2018.

overreaction to infection (Hunt, 2019). Patients with sepsis continue to experience significant morbidity and mortality, and sepsis has now been defined as "life-threatening organ dysfunction caused by a dysregulated host response to infection" (Surviving sepsis campaign, 2016) in which septic shock is now defined as a subset of this (Seckel, 2017)

Risk factors for sepsis include the following:

- The very young (under 1 year) and older people (over 75 years) or people who are very frail
- People who have impaired immune systems because of illness or drugs, including:
  - People being treated for cancer with chemotherapy (suspect neutropenic sepsis in patients having anticancer treatment who become unwell)
  - People who have impaired immune function (for example, people with diabetes, people who have had a splenectomy or people with sickle cell disease)
  - People taking long-term steroids
  - People taking immunosuppressant drugs to treat non-malignant disorders such as rheumatoid arthritis
  - People who have had surgery, or other invasive procedures, in the past 6 weeks
  - People with any breach of skin integrity (for example, cuts, burns, blisters or skin infections)
  - People who misuse drugs intravenously
  - People with indwelling lines or catheters
  - Take into account that women who are pregnant, have given birth or had a termination of pregnancy or miscarriage in the past 6 weeks are in a high-risk group for sepsis. In particular, women who:
  - Have impaired immune systems because of illness or drugs
  - Have gestational diabetes or diabetes or other comorbidities
  - Needed invasive procedures (for example, caesarean section, forceps delivery, removal of retained products of conception)
  - Had prolonged rupture of membranes
  - Have or have been in close contact with people with group A streptococcal infection, for example, scarlet fever
  - Have continued vaginal bleeding or an offensive vaginal discharge

(NICE, 2016 updated 2020)

Red flag

Prevention of toxic shock syndrome

Toxic shock syndrome (TSS) is a form of septic shock that can occur in women who use tampons during menstruation or in individuals who have body piercings. It is caused by the bacteria *Staphylococcus aureus* and *Streptococcus pyogenes* which normally reside harmlessly on the skin but if introduced into the bloodstream produce toxins that cause extensive vasodilatation, leading to a drop in blood pressure, dizziness and confusion. In addition, the toxins attack the skin and organs of the body and can cause death if left untreated.

Although TSS does not solely affect women, the first cases of the syndrome were reported in women who used tampons during menstruation, and infection could occur if tampons were left *in situ* for more than six hours (Eckert and Lentz, 2012). Therefore, at the time of admission, it is important that nurses ask female patients if they are menstruating and advise them to use external sanitary protection (sanitary towels) if undergoing surgery.

Table 6.3   Types of shock and common causative factors.

Type of shock	Common causative factors
Hypovolaemic shock	External and internal fluid volume loss
Anaphylactic shock	Repeated exposure to an antigen
Septic shock	Gram-negative bacteria Gram-positive bacteria
Neurogenic shock	Spinal cord injury Spinal anaesthetic Brain injury Vasomotor depression Drug overdose Severe pain
Cardiogenic shock	Myocardial infarction Cardiomyopathy Valvular disease Structural defects Cardiac arrhythmias
Obstructive shock	Cardiac tamponade Pulmonary embolism

Neurogenic (vasogenic) shock

This is a rare form of shock which can occur following major brain or spinal trauma, emotional trauma, severe pain or following a drug overdose or incorrectly administered spinal anaesthesia. The loss of sympathetic impulses causes a significant decrease in peripheral vascular resistance. This results in massive vasodilatation, which affects venous return to the heart, leading to a decrease in cardiac output, low blood pressure and a reduction in blood flow (see Table 6.3).

Pathophysiology of shock

Shock is a severe, life-threatening clinical syndrome that can result in death and is characterised by inadequate tissue perfusion that results in impaired cellular metabolism. Shock manifests itself as a syndrome within many diseases or traumatic injuries that may be life-threatening and is a state of insufficient oxygenation and perfusion to vital organs and tissues throughout

Table 6.4   A summary of clinical presentation of different types of shock.

Manifestation	Hypovolaemic	Anaphylactic	Septic	Neurogenic
Heart rate	Tachycardia	Tachycardia	Tachycardia	Bradycardia
Respiratory rate	Tachypnoea	Tachypnoea and dyspnoea	Tachypnoea	Rapid and shallow
Blood pressure	Hypotension	Hypotension	Hypotension	Hypotension
Urine output	Decreased urine production	Decreased urine production	Increased initially, then oliguria	Decreased urine production
Temperature	Temperature within normal range	Temperature within normal range	Temperature initially raised and then within normal range	Temperature regulation disrupted; therefore may be experiencing hypo/hyperthermia
Skin	Cool, pale skin	Cyanosis, swollen oedematous face, hands	Skin is initially flushed and warm (warm shock) then cool and pale	Cool, pale skin
Mental state	Restless and anxious	Restless and anxious	Restless and anxious	May be unconscious due to fainting or head injury

the body. Therefore, whilst the causes of shock are varied and the individual's presentation may differ according to this (see Table 6.4), the end results (at a cellular level), e.g. cellular hypoxia/damage, are the same (Tortora and Derrickson, 2017).

Stages of shock

Although the patient's initial response to shock may vary, as it is dependent on the individual's age and general state of health prior to the event leading to the shock state, three distinct stages of shock are recognised and occur regardless of the type of shock experienced (Sole *et al.*, 2016).

Stage 1: compensatory (non-progressive) stage of shock

A sufficient blood pressure is essential to adequately perfuse cells with oxygen and nutrients. Shock begins when the blood pressure is unable to do this, and the body then initiates a series of compensatory mechanisms. During this stage, although the individual will be experiencing symptoms of shock, he/she is not at imminent risk of death and shock may be reversed if appropriate interventions are initiated (Foster and Prevost, 2012). In the early stages of compensatory shock, a set of neural, hormonal and chemical compensatory mechanisms are initiated in an attempt to restore homeostasis and maintain blood flow to vital organs such as the heart, brain and kidneys.

Neural compensatory mechanisms

The sympathetic nervous system regulates blood flow and pressure through its ability to increase heart rate and total peripheral resistance. In the shock state, the baroreceptors and chemoreceptors located in the carotid sinus and aortic arch detect the reduction in blood pressure, and impulses are relayed to the vasomotor centre in the medulla oblongata.

Hormonal compensatory mechanisms

Stimulation of the sympathetic nervous system causes the adrenal medullae to release the catecholamines (epinephrine and norepinephrine), which increase the heart rate and force of contractions to improve cardiac output. The coronary arteries vasodilate to increase blood flow to the heart and meet its increasing demands for oxygen. The rate and depth of respirations will also increase to try and increase gaseous exchange and oxygen levels in the blood (Sole *et al.*, 2016).

Medications management

Oxygen

Oxygen therapy can be life-saving; however, without appropriate assessment and ongoing evaluation, it can also be harmful. Oxygen is a drug that must be prescribed.
   Oxygen therapy is indicated in acute illness for:

- Cardiac/respiratory arrest or peri-arrest
- Hypoxaemia
- Shock, sepsis, major trauma, anaphylaxis
- Carbon monoxide poisoning.

Venturi valves are colour-coded to signify the fixed percentage of delivery:

- 24% Blue
- 28% White
- 35% Yellow
- 40% Red
- 60% Green

(Olive, 2017)

A fall in cardiac output will also impact the renal system, which detects a decrease in blood flow and pressure to the kidneys. This causes the kidneys to release renin, which converts angiotensinogen into angiotensin I, which is metabolised into angiotensin II – a powerful vasoconstrictor. The presence of angiotensin II leads to the release of the hormone aldosterone from the adrenal gland, which causes the reabsorption of sodium from the renal tubule. This leads to the retention of water with the aim of increasing the falling blood volume (see Figure 6.4). Stimulation of the posterior pituitary gland causes the release of antidiuretic hormone (ADH), also known as vasopressin hormone, which increases the amount of water reabsorbed by the kidney tubules; hence, the patient may produce small volumes of concentrated urine, or in more severe cases, no urine (anuria).

Red flag

Fluid balance monitoring

The Nursing and Midwifery Council (NMC) Code (NMC, 2018) requires that nurses keep accurate and clear records, including fluid balance charts. An understanding of the physiological mechanisms of fluid balance is necessary if nurses are to not only carry out charting with knowledge and thought, but also to quickly and accurately detect or anticipate imbalances (NICE, 2013 updated 2017). In addition, NICE (2013 updated 2017) recommends that all patients receiving vIV fluids require, as a minimum, a daily assessment of their fluid status including the nature of the electrolyte content of the IV fluids clinicians prescribe.

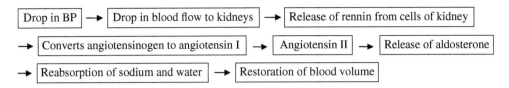

Figure 6.4   Renin angiotensin mechanism.

143

Chemical compensatory mechanisms

A reduction in cardiac output leads to a decrease in blood flow to the lungs, which is detected by the chemoreceptors located in the aorta and carotid arteries. This leads to an increase in the rate and depth of respirations; however, this hyperventilation causes a reduction in carbon dioxide which impacts blood flow and oxygen levels to the brain, which can lead to confusion and restlessness. The individual will move to the next stage of shock if the physiological adaptations that the body has initiated to overcome shock start to fail.

Stage 2: progressive (decompensated) stage of shock

Progressive shock occurs when the body's initial compensatory responses fail to restore an adequate blood pressure and tissue perfusion (Foster and Prevost, 2012). In the early stages of progressive shock, the individual's life can usually be saved if treatment is timely and appropriate. However, if the originating problem, e.g. haemorrhage, has not been corrected, the body's compensatory mechanisms can no longer cope with the continuing decreased cardiac output and blood pressure; consequently, vital organs are not sufficiently perfused (hypoperfusion), and tissue damage can occur. The systemic circulation continues to vasoconstrict with the aim of shunting blood to vital organs; however, this is at the expense of the microcirculation, resulting in ischaemia of the extremities. Impaired cellular metabolism occurs as a result of an inadequate supply of oxygen and nutrients, and the decreased levels of oxygen cause the cells to switch from aerobic metabolism to anaerobic metabolism, which results in the production of lactic acid and leads to metabolic acidosis.

Prolonged anaerobic metabolism results in a reduction in the production of adenosine triphosphate (ATP), which leads to failure of the sodium-potassium pump, causing sodium ions to accumulate inside the cell, resulting in swelling and a deterioration in the cell's function.

As shock progresses, histamine and bradykinin (both of which have vasodilating properties) are released and decrease the peripheral vascular resistance further, resulting in a continued reduction in blood returning to the heart. This leads to a further decrease in cardiac output and blood pressure, leading to cellular hypoxia.

Hypoxia can lead to depression of the vasomotor centre in the medulla and the sympathetic nervous system. Levels of consciousness decrease, and the patient may become restless, disorientated and confused. Abdominal distension and paralytic ileus are common, and the pancreas may become ischaemic (Foster and Prevost, 2012).

Clinical investigation

Arterial Blood Gas (ABG)

The collection of blood from an artery is indicated when there is a clinical need to determine the acid/base balance and electrolyte and haemoglobin levels, The blood is usually drawn from the radial artery in the wrist but may also be drawn from an artery in the groin or on the inside of the elbow. Indications for the test are summarised below:

- Monitoring of acid/base status
- Measurement of the partial pressures of respiratory gases involved in oxygenation and ventilation

- Assessment of response to a therapeutic intervention e.g. ventilation
- Determination of arterial respiratory gases for diagnostic and evaluation purposes
- In an emergency situation when a blood sample is required and venous sampling is not possible.

Stage 3: irreversible (refractory) stage of shock

At this stage, the continued decrease in blood pressure and heart rate means that the inadequate tissue perfusion leads to the subsequent failure of the body to respond to any form of therapy, which results in multiple organ failure and death within a matter of hours (Foster and Prevost, 2012).

Red flag

Disseminated intravascular coagulation
Disseminated intravascular coagulation (DIC) is characterised by widespread coagulation and bleeding in the vascular compartment and occurs as a complication of a wide variety of conditions, e.g. infection, injury and severe tissue damage, that cause the body's normal blood clotting process to become overactive. Signs and symptoms may include, bruising, bleeding, low blood pressure, breathlessness and confusion.

Table 6.5 summarises the stages of shock, the physiological changes that occur and how the individual may present clinically.

Table 6.5   Physiological changes that occur at each stage of shock.

Stage of shock	Physiological changes	Clinical presentation
1. Compensatory	Neural and hormonal compensation. Mild to moderate vasoconstriction. Some anaerobic metabolism.	Normal blood pressure. Increased pulse rate (tachycardia) and respiratory rate (tachypnoea). Increased thirst. Decreased urinary output. Altered level of consciousness/dilated pupils
2. Progressive	Overall aerobic metabolism. Decrease oxygen levels (hypoxia) to vital organs. Little or no oxygen (anoxia) to non-vital organs. Impaired blood flow (ischaemia) to tissues. Failure of sodium-potassium pump.	Low blood pressure (hypotension). Raised pulse rate. Tachypnoea. Pulmonary oedema. Peripheral oedema. Decreased urinary output. Altered level of consciousness. Abdominal distension. Paralytic ileus. Cold, ashen skin.
3. Irreversible	Severe tissue hypoxia, ischaemia and necrosis (tissue death). Build-up of toxic metabolites.	Severe hypotension. Respiratory failure. Acidosis. Peripheral oedema. Acute renal failure (oliguria). Alterations in the blood clotting cascade.

Source: Adapted from Sole *et al.*, 2016.

Care of the patient in shock

Due to the life-threatening nature of shock, it is essential that the condition is recognised and treated in a prompt manner if inadequate tissue perfusion and subsequent organ failure is to be avoided. Therefore, the patient in shock requires close and careful monitoring within an intensive care or high-dependency unit. Common interventions include oxygen, fluid and/or drug therapy, and care should be focused on the care of the patient whilst they are undergoing these restorative measures. Key clinical considerations include the following:

145

- Close monitoring of vital signs (blood pressure, pulse, temperature, respiratory rate) to ensure the early detection of any deterioration in the patient's condition. The frequency of monitoring will be determined by the patient's progress; however, half-hourly observations should be considered in the first instance unless the patient is at risk of deteriorating rapidly, in which case continuous monitoring should be instigated. Where there is a risk of neurological deterioration, e.g. if the patient is in neurogenic shock or experiencing fluctuations in levels of consciousness, then assessment of the patient's neurological status using the Glasgow Coma Scale (see Chapter 7) may also be required.
- Administration of oxygen therapy as an imbalance between oxygen supply and tissue demand is fundamental to the nature of shock (British Thoracic Society, 2017). For patients who are conscious and able to breathe spontaneously, oxygen should be administered via a face mask or nasal cannulae. However, if the patient is unable to maintain their airway/ sufficient oxygen levels in the blood, then they may have to be intubated and ventilated. The rate/percentage of oxygen required should initially be at 15 L/min and aim at a saturation of 94–98% or 88–92% for those at risk of hypercapnic respiratory failure (British Thoracic Society, 2017). Ongoing treatment should be guided by regular measurements of pulse oximetry and blood gas analysis. As oxygen therapy is wvery drying to the mucosa, it should be humidified with sterile water, and the patient should be given regular mouth care.
- Administration of prescribed intravenous fluid to improve the patient's blood pressure and cardiac output, as an adequate cardiac output and a systemic blood pressure that is sufficient to maintain perfusion of vital organs is essential to meet the body's metabolic requirements. Therefore, the patient will require intravenous fluid replacement to correct the decreased circulating volume (hypovolaemia).
- If the patient has lost blood, e.g. through a haemorrhage, then a blood transfusion is indicated to raise the haemoglobin level to a point that ensures that there is adequate oxygen-carrying capacity in the blood. Whilst the choice and volume of fluid given, e.g. blood, colloid or crystalloid infusion, is dependent on the type of shock the patient is experiencing, strict monitoring of fluid balance is required to ensure the effectiveness of the fluid therapy and early detection of its complications, e.g. fluid overload. This will require the insertion of a urinary catheter and hourly monitoring of urine output to ensure that an output of at least 30 mL of urine per hour is being produced and regular monitoring of vital signs (see above) for early detection of any adverse reactions.
- In the case of the suspected septic shock, the Surviving Sepsis Campaign Guidelines (2016) recommend a resuscitation care bundle which should be implemented within the first one hour where there is suspected or confirmed red flag sepsis (Rhodes *et al.*, 2016), and all NHS trusts are required to have protocols in place which meet the guidelines – see Table 6.6.
- Psychological care for the patient and their family. The patient in shock is a medical emergency and very frightening for both the patient and their family. Therefore, they

Table 6.6   Sepsis Six care bundle.

To be completed within one hour	Give oxygen Take blood cultures Give IV antibiotics Give IV fluids Check serial lactates Measure urine output
To be completed within three hours	• Give oxygen • Maintain lactate levels • Obtain blood culture sample before administering antibiotics • Administer broad-spectrum antibiotics
To be completed within six hours	• If low blood pressure does not respond to fluid resuscitation, vasopressors should be given • Central venous pressure (CVP) should be measured and maintained at 8 mmHg if hypotension persists or if lactate is >4 mmol/L • Lactate levels should be measured if the initial lactate is raised • Central venous oxygen saturation should be measured if hypotension persists or if lactate levels are >4 mmol/L.

The mnemonic **BUFALO** (**B**lood cultures, **U**rine output, **F**luids, **A**ntibiotics, **L**actate and Hb, **O**xygen) can be used for Implementation of the Sepsis Six bundle, and the steps outlined will normally require admission to a critical care unit.
Source: Rhodes *et al.*, 2016.

should be kept fully informed about any changes/progress in the patient's condition, the purpose of any equipment used and any interventions given, as this will help to reduce anxiety and alleviate fear.

- Maintaining adequate nutrition, as the patient in shock will have increased demand for energy to support metabolic processes. Additionally, the patient may be nil by mouth due to their need for possible surgery or due to impairment in digestive function, e.g. paralytic ileus. Therefore, enteral or total parenteral feeding may be required, depending on the patient's condition.
- Ensuring the skin remains intact as due to poor tissue perfusion and immobility, the patient will be at increased risk of pressure sore formation. The patient will require regular pressure area care and should be nursed on a pressure relief mattress.

Pharmacological management of shock

In the patient in shock, drug therapy is primarily directed at enhancing the heart's ability to pump and to improve tissue perfusion (Foster and Prevost, 2012), and common drugs used to manage the patient in shock are summarised in Table 6.7.

Table 6.8 provides additional measures that may be taken according to the type of shock being experienced.

Table 6.7   Common drugs used to manage shock.

Drug	Action
Dopamine	Increase the heart's ability to contract
Dobutamine	
Amrinone	
Norepinephrine	
Epinephrine	Increases venous return to the heart by causing vasoconstriction
Norepinephrine	
Atropine	Increases heart rate and force of contraction
Isoproterenol	

Table 6.8 Additional management of shock according to type.

Classification		Management
Hypovolaemic		Eliminate and treat cause of hypovolaemia
Distributive	Anaphylactic	Antihistamines
		Steroids
		Bronchodilators
	Septic	Establish and treat source of infection with appropriate antimicrobial agents.
	Neurogenic	Treat cause
		Adequate pain relief

Conclusion

Shock is a common threat to all patients and represents a medical emergency, and the causes and treatment of the patient in shock are varied and complex. The overall aim of this chapter has been to explore the different types of shock and the resulting pathophysiology this creates. The prompt recognition of the signs and symptoms of shock is critical to the patient's prognosis, and healthcare professionals play a central role in the early detection of any deterioration in the patient's condition.

Test your knowledge

1. Outline the mechanisms the body uses to regulate and maintain blood pressure.
2. Compare and contrast the signs and symptoms of hypovolaemic and distributive shock.
3. Describe the mode of action of three pharmaceutical agents used in the treatment of circulatory shock.
4. Outline a plan of care for the patient in circulatory shock.
5. Which patients are at most risk of developing septic shock and why? Describe how these risks can be prevented.

Activities

Here are some activities and exercises to help test your learning. For the answers to these exercises, as well as further self-testing activities, visit our website at www.wiley.com/go/fundamentalsofappliedpathophysiology/student4e

Multiple choice questions

1. Hypoxia is
   (a) High carbon dioxide level
   (b) Low oxygen level
   (c) High red blood cell count
   (d) Low white cell count

2. Hypovolaemic shock is divided into
   (a) Two stages
   (b) Three stages
   (c) Four stages
   (d) Six stages

3. Anaphylactic shock is associated with which type of hypersensitivity?
   (a) Type 1
   (b) Type II
   (c) Type III
   (d) Type IV

4. Shock can be caused by:
   (a) Pleural effusion
   (b) Decreased peripheral vascular resistance
   (c) Low intravascular volume
   (d) Low cardiac output

5. Distributive shock is also known as
   (a) Septic shock
   (b) Neurogenic shock
   (c) Anaphylactic shock
   (d) All of the above

6. A 30-year-old man presents to the emergency department with shortness of breath, wheezing, BP 70/30, pulse rate 100 bpm. He started to feel unwell soon after eating a takeaway. What is the likely cause?
   (a) Myocardial infarction
   (b) Anaphylaxis
   (c) Tension pneumothorax
   (d) Pulmonary embolism

7. Which stage of shock is associated with the worsening of tissue hypoperfusion and onset of worsening circulatory and metabolic imbalances?
   (a) Initial non-progressive phase
   (b) Developing phase
   (c) Progressive stage
   (d) Irreversible stage

8. The release of renin from the kidneys;
   (a) Is a response to a rise in cardiac output
   (b) Causes increased urine production
   (c) Converts angiotensinogen to angiotensin I
   (d) A reduction in blood volume

9. Which of the following are a sepsis 'red flag'?
   (a) Respiratory rate less than 25 per minute
   (b) Oxygen saturation level of 95% on room air
   (c) Urine production of less than 30 mL per hour
   (d) Heart rate of 90 bpm

10. Dopamine;
    (a) Decreases the heart's ability to contract
    (b) Increases venous return
    (c) Decreases venous return
    (d) Increases the heart's ability to contract

11. Name two causes of neurogenic shock.
    (a) Spinal cord injury and improperly administered anaesthesia
    (b) Road traffic collision and post-operative infection
    (c) Sepsis and trauma to the back of the body
    (d) An overdose of beta blocker medication
12. In a patient presenting with low body temperature, cold and clammy skin, low urine output and raised levels of lactate, the most likely cause of shock is
    (a) Heart failure
    (b) Lung disease
    (c) Deep vein thrombosis
    (d) Sepsis
13. An arterial blood gas (ABG) test:
    (a) Is measured using blood from a vein
    (b) Measure how alkaline the blood is
    (c) Has six components
    (d) Requires a large volume of blood to be drawn
14. Which part of the nervous system is involved in neurogenic shock?
    (a) Peripheral
    (b) Somatic
    (c) Sympathetic
    (d) Parasympathetic
15. 40% Oxygen therapy should be administered using a Venturi valve of which colour?
    (a) Blue
    (b) Red
    (c) Green
    (d) Yellow

149

Conditions

The following is a list of conditions that are associated with shock. Take some time and write notes about each of the conditions. You may make the notes taken from textbooks or other resources (e.g. people you work with in a clinical area), or you may make the notes based on the people you have cared for. If you are making notes about people you have cared for, you must ensure that you adhere to the rules of confidentiality.

Hypoxia	
Sepsis	

Stages of Shock	
Disseminated Intravascular Coagulation	
Hypovolaemia	

Further resources

Resuscitation Council (UK)

http://www.resus.org.uk/pages/guide.htm

A useful resource for students wishing to understand more about the treatment of anaphylactic reactions and basic life support. The website is free and contains the latest guidance as well as links to other useful medical information, science worksheets and an application for the iPhone called iResus.

The UK Sepsis Trust Professional Resources (2016)

http://sepsistrust.org/professional-resources/

This charity was set up in 2012 and provides many useful resources for the public and health professionals who wish to know more about sepsis, its impact and management. The website provides free contemporary guidance and links to useful medical information relating to sepsis.

Sepsis Six Saving Lives video (15 minutes duration)

www.youtube.com/watch?v=CrUHnY1ZbpM

NICE guideline on Sepsis: recognition, diagnosis and early management (2016)

www.nice.org.uk/guidance/ng51

NHS Clinical Knowledge Summaries

Podcast on the treatment and management of anaphylaxis

http://www.cks.nhs.uk/knowledgeplus/podcasts/anaphylaxis#-350698

This is a useful website for students wishing to understand more about the treatment and management of anaphylaxis. The *NHS Clinical Knowledge Summaries* (formerly PRODIGY) are a reliable source of evidence-based information and practical 'know how' about the common conditions managed in primary care. This link provides two podcasts on anaphylactic shock.

Trauma and shock factsheet

http://www.nigms.nih.gov/Publications/Factsheet_Trauma.htm

A useful resource that provides fact sheets on the different kinds of trauma and shock that health professionals may encounter, including symptoms and causes. It is one in a series of fact sheets published by the National Institute of General Medical Sciences (NIGMS), which supports basic biomedical research to aid advances in the diagnosis, treatment and prevention of disease.

Toxic shock syndrome

http://www.mckinley.illinois.edu/Handouts/toxic_shock_syndrome.html

Part of a series that students will find useful for information resources on common medical conditions and diseases. This resource focuses on toxic shock syndrome (TSS) and tampons. It provides details of the causes, symptoms, treatment and prevention of TSS.

Food Allergy and Anaphylaxis Network (FAAN)

http://www.foodallergy.org/

A useful resource for students wishing to understand more about food allergies and anaphylaxis. The FAAN website includes information about FAAN and their work; information about common food allergens and anaphylaxis; hot topics; allergy alerts; and resources aimed at managing food allergies and details of food allergy research.

British Society for Allergy and Clinical Immunology

http://www.bsaci.org/index.php?option=com_content&task=view&id=117&Itemid=1

A useful website containing guidance on a range of allergens, most of which is freely accessible. Also contains links to other useful resources relating to allergy.

Glossary of terms

Aerobic   Requiring the presence of oxygen.

Anaerobic   Without oxygen.

Allergen   A compound that produces a hypersensitivity response.

Anaphylaxis   A sudden, acute allergic reaction to a material, e.g. food, environment, drug or biological substance.

Antibody   A substance in the blood which destroys or neutralises various toxins.

Antigen   A substance which causes the formation of antibodies.

Anuria   A condition in which no urine is produced.

Bacteraemia   The presence of bacteria in the bloodstream.

Bradykinin   A substance derived from plasma proteins – its prime action is in producing dilatation of arteries and veins.

Dyspnoea   Difficulty in breathing.

Histamine   A substance that causes constriction of smooth muscle, dilates arterioles and capillaries and stimulates gastric juices.

Homeostasis   Maintenance of relatively constant conditions within the body's internal environment.

Hypersensitivity reaction   An overreaction to an allergen that results in inflammation and tissue damage.

Hyperventilation   Abnormally deep and prolonged breathing.

Hypoperfusion   Abnormally low blood flow through a tissue.

Hypoxia   A low tissue oxygen concentration.

Immunoglobulin   Protein in the blood that carries the antibody activity of the blood against infectious microorganisms.

Interstitial fluid   The fluid in the tissues that fills the spaces between cells.

Ischaemia   Lack of blood to a part of the body due to constriction or blockage of the artery.

Peripheral Vascular Resistance   Refers to the resistance blood encounters at it flows through the systemic circulation.

Vasoconstriction   A decrease in the diameter of a blood vessel due to relaxation of smooth muscle in the vessel wall which may occur as a result of hormones or after stimulation of the vasomotor centre, leading to increased peripheral resistance.

Vasodilatation   An increase in the diameter of a blood vessel due to relaxation of smooth muscle in the vessel wall which may occur as a result of hormones or after decreased stimulation of the vasomotor centre, leading to decreased peripheral resistance.

References

British Medical Journal (2015). Sepsis in adults. *BMJ Best Practice Monograph*, 245.

British Thoracic Society Emergency Oxygen Guideline Development Group (2017). BTS guideline for Oxygen use in adults in healthcare and emergency settings. *Thorax*, 72: i1–i90. DOI:10.1136/thoraxjnl-2016-209729

Dellinger, R.P., Levy, M.M., Rhodes, A. *et al*. (2013). Surviving sepsis campaign: International guidelines for management of severe sepsis and septic shock. *Critical Care Medicine*, 41(2): 580–637. DOI: 10.1097/CCM.0b013c31827c83af

Eckert, L.O. and Lentz, G.M. (2012). Infections of the lower genital tract: vulva, vagina, cervix, toxic shock syndrome, endometritis, and salpingitis. In: Lentz, G.M., Lobo, R.A., Gershenson, D.M. and Katz, V.L. (eds), *Comprehensive Gynecology*, 6th edn. Philadelphia: Mosby Elsevier, Chapter 23.

Foster, J.G. and Prevost, S.S. (2012). *Advanced Nursing Practice Care of Adults in Acute Care*. Philadelphia: F.A. Davis Company.

Hunt, A. (2019). Sepsis: An overview of the signs, symptoms, diagnosis, treatment and pathophysiology. *Emergency Nurse*. DOI:10.7748/en.2019.e1926

Kanaparthi, L.K. and Pinsky, M.R. (2011). *Distributive Shock*. www.emedicine.com/med/article/168689

Lewis, S.L., Dirksen, S.R. and Heitkemper, M.M. (2014). *Clinical Companion to Medical-Surgical Nursing*. St Louis: Elsevier Health Sciences.

Martini, F. (2017). *Fundamentals of Anatomy and Physiology*, 11th edn. London: Pearson.

National Institute for Health and Care Excellence (NICE) (2013 updated 2017). *Intravenous Fluid Therapy in Adults in Hospital CG174*. Available at: www.nice.org.uk/guidance/cg174.

NICE (2011). *Anaphylaxis: Assessment and Referral after Emergency Treatment CG 134*. Available at: www.nice.org.uk/guidance/cg134.

NICE (2014). *Drug Allergy: Diagnosis and Management*. Available at: https://www.nice.org.uk/guidance/cg183/resources/drug-allergy-diagnosis-and-management-35109811022821 Accessed March 2017.

NICE (2016 updated 2020). *Sepsis: Recognition, Diagnosis and Early Management*. Available from: www.nice.org.uk/guidance/NG51.

Nishikawa, K., Takasu, A., Morita, K., Tsumori, H. and Sakamoto. T. (2010). Deposits on the intraluminal surface and bacterial growth in central venous catheters. *Journal of Hospital Infection*, 75: 19–22.

Nursing and Midwifery Council (NMC) (2018). *The Code: Professional Standards of Practice and Behavior for Nurses, Midwives and Nursing Associates*. London: NMC. Available at https://www.nmc.org.uk/globalassets/sitedocuments/nmc-publications/nmc-code.pdf.

Norris, T.L. (2019). *Porth's Essentials of Pathophysiology: Concepts of Altered Health Status*, 4th edn. Philadelphia: Lippincott, Williams & Wilkins.

Olive, S. (2017). Emergency oxygen therapy. In: Preston, W. and Kelly, C. (eds), *Respiratory Nursing at a Glance*. Oxford: Wiley. Chapter 46, pp. 98–99.

Resuscitation Council UK (2012). *The Emergency Medical Treatment of Anaphylactic Reactions – Guidelines for Healthcare Providers*. London: Resuscitation Council (UK).

Rhodes, A., Evans, L.E., Alhazzani, W. *et al*. (2016). Surviving Sepsis Campaign: International guidelines for management of sepsis and septic shock: 2016. *Critical Care Medicine*, March 2017, 45(3): 486–552. DOI: 10.1097/CCM.0000000000002255

Seckel, M.A. (2017). Sepsis-3 The new definitions. *Nursing Critical Care*, 12(2): 37–45.DOI: 10.1097/01.CCN.0000511827.42216.0e

Smeltzer, S. and Bare, B. (2013). *Brunner and Suddarth's Textbook of Medical-Surgical Nursing*, 13th edn. Philadelphia: Lippincott, Williams & Wilkins.

Sole, M.L., Klein, D.G. and Moseley, M.J. (eds) (2016). *Introduction to Critical Care Nursing*, 7th edn. St Louis: Saunders.

Surviving Sepsis Campaign. (2016). *Surviving Sepsis Campaign responds to Sepsis-3. 2016*. www.survivingsepsis.org/SiteCollectionDocuments/SSC-Statements-Sepsis-Definitions-3-2016.pdf.

Tortora, G.J. and Derrickson, B.H. (2017). *Principles of Anatomy and Physiology*, 15th edn. England: Wiley.

Turner, P.J., Gowland, M.H., Sharma V. *et al*. (2015). Increase in anaphylaxis-related hospitalizations but no increase in fatalities: An analysis of United Kingdom anaphylaxis data, 1992-2012. *Journal Allergy Clinic* 135(4): 956–963. https://doi.org/10jaci.2014.10.021.

Chapter 7

The nervous system and associated disorders

Janet G. Migliozzi

Senior Lecturer, Department of Nursing, Health and Wellbeing, School of Health and Social Work, University of Hertfordshire, Hatfield, Hertfordshire, UK

Contents

Introduction 154
Structure of the nervous system...................155
Disorders of the nervous system 161
Conclusion 179
Test your knowledge...179

Multiple choice questions...............................180
Conditions..181
Further resources..182
Glossary of terms..182
References..183

Key words

- Cranial nerves
- Spinal nerves
- Sympathetic nervous system
- Parasympathetic nervous system
- Brain stem
- Cerebrospinal fluid
- Blood–brain barrier
- Peripheral nervous system
- Intracranial pressure
- Glasgow Coma Scale
- Cerebrovascular accident
- Alzheimer's
- Multiple sclerosis
- Seizures

Fundamentals of Applied Pathophysiology: An Essential Guide for Nursing and Healthcare Students, Fourth Edition. Edited by Ian Peate.
© 2021 John Wiley & Sons Ltd. Published 2021 by John Wiley & Sons Ltd.
Student companion website: www.wiley.com/go/fundamentalsofappliedpathophysiology/student4e
Instructor companion website: www.wiley.com/go/fundamentalsofappliedpathophysiology/instructor4e

Test your prior knowledge

- List the structures of the central nervous system (CNS) and peripheral nervous system (PNS).
- What is the difference between the sympathetic and parasympathetic division of the autonomic nervous system?
- Explain the term *blood–brain barrier*.
- Explain the role of cerebrospinal fluid.
- Discuss the role of the meninges in protecting the brain.

Learning outcomes

On completion of this section, the reader will be able to:

- Describe the areas of the brain and how nerves transmit information around the body.

- Understand the roles of the CNS and the PNS.

- Understand assessment of neurological function and its relationship to pathological changes in the brain.

- Understand the care of the patient with a common disorder of the nervous system.

Don't forget to visit the companion website for this book (www.wiley.com/go/fundamentalsofappliedpathophysiology/student4e) **where you can find self-assessment tests to check your progress, as well as lots of activities to practise your learning.**

Introduction

The nervous system is the body's 'computer', as it is responsible for and controls all aspects of voluntary and involuntary action. It is a network of specialised cells and fibres that transmit messages between different parts of the body. This enables functions such as walking, temperature control and identification of pain as a few examples. These highly specialised cells are called neurons and through electrical impulses they transmit messages to other cells. This relay of information enables modification of behaviour or responses to the signals. These cells are an essential component in maintaining homeostasis.

This chapter will discuss the structure and function of the central and peripheral nervous systems. Common disorders of the nervous system – multiple sclerosis, stroke, Parkinson's disease, Alzheimer's disease, epilepsy and traumatic head injury will also be explored and their management outlined. Snapshots will be used to explore the signs and symptoms associated with the pathophysiology of disease.

Structure of the nervous system

The nervous system is divided into two major sections, the central nervous system (CNS) and the peripheral nervous system (PNS):

1. The CNS consists of the brain and spinal cord.
2. The PNS consists of the cranial and spinal nerves. These nerves carry impulses to and from the spinal cord; it includes the cranial nerves from the brain and the spinal nerves from the spinal cord. The PNS can also be divided into the somatic and autonomic nervous system, which is divided further into the parasympathetic and sympathetic divisions (Figure 7.1).

Central nervous system

Brain

The brain or encephalon, which is encased in the cranium (or skull), is the body's control system and can be divided into four main parts (Figure 7.2):

1. Cerebrum
2. Cerebellum
3. Diencephalon
4. Brainstem.

Cerebrum

The cerebrum (or cerebral cortex) makes up the largest part of the brain and lies uppermost in the skull. The surface of the cerebrum appears wrinkled due to the numerous convolutions or gyri – raised areas that fold in on each other to increase the brain's surface area. The outer surface of the cerebrum is known as the cerebral cortex and is composed of a thin

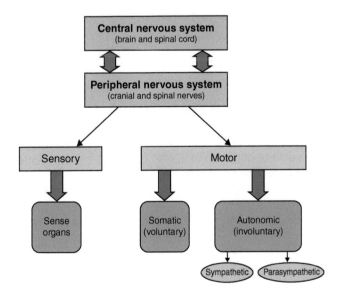

Figure 7.1   Divisions of the human nervous system.

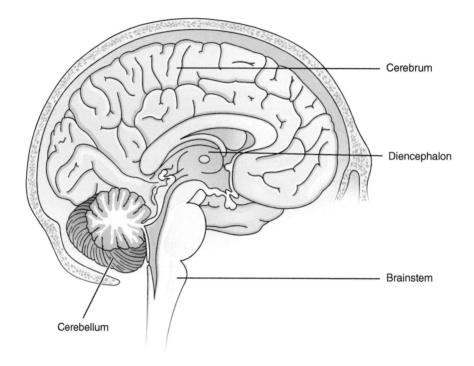

Figure 7.2   The four main parts of the human brain.

Table 7.1   The lobes of the cerebral hemispheres.

Lobe	Function
Frontal lobe	Conscious thought, personality, abstract thinking, affective reactions, memory, judgement and initiation of motor activity
Parietal lobe	Spatial awareness and receiving and interpreting stimuli from sensory neurons
Temporal lobe	Processing of language and understanding (Wernicke's area) memory
Occipital lobe	Visual stimuli interpretation

Source: Adapted from Douglas and Platt, 2013.

layer of nerve cell bodies known as grey matter. Beneath the cerebral cortex is the white matter which is made up of myelinated nerve axons. The cerebrum is divided into two hemispheres, and each hemisphere has four lobes: the frontal, parietal, occipital and temporal. Each hemisphere is able to communicate with the other hemisphere via the corpus callosum, which is a thick area of nerve fibres.

The basal ganglia plays an important role in producing automatic movements and the body's posture.

The cerebrum is divided into four lobes, each of which has a specific function (Table 7.1).

Cerebellum

The cerebellum lies under the occipital lobe of the cerebrum and is the second largest part of the human brain. It consists of an inner layer of white matter and an outer layer of grey matter, and its surface is convoluted like the surface of the cerebrum. It receives input from peripheral nerves and plays a major role in balance, posture, fine movement and coordination.

Diencephalon

The diencephalon, or interbrain, lies between the brainstem and the cerebrum, where it encircles the third ventricle (small cavity). It consists of the thalamus and hypothalamus. The pineal gland, which is responsible for the secretion of the hormone melatonin, is also located in the diencephalon.

The thalamus consists of grey matter and is a dumbbell-shaped structure that encloses the third ventricle of the brain. It acts as a relay centre that receives information from the body via the spinal cord and forwards this on to the appropriate areas of the brain. The thalamus plays a crucial role in the conscious awareness of pain as well as driving circadian rhythms. The thalamus has connections with the limbic system of the brain, which controls instinctual and emotional drives, e.g. hunger, fear, sexual drive and short-term memory.

The hypothalamus is located just below the thalamus (as its name suggests) and is the major link between the body's endocrine and nervous system, where it has many roles to play in the regulation of homeostasis (Coe, 2019). Some of the functions of the hypothalamus include maintenance of autonomic nervous system, water balance, appetite and acid base balance. The hypothalamus also forms part of the limbic system of the brain.

Brainstem

The brainstem connects the spinal cord to the remainder of the brain and is responsible for many essential functions, including the entry to and exit from the brain of 10 of the 12 cranial nerves (Table 7.2).

The brainstem contains the midbrain, the pons and the medulla oblongata. In the brainstem, a collection of nerve cell bodies known as the reticular formation controls vital reflexes. The reticular formation is essential for controlling cardiovascular and respiratory function as well as for maintaining wakefulness, and plays a key role in consciousness. It is therefore known as the reticular activating system.

The midbrain or mesencephalon is a short section of the brainstem between the diencephalon and the pons, and is involved in the control of eye movement (both voluntary and involuntary) and is responsible for the startle reflex (Douglas and Platt, 2013). The midbrain consists of bundles of nerve fibres that join the lower parts of the brainstem and the spinal

Table 7.2 Cranial nerves.

Nerve	Brain location	Transmits nerve impulses to and from
I Olfactory	Olfactory bulb	Olfactory receptors for sense of smell
II Optic	Thalamus	Retina (sight)
III Oculomotor	Midbrain	Eye muscles (including eyelids, lens, pupil)
IV Trochlear	Midbrain	Eye muscles
V Trigeminal	Pons	Teeth, eyes, skin, tongue
VI Abducens	Pons	Jaw muscles (chewing). Eye muscles
VII Facial	Pons	Taste buds. Facial muscles, tear and salivary glands
VIII Vestibulocochlear	Pons	Inner ear (hearing and balance)
IX Glossopharyngeal	Medulla oblongata	Pharyngeal muscles (swallowing)
X Vagus	Medulla oblongata	Internal organs
XI Spinal accessory	Medulla oblongata	Neck and back muscles
XII Hypoglossal	Medulla oblongata	Tongue muscles

157

cord with the higher parts of the brain, and also plays a role in the control of the wakefulness of the brain. The basal ganglia is also found within this region.

The pons is Latin for 'bridge' (Coe, 2019), and its role is to relay information between the two cerebral hemispheres as well as transmitting information from the cerebellum to the brainstem. The cranial nerves (V–VIII) pass through this region. The pons plays an important role in the control of the rate and length of respiration.

The medulla oblongata, which consists of grey and white matter, is approximately 3 cm long and is, arguably, an extension of the spinal cord as it lies just inside the cranial cavity above the large hole in the occipital bone called the foramen magnum. Within it are contained a number of reflex centres for control of blood vessel diameter, heart rate, breathing, coughing, swallowing, vomiting and sneezing. On either side of the medulla oblongata is a round oval protrusion called the olive, which plays a part in controlling balance, coordination and the intonation of sound impulses from the middle ear.

Blood supply to the brain

The brain receives approximately 15–20% of the body's total circulating volume of blood, which is equivalent to 800 mL of blood per minute (Sugerman and Huether, 2019). The brain requires a constant supply of oxygen and glucose and therefore through a process of autoregulation the blood flow needs to be maintained. The blood supply to the brain is supplied by the vertebral and internal carotid arteries. The internal carotid is a branch of the common carotid, which is where the pressoreceptors and baroreceptors that identify changes in blood pressure are located. Chemoreceptors are also found here, and these detect changes in oxygen levels and blood pH (VanMeter and Hubert, 2014).

The vertebral and internal carotid arteries interconnect at the base of the brain to form the cerebral arterial circle or circle of Willis (Figure 7.3), which provides a collateral supply of blood to the whole of the brain in the event that one of the carotid arteries becomes compromised.

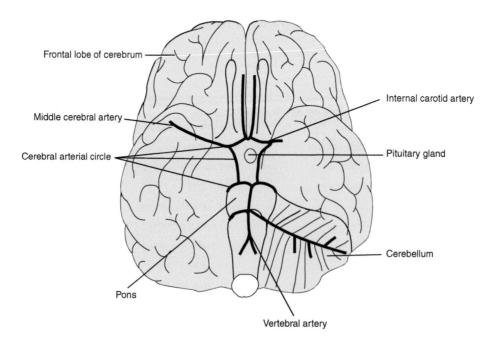

Figure 7.3   The circle of Willis.

Blood–brain barrier

The brain (unlike other organs) is unable to withstand changes in levels of circulating nutrients, hormones and ions. Therefore, maintenance of a constant environment is crucial to the brain's ability to function, and the blood–brain barrier, which is an impermeable network of brain capillaries, acts as a 'filter' between the brain tissue and blood-borne substances to provide the brain with some protection against harmful toxins and metabolites. However, the blood–brain barrier provides little protection against fat-soluble molecules and respiratory gases (Marieb and Keller, 2017); consequently, some substances, e.g. nicotine, anaesthetic gases and alcohol, can cross the barrier and affect the brain.

Cerebrospinal fluid

Cerebrospinal fluid is a fluid that is similar in composition to blood plasma. It is clear and colourless and consists of water, glucose, protein and electrolytes. It is produced by specialised epithelial cells called the choroid plexus, mainly found within the ventricles of the brain. The cerebrospinal fluid (CSF) is mainly found circulating within the ventricles (cavities) of the brain and within the subarachnoid space.

CSF helps absorb any shocks and jolts by surrounding the brain in a cushion of fluid and keeping the brain buoyant. This helps prevent damage from occurring to nerve roots, meninges and blood vessels when a change in motion occurs.

Meninges

The brain and spinal cord have added protection by being surrounded by three layers of connective tissue. These consist of the dura mater, arachnoid mater and pia maters and are known as the meninges.

Spinal cord

The spinal cord is located in the vertebral column and provides the communication route between the brain and parts of the body not supplied by cranial nerves. It is protected from damage by the vertebral column, which consists of 33 vertebrae that are subdivided into cervical, thoracic, lumbar, sacrum and coccyx. In between each disc, there is an intervertebral disc which helps absorb shock and prevents damage to the vertebrae.

Peripheral nervous system

The peripheral nervous system consists of the cranial and spinal nerves, which connect the brain and spinal cord to other parts of the body (Figure 7.4). Each nerve is made up of an axon which is covered by a myelin sheath, and these are arranged in bundles. There are 31 pairs of spinal nerves, which are grouped as either the cervical (8), thoracic (12), lumber (5), sacral (5) and coccygeal (1) according to their location along the vertebral column (Figure 7.4).

Spinal nerves have both sensory and motor neurons, and relay information from and to peripheral structures, e.g. the skin and skeletal muscles. Cranial nerves connect to the brain and brain stem and are also a mixture of sensory and motor neurons (Table 7.2).

The PNS is divided into the somatic and autonomic nervous systems, of which the autonomic nervous system has two divisions – the parasympathetic and sympathetic divisions.

Somatic nervous system

The somatic nervous system consists of motor neurons that connect the CNS to the skin and skeletal muscles, and plays a major role in the regulation of skeletal muscle contractions and conscious activities.

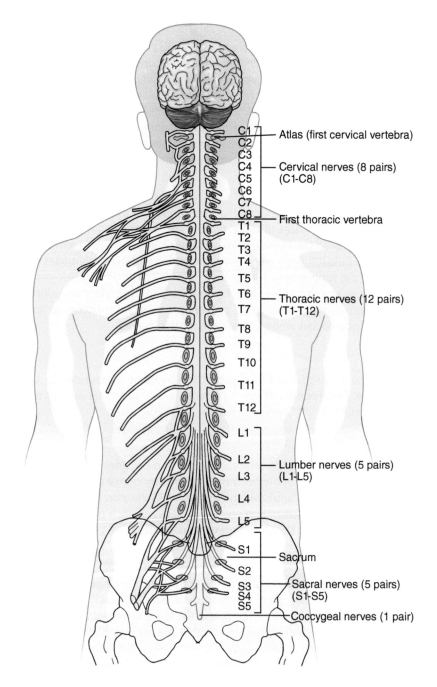

Figure 7.4   The spinal cord and the location of the 31 pairs of spinal nerves.

Autonomic nervous system

The autonomic nervous system (ANS) plays a major role in the maintenance of homeostasis by regulating the body's automatic, involuntary functions. In common with the rest of the nervous system, it consists of neurons, neuroglia and other connective tissue. However, its structure is unique in that it is divided in two – the sympathetic division and the parasympathetic division.

Table 7.3 Physiological effects of the sympathetic and parasympathetic nervous systems.

Organ/system	Sympathetic effects	Parasympathetic effects
Cell metabolism	Increases metabolic rate, stimulates fat breakdown and increases blood sugar levels	No effect
Blood vessels	Constricts blood vessels in viscera and skin. Dilates blood vessels in the heart and skeletal muscle	No effect
Eye	Dilates pupils	Constricts pupils
Heart	Increases rate and force of contraction	Decreases rate
Lungs	Dilates bronchioles	Constricts bronchioles
Kidneys	Decreases urine output	No effect
Liver	Causes the release of glucose	No effect
Digestive system	Decreases peristalsis and constricts digestive system sphincters	Increases peristalsis and dilates digestive system sphincters
Adrenal medulla	Stimulates cells to secrete epinephrine and norepinephrine	No effect
Lacrimal glands	Inhibits the production of tears	Increases the production of tears
Salivary glands	Inhibits the production of saliva	Increases the production of saliva
Sweat glands	Stimulates to produce perspiration	No effect

The sympathetic division controls many internal organs when a stressful situation occurs. This can take the form of physical stress, e.g. if undertaking strenuous exercise, or emotional stress, e.g. at times of anger or anxiety. In emergency situations, the sympathetic nervous system releases norepinephrine, which assists in the 'fight or flight' response.

The parasympathetic division utilises acetylcholine to control all the internal responses associated with a state of relaxation and therefore has the opposite effect on the body to the sympathetic nervous system.

Table 7.3 provides a summary of the physiological effects of the sympathetic and para-sympathetic divisions of the nervous system.

Disorders of the nervous system

Learning outcomes

At the end of this section, the reader will be able to:

- List some of the common diseases associated with disorders of the CNS.

- Describe the pathophysiological processes related to some specific CNS disorders.

- Outline the management and interventions related to the disorders described.

- Discuss some of the non-pharmacological interventions used in the treatment of the disorders.

Snapshot   Road traffic collision

Julian Abbas is a 23-year-old man who was brought into the ED following an accident on his motorbike. His bike had skidded on a corner during a brief downpour, and he had fallen off the bike. The exact nature of his accident was unclear as he was found unconscious and help was called. He arrived with a neck brace *in situ* and was conscious on admission. His Glasgow Coma Scale (GCS) was 13, and his pupils were equal and reacting to light. He had a laceration on the front of his skull and skin abrasions on his thigh and lower leg with a suspected fractured collar bone (clavicle). He was sent to have an Magnetic Resonance Imaging (MRI) to detect any damage to the brain, and he was given pain relief for his fractured clavicle. On his return to the ward, it was identified that Julian's GCS had fallen to 11 and his left pupil was sluggish when reacting to light. The MRI confirmed a fractured skull, and a CT scan was organised.

Vital signs

The following vital signs were noted and recorded:

Vital sign	Observation	Normal
Temperature	36.5°C	36.0–37.9°C range
Pulse	73 beats per minute	60–100 beats per minute
Respiration	12 breaths per minute	12–20 breaths per minute
Blood pressure	140/80 mmHg	100–139 mmHg (systolic) range
O$_2$ saturation	98%	94–98%
Alert/Voice/Pain/Unresponsive AVPU	Voice	Alert

A full blood count was performed.

Test	Result	Guideline normal values
White blood cells (WBC)	4.6×10^9/L	4 to 11×10^9/L
Neutrophils	6.2×10^9/L	2.0 to 7.5×10^9/L
Lymphocytes	3.0×10^9/L	1.3 to 4.0×10^9/L
Red blood cells (RBC)	4.7×10^9/L	4.5 to 6.5×10^9/L
Haemoglobin (Hb)	118 g/L	130–180 g/L
Platelets	332×10^9/L	150 to 440×10^9/L

Reflect on this case and consider the following:

1. Consider what may be causing Julian's falling GCS?
2. Discuss the role of the GCS in identifying possible brain trauma.
3. What could a sluggish reaction to light indicate in a pupil?
4. What treatment options are available to avoid secondary complications from Julian's head injury?

Traumatic brain injury

Brain injuries range from mild bruising of the tissue or can be severe and life-threatening. It can include skull fractures, swelling, haemorrhage or direct injury to the brain.

Damage from brain trauma can be focal or it can be diffuse, depending on what caused the damage. Traumatic brain injury can occur from traffic accidents, falls, sporting accidents and violence and can cause significant morbidity and devastating changes in functionality (Book, 2019).

Primary brain trauma

These are direct injuries to the brain and occur at the time of the incident. They can be a result of an impact with an object in a precise location. In injuries caused by road traffic accidents or falls, it is important to consider the point of impact as well as the rebound effect within the skull. This is known as coup or contrecoup. The brain is held in fluid which can shift or rotate inside the skull, causing shearing of blood vessels and stretching of nerve fibres within the brain.

Secondary brain trauma

This develops from the initial injury, and the aim of management of patients is to reduce damage caused after the primary damage. Damaged cells and bleeding lead to inflammation and an increase in intracranial pressure. This can lead to further ischaemia and death of cells surrounding the initial injury. Contributory factors that can increase secondary brain insults include decreased cerebral perfusion, hypoxia, hypercapnia, hypocapnia and hypotension.

Raised intracranial pressure

Intracranial pressure (ICP) is the recordable pressure within the skull caused by three intracranial components – brain tissue, cerebrospinal fluid (CSF) and blood. As the skull is a rigid structure, any increase in volume in any of the three components will lead to an increase in ICP. Several conditions can lead to an increase in ICP, including bleeding in the brain due to a head injury, a space-occupying lesion, e.g. a brain tumour, or infection, e.g. a brain abscess. Left untreated, raised ICP can lead to poor perfusion of the brain as the cerebral arteries and veins become compressed and the brain herniates or shifts as it becomes compressed within the skull. Common signs and symptoms of increased ICP in the early stages are the following:

- Decreasing levels of consciousness
- Headache
- Sluggish pupil reaction
- Visual disturbances
- Abnormal breathing patterns
- Impaired motor responses.

Red flag

Increased blood pressure with widening pulse pressure, bradycardia and a decreased respiratory rate could indicate an increase in intracranial pressure.

As the ICP increases, the rigid skull prevents the pressure from being dissipated, and the pressure is exerted upon the brain stem. The vital centres (Coe, 2019) are located here, and therefore there are observable effects of increased ICP. In the later stages, the individual may experience the following:

- Further deterioration in level of consciousness
- A rise in systolic blood pressure
- A fall in diastolic blood pressure
- Irregular shallow, slow breathing
- Slow pulse
- A high temperature.

Care and management of the patient at risk of increased intracranial pressure

Patients at risk of neurological deterioration require frequent, accurate neurological assessment in order to detect problems early. A method of assessing neurological status known as the Glasgow Coma Scale (GCS) was developed more than 40 years ago by two neurosurgeons in Glasgow and is widely applied today (Mehta and Chinthapalli, 2019). It is a systematic approach to performing part of a neurological assessment.

A neurological assessment should include the following(NICE, 2014 updated 2019):

- GCS
- Pupil size and reactivity
- Vital signs, e.g. temperature, heart rate, respiratory rate, blood pressure and blood oxygen saturation
- Limb movements.

Red flag

A decrease in GCS from baseline assessment could mean that the injury may be evolving.

Glasgow Coma Scale

The National Institute for Health and Care Excellence (NICE, 2014 updated 2019) advocates the use of the Glasgow Coma Scale (GCS) for assessment and classification of all head-injured patients.

The GCS was specifically designed as a tool for detecting and monitoring changes in the patient's neurological status (Teasdale *et al.*, 2014) by evaluating three categories of behaviour: eye opening, verbal response and best motor response (Table 7.4). Within each category, each level of response is allocated a numerical value (Mehta and Chinthapalli, 2019), and the lower the patient scores on the scale, the more serious the neurological condition; e.g. a score of 15 indicates a fully conscious, alert, responsive patient, whereas a score of 3 means that the patient is deeply unconscious.

Vital signs

AVPU is a quick assessment of consciousness which can be made with every interaction with a patient:

Alert
Voice
Pain
Unresponsive

Table 7.4   The Glasgow Coma Scale.

GLASGOW COMA SCALE: DO IT THIS WAY
Institute of Neurological Sciences Glasgow

? → **Check**
For factors Interfering with communication, ability to respond and other injuries

👁 → **Observe**
Eye opening, content of speech and movements of right and left sides

◎ → **Stimulate**
Sound : spoken or shouted request
Physical : pressure on fingertip, trapezius or supraorbital notch

☑ → **Rate**
Assign according to highest response observed

Eye opening

Criterion	Observed	Rating	Score
Open before stimulus	✓	Spontaneous	4
After spoken or shouted request	✓	To sound	3
After fingertip stimulus	✓	To pressure	2
No opening at any time, no interfering factor	✓	None	1
Closed by local factor	✓	Not testable	NT

Verbal response

Criterion	Observed	Rating	Score
Correctly gives name, place and date	✓	Orientated	5
Not orientated but communication coherent	✓	Confused	4
Intelligible single words	✓	Words	3
Only moans/groans	✓	Sounds	2
No audible response, no interfering factor	✓	None	1
Factor interfering with communication	✓	Not testable	NT

Best motor response

Criterion	Observed	Rating	Score
Obey 2-part request	✓	Obeys commands	6
Brings hand above clavicle to stimulus on head neck	✓	Localising	5
Bends arm at elbow rapidly but features not predominantly abnormal	✓	Normal flexion	4
Bends arm at elbow, features clearly predominantly abnormal	✓	Abnormal flexion	3
Extends arm at elbow	✓	Extension	2
No movement in arms/legs, no interfering factor	✓	None	1
Paralysed or other limiting factor	✓	Not testable	NT

Sites for physical stimulation

Fingertip pressure   Trapezius pinch   Supraorbital notch

Features of flexion responses

Modified with permission from Van Der Naalt 2004 Ned Tijdschr Geneeskd

Abnormal flexion
Slow Sterotyped
Arm across chest
Forearm rotates
Thumb clenched
Leg extends

Normal flexion
Rapid
Variable
Arm away from body

For further information and video demonstration visit www.glasgowcomascale.org

Source: https://www.nursingtimes.net/Journals/2014/10/10/n/p/l/141015Forty-years-on-updating-the-Glasgow-coma-scale.pdf. Reproduced with permission of EMAP.

Red flag

The airway needs to be protected when there is evidence of reduced consciousness or coma (GCS of 8 or below).

Vital signs recording

The National Institute for Health and Care Excellence (NICE, 2014 updated 2019) recommends that the head-injured patient with a GCS of less than 15 should have their vital signs monitored half-hourly until a GCS of 15 is achieved. After the initial assessment (usually in the Emergency Department), the frequency of observations of patients with a GCS of 15 should be:

- Half-hourly for 2 hours
- Then 1-hourly for 4 hours
- Then 2 hourly thereafter.

If the patient with a GCS of 15 deteriorates at any time after the initial 2-hour period, observations should revert back to half-hourly and follow the schedule outlined above. Additionally, the patient should undergo an urgent reappraisal by medical staff if they experience any of the following:

- Development of agitation or abnormal behaviour
- Development of severe or increasing headache or persistent vomiting
- A sustained (at least 30 minutes) drop of one point in the GCS (a drop of one point in the motor response score requires more urgent attention)
- A drop of three or more points in the eye-opening or verbal response scores of the GCS or two or more points in the motor response score
- New or evolving neurological signs or symptoms, e.g. pupil inequality or loss of movement/strength to one side of the body or face (NICE, 2014 updated 2019: 34).

Management of a patient with a head injury

The main aim of managing a patient with a head injury is to prevent further injury to the brain, known as secondary injury. Certain physiological factors need to be managed, and these include managing ICP, hypoxia, hypotension and any seizures.

Management strategies include the following:

- The use of hypertonic solution to draw fluid and reduce ICP.
- Oxygen therapy may be used to aid with respiration and reduce carbon dioxide, which is a powerful vasodilator and can increase ICP.
- The use of IV fluids to ensure blood pressure is maintained and to minimise reduced blood flow to the brain.
- Catheterisation and fluid balance management to identify any problems that could occur.
- Blood glucose is found to be elevated in head-injury patients due to the secretion of adrenaline, and this needs to be managed.
- Anticonvulsants can be used to prevent seizures, such as carbamazepine and phenytoin.
- Feeding patients with head injury is linked to improved outcome.

Snapshot Cerebrovascular accident

Mrs Alli is a 68-year-old woman who presented in the Emergency Department after falling at a wedding reception. Small cuts and grazes were sustained, but Mrs Alli's son noticed his mother appeared slightly muddled and confused and was unable to smile. Her mouth appeared to droop slightly on the right side. Mrs Alli was admitted to the ward, and an imaging scan confirmed that she has had a cerebrovascular accident.

Mrs Alli has a history of high blood pressure (hypertension) which she controls with antihypertensives. She smokes around 2–3 cigarettes a day, but she does not drink alcohol. She has no known allergies and occasionally takes painkillers for backache. Her weight is 74.4 kg, and her height is 162 cm with a BMI of 28.

Vital signs Physical and bloods

The following vital signs were noted and recorded:

Vital sign	Observation	Normal
Temperature	37.2°C	36.0–37.9°C range
Pulse	112 beats per minute	60–100 beats per minute
Respiration	24 breaths per minute	12–20 breaths per minute
Blood pressure	164/104 mmHg	100–139 mmHg (systolic) range
O_2 saturation	94%	94–98 %

A full blood count was performed.

Test	Result	Guideline normal values
White blood cells (WBC)	6.9×10^9/L	4 to 11×10^9/L
Neutrophils	3.0×10^9/L	2.0 to 7.5×10^9/L
Lymphocytes	3.7×10^9/L	1.3 to 4.0×10^9/L
Red blood cells (RBC)	4.9×10^9/L	4.5 to 6.5×10^9/L
Haemoglobin (Hb)	129 g/L	130–180 g/L
Platelets	225×10^9/L	150 to 440×10^9/L

- A on the AVPU scale
- Her National Early Warning Score (NEWS) Score was 5 on admission

On examination Mrs Alli was alert, but was quiet and uncommunicative.
Take some time to reflect on this case and then consider the following:

1. What type of stroke has Mrs Alli experienced?
2. Discuss Mrs Alli's risk factors for stroke.
3. Consider what action you would take in regard to Mrs Alli's NEWS score.
   Outline the immediate care that Mrs Alli will require.

NEWS 2

Mrs Alli

Physiological parameter	3	2	1	0	1	2	3
Respiration rate						24 breaths/ min	
Oxygen saturation %			94%				
Supplemental oxygen				No			
Temperature °C				37.2			
Systolic BP mmHg				164/104 mmHg			
Heart rate						112 b/min	
Level of consciousness				Alert			
Score	0	0	1	0	0	4	
Total	5						

Stroke (cerebrovascular accident)

A cerebrovascular accident (CVA), or 'stroke', occurs as a direct result of impaired blood flow to the brain, either because of vessel occlusion or haemorrhaging due to a ruptured vessel. The nature and extent of neurological impairment that the patient may suffer is dependent on the amount and location of oxygen starvation that the brain tissue has experienced and/ or the severity of cerebral bleeding that has occurred.

There are more than 100,000 strokes in the UK each year, and it is the fourth leading cause of death and disability, accounting for 38,000 deaths each year (NICE, 2019), with approximately 85% being caused from cerebral infarction. Stroke is also the single largest cause of complex disability (Stroke Association, 2018). Whilst stroke is primarily a disease experienced by older people and is more likely to be experienced by men (although women who experience a stroke are more likely to die), other factors exist that make certain groups more at risk of having a stroke (Book, 2019):

- Smoking
- Obesity
- History of heart disease or high blood pressure (hypertension)
- High cholesterol (hyperlipidaemia)
- Diabetes
- Afro-Caribbean or South Asian descent
- A family history of stroke at a young age (less than 50 years of age).

Pathophysiology

The brain is unable to store nutrients or glucose for use and is therefore dependent on a steady supply of these from the circulation of blood via the internal carotid and vertebral arteries. Any interruption of blood supply to the brain tissue will result in ischaemia and if prolonged, results in the death of brain cells. There are two main types of stroke: ischaemic stroke and haemorrhagic stroke.

Ischaemic stroke occurs when a blood clot blocks an artery to the brain, causing an interruption of blood flow to the brain cells. A high cholesterol level causing a 'furring' of the arteries is a common cause of this type of stroke.

Table 7.5 Signs and symptoms of stroke according to side of brain affected.

Damage to left side of brain	Damage to right side of brain
Loss of motor function to the right side of the body	Loss of motor function to the left side of the body
Language impairment – either an inability to express self – expressive aphasia, or difficulty in understanding or using speech appropriately although able to speak fluently – receptive aphasia	Language centres not affected
Right visual field deficit	Left visual field deficit
Frustration and depression over loss of independence	Apparent unconcern over loss of independence
Intellectual impairment	Poor judgement and impulsive behaviour

Haemorrhagic stroke occurs when a blood vessel in or around the brain bursts, causing bleeding and increased pressure in the skull, resulting in compression and eventual ischaemia to brain tissue. Untreated high blood pressure (hypertension) is a common cause of this type of stroke.

Following a stroke, it is possible to determine the area of the brain that has been damaged by observing the signs and symptoms the patient may experience (Table 7.5). An imaging scan should be undertaken to determine whether stroke is ischaemic or haemorrhagic.

Transient ischaemic attack

A transient ischaemic attack (TIA) or 'mini' stroke is a temporary interruption in blood flow to the brain which can result in numbness, temporary paralysis and impaired speech. Whilst the symptoms experienced are not permanent and by definition resolve within 24 hours, a TIA is often a warning of an impending, more serious cerebrovascular accident.

Pharmacological management

The pharmacological treatment of stroke aims to reduce the effects of and prevent the reoccurrence of stroke or TIA, whilst also taking into consideration the cause of the stroke. NICE (2019) have provided guidance on best practice:

- In ischaemic stroke:
  - Thrombolytic agents such as alteplase are advocated within the first 3 hours and up to 4.5 hours in patients under 80.
  - Aspirin may be prescribed to reduce platelet aggregation in the case of TIA or ischaemic stroke.
- Preventative medications include the following:
  - Antihypertensives may be prescribed for patients who have high blood pressure.
- Cholesterol-reducing drugs such as simvastatin should be prescribed to prevent recurrent ischaemic stroke or TIA.

Non-pharmacological management

- Carotid endarterectomy (removal of fatty plaques from the wall of the carotid artery) may be performed in patients with stenosis (narrowing) of the carotid arteries that supply blood to the brain.
- Thrombectomy (alongside intravenous thrombolysis) is indicated within 6 hours of symptom onset to individuals who have had an ischaemic stroke and confirmed occlusion of a major cerebral artery (NICE, 2019).
- The patient should be educated as to the importance of a varied diet that is low in fat in order to keep their blood cholesterol within safe limits. Patients who are overweight or obese need support to lose weight and be encouraged to take regular exercise.

Orange flag

Psychological support following a cerebrovascular accident

Mood disturbance is common following a stroke and may present as anxiety or depression. 30% of patients will suffer from depression at some point post stroke, and a significant number of these will remain undiagnosed or inadequately treated. However, psychological mood disturbance is associated with higher rates of mortality, suicide, long-term disability, higher rates of hospital readmission and increased usage of outpatient and community services. In addition, carers of people with stroke are more likely to experience serious psychological problems and strain. Significant improvements in psychological and emotional care after stroke can be made by ensuring that psychological support is considered by the Multi-Disciplinary Team to be as critical to recovery from stroke as physical rehabilitation (NHS Improvement, 2020).

- Patients should be offered support to stop smoking and reduce alcohol intake.
- Regular monitoring of blood pressure is important to ensure that it is kept within safe limits, and patients should be encouraged to reduce their salt intake.
- Maintenance of blood sugar concentration between 4 and 11 mmol/litre.

Care and management

Management of a patient who has suffered a stroke varies according to the area of the brain affected and the neurological and functional deficits that the individual experiences. However, the care of the patient during the acute phase of stroke will differ from the care required once the patient has stabilised and is in the rehabilitative phase.

Key considerations during the acute phase focus on early detection and prevention of neurological deterioration and life-threatening complications:

- Frequent monitoring of the patient's vital signs using the NEWS score. Maintain the blood pressure within specific limits. Blood glucose needs to be monitored as 78% of acute stroke patients are hyperglycaemic on admission (Pierce and Braine, 2014), and this increases mortality and morbidity.
- Neurological function during the acute phase using an appropriate assessment tool, e.g. the GCS, to detect any deterioration in the patient's level of consciousness.
- Keeping the patient nil by mouth until an assessment of the swallowing reflex can be carried out.
- Undertaking a nutritional status assessment within the first 48 hours of admission.
- Protecting the patient from injury due to possible seizures, motor and visual deficits.
- Preventing pressure sore formation as immobility and incontinence place the patient at increased risk.
- Providing explanations to the patient and their family concerning treatment and care interventions in order to alleviate anxiety and fear.

During the rehabilitative phase of stroke, care is geared towards maximising the patient's independence and key considerations include the following:

- Collaborating with other healthcare professionals to teach the patient adaptive measures to enable them to carry out their activities of daily living, e.g. bathing, eating, dressing and toileting, as independently as possible.

- Minimising the risk of injury and complications associated with impaired mobility.
- Involving a speech therapist to ensure that the patient who has impaired communication is able to express themselves effectively.
- Providing information and support for the patient and their carers/family.
- Liaising with other healthcare professionals and social services prior to the patient's discharge from hospital to ensure that the patient's home environment is suitably adapted to deal with any residual disabilities that the patient may have.

Clinical investigation

MRI scan

An MRI scan can be used to look at soft tissue structures within the body. It does not use radiation (unlike X-rays and CT scans) and therefore can be used repeatedly. An MRI works by using a magnetic field and radio waves that can produce a 2- or 3-dimensional image of part of the body being imaged.

Indications for use are as follows:

- To scan the brain to identify any abnormal pathology such as tumours, stroke and meningeal disease.
- To look at the spinal cord and identify any tumours, degenerative disease and infection.
- Liver
- Breast
- Pelvic anatomy
- Musculoskeletal system.

Full body scans can take place as well as targeted areas. An MRI is not usually undertaken in trauma.

Contraindications

Individuals with non-MRI-compatible implanted devices such as cardiac pacemakers, stents and cochlear implants must not be scanned.

Pre-procedural considerations

A contrast agent may be used to aid in scanning, and this is usually an agent known as gadolinium-based contrast. It is contraindicated in patients with kidney disease. An antispasmodic may be used to relax the bowel when scanning the pelvic area. Sedatives may also be used to relax an individual. It is very noisy in the scanner, so ear muffs should be used. To avoid movement during the scan, individuals may be asked to avoid drinking prior to the scan.

There are no post-procedural concerns.

Parkinson's disease (paralysis agitans)

Parkinson's disease (PD) is a disease of the brain that mainly occurs over the age of 50 years of age, with increasing prevalence over the age of 85 years (Porth, 2019). It is a progressive degenerative disease, which means that there is a continual loss of neurons and their function. It primarily affects part of the basal ganglia known as the substantia nigra, which is an important area for controlling voluntary movement. In PD, the nerves that use dopamine as a neurotransmitter (dopaminergic neurons) start to die, and this leads to the signs and symptoms of PD. Its cause is unknown, but it is thought that it may be linked to an interaction of genetics and environmental factors.

Pathophysiology

The symptoms of PD are directly attributable to the loss of the neurotransmitter dopamine, and as the neurons die the symptoms a patient experience worsens. Symptoms of Parkinson's include the following:

- Slow movements (bradykinesia)
- Tremors (initially in the hand but also seen in the limbs, head, face and jaw)
- Muscle stiffness and rigidity
- Tendency to walk forwards on the toes with small, shuffling steps
- Changes in balance
- Stooped posture
- Confusion
- Depression
- Difficulty with fine motor functions, e.g. writing and eating
- 'Mask'-like face
- General weakness and muscle fatigue.

Typical disease progression of Parkinson's is around 10–15 years until it reaches the end stage, with approximately 20–30% of these patients developing dementia (Porth, 2019).

Pharmacological management

Treatment for PD is individualised and includes non-pharmacological as well as pharmacological and possible surgical methods for reducing symptoms.

Pharmacological approaches are aimed at increasing dopamine levels within the brain in order to minimise the effects of the disease. Drugs commonly used include the following:

- L-dopa, or levodopa, is a drug which can cross the blood–brain barrier (unlike dopamine). It is converted to dopamine within the brain and is the main treatment for PD. However, when levodopa is converted to dopamine in the rest of the body, it causes side effects such as nausea and vomiting. To prevent this conversion outside of the brain, it is administered with either carbidopa (Sinemet) or benserazide (Madopar), which cannot cross the blood–brain barrier but prevents conversion to dopamine systemically.
- Selegiline (Eldepryl) and rasagiline are commonly prescribed for patients who are newly diagnosed with PD, as it delays the progression of the disease by slowing the breakdown of dopamine and therefore improves motor control.
- Amantadine (Symmetrel) – an antiviral agent that is also used in the early stages of PD, as it acts by allowing more dopamine to accumulate at and enter the nerve synapse, which delays the need for $_L$-dopa.
- Dopamine agonists such pramipexole, rotigotine and ropinirole work by directly stimulating the receptors and imitating the effects of dopamine.

Medication alert

It is important that medication should be given on time to patients with PD to ensure that there is no fall in therapeutic levels. Symptoms may start to occur with delayed doses, in particular dopamine agonists.

Non-pharmacological management

- Education and support may be offered to help individuals understand the symptoms they are experiencing and managing the disease progression. Daily exercise and nutritional support can also form part of the care plan for the patient.
- More recent therapy has involved the use of deep-brain stimulation to send impulses deep into the brain and block the signals that cause Parkinsonian movements (Porth, 2019).
- The use of stem cells from the umbilical cords of the newborn or the creation of the patient's genetically identical cells using donor eggs are experimental treatments being currently explored (Boss and Huether, 2019).

Care and management

Whilst the majority of patients with PD are managed in the community, as the disease progresses to the later stages, the patient may require residential/nursing home care. Key considerations include the following:

- Reducing the threat of injury from falls; due to physical immobility, weakness, rigidity and slow movement, the patient with PD is at greater risk. This may also require undertaking a risk assessment of the patient's home environment to ensure that any potential hazards are removed.
- Ensuring that the patient is able to express themselves effectively; due to vocal changes and difficulty with writing, the patient's ability to communicate may be affected. Therefore, it might be necessary to involve a speech therapist and other support measures to ensure that the patient will be able to communicate effectively.
- Monitoring the patient's body weight and the provision of adequate nutrition that the patient is able to tolerate; due to possible difficulties with swallowing (dysphagia), there is a risk of malnutrition and weight loss.
- Assisting the patient with meeting their hygiene needs as necessary.

Dementia

Dementia is a condition which is a progressive and irreversible destruction of cerebral function.

The term 'dementia' describes a set of symptoms that include loss of memory, mood changes and problems with communication and reasoning. These symptoms occur when the brain is damaged by certain diseases, including Alzheimer's disease (AD), or by a series of small strokes.

Alzheimer's disease

AD is one of the most common types of dementia. The risk of developing AD increases with age and is relatively uncommon under the age of 65, although early onset, in particular familial AD, can occur. Initial diagnosis may be missed and may be attributed to forgetfulness. As the disease progresses, forgetfulness, short-term memory loss, lack of concentration, disorientation and confusion can occur. Personality changes and mood changes may also be evident as the disease progresses.

Pathophysiology

The cause of AD remains unclear, although there is research underway to identify factors that may trigger the development of Alzheimer's (VanMeter and Hubert, 2014). Within the affected part of the brain, senile plaques and tangles in the neurons are found, as well as atrophy of the

Table 7.6 Stages of Alzheimer's disease.

Stage of disease	Common signs and symptoms
1 (2–4 years)	Loss of interest in people, environment and present affairs. Hesitant in using own initiative, becomes uncertain about making decisions/actions and is forgetful.
2 (2–12 years)	Memory loss becomes more apparent, has difficulty in undertaking simple tasks or carrying out simple instructions. Loses documents, forgets to pay bills or undertake household chores. Unable to meet own needs, loses inhibitions, has periods of irritability, paranoia and anxiety. Prone to wandering, particularly at night, becomes lost in familiar surroundings and may forget way home.
3 (Final stage)	Loses the ability to communicate verbally or in writing. Becomes bedridden and incontinent of urine and faeces. Does not recognise loved ones. Becomes emaciated due to lack of eating.

cerebral cortex and enlargement of the ventricles of the brain. Additionally, the disease has also been associated with a shortage of acetylcholine, loss of nerve cells and structural changes in the memory and cognition areas of the brain. Therefore, the sufferer exhibits memory loss, poor judgement, disorientation, confusion, changes in personality that can lead to mood swings, and sometimes violent outbursts. Inability to maintain self-care, wandering and hallucinations are common in the later stages. Table 7.6 outlines the stages of the disease. Diagnosis is usually made by excluding all other possibilities and involves history taking, cognitive and mental state exam, physical examination and medication review (NICE, 2018).

Pharmacological management

Whilst there is no cure for AD, there are a number of drugs that can alleviate or slow down the symptoms of the disease:

- Donepezil (Aricept), rivastigmine tartrate (Exelon) and galantamine (Reminyl) work by maintaining existing levels of acetylcholine in patients with mild to moderate dementia.
- Memantine (Ebixa) can be used in patients with middle to late stage dementia; it prevents excess entry of calcium ions into brain cells. Excess calcium is known to damage brain cells and prevent them from receiving messages from other brain cells.

In addition, drug therapy can be used to manage behavioural changes associated with the disease. These include:

- Antidepressant medication to treat depressive symptoms
- Neuroleptic drugs to treat psychosis and delusional behaviour
- Sedatives to treat agitation.

Non-pharmacological management

Patients with mild to moderate disease should be offered the opportunity to participate in a structured group cognitive stimulation programme (NICE, 2006 updated 2016).

Care and management

The progressive nature of AD, which results in the patient's loss of independence, personality and cognitive function, presents the healthcare professional and the patient's family with many challenges. Key considerations include the following:

- Maintenance of a safe environment: Due to loss of judgement, cognitive decline and poor memory, the patient is at increased risk of injury.

- Maintenance of hygiene and nutritional needs: Due to loss of independence and the inability to make decisions, the patient is unable to meet or plan for their own needs.
- Promotion of restful sleep: As the patient is likely to be awake at night and prone to wandering.

Multiple sclerosis

Multiple sclerosis (MS) is a chronic degenerative disease where demyelination of the brain, spinal cord and cranial nerves occurs. This loss of myelin blocks conduction of the nerve fibres, resulting in loss of function in the affected area. The disease is progressive; however, the patient may experience periods of remission before relapsing again. There are a number of types of MS which vary in progression, relapse and severity.

Whilst the cause of MS is unclear, it is thought that genetics, immunology and environmental factors influence its development. MS is found more frequently in people who reside in northern latitudes, particularly before the age of 15 (Porth, 2019). Low vitamin D levels have been linked to MS as well as viral infections and having a close relation with MS.

Pathophysiology

MS primarily affects the white matter of the brain and spinal cord by causing areas of demyelination and a breakdown of the myelin sheath that surrounds the nerve fibres and axons (Figure 7.5). This prevents conduction of normal nerve impulses. Sensory, motor and autonomic nerves can be affected, and this demyelination occurs in diffuse patches. The lesions occur after an acute period of inflammation in the area, which permits cells to enter that do not normally enter the brain or spinal cord. As this develops, plaques, which are areas of inflammation and demyelination, form, which eventually become firm. As the inflammation subsides, some function may return until a further exacerbation occurs. With each exacerbation, further neurons are lost, and function is lost permanently.

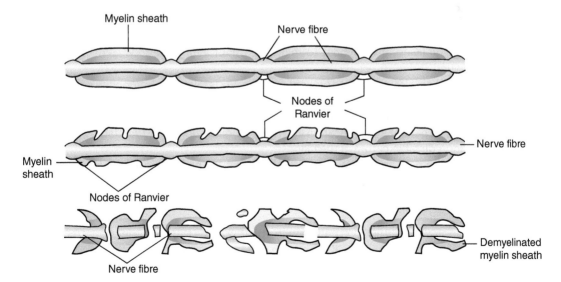

Figure 7.5   The process of demyelination.

Signs and symptoms

The signs and symptoms of MS vary greatly from patient to patient and may vary over time in the same patient (Hickey, 2019). Common signs and symptoms are:

- Muscular weakness/feeling of heaviness to the legs
- Numbness to face or extremities
- Loss of short term memory
- Visual field defects
- Bladder and bowel dysfunction
- Sexual dysfunction
- Fatigue
- Depression.

Pharmacological management

MS is an incurable, extremely debilitating disease, and drug therapy can help with the management of the condition. Drug therapy falls into two broad categories:

1. Treatment to slow or arrest the disease process – includes the use of interferon and steroids, e.g. prednisolone, to treat acute relapses and aid recovery.
2. Treatment to manage the symptoms of MS:
    - Baclofen or diazepam to treat muscle spasticity
    - Stool softeners and laxatives to manage constipation
    - Oxybutynin (Ditropan) to manage bladder function
    - Fluoxetine (Prozac), amitriptyline (Elavil) or imipramine (Tofranil) to treat depression.

Care and management

Due to the unpredictable nature of its progression, MS presents the healthcare professional, the patient and their family with many challenges. Therefore, the care of the patient with MS will require a multidisciplinary approach to ensure that all aspects of care are met. The healthcare professional plays a key role in this process and key considerations include the following:

- Adapting the living environment to minimise risk of injury due to weakness, impaired coordination and sensory deficits.
- Exercise and physical therapy to prevent complications related to immobility and physical weakness.
- Ensuring that the patient's activities of daily living are met.
- Providing the patient with education and psychological support to understand and adapt to the unpredictable nature of their illness.
- Educating the patient on how to avoid relapses where possible, e.g. keeping stress to a minimum, reducing the risk of infection.

Epilepsy

There are approximately 600 000 people with epilepsy in the UK; i.e. one in every 103 people has epilepsy (Epilepsy Research UK, 2020). The disease affects all age groups, and 32 000 new cases are treated each year. The term *epilepsy* describes a range of conditions, and it is classified depending upon where the seizure starts and what part of the brain it occurs in, as well as the triggers and age of the person.

Pathophysiology

A seizure, or 'fit', is caused by an abnormal electrical discharge in the brain in either the sensory system, motor system or ANS. Normal function of the neurons allows messages to be transmitted through electrical impulses in a coordinated way. In a person with epilepsy, a sudden electrical discharge results in large groups of neurons randomly firing in an uncoordinated way. This results in an epileptic seizure. The symptoms the patient will exhibit depend upon where this electrical discharge occurs (Book, 2019).

A seizure can occur without a diagnosis of epilepsy and may be a result of hypoglycaemia, hypoxia, hyponatraemia, fever and due to drugs and alcohol. A diagnosis of epilepsy can be made if the seizures happen repeatedly. Any damage sustained to the brain can also cause epilepsy.

The part of the brain where the abnormal discharge occurs is the epileptogenic focus. These neurons are particularly sensitive and more easily activated by triggers. These triggers could be physical such as loud noises and flashing lights, or internal changes such as sleep deprivation, stress, hypoxia, hyperthermia and hypoglycaemia (VanMeter and Hubert, 2014). When the focal cells become irritated, they produce an excitable discharge which stimulates the surrounding normal cells, and this can spread. Consequently, a seizure may take many different forms, depending on the area and amount of the brain involved. The International League against Epilepsy has developed a widely used system of classifying seizures (Table 7.7).

Status epilepticus

Status epilepticus is an episode of seizure activity that does not spontaneously stop, or it occurs repeatedly without a full recovery period in between (Book, 2019). Prolonged seizures can be life-threatening as they lead to cellular destruction and death if not stopped, and should be treated as a medical emergency.

Table 7.7 Classification of seizures.

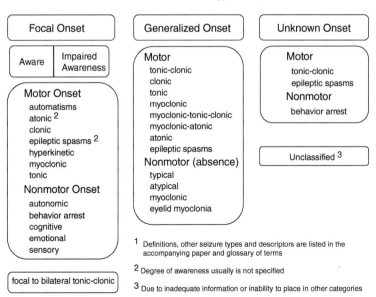

ILAE 2017 Classification of Seizure Types Expanded Version [1]

Source: http://www.ilae.org/Visitors/Centre/documents/ClassificationSeizureILAE-2017.pdf Fisher *et al.*, 2017.

Orange flag

Psychosocial impact of epilepsy

Having epilepsy does not necessarily stop a sufferer from doing the job they want, but there are factors that can affect them at work such as the nature and frequency of seizures, the type of work an individual does and the risk that having seizures at work might bring. This does not mean that the sufferer cannot still work in their chosen field, but it may mean that there are aspects of their work that they can no longer do as it may risk the safety of the individual or the safety of other people in the work environment. Under the Health & Safety at Work Act (1974), employers have to make sure all their employees are safe at work buy undertaking a risk assessment and if required, make reasonable adjustments for the employee (Equality Act 2010) that may include making their workspace safer in case of a seizure, avoiding lone working so that another can help if the sufferer has a seizure, exchanging some tasks of the job with another employee's tasks and adapting or providing equipment or support to help the individual work.

Care and management of the patient with seizures

Healthcare professionals need to act quickly when a patient has a seizure. Key considerations include the following:

- Easing the patient to the floor if seated when the seizure occurs.
- Protecting the patient from injury by moving nearby furniture or objects out of the way and putting a pillow under the head.
- Not restraining the patient or forcing anything into the patient's mouth.
- When the seizure has stopped, ensuring that the airway is clear and administering oxygen if necessary.
- Documenting the duration and type of seizure, as well as how long it takes for the patient to become fully responsive to their surrounding (post-ictal phase).
- Staying with the patient throughout the seizure and orientating/informing the patient about the event once they are awake.

Care and management of the patient with status epilepticus

As status epilepticus is a medical emergency, key considerations include the following:

- Maintenance of the patient's airway to ensure adequate ventilation – this may include suction of the airway to prevent obstruction.
- Providing oxygen therapy via nasal cannulae as prescribed.
- Protecting the patient from injury.
- Administering prescribed medication, usually diazepam or lorazepam, until the seizures stop.

Clinical investigation

Electroencephalogram EEG

An EEG involves the non-invasive recording the electrical activity of the brain and can be used to support a diagnosis of epilepsy. In addition, an EEG can help determine the seizure type and epilepsy syndrome that the individual is suffering from and aid prognosis.

Pharmacological management

Up to two-thirds of people with epilepsy have the condition controlled with anti-epileptic (also known as anticonvulsant) drugs. Other options may include surgery. NICE guidelines provide guidance on drug administration to control epilepsy (NICE, 2012 updated 2016).
Commonly drugs used include:

- Carbamazepine (Tegretol)
- Sodium valproate (Epilim)
- Phenytoin (Dilantin).

179

Medicines management

There are many drug interactions with epileptic drugs, and this aspect needs to be managed. Grapefruit juice can increase toxicity of the drug carbamazepine.

Non-pharmacological management

- Surgical intervention, such as removal of the temporal lobe (temporal lobectomy), and vagal nerve stimulation may be performed for patients who do not respond to medication.
- As treatment for epilepsy is usually long-term or lifelong, the patient needs to be educated as to the importance of compliance with drug therapy.
- The patient needs to be educated as to lifestyle changes that may be required as a result of having epilepsy, e.g. occupation and driving.
- Women of child-bearing age need to have careful management of medication due to increased risk of congenital defects.

Conclusion

The neurological system is a highly complex control system that is able to transmit messages to, and receive them from, all parts of the body. When acute damage occurs, this can lead to loss of function that can present as either a motor, cognition or sensory deficit. Regeneration of neurons does not occur within the CNS, so when damage occurs, the main aim is to limit further damage. Diseases affecting the nervous system can lead to progressive dysfunction and significant morbidity. With the use of pharmacological management and care planning, patients can reduce the progression or manage the symptoms of the disease.

Test your knowledge

1. What does a falling GCS mean?
2. Discuss the meaning of secondary brain trauma.
3. In ischaemic stroke, what is the time frame for receiving thrombolytic agents?
4. What can be a cause of a seizure?
5. Describe what the term *dementia* means.
6. What neurotransmitter is deficient in Parkinson's disease?

Activities

Here are some activities and exercises to help test your learning. For the answers to these exercises, as well as further self-testing activities, visit our website at **www.wiley.com/go/fundamentalsofappliedpathophysiology/student4e**

Multiple choice questions

1. The amount of blood supplied to the brain is approximately:
   - (a) 400 mL/min
   - (b) 1000 mL/min
   - (c) 750 mL/min
   - (d) 600 mL/min
2. An abnormally raised volume of cerebrospinal fluid is known as:
   - (a) Herniation
   - (b) Cerebral oedema
   - (c) Papilloedema
   - (d) Hydrocephalus
3. The vital centres lie in the:
   - (a) Pons
   - (b) Midbrain
   - (c) Hypothalamus
   - (d) Medulla oblongata
4. When bright light reaches the eye, the pupil constricts. This is an example of:
   - (a) A stretch reflex
   - (b) An autonomic reflex
   - (c) A spinal reflex
   - (d) A voluntary movement
5. Altered level of consciousness can be assessed using a simple assessment tool. This is known as AVPU. What does AVPU stand for?
   - (a) Alert, Voice, Pain, Unresponsive
   - (b) Alert, Voice, peripheries, Unable
   - (c) Assess, Voice, Pain Unresponsive
   - (d) Assess, Voice, Peripheries, Unresponsive
6. What are two effects of ageing on the nervous system?
   - (a) Slowed conduction times
   - (b) Memory changes
   - (c) Both a and b
   - (d) Neither a or b
7. Identify causes of raised intracranial pressure (highlight all that are relevant)
   - (a) Brain tumour
   - (b) Skull fracture
   - (c) Gastrointestinal infection
   - (d) Meningitis
8. What are the two divisions of the nervous system?
   - (a) Central and peripheral
   - (b) Motor and sensory
   - (c) Central and functional
   - (d) Sympathetic and parasympathetic
9. Nerve impulses:
   - (a) Travel more quickly in unmyelinated neurones
   - (b) Can travel either way along a neurone
   - (c) Travel during the refractory period
   - (d) Travel by saltatory conduction in myelinated neurones

10. Diagnostic dyes, local anaesthetics and analgesic drugs are injected into the:
    (a) Subdural space
    (b) Filum terminale
    (c) Subarachnoid space
    (d) Epidural space
11. Epilepsy is a common neurological disorder. Identify potential triggers in a person that may increase the likelihood of a seizure (highlight all that are relevant).
    (a) An elevated temperature
    (b) Stress and anxiety
    (c) Exercise
    (d) Alcohol and/or drugs
12. The fibrous tissue that encloses bundles of nerve fibres is called:
    (a) Myelin
    (b) Epineurium
    (c) Perineurium
    (d) Endoneurium
13. What is a transient ischaemic attack (TIA)?
    (a) It is an infection in the brain
    (b) It is a small bleed on the brain
    (c) It is a small temporary clot in the brain
    (d) It is total occlusion of a blood vessel in the brain
14. Which of the following is NOT an effect of sympathetic stimulation?
    (a) Goosebumps
    (b) Greatly increased metabolic rate
    (c) Fight or flight response
    (d) Increased motility and secretion in stomach and small intestine
15. Wernicke's area is concerned with:
    (a) Speech
    (b) Hearing
    (c) Smell
    (d) Taste

Conditions

The following is a list of conditions that are associated with the nervous system. Take some time and write notes about each of the conditions. You may make the notes taken from textbooks or other resources (e.g. people you work with in a clinical area), or you may make the notes based on people you have cared for. If you are making notes about people you have cared for, you must ensure that you adhere to the rules of confidentiality.

Cerebrovascular accident	
Alzheimer's Disease	

Raised intracranial pressure	
Epilepsy	
Multiple sclerosis	

Further resources

National Institute for Health and Care Excellence (NICE)

NICE provides guidance, sets quality standards and manages a national database to improve people's health and prevent and treat ill health. There are many excellent resources on this website that can help guide and inform practice.

http://www.nice.org.uk/

SIGN: Health Improvement Scotland

Provide guidelines and resourced to support patient care including management of patients with head injuries, epilepsy and Parkinson's http://www.sign.ac.uk/guidelines/published/numlist.html

Stroke Association

The Stroke Association provides specialist support and funds critical research to make sure individuals affected by stroke get the very best care and support to rebuild their lives. There are many good resources on this website that can help with understanding the impact that stroke has on the individual and the support services available.

http://stroke.org.uk/

Glasgow Coma Scale

This website provides a comprehensive explanation of how to undertake a Glasgow Coma Scale and the elements involved in performing this task.

http://www.glasgowcomascale.org/

Royal College of Physicians

This website has a wealth of resources to support management of patients. These include traumatic brain injury, stroke as well as resources for the National Early Warning Score (NEWS).

https://www.rcplondon.ac.uk/guidelines-policy/stroke-guidelines

Glossary of terms

Acetylcholine   A neurotransmitter found widely in the central and peripheral nervous system.

Blood–brain Barrier   An impermeable network of brain capillaries which acts as a filter between the brain tissue and blood-borne substances. It provides the brain with some protection from harmful toxins and metabolites.

Cerebrovascular accident Occurs as a direct result of impaired blood flow to the brain. Also known as stroke.

Choroid plexus The tissue in the ventricles of the brain which produces cerebrospinal fluid.

Dementia The loss of mental ability.

Demyelination The loss of the myelin sheath from around the axon of the nerve cell.

Dopamine A neurotransmitter found in the central nervous system.

Foramen magnum A large hole in the occipital bone through which the vertebral column and spinal cord pass.

Glasgow Coma Scale (GCS) A tool designed for detecting and monitoring changes in a patient's neurological status.

Intracranial pressure The recordable pressure within the skull.

Norepinephrine (noradrenaline) A neurotransmitter in the central and peripheral nervous system.

Parasympathetic nervous system (PNS) Part of the nervous system which utilises acetylcholine to moderate internal responses. Associated with a state of relaxation.

Peripheral nervous system Cranial and spinal nerves which connect the brain and spinal cord to other parts of the body.

Schwann cell A cell that forms myelin around the axon of a nerve cell.

Substantia nigra The part of the midbrain that connects to the basal ganglia.

Sympathetic nervous system Part of the nervous system which initiates response to stress through the release of norepinephrine. This assists in the 'Fight or flight' response.

Ventricle A cavity filled with cerebrospinal fluid.

References

Book, D. (2019). Disorders of brain function. In: C.M. Porth (ed.), *Essentials of Pathophysiology*, 5th edn. Philadelphia: Wolters Kluwer.

Boss, B. and Huether, S. (2019). Alterations in cognitive systems, cerebral hemodynamics and motor function. In: S. Huether and K. McCance (eds), *Understanding Pathophysiology*, 7th edn. Missouri: Elsevier Mosby.

Coe, F. (2019). Organisation and control of neural function. In: Norris, T.L. (ed.), *Porth's Essentials of Pathophysiology*, 5th edn. Philadelphia: Wolters Kluwer.

Douglas, M. and Platt, S. (2013). Assessment and monitoring of neurological status. In: J. Mallett, J. Albarran and A. Richardson (eds), *Critical Care Manual of Clinical Procedures and Competencies, 1st edn*. London: John Wiley & Sons.

Fisher, R.S., Cross, J.H., French, J.A., Higurashi, N., Hirsch, E. *et al.* (2017). Operational classification of seizure types by the International League Against Epilepsy. *Epilepsia*, 58(4): 522–530.

Hickey, J. (2019). *The Clinical Practice of Neurological and Neurosurgical Nursing*, 8th edn. Philadelphia, Wolters Kluwer.

Epilepsy Research UK (2020). *Epilepsy Statistics*. Available at: https://www.epilepsyresrach.org.uk/about-epilepsy/epilepsy-statistics/

Marieb, E.N. and Keller, S.M (2017). *Essentials of Human Anatomy and Physiology, Global Edition*, 12th edn. Harlow: Pearson.

Mehta, R. and Chinthapalli, K. (2019). Glasgow Coma Scale explained. *BMJ*, 365: I1296. DOI: 10.1136/bmj.l1296

National Institute for Health and Care Excellence (NICE) (2018). *Dementia: Assessment, Management and Support for People Living with Dementia and Their Carers*. Clinical Guideline NG97. London: NICE.

NICE (2019). *NICE Impact stroke*. Manchester, NICE

NICE (2012 updated 2020). *Epilepsies: Diagnosis and Management*. Available at: https://www.nice.org.uk/ guidance/cg137

NICE (2014 updated 2019). *Head Injury: Assessment and Early Management (CG176)*. Available at: nice.org.uk/guidance/ cg176

NHS Improvement (2020). *Stoke – Psychological Care After Stroke – Improving Stroke Services for People with Cognitive and Mood Disorders*. Available at https://www.england.nhs.uk/improvement-hub/wp-content/uploads/sites/44/2017/11/Psychological-Care-after-Stroke.pdf

Pierce, E. and Braine, M. (2014). Nursing care of conditions related to the neurological system. In: A.-M. Brady, C. McCabe and M. McCann (eds), *Medical-Surgical Nursing: A Systems Approach, 1st edn*. Chichester: Wiley Blackwell.

Porth, C.M. (2019). Disorders of Neuromuscular function. In: Norris, T.L. (ed.), *Porth's Essentials of Pathophysiology*, 5th edn. Philadelphia: Wolters Kluwer.

Stroke Association (2018). *State of the Nation: Stroke Statistics*. Available from: https://www.stroke.org.uk/system/files/sotn_2018.pdf

Sugerman, R. and Huether, S. (2019). The neurological system. In: S. Huether and K. McCance (eds), *Understanding Pathophysiology*, 7th edn. Missouri: Elsevier Mosby.

Teasdale, G., Allen, D., Brennan, P., McElhinney, E. and Mackinnon, L. (2014). The Glasgow Coma Scale: An update after 40 years. *The Nursing Times*, 110, 12–16.

VanMeter, K. and Hubert, R. (2014). *Gould's: Pathophysiology for the Health Professions*, 5th edn. Missouri: Elsevier.

184

Chapter 8

The heart and associated disorders

Valerie Nangle

Assistant Professor, Coventry University (London), Spitalfields, London, UK

Contents

Introduction 186	Conclusion 210
Location of the heart............................186	Test your knowledge...........................210
Structures of the heart 187	Multiple choice questions....................211
Blood flow through the heart.................190	Further resources...............................212
Conducting systems of the heart 190	Glossary of terms...............................213
Nerve supply of the heart 192	References..215
Diseases of the heart...........................193	

Key words

- Pericardium
- Chambers
- Systemic circulation
- Atria
- Myocardium
- Valves
- Pulmonary circulation
- Ventricles
- Endocardium
- Impulses
- Conducting systems
- Pacemaker

Fundamentals of Applied Pathophysiology: An Essential Guide for Nursing and Healthcare Students, Fourth Edition. Edited by Ian Peate.
© 2021 John Wiley & Sons Ltd. Published 2021 by John Wiley & Sons Ltd.
Student companion website: www.wiley.com/go/fundamentalsofappliedpathophysiology/student4e
Instructor companion website: www.wiley.com/go/fundamentalsofappliedpathophysiology/instructor4e

Test your prior knowledge

- What are the three different layers of the heart muscle called?
- How many chambers does the heart have? Can you name them?
- Can you trace the blood flow through the heart?
- Name the conducting systems of the heart.
- List the possible modifiable and non-modifiable risk factors of coronary heart disease.

Learning outcomes

On completion of this section, the reader will be able to:

- Describe the structure and functions of the heart.

- Describe the blood flow through the heart.

- Trace the systemic and pulmonary circulations.

- Outline the conducting system(s) of the heart.

- Understand various cardiac diseases and conditions and the appropriate investigations and treatment.

Don't forget to visit the companion website for this book (www.wiley.com/go/fundamentalsofappliedpathophysiology/student4e) where you can find self-assessment tests to check your progress, as well as lots of activities to practise your learning.

Introduction

The heart is a muscular organ that continuously pumps blood throughout the body. Through a cycle of contraction and relaxation, this synchronised double pump pumps oxygen-rich blood and nutrients to all the cells in the body while carrying metabolic waste away to the lungs. A healthy and efficient heart is essential for cellular function. This chapter discusses the structure and functions of the heart, the conduction system and the blood flow through the heart. It also includes cardiac diseases such as myocardial infarction (MI), heart failure (left and right heart failure), cardiogenic shock and angina and the related care and management of these common cardiac conditions.

Location of the heart

The heart position is posterior to the sternum in the mediastinum. The mediastinum refers to the space in the centre of the thorax between the right and the left lungs. It is positioned slightly more to the left than the right side of the chest, and the base of the heart is superior to its apex (Figure 8.1).On average, an adult heart weighs approximately 250–305 g and is approximately 12–14 cm in length and 9–11 cm in diameter (Knight *et al.* 2020).

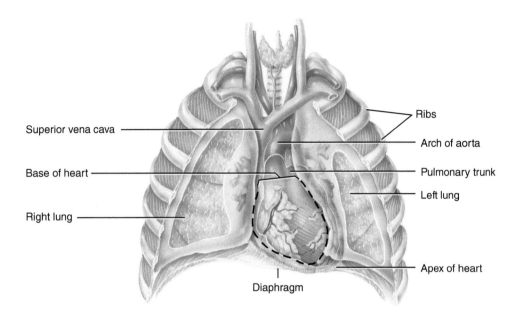

Superior vena cava

Base of heart

Right lung

Ribs

Arch of aorta

Pulmonary trunk

Left lung

Apex of heart

Diaphragm

Figure 8.1   Location of the heart.

Structures of the heart

The heart is composed of three layers of specialised cardiac muscle: the pericardium, the myocardium and the endocardium.

The pericardium is a protective membrane that surrounds and protects the heart. The pericardium is divided into two layers called the parietal and visceral pericardium. The parietal pericardium, which is the outer layer, is a fibrous sac. The fibrous pericardium protects the heart and anchors it to the mediastinum.

The inner layer, called the visceral pericardium or the epicardium, is a serous membrane, which adheres to the myocardium (Figure 8.2). Within these two layers is <50 mL of serous fluid, which lubricates the surface of the heart (Rodiquez and Tan 2017); this pericardial fluid prevents any friction during heartbeats so the heart can move freely.

The cardiac muscle is called the myocardium, and this type of muscle is unique and specific to the heart. The bulk of the heart is composed of myocardial muscle, which is responsible for the pumping action of the heart. The fibres of the myocardium are involuntary, striated and branch and join with each other to allow contraction of the myocardial fibres, which in turn results in contraction of the heart (Figure 8.2).

The endocardium lines the chambers, and the valves of the heart are made up of epithelial cells. It is a thin, smooth and shiny membrane which allows the smooth flow of blood (Waugh and Grant, 2018).

Thus, the heart can be described as having three layers:

- Pericardium – the outer layer
- Myocardium – the middle layer
- Endocardium – the inner layer.

Chambers of the heart

The heart is divided into two sides, right and left, which are separated by a muscular wall called the septum. The septum ensures that the oxygen-rich blood from the left side of the

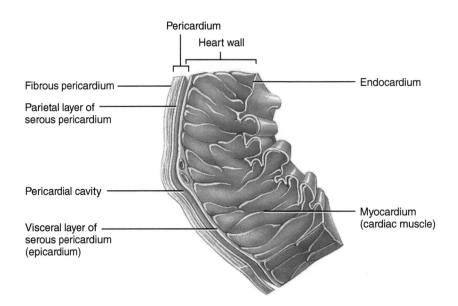

Figure 8.2   The cardiac muscle.

heart does not mix with the oxygen-depleted blood on the right side (Tortora and Derrickson, 2016). Each side of the heart is further divided into two chambers. The upper chambers are called the atria (the right and left atrium), and the lower chambers are called the ventricles (the right and left ventricle) (Figure 8.3). The thickness of the wall of the heart chamber is dependent on its function.

The walls of the atria are much thinner than the walls of the ventricles. The left ventricle has a thicker muscular wall than the right ventricle due to its requirement and function of pumping blood through the systematic circuit at high pressure, whereas the right ventricle pumps blood at a lower pressure through the pulmonary circuit.

Valves of the heart

There are four valves which are responsible for directing blood flow through the heart. The valves between the atria and the ventricles are called the atrioventricular valves. The right atrioventricular valve is known as the tricuspid valve because it has three cusps, and the left valve has two cusps and is also known as the bicuspid or mitral valve (McCance *et al.*, 2017). These valves only allow the blood to flow from the atria to the ventricles and prevent the blood from flowing in the opposite direction, or the backflow of blood. Similarly, there are valves in the aorta and pulmonary artery, and these are semilunar valves known as the aortic valve and the pulmonary valve (Figure 8.3).

Vessels of the heart

Blood flows both into the heart through several large vessels called the vena cavae. The right atrium receives venous blood through the superior and inferior venae cavae. This oxygen-depleted blood then travels to the right ventricle and onwards to the lungs via the pulmonary artery. The pulmonary veins return oxygen-rich blood from the lungs to the left atrium. The aorta transports oxygenated blood from the left ventricle to the whole body (McCance *et al.*, 2017). In addition, the heart requires its own blood supply, which this is delivered by the coronary arteries, and the coronary veins return oxygen-depleted blood from the heart tissue to the right atrium (Figure 8.4). Table 8.1 summarises the vessels and their functions.

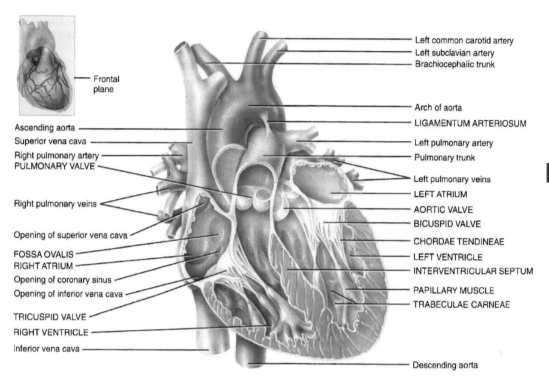

Figure 8.3   The chambers and valves of the heart.

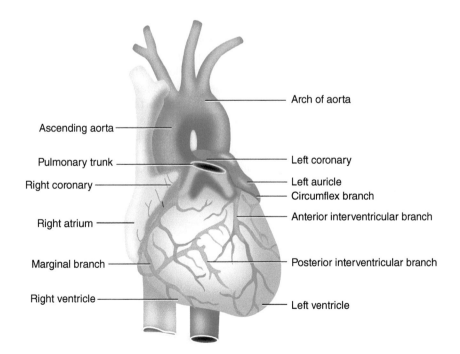

Figure 8.4   The vessels of the heart.

Table 8.1   Summary of the vessels and their functions (Nair and Peate, 2017).

Vessel	Function
Superior vena cava	Returns oxygen-depleted blood to the right atrium from the thoracic organs, head, neck and both arms
Inferior vena cava	Returns oxygen-depleted blood to the right atrium from the rest of the body
Pulmonary artery (divides into the right and left pulmonary artery)	Takes oxygen-depleted blood from the right ventricle to the lungs
Pulmonary veins (two from the right lung and two from the left lung)	Returns oxygen-rich blood from the lungs to the left atrium
Aorta	Takes oxygen-rich blood from the left ventricle to the whole body
Coronary arteries	Takes oxygen-rich blood to the heart tissues
Coronary veins	Returns oxygen-depleted blood from the heart tissues to the right atrium via the coronary sinus

Blood flow through the heart

The right atrium receives deoxygenated blood via the superior and inferior venae cavae and the coronary sinus. From the right atrium, deoxygenated blood flows into the right ventricle via the tricuspid valve. The right ventricle then pumps the blood to the lungs via the right and left pulmonary arteries by opening the pulmonary semilunar valve. In the lungs, gaseous exchange occurs, where carbon dioxide is exchanged for oxygen molecules. The blood returning to the lungs has a higher content of carbon dioxide, which diffuses out of the lung capillaries into the alveolar sac and is disposed of during expiration.

During inspiration, oxygen diffuses from the alveolar sac into the lung capillaries, where it attaches itself to the haemoglobin molecules in the red blood cells. The oxygen-rich red blood cells are then transported in the blood to the left atrium by four sets of pulmonary veins. The short circulation from the right ventricle to the lungs and from the lungs to the left atrium is called the pulmonary circulation (Marieb and Hoehn 2018).

From the left atrium, the blood is then pumped into the left ventricle via the bicuspid (mitral) valve. From the left ventricle, the blood is then transported to the whole body via the aorta through the semilunar (aortic) valve (Figure 8.5). The aorta and its branches then transport the oxygen-rich blood to all parts of the body. The blood is then returned to the right atrium via the venae cavae. This loop is called the systemic circulation (Marieb and Hoehn, 2018). The role of the systemic circulation is to transport oxygen and nutrients throughout the body, and to remove waste products, e.g. carbon dioxide, from the tissues.

Conducting systems of the heart

The heart has a natural conduction system which is responsible for producing a coordinated myocardial contraction of the four chambers of the heart. The cardiac conducting system (Figure 8.6) comprises the following:

- Sinoatrial (SA) node
- Atrioventricular (AV) node
- Bundle of His
- Right and left bundle branches
- Purkinje fibres.

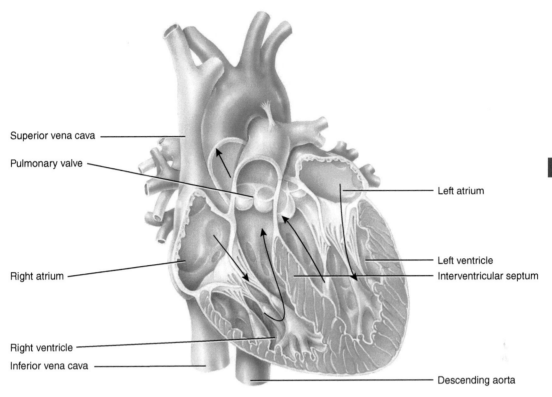

Superior vena cava

Pulmonary valve

Left atrium

Right atrium

Left ventricle
Interventricular septum

Right ventricle

Inferior vena cava

Descending aorta

Figure 8.5 Blood flow through the heart. The arrows indicate the direction of blood flow.

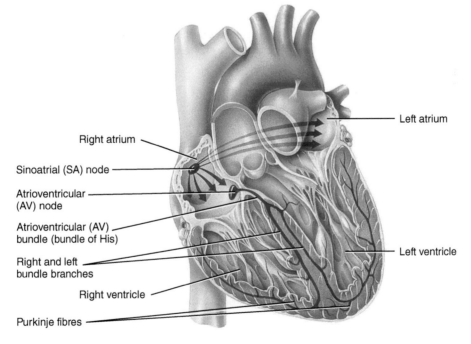

Right atrium

Sinoatrial (SA) node

Atrioventricular (AV) node

Atrioventricular (AV) bundle (bundle of His)

Right and left bundle branches

Right ventricle

Purkinje fibres

Left atrium

Left ventricle

Figure 8.6 The conducting system of the heart.

The SA node

The SA node is situated in the right atrium just below the opening of the superior vena cava. It is also known as the cardiac pacemaker, so called because it initiates impulses much faster than other groups of neuromuscular cells (Waugh and Grant, 2018). Impulses from the SA node are responsible for contraction of the atria.

The AV node

The AV node is situated at the base of the right atrium. This is the final region of the atria to be stimulated, thus allowing time for the atria to empty the blood into the ventricles before the ventricles start to contract again. Electrically, it forms a connection between the atria and ventricles. This ensures that the blood will flow in one direction only.

Bundle of His

This is a set of fibres that originate from the AV node, and they further divide into the left and right bundle branches.

Right and left bundle branches

The left and right bundle branches run down each side of the muscular interventricular septum. The right bundle branch runs down the right side to supply the right ventricle, and the left bundle branch runs down the left side to supply the left ventricle.

Purkinje fibres

These fibres distribute rapid electrical impulses to the endocardial cells of the heart.

Nerve supply of the heart

The pumping action of the heart is rhythmic. In other words, the cardiac muscle has the inherent ability of automatic rhythmic contraction, independent of its nerve supply. However, the rate of contraction is influenced by the nerve supply to the heart.

The nerve supply originates from the cardio regulatory centre in the medulla oblongata in the brainstem (Figure 8.7). These nerves are a branch of the autonomic nervous system and are called the sympathetic and parasympathetic nerves (Waugh and Grant 2018).

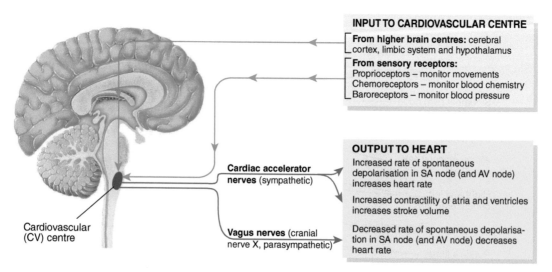

Figure 8.7   The cardioregulatory centre.

The sympathetic nerve increases heart rate; it innervates the SA node, AV node and the myocardium of the atria and ventricles. The parasympathetic (vagus) nerve slows down the heart rate; it supplies the SA and AV nodes, and the atria muscles. Factors affecting heart rate include the following (Waugh and Grant, 2018):

- Hormones such as epinephrine, steroids
- Stress
- Age
- Drugs such as propranolol, dopamine, cocaine
- Body temperature
- Electrolyte imbalance
- Overactive thyroid gland
- Heart disease
- Smoking
- Exercise
- Autonomic nervous system
- Circulating volume of blood
- Levels of oxygen and carbon dioxide in the blood.

Diseases of the heart

Learning outcomes

On completion of this section, the reader will be able to:

- Know about commonly diagnosed cardiac conditions.

- Describe the pathophysiology of the common diagnosed cardiac conditions.

- List possible cardiac investigations used to diagnose cardiac conditions.

- Outline the care and management of some cardiac conditions.

Snapshot   Chest pain and hypertension

Mr Ahmed is a 52-year-old married man who works as a heavy goods vehicle driver. This morning, while he was having breakfast, he complained of severe central chest pain and shortness of breath. His wife called for an ambulance. He is admitted to the local emergency department and is receiving oxygen therapy via a high flow oxygen mask. Mr Ahmed indicated to the nurse that the pain was spreading to his shoulders, neck and down both arms. His wife states that he complained of not feeling well when he got up that morning and that he vomited a couple of times in the toilet. His wife reports that generally he is a fit man but has recently been diagnosed with hypertension and has been commenced on antihypertensive medications. His wife informs the nurse that Mr Ahmed has a family history of both heart disease and hypertension. He has been suffering from stress lately as he fears he will lose his job because of redundancy, and they have two small children and she does not work.

Vital signs

On admission to the emergency department, the following vital signs were noted and recorded according to NEWS2 scoring system (2017):

Vital sign	Observation	Normal
Temperature	37.2°C	36.0–37.9°C range
Pulse	88 beats per minute (regular)	60–100 beats per minute
Respiration	22 breaths per minute	12–20 breaths per minute
Blood pressure	112/65 mmHg	100–139 mmHg (systolic) range
O_2 saturation	98% on O_2 therapy	94–98%

A full blood count and urea and electrolytes was performed.

Test	Result	Guideline normal values
White blood cells (WBC)	10×10^9/L	4 to 11×10^9/L
Neutrophils	7.2×10^9/L	2.0 to 7.5×10^9/L
Lymphocytes	4.0×10^9/L	1.3 to 4.0×10^9/L
Red blood cells (RBC)	6.7×10^{12}/L	4.5 to 6.5×10^{12}/L
Haemoglobin (Hb)	160 g/L	130–180 g/L
Platelets	298×10^9/L	150 to 440×10^9/L
C-reactive protein	5.2 mg/L	<5 mg/L
Urea	6.5 mmol/L	2–6.6 mmol/L
Potassium	5.1 mmol/L	3.4–5.6 mmol/L
Sodium	138 mmol/L	135–147 mmol/L
Troponin T	1.0 ng/mL	0.00–0.4 ng/mL

Take some time to reflect on this case and then consider the following:

1. What is the possible diagnosis for Mr Ahmed?
2. List the investigations that may be carried out and the rationale to confirm diagnosis.
3. Discuss the assessment activity needed to confirm diagnosis.
4. Identify Mr Ahmed's modifiable and non-modifiable risk factors for cardiovascular disease.

NEWS 2

Mr Ahmed

Physiological parameter	3	2	1	0	1	2	3
Respiration rate						22	
Oxygen saturation %				98			
Supplemental oxygen		Yes					
Temperature °C				37.2			
Systolic BP mmHg				112			
Heart rate				88			
Level of consciousness				A			
Score	0	2	0	0	0	2	0
Total	4						

Clinical diagnostic investigations

12-lead ECG

A 12-lead electrocardiogram (ECG) is a quick valuable test which measures the rate, rhythm and electrical activity of the heart and is performed routinely by nurses.

A 12-lead ECG records the heart's rhythm, rate, and activity on a moving strip of paper or on a screen. The healthcare professional performing the procedure can read and interpret the waves on special ECG graph paper or screen to determine any abnormalities or unusual activity.

So why is a 12-lead ECG carried out?

- Record the rate, rhythm and electrical activity of the heart.
- Diagnose cardiac arrhythmias such as heart blocks, atrial and ventricular fibrillations, bradycardias and tachycardias.
- Investigate causes of loss of consciousness (syncope).
- Determine the cause of unexplained chest pain or pressure experienced in the chest. This could potentially be caused by angina, myocardial infarction or inflammation of the sac surrounding the heart (pericarditis).
- Investigate the cause of symptoms of heart disease. Symptoms may include shortness of breath, dizziness, sweating, fainting, and heartbeats that are rapid and irregular (palpitations).
- As an examination to diagnose cardiac hypertrophy (enlargement of the heart chamber).
- Monitor the effectiveness of prescribed medications and determine if they are adversely affecting cardiac functioning.
- Check the effectiveness of implanted mechanical cardiac devices, such as pacemakers and implantable cardioverter defibrillator (ICD). These devices help to control and regulate the electrical activity of the heart.
- Assess the functioning of the heart in the presence of other diseases or conditions. These can include heart failure, cardiomyopathy, hypertension, hypercholesterolemia, diabetes mellitus, genetic predisposition to cardiac disease as well as lifestyle choices such as smoking, recreational drug use and excessive alcohol abuse.

Prior to the ECG, the procedure must be explained to the patient and verbal consent obtained. Nurses must adhere to local and professional guidelines when undertaking this procedure to include local policies on chaperoning. There may be a need to assist the patient pre, peri and post procedure; at all times dignity and comfort must be maintained.

Red flag

An ECG is an easily obtained cardiac investigation. As it is non-invasive, it can be repeated as often as required. It can be a useful diagnostic tool and can detect a heart problem. However, a normal ECG does not rule out serious heart disease.

For example, with an irregular heart rhythm that is intermittent, the recording can be normal between episodes. Also, not all heart attacks can be detected by ECG; non-ST elevated myocardial infarctions and angina cannot usually be detected by a routine ECG. Raised Troponin blood levels are more reliable in diagnosing a myocardial infarction as this blood test is specific to cardiac injury.

Myocardial Infarction

MI is commonly referred to as a 'heart attack', or a 'coronary' (Figure 8.8). When the coronary blood flow is occluded because of a blood clot or fatty deposits (atheromatous plaque) over a period of time, death of the myocardium will take place (McCance *et al.*, 2017), resulting in an MI.

Aetiology

MI is a medical emergency that requires urgent intervention; it is a major cause of death for both men and women (Bullock and Henze, 2020). Individuals at risk include the following:

- People who have a medical history of vascular disease such as atherosclerosis, a condition where fatty deposits build up in the arteries, causing them to narrow and restrict the blood flow to the tissues.
- Previous past medical history of MI or cerebrovascular accident (CVA)
- Family history of cardiovascular disease
- Certain ethnic populations – South Asians
- Older age group – risk increases for men after the age of 45 and for women after the age of 55, or after menopause
- Smokers, because the two main ingredients, nicotine and tar, lead to atherosclerosis, causing narrowing of the arteries
- Excessive alcohol intake due to risk of increasing the level of low-density lipoprotein (LDL)
- Recreational drug use such as cocaine
- Hypertensives
- Diabetics with or without insulin resistance
- People with hyperlipidemia and obesity
- Inactivity

Investigations

The following investigations may be carried out to confirm diagnosis:

- Chest X-ray
- Blood chemistry (troponin, urea and electrolytes, cardiac enzymes, e.g. creatine kinase, full blood count)
- Electrocardiogram (ECG) to detect any abnormal changes in the rate, rhythm or electrical activity
- Angiogram, an invasive test to determine the location and severity of any blockages or narrowing in the coronary arteries
- Echocardiogram, a non-invasive scan to determine the shape, size and left ventricular function of the heart
- Cardiac MRI

Pathophysiology

Myocardial ischaemia results from of an occlusion of the coronary artery and oxygen deprivation of the myocardial cells. If the heart muscle is deprived of oxygen for a prolonged period, approximately 20–45 minutes, this can lead to necrosis distal to the occlusion (Figure 8.8) (Hogan *et al.*, 2014). The extent of the ischaemia depends on the location, the extent of the occlusion, amount of heart tissue supplied by the blood vessel and duration of the occlusion. It may affect one of the three layers of the heart (pericardium, myocardium, and endocardium) or a combination of these layers (Porth, 2018).

A collagen scar forms at the position of the infarct and results in the damaged muscle's inability to contract efficiently. Collagen is a bundle of inelastic fibres that do not stretch or contract effectively. Damaged heart tissue conducts electrical signals much more slowly

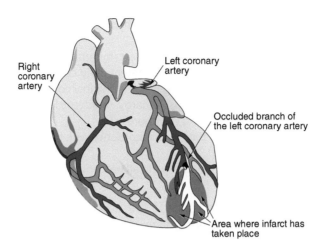

Figure 8.8   Myocardial infarction.

than normal heart tissue, which can result in inefficient contraction of the myocardium. This can result in decreased:

- Volume of blood ejected by the left ventricle with each heartbeat
- Cardiac output (volume of blood pumped out by the left ventricle each minute)
- Blood pressure
- Tissue perfusion

Signs and symptoms

- Chest pain that radiates to the left arm, the lower jaw, shoulders, neck, back and right arm. The pain may be described as crushing, stabbing, pressure or tightness in the chest. Pain is usually prolonged and is not usually relieved by rest.
- Rapid, irregular pulse, hypotension and dyspneoa (shortness of breath).
- Diaphoresis (excessive sweating), nausea, vomiting, palpitations, loss of consciousness and even cardiac arrest and sudden death.
- Signs of shock.
- Cyanosis.
- Anxiety.
- Women often experience markedly different symptoms compared to men. Symptoms such as dyspnoea, fatigue, sleep disturbances and weakness are more common in women than in men (http://www.heart.org/HEARTORG/Conditions/HeartAttack/Warning Signsof aHeartAttack/Heart-Attack-Symptoms-in-Women_UCM_436448_Article.jsp).

Care and management

Management of a patient with acute myocardial infarction (AMI) is a medical emergency. Local guidelines for the management of MI should be followed where they exist. Key care considerations include the following:

- Prioritise pain control to ensure that the patient is pain free as a result of myocardial ischaemia. Accurate pain assessment should be carried out using pain assessment tools such as the Numerical Rating Scale or the Verbal Rating Scale (Peate 2019). Patients should be encouraged to report their pain as it occurs.
- Ensure that the patient is attached to a cardiac monitor and that resuscitation equipment is close at hand and easily accessible.

- Administer prescribed oxygen to treat tissue hypoxia, which helps to reduce ischaemia and pain (LeMone *et al.*, 2015).
- Monitoring of all the vital signs (heart rate, heart rhythm, blood pressure, temperature, O_2 saturation and respiration) is important to detect early complications or changes in the patient's condition. Regularity depends on the individual condition of the patient.
- Observe for signs of shock, such as lethargy, bradycardia or tachycardia, cyanosis, hypotension and excessive sweating (diaphoresis).
- Document any care given to the patient in accordance with the local policy and procedure and the NMC Code (NMC, 2018).
- Reassure the patient and family, and explain all procedures to them.

Pharmacological and non-pharmacological treatment

Some of the pharmacological and non-pharmacological interventions are as follows:

- Initially with high dose antiplatelet medication – aspirin 300 mg orally.
- Prompt angiography and revascularisation with appropriate treatment is necessary to achieve myocardial perfusion and preservation of the myocardial. This involves insertion of a catheter into the obstructed coronary artery under local anaesthesia. The balloon in the catheter is then inflated for 15 seconds to 2 or 3 minutes (Porth, 2018), which dilates the artery, and a percutaneous coronary intervention (PCI) is inserted if indicated.
- Continuous ECG monitoring is carried out to detect abnormal cardiac rhythms and to allow prompt action to be taken.
- Strict fluid balance chart is necessary to record urine output.
- Drugs such as morphine or morphine derivatives are administered to control pain. Sublingual or intravenous nitrates such as glyceryl trinitrate (GTN) are also considered (Adams *et al.*, 2019).

All patients who have had an acute MI treatment should be treated with the following drugs unless contraindicated:

- Dual antiplatelet therapy (aspirin plus a second antiplatelet agent)
- Beta blocker
- ACE (angiotensin-converting enzyme) inhibitor
- Statin.

Red flag

Nurses need to be aware that oxygen, that is to be administered, must be prescribed by a recognised prescriber (i.e. independent prescriber, doctor). Failure to administer oxygen appropriately can potentially result in serious harm to the patient. The device and flow rate of administered oxygen should be recorded.

Orange flag

Studies have shown that in patients with coronary heart disease, the prevalence of anxiety disorders is as high as 40% to 70%. (Gu et al 2016). This can impact their recovery and return to normal familial, vocational and leisure activities. Psychological counselling should be included in post MI management.

Medicines management

Sublingual glyceryl trinitrate

Although the mucous membrane is not highly vascular, certain drugs such as glyceryl trinitrate are administered using the sublingual route. The drug is absorbed quickly and is available for action within a short time. The advantage of this route is that drugs administered through the route bypass the first pass metabolism. Nurses need to advise the patient to avoid drinking alcohol while taking glyceryl trinitrate, because it can make the side effects worse. If they experience dizziness, they should avoid driving and operating complex or heavy machinery. Other side effects include the following:

- Headaches
- Postural hypotension (lowered blood pressure especially on standing or sitting up)
- Tachycardia
- Feeling drowsy
- Hypotension
- Vertigo
- Lethargy

Secondary prevention

All patients who have experienced an MI or are diagnosed with cardiovascular disease are recommended to attend a structured cardiac rehabilitation programme. These multifaceted multidisciplinary programmes consist of symptom monitoring, risk factor modification, psychological support, and supervised exercise. The overall aim of cardiac rehabilitation and secondary prevention is to return the individual to their optimal health and well-being and prevent further cardiac events.

Heart failure/congestive heart failure

Heart failure (HF) is an umbrella term used to describe the inability of the heart to sustain a normal cardiac output that ultimately leads to poor perfusion of tissues. HF may affect either side of the heart; however, as all the chambers are part of the heart structure, if one side fails, the other side is affected (Waugh and Grant, 2018). Nevertheless, left heart failure (LHF) is more common than right heart failure (RHF).

Red flag

Congestive heart failure is a progressive and debilitating disease that is accompanied by congestion of body tissues. Heart failure can develop at any age but clearly becomes more common with increasing age. Around 1% of people under 65 years of age have heart failure, but 7% of 75–84-year-olds have heart failure, and this increases to 15% in people older than 85. It is the most common cause of hospitalisation in patients over 65 years of age. Heart failure is a problem globally, and in the UK, it is estimated that more than half a million people are living with a diagnosis of heart failure (Townsend et al 2015). This accounts for 1–2 % of the total NHS budget annually.

Orange flag

Patient with long-term conditions such as heart failure are at increased risk of depression, and routine psychological screening and interventions should be available to patients and their families and carers.

Snapshot – collapse and breathlessness

Mr Martin Goldsmith, a 58-year-old married man with two children, collapsed whilst walking his dog. A passer-by went to his aid and called for an ambulance to take him to the local hospital. At the local hospital, Mr Goldsmith was examined by the emergency department nurse practitioner. During the assessment, the nurse practitioner noticed that Mr Goldsmith was breathless with bilateral ankle oedema. Mr Goldsmith refused to lie down and insisted that he would rather sit in the chair. The nurse in charge rang his wife to inform her that her husband had been admitted to the hospital after collapsing on the road. Mrs Goldsmith rang one of her children, and they went immediately to the hospital.

Vital signs

On admission to the emergency department, the following vital signs were noted and recorded:

Vital sign	Observation	Guideline normal values
Temperature	37.8°C	36.0–37.9°C range
Pulse	102 beats per minute	60–100 beats per minute
Respiration	24 breaths per minute	12–20 breaths per minute
Blood pressure	172/110 mmHg	100–139 mmHg (systolic) range
O_2 saturation	94%	94–98 %

A full blood count and urea and electrolytes was performed.

Test	Result	Guideline normal values
White blood cells (WBC)	15×10^9/L	4 to 11×10^9/L
Neutrophils	8.5×10^9/L	2.0 to 7.5×10^9/L
Lymphocytes	5.0×10^9/L	1.3 to 4.0×10^9/L
Red blood cells (RBC)	5.3×10^{12}/L	4.5 to 6.5×10^{12}/L
Haemoglobin (Hb)	158 g/L	130–180 g/L
Platelets	298×10^9/L	150 to 440×10^9/L
C-reactive protein	5.0 mg/L	<5 mg/L
Urea	5.9 mmol/L	2–6.6 mmol/L
Potassium	5.1 mmol/L	3.4–5.6 mmol/L
Sodium	138 mmol/L	135–147 mmol/L
Troponin T	0.01 ng/mL	0.00–0.4 ng/mL

Take some time to reflect on this case and then consider the following:

1. What are the possible reasons why Mr Goldsmith collapsed on the road?
2. What assessments procedures should be carried out to confirm diagnosis?
3. During the assessment, the nurse practitioner noticed that Mr Goldsmith was breathless, and his ankles were swollen. Explain.
4. Discuss the nursing care for Mr Goldsmith in the emergency department.

Aetiology

HF may be caused by a variety of conditions:

- Acute MI and coronary artery disease where there is a loss of myocardial muscle, which can lead to poor contraction
- Cardiomyopathy
- Hypertension
- Valvular heart disease
- Inadequate emptying from the left ventricle due to poor contraction of the myocardium
- Anaemia resulting from reduced red blood cells.

Pathophysiology

The onset of HF may be acute or chronic. It is often associated with systolic and diastolic congestion and with myocardial weakness. This weakness impairs the ability of the heart to pump efficiently. In acute HF, there is a sudden decrease in the amount of blood pumped out from both ventricles, which reduces oxygen supply to the tissues. However, in chronic HF, the progression of the disease is gradual, and in the early stages there may be no symptoms of heart failure.

Investigations

The following investigations may be carried out to confirm diagnosis:

- Electrocardiogram
- Chest X-ray
- Full blood chemistry and troponin T
- N-terminal pro-B-type natriuretic peptide (NT-proBNP) blood test
- Physical examination
- Echocardiogram
- Cardiac MRI
- Transesophageal echocardiogram.

Red flag

NT-proBNP is a diagnostic blood test to diagnose and measure heart failure. The normal values differ according to gender and age.

Clinical investigations

Echocardiograph

Echocardiography is a safe and relatively inexpensive investigation which is commonly used to diagnose heart failure and determine the causation of heart failure. It is a non-invasive procedure using ultrasound waves. There are no known risks from the ultrasound waves. It provides a semi-quantitative assessment of left ventricular systolic and diastolic function, valvular disorders can usually be accurately delineated, and pulmonary artery systolic pressure can be estimated. The limitation of poor image quality due to obesity or lung disease is minimised by the skilled use of modern imaging equipment and up-to-date technology.

Nurses should advise the patient as follows:

- Eat and drink as usual.
- Take all prescribed medications as usual.
- Before the test, the examination will be explained, and questions encouraged.

Pathophysiology of RHF

RHF is associated with the right ventricle's impaired ability to pump the blood to the pulmonary artery and to the lungs. This leads to an increase in volume of the right ventricle during the end-diastolic phase, which causes an increase in volume of the right atria (Bullock and Henze, 2020). This results in an increase in the volume of blood and pressure in the systemic venous system. There is accumulation of blood in some of the major organs: the liver, the kidneys and the spleen (Nowak and Handford, 2010), resulting in hypertrophy of these organs, which can lead to failure.

Signs and symptoms of RHF

- Pitting oedema may be observed in the sacral area of a patient confined to bed, as well as on the feet and legs when the patient is sitting. This is due to the impaired pumping ability of the heart, and as a result fluid accumulates in the tissues, resulting in weight gain.
- Enlargement of the organs such as the liver (hepatomegaly) and the spleen (splenomegaly) can cause pressure on the surrounding organs such as the stomach.
- Pleural effusion may occur due to the increased capillary pressure.
- Distended jugular veins are a visible sign in patients who experience RHF.
- Patients have difficulty in breathing.
- Nausea and anorexia.
- Fatigue.
- Jaundice and coagulation problems may be present due to liver damage.

Pathophysiology of LHF

LHF results from damage to the left ventricular myocardium. The contraction of the left ventricle is ineffective, and it cannot pump out all the blood it receives from the left atrium (Hogan and Hill, 2014). This results in a pooling of blood in the left atrium and raised pressure in the pulmonary veins, which leads to pulmonary oedema. Common symptoms of pulmonary oedema include dyspnoea, orthopnoea, productive cough, frothy sputum and changes in pallor. Failure of the left ventricle results in poor cardiac output. As the cardiac output decreases, perfusion to the tissues also diminishes, resulting in poor delivery of oxygen and nutrients to the tissues (McCance *et al.*, 2017).

LHF (backward effects)
- Emptying of the left ventricle is diminished.
- There is an increase in volume and end-diastolic pressure of the left ventricle.
- Pressure in the left atrium increases.
- Volume and pressure in the pulmonary veins increase.
- Volume of fluid in the pulmonary capillary bed increases.
- Movement of fluid from the lung capillaries to the interstitial space of the alveoli.
- Rapid filling of alveoli spaces with fluid leading to pulmonary oedema.

LHF (forward effects)
- Cardiac output decreases.
- Perfusion to tissues of the body decreases.
- Blood flow to the kidneys and other organs decreases.
- This leads to reabsorption of sodium and water by the kidneys to increase the circulating fluid volume.

Signs and symptoms of LHF
- Patients with LHF may develop dyspnoea in the early stages due to fluid accumulation in the pulmonary capillary bed, resulting in poor exchange of gases (oxygen and carbon dioxide) in the lungs.
- Dizziness, fatigue and weakness due to the poor oxygenation of the body tissues, resulting from the low cardiac output and oxygen saturation. Reduced oxygen travelling to the brain may result in symptoms of dizziness, disorientation, confusion and unconsciousness.
- Orthopnoea – difficulty in breathing in a supine position.
- Peripheral oedema.
- Productive cough and frothy sputum.
- Tachycardia.
- Cyanosis – the bluish discoloration of the mucous membranes around the lips and in the nail bed.
- Wheezing due to bronchospasm.
- Crackles at the lung bases due to pulmonary oedema.

Care and management
In order to provide high-quality care, healthcare professionals need to undertake a full and accurate assessment and to devise a care plan for all the problems identified. Vital signs are monitored regularly, and frequency is individualised according to the patient's condition. Early detection of changes in vital signs and the patient's condition with prompt reporting and treatment may save the patient's life. Key care considerations are the following:

- Patients with HF may experience respiratory symptoms such as breathlessness, especially on exertion. Prescribed oxygen should be administered to improve oxygenation of the blood with close monitoring of oxygen saturations.
- Patients with LHF may expectorate large amounts of frothy sputum due to pulmonary oedema; therefore, they will need access to a sputum mug/carton to expectorate into and tissues and a waste receptacle to dispose of used tissues. Local infection prevention and control procedures must be adhered to.

- The patient should be nursed in the upright position in bed supported by pillows to assist breathing unless contraindicated.
- Accurate monitoring of daily fluid intake and output is important in patients with HF. Output should be in excess of 30 mL/hour (Kozier *et al.*, 2020), and this should be recorded hourly (if a urinary catheter is *in situ*) and any changes in output reported immediately.
- The patient should be encouraged to reduce salt intake in the diet, as salt promotes fluid retention.
- Patients may require assistance with everyday activities.
- All treatment and care must be explained to the patient and family in appropriate terms that will be understood.
- Patients may need aperients to avoid straining when defaecating.

Pharmacological and non-pharmacological treatment

The treatment of HF focuses on treating the signs and symptoms and improving the quality of life and requires self-management techniques. Such measures include the following:

- Moderate physical activity as the condition allows.
- Weight reduction is important through physical activity and healthy eating to reduce BMI.
- Reduction in salt intake is essential, as excessive intake can cause fluid retention and lead to an exacerbation of cardiac problems.
- Patients with HF will need their fluid intake monitored carefully to prevent fluid overload and may be placed on a fluid restriction as directed by for example, their Heart Failure Specialist Nurse.
- Daily weights with any sudden increases in weight reported and documented.

The recommended pharmacological interventions for HF unless otherwise contraindicated include the following:

- ACE inhibitors and beta blockers commenced at a low dose and then titrated until target dose is achieved or tolerated dose is reached. Blood pressure, pulse, urea and electrolytes are measured before and after starting ACE inhibitors and beta blockers, and after each dose increment.
- Diuretics such as furosemide are used to decrease fluid load in patients with HF.
- Anticoagulants and anti-arrhythmia medication will be used in patients with HF with arrhythmias, e.g. atrial fibrillation.

Medicine management

ACE inhibitors

These work by dilating the blood vessels, which makes the blood flow more easily and reduces blood pressure. This makes it easier for the heart to pump blood around the body. ACE inhibitors often have a positive impact on the heart's performance and may improve the quality of life. They reduce the risk of hospitalisation and prolong life.

Some examples of ACE inhibitors include ramipril, captopril, enalapril, lisinopril and perindopril. Nurses need to be aware that ACE inhibitors can excessively lower the blood pressure, and too low a pressure can affect renal function. Regular monitoring and documentation of the blood pressure is essential for patients who are taking ACE inhibitors or other forms of antihypertensives

Devices and procedures

ICDs and resynchronisation therapy for patients with ejection fractions of 35% or less (NICE 2014) to help improve symptoms of HF and prevent sudden death.

Cardiogenic shock

Cardiogenic shock occurs due to the impaired pumping ability of the cardiac muscle. It is a complex physiological state in which inadequate tissue perfusion occurs from failure of the pumping system of the heart. It is a medical emergency, and prognosis for patients with cardiogenic shock is poor, with high mortality rates estimated at 50% (Diehl 2017). Early recognition and treatment of cardiogenic shock in the clinical setting is vital to improve outcomes for patients.

Aetiology

There are numerous causes of cardiogenic shock, but the most common cause is acute MI. The severity of the shock is associated with the extent of the myocardial damage. Low cardiac output due to cardiogenic shock also impairs perfusion of the coronary arteries and the myocardium, thus further increasing myocardial damage. Although MI is the most common cause of cardiogenic shock, several other factors may be implicated:

- Acute pulmonary embolism
- Myocarditis
- Acute mitral valve regurgitation
- Right ventricular infarction
- Septic shock
- Mitral stenosis
- Complications of cardiac surgery
- Valvular heart disease.

Investigations

The following investigations may be carried out to confirm diagnosis:

- Chest X-ray
- ECG
- Arterial blood gas analysis
- Full blood chemistry
- Cardiac enzymes, e.g. troponin
- Echocardiogram
- Cardiac perfusion scan

Pathophysiology

Cardiogenic shock results from the diminished ability of the heart to function effectively. In MI, cardiogenic shock usually develops when approximately 40% of the myocardium is damaged. This leads to decreased blood pressure, poor cardiac output and inadequate perfusion to the tissues (Peate 2019). The sympathetic nervous system's response is to increase the heart rate and induce vasoconstriction. This causes unwanted stress on the heart, which results in further damage to the cardiac muscle, leading to poor cardiac output and hypotension, and it becomes a vicious cycle of cardiogenic shock (Figure 8.9). Poor cardiac output reduces blood flow to essential body organs, thus affecting their functions. The

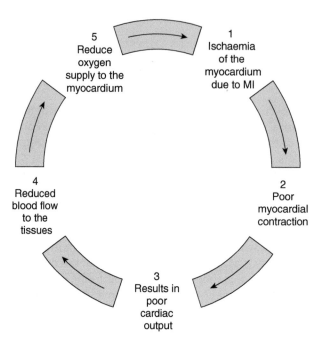

Figure 8.9 Vicious cycle of cardiogenic shock.

sympathetic stimulation also causes decreased renal blood flow, which could lead to acute renal failure.

As the perfusion to the tissues is reduced, the peripheral cells utilise anaerobic metabolism to produce energy. Anaerobic metabolism is the process in which cells use carbohydrates to produce energy in the absence of oxygen. The effect of this energy production is to keep the cells functioning; however, the production of lactic acid leads to metabolic acidosis, which in turn depresses cardiac function.

Signs and symptoms

Signs and symptoms of cardiogenic shock include the following:

- Pulmonary oedema
- Severe hypotension
- Oliguria/anuria
- Pale and cold skin
- Raised jugular venous pressure
- Chest pain
- Nausea and vomiting
- Dyspnoea
- Profuse sweating
- Confusion/disorientation.

Care and management

Patients in cardiogenic shock will require precise and immediate care and management; if the condition is not treated immediately, it could lead to severe complications and the death of the patient. The priority in the management of cardiogenic shock is to prevent further damage to the myocardium:

- Maintaining a clear airway and monitoring respiration is important in patients with cardiogenic shock. Health professionals should observe the patient for signs of restlessness, breathlessness, dyspnoea and confusion. Oxygen must be administered as prescribed either by nasal cannula or a Ventimask.
- Patients in cardiogenic shock and their relatives are very anxious and frightened. They will need support and reassurance from healthcare professionals.
- Vital signs must be monitored hourly, and they include temperature, heart rate, blood pressure, capillary refill test, oxygen saturation and respiratory rate. Any changes in the vital signs must be reported immediately to allow prompt action to be taken.
- Health professionals must observe the effectiveness of drugs administered and report any side effects.

Pharmacological interventions
Some of the medications include:

- Analgesia for pain relief
- Antihypertensive drugs to treat hypertension and decrease effort on the heart
- Diuretics to decrease fluid load
- Inotropic drugs to increase contractibility and increase cardiac contractibility.

Angina

Angina is characterised by chest pain that occurs when the heart muscle does not receive enough oxygenated blood. It can described as a crushing pain, a tightness or a sharp pain in the chest. The pain can radiate through to the back and shoulder, or to one or both arms, into the neck and jaw. The description of pain and symptoms differ from individual to individual.

Investigations
These include the following:

- Physical examination
- Medical history
- ECG
- Full blood analysis to include haemoglobin, urea and electrolytes and lipid profile
- Stress test
- Angiogram
- Echocardiogram
- Stress perfusion cardiac magnetic imaging

Pathophysiology
Angina pain closely resembles the signs and symptoms of MI; thus, it is vital that healthcare professions are able to differentiate between the two conditions, as the treatment differs in both cases. Angina pain can often respond positively and be relieved by vasodilators, e.g. GTN.

Angina results from a narrowing in the coronary arteries, which reduces blood supply to the affected part of the heart muscle (Figure 8.10). At rest the blood supply may be sufficient

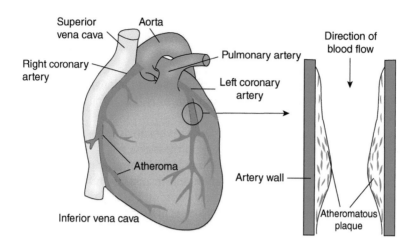

Figure 8.10   Blockage of the coronary arteries.

to provide nutrients and oxygen to the heart muscle; however, during activity, e.g. walking or running, or emotional distress, the heart rate increases, which puts more strain on the heart. During exertion, if the blood flow to the heart muscle is inadequate, the oxygen supply is also diminished, leading to anginal pain. Angina symptoms may also be precipitated by cold weather or after eating a heavy meal. The patient may present with dyspnoea, cyanosis, diaphoresis and tachycardia (Adams *et al.*, 2019).

Types of angina

There are three types of angina:

1. Stable angina
2. Unstable angina
3. Variant angina.

Stable angina is the most common type, and it occurs on exertion when there is a greater demand has been placed. It is estimated that almost 2 million people in England currently have or have had angina (NICE 2016). Stable angina is mainly caused by myocardial ischaemia. The pain usually lasts about 3–5 minutes. If the blood flow is restored by immediate treatment, no permanent damage results (McCance *et al.*, 2017).

Unstable angina (also known as crescendo angina) is characterised by a change in the frequency, intensity and duration of pain. It is more serious than stable angina and is unpredictable. It can also occur when the person is at rest, and it is not relieved by rest or medication. Patients who develop unstable angina are at risk of having an MI (Hogan *et al.*, 2014).

Red flag

Most cases of angina are caused by atherosclerosis, which is the hardening and narrowing of arteries as a result of a build-up of fatty substances known as plaques. This can restrict the blood supply to the heart and trigger the symptoms of angina. Advanced age, ethnicity, family history of heart disease, hypertension, hypercholesteremia, diabetes mellitus, stress, smoking, obesity and high alcohol intake and sedentary lifestyles all increase the risk of developing atherosclerosis.

Variant angina is a rare form of angina. It is thought to occur as a result of coronary artery vasospasm, resulting in diminished blood flow. Variant angina is very painful and occurs from midnight to early morning. It usually occurs at rest and at the same time each day (Hogan *et al.*, 2014).

Signs and symptoms
- Crushing pain in the chest
- Pain radiates to arms, jaw, neck and back
- Shortness of breath on exercise
- Sweating
- Light-headedness
- Hypotension
- Irregular pulse
- Indigestion.

Care and management
Healthcare professionals play a vital role in the management of patients with angina. An accurate assessment of the patient must be carried out to ascertain the location, duration and intensity of the pain. Risk factors must be identified to provide high-quality care. The care will include:

- Controlling pain
- Reducing anxiety
- Advising the patient on the possible risks and preventative measures
- Providing health promotion and education.

Non-pharmacological interventions
- Secondary prevention and modification of risk factors through a healthy lifestyle is recommended.
- Dietary counselling to encourage a cardioprotective diet should be available. This will help lower cholesterol and lower body mass index.
- Encourage the patient to engage in moderate intensity cardiovascular exercise such as walking and swimming, as physical activity aids circulation and improves cardiac and respiratory function unless contraindicated.
- Patients who are overweight should be encouraged to lose weight through individual programmes of diet and physical activity, unless contraindicated, to reach their target body mass index.
- Advice on the excessive alcohol consumption and smoking cessation should be offered, as these are risk factors associated with cardiac problems.
- Regular monitoring of blood pressure, cholesterol, waist circumference and body mass index is advised.

Pharmacological interventions
Anti-anginal medications are recommended plus medications for secondary prevention of cardiovascular disease. Registered healthcare professionals who administer medicines, or when appropriate delegate the administration of medicines, are accountable for their actions, non-actions and omissions, and exercise professionalism and professional judgement at all times (Royal Pharmaceutical Society and Royal College of Nursing 2019).

The following medications could be prescribed for angina:

- GTN is administered as tablets (sublingual), intravenous, patches and spray. It is a quick-acting anti-anginal medicine that dilates blood vessels and improves blood flow.
- First-line treatment of beta blockers or calcium channel blockers are recommended for angina patients.
- All patients with stable angina due to atherosclerotic disease should receive long-term standard aspirin and statin therapy.

Other treatments such as bypass surgery and balloon angioplasty may be performed if the medications are ineffective in controlling the angina or if the condition becomes progressively worse.

Conclusion

The overall aim of this chapter is to provide the reader with an insight into conditions related to the heart. In order to help patients with cardiac problems, healthcare professionals need an in-depth knowledge of the normal anatomy and physiology of the heart to allow them to recognise the related dysfunctions and to provide the appropriate care. There are numerous conditions associated with the heart, and it is not the remit of this chapter to address all of them. Some of the common conditions were discussed, along with their associated care and management.

Healthcare professionals are often in the forefront in delivering high-quality care for patients with cardiac problems, and it is their duty to ensure that they have a sound knowledge base and are confident of delivering safe and effective individualised care in both hospital and community settings. Therefore, they need to recognise various signs and symptoms quickly and take immediate action to prevent any further complications arising from the illness. Ongoing assessment and evaluation of interventions are important in order to respond to the changing requirements of the patient, which may have implications for patient outcomes.

Test your knowledge

1. How does the heart rate affect the cardiac output?
2. Explain the differences between ischaemia and infarction.
3. Explain how the backward effect causes pulmonary oedema.
4. Define cardiogenic shock and list the possible causes.
5. What advice would you give a patient with congestive heart failure?

Activities

Here are some activities and exercises to help test your learning. For the answers to these exercises, as well as further self-testing activities, visit our website at **www.wiley.com/go/fundamentalsofappliedpathophysiology/student4e**

Multiple choice questions

1. The heart is positioned . . . . to the sternum
   (a) Lateral
   (b) Anterior
   (c) Posterior
   (d) Vertical
2. The heart consists of three layers of specialised heart muscle.
   (a) Myocardium
   (b) Pericardium
   (c) Skeletal
   (d) Endocardium

3. The heart is divided into two sides by a muscular wall called the
   (a) Ventricular wall
   (b) Pulmonary artery
   (c) Septum
   (d) Mitral valve
4. The right side of the heart receives deoxygenated blood from .
   (a) Inferior vena cava
   (b) Superior vena cava
   (c) Coronary arteries
   (d) Atrioventricular node
5. The SA node is also known as the
   (a) Cardiac output
   (b) Pacemaker
   (c) Bicuspid valve
   (d) Left ventricle
6. A 12-lead ECG measures
   (a) The electrical activity in the heart
   (b) Rate of the heart
   (c) Rhythm of the heart
   (d) Respiration rate
7. Risk factors for heart disease include
   (a) Hypertension
   (b) Ethnicity
   (c) Hypercholesterolemia
   (d) Diabetes mellitus
8. Common symptoms of heart failure include
   (a) Ankle swelling
   (b) Orthopnoea
   (c) Hypoglycaemia
   (d) Anxiety
9. Which of the following blood tests are used to diagnose a myocardial infarction?
   (a) Glucose
   (b) Haemoglobin
   (c) Troponin
   (d) White blood count

10. Coronary angiogram is an invasive procedure used to
    (a) Assess the blood flow in the coronary arteries
    (b) Assess the site and severities of any narrowing or blockages in the coronary arteries
    (c) To decide on appropriate treatment e.g angioplasty or coronary artery bypass
    (d) To treat electrolyte imbalances
11. Symptoms of stable angina can be exacerbated by
    (a) Physical exertion
    (b) Eating a heavy meeting
    (c) Strong emotional responses e.g. excitement or anxiety
    (d) Cold weather
12. Angiotensin-converting enzyme inhibitors (ACE inhibitors) can have an adverse effect on
    (a) Blood pressure
    (b) Temperature
    (c) Renal function
    (d) Body mass index
13. N-T pro BNP is used to diagnose
    (a) Valvular disease
    (b) Heart failure
    (c) Peripheral vascular disease
    (d) Angina
14. Cardiogenic shock occurs due to
    (a) Impaired pumping ability of the heart
    (b) Stenosis of the atrial valve
    (c) Hypoglycaemia
    (d) Hyperthyroidism
15. Raised jugular venous pressure (JVP) can be seen in the
    (a) Groin area
    (b) Radial area
    (c) Neck
    (d) Pedal area of the foot

Further resources

BUPA
http://www.bupa.co.uk/individuals/health-information/directory/h/heartfailure
This is a useful website for students to browse for health-related topics. Like the NHS Choice site, it gives a quick overview of health-related topics.

British Heart Foundation
www.bhf.org is a national charity that has useful resources and information for health professionals and patients.

National Institute for Health and Care Excellence (NICE)
https://www.nice.org.uk/guidance
Here students should find evidence-based guidelines related to healthcare issues, such as heart failure, pharmacology and care in the community.

NHS Choices
http://www.nhs.uk/conditions/heart-failure/Pages/Introduction.aspx
Students will find this NHS website useful. This site discusses heart failure, symptoms, causes, diagnosis, treatment and prevention

Department of Health and Social Care– Policy, guidance and publications for NHS and social care professionals

https://www.gov.uk/government/organisations/department-of-health-and-social-care
This is a useful website for students and healthcare professionals to browse. Policy, guidance and publications for NHS and social care professionals can be found on this website.

NHS Choices

http://www.nhs.uk/conditions/Angina/Pages/Introduction.aspx Accessed 25/07/2020.
Students will find this NHS website useful. This site discusses angina, symptoms, causes, diagnosis, treatment and prevention.

Pumping marvellous

https://pumpingmarvellous.org is a resource for both heart failure patients and professionals working with patients with heart failure or who have a special interest in this area

Glossary of terms

Aetiology   The cause of a disease.

Alveolar sac   A small sac structure in the lungs where gas exchange takes place.

Anaerobic metabolism   Metabolism by the body cells in the absence of oxygen.

Angiogram   An invasive investigation to detect narrowings and blockages in the coronary arteries.

Antidiuretic hormone   A protein hormone produced in the hypothalamus and stored in the posterior pituitary gland; it aids reabsorption of water by the kidneys.

Artery   A blood vessel that carries blood away from the heart.

Ascites   Accumulation of fluid in the peritoneal cavity.

Atherosclerosis   A condition where cholesterol and lipid deposits accumulate on the inner layer of the medium and large blood vessels, leading to narrowing of these vessels.

Atheromatous plaque   A collection of lipids and cholesterol that accumulates in large- and medium-sized vessels.

Atria   The upper chambers of the heart.

Atrioventricular valve   A heart valve made up of membranous flaps that allow blood to flow in one direction only: also known as the bicuspid valve.

Atrioventricular node   A component of the electrical conduction system that connects the atria and ventricles.

Automated implantable cardioverter defibrillator (AICD)   An implanted devise with the ability to cardiovert, defibrillate and act as a pacemaker.

Bicuspid valve   As its name suggests, it contains two cusps: also known as the atrioventricular valve.

Bronchospasm   Constriction of the walls of the bronchi.

Cardiac magnetic resonance imaging (CMR)   A non-invasive investigation that uses magnetic fields and radiofrequency pulses to assess the function and structures of the heart.

Cardiac output   The amount of blood the heart pumps in 1 minute; it is calculated by multiplying the heart rate and the stroke volume.

Coronary arteries   Supply oxygenated blood to the heart muscle.

Collagen   A protein that is the main organic component of connective tissues.

Dyspnoea   Shortness of breath; laboured breathing.

Echocardiogram   An ultrasound scan that measures the function and structure of the heart.

Electrocardiogram   Records the electrical activity of the heart

Endocardium   The endothelial membrane that lines the inner surface of the heart.

Hypertrophy   An increase in muscle mass.

Inferior vena cava   The large vein that returns oxygen-depleted blood from all parts of the body below the diaphragm to the right atrium.

Interstitial space   The space between the cells.

Intracellular space   The space found within the cell.

Lactic acid   The product of anaerobic metabolism, especially in the muscle.

Mediastinum   A subdivision of the thoracic cavity.

Medulla oblongata   The lowest portion of the brain; concerned with the control of internal organs.

Mitral valve   The left atrioventricular valve.

Molecule   A particle containing two or more atoms joined together by chemical bonds.

Myocardial infarction   Death of an area of heart muscle due to an interruption of the blood supply to the affected area.

Myocardium   The middle layer of the heart.

National Early Warning Score (NEWS)   A scoring system to improve the detection on acutely ill patients based on assessment of vital signs.

Natriuretic Peptide Test (NT-proBNP)   Measure the levels of NT-proBNP in the blood used to diagnose heart failure

Oliguria   Deficient secretion of urine; less than 30 mL per hour.

Orthopnoea   Difficulty in breathing unless in an upright position.

Pacemaker   The sinoatrial node.

Parasympathetic nerve   A division of the autonomic nervous system.

Parietal   Pertaining to the walls of a cavity.

Pericardium   A double-layered sac that encloses the heart.

Pericarditis   Infection of the pericardium.

Pulmonary artery   The vessel that takes oxygen-depleted blood from the right ventricle to the lungs.

Pulmonary circulation   The flow of blood from the right ventricle to the lungs.

Pulmonary oedema   The abnormal collection of fluid in the tissue space and the alveolar sac.

Pulmonary vein   The vessel that returns oxygenated blood from the lungs to the left atrium.

Semilunar valve   A valve that prevents the backflow of blood to the ventricles after contraction.

Septum   A wall dividing the two cavities.

Sinoatrial node   Also known as the pacemaker of the heart.

Superior vena cava   The large vein that returns oxygen-depleted blood superior to the diaphragm to the right atrium.

Sympathetic nerve   A division of the autonomic nervous system.

Systemic circulation   The flow of blood from the left ventricle to all parts of the body.

Tissue perfusion   Blood flow through the body tissues and organs.

Transesophageal Echo   An ultrasound of the heart where a probe is inserted into the oesophagus which allows for detailed examination of the heart.

Tricuspid valve   The right atrioventricular valve.

Troponin   A protein found in the fibres of cardiac and skeletal muscle and blood levels are used to detect cardiac injury

Vasoconstriction A decrease in the diameter of a blood vessel due to the relaxation of smooth muscle in the vessel wall; may occur as a result of hormones or after stimulation of the **vasomotor centre leading to increased peripheral resistance.**

Ventricle The two larger lower cavities of the heart.

References

Adams, M.P., Holland, L.N. and Urban, C. (2019). *Pharmacology for Nurses: A Pathophysiologic Approach*, 6th edn. New Jersey: Pearson Prentice Hall.

Bullock, B.A. and Henze, R.L. (2020). *Focus on Pathophysiology*. Philadelphia: Lippincott.

Diehl, A. (2017). Ischaemic cardiogenic shock. *Anaesthesia and Intensive Care Medicine*, 18(3), 122–125.

Gu, G., Zhou, Y., Zhang Y. *et al.* (2016). Increased prevalence of anxiety and depression symptoms in patients with coronary artery disease before and after percutaneous coronary intervention treatment. *BMC Psychiatry*, 16: 259.

Hogan, M., Gingrich, M., Hill, K., Scialdo, T. and Wolf, L. (2014). *Pathophysiology: Reviews and Rationales*, 3rd edn. Upper Saddle River, NJ: Pearson Education, Inc. http://www.heart.org/HEARTORG/Conditions/HeartAttack/WarningSignsofaHeartAttack/Heart-Attack-Symptoms-in-Women_UCM_436448_Article.jsp. Accessed 25/07/2020.

Knight, J., Nigam, Y. and Cutter, J. (2020). *Understanding Anatomy and Physiology in Nursing*. London: Sage, pp. 47–82.

Kozier, B., Erb, G., Berman, A., Snyder, S.J., Harvey, S. and Morgan Samuel, H. (2020). *Fundamentals of Nursing. Concepts, Processes and Practice*, 11th edn. Harlow: Pearson Education.

LeMone, P., Burke, K. and Bauldoff, G. (2015). *Medical – Surgical Nursing; Critical Thinking in Client Care*, 6th edn. New Jersey: Pearson.

Marieb, E.N. and Hoehn, K. (2018). *Human Anatomy and Physiology*, 11th edn. San Francisco: Pearson Benjamin Cummings.

McCance, K.L., Huether, S.E., Brashers, V.L. and Rote, N.S. (2017). *Pathophysiology: The Biologic Basis for Disease in Adults and Children*, 8th edn. St Louis: Mosby.

Nair, M. and Peate, I. (2017). *Fundamentals of Applied Pathophysiology: An Essential Guide for Nursing and Healthcare Students*, 3rd edn. Chichester, UK: John Wiley & Sons, p. 120.

NICE (2014). https://www.nice.org.uk/guidance/cg187/chapter/1-Recommendations#mechanical-assist-devices Accessed 25/07/2020.

NICE (2016). https://www.nice.org.uk/guidance/cg126/chapter/Introduction Accessed 25/07/2020.

Nowak, J. and Handford, A.G. (2010). *Essentials of Pathophysiology: Concepts and Applications for Health Care Professionals*, 3rd edn. Boston: McGraw-Hill.

Nursing and Midwifery Council (2018). *The Code. Professional Standards of Practice and Behaviour for Nurses and Midwives*. http://www.nmc.org.uk/globalassets/siteDocuments/NMC-Publications/revised-new-NMC-Code.pdf Accessed 04/07/2020.

Peate, I. (2019) *Alexander's Nursing Practice, Hospital and Home*, 5th edn. Edinburgh: Churchill Livingstone.

Porth, C.M. (2018). *Pathophysiology: Concepts of Altered Health States*, 10th edn. Philadelphia: Lippincott Williams & Wilkins.

Rodriquez, E.R., Tan, C.D. (2017). Structure and anatomy of the human pericardium. *Progress in Cardiovascular Disease*, 59(4): 327–340.

Royal College of Physicians. (2017). *National Early Warning Score (NEWS) 2: Standardising the Assessment of Acute-Illness Severity in the NHS*. Updated report of a working party. London: RCP. https://www.rpharms.com/Portals/0/RPS%20document%20library/Open%20access/Professional%20standards/SSHM%20and%20Admin/Admin%20of%20Meds%20prof%20guidance.pdf?ver=2019-01-23-145026-567. Accessed 05/07/2020.

Scottish Intercollegiate Guidelines Network (SIGN). *Risk Estimation and the Prevention of Cardiovascular Disease*. Edinburgh: SIGN; 2017. (SIGN publication number 149). Available from url: http:// www.sign.ac.uk/sign-149-risk-estimation-and-the-prevention-ofcardiovascular-disease.html Accessed 05/07/2020

Tortora, G.J. and Derrickson, B. (2016). *Principles of Anatomy and Physiology*, 15th edn. New Jersey: John Wiley & Sons.

Townsend, N., Bhatnagar, P., Wilkins, E., Wickramasinghe, K. and Rayner, M. (2015). *Cardiovascular Disease Statistics*. London: British Heart Foundation (available at https://www.bhf.org.uk/publications/statistics/cvd-stats-2015). Accessed on 24/07/2020.

Waugh, A. and Grant, A. (2018). *Ross and Wilson Anatomy and Physiology in Health and Illness*, 13th edn. Edinburgh: Elsevier.

Chapter 9

The vascular system and associated disorders

Jim Blanchflower[1] and Ian Peate[2]

[1]Senior Lecturer, University of Salford, Manchester, UK

[2]Principal, School of Health Studies, Gibraltar

Contents

Introduction 218
Overview of blood vessels 218
Structure of the blood vessels 219
Blood pressure...224
Diseases of the blood vessels........................224
Conclusion 245

Test your knowledge...246
Multiple choice questions...............................246
Conditions...248
Further resources..248
Glossary of terms..249
References..250

Key words

- Arteries
- Arterioles
- Tunica media
- Vasodilatation
- Veins
- Venules
- Tunica intima
- Vasoconstriction
- Capillaries
- Tunica externa
- Aorta

Fundamentals of Applied Pathophysiology: An Essential Guide for Nursing and Healthcare Students, Fourth Edition. Edited by Ian Peate.
© 2021 John Wiley & Sons Ltd. Published 2021 by John Wiley & Sons Ltd.
Student companion website: www.wiley.com/go/fundamentalsofappliedpathophysiology/student4e
Instructor companion website: www.wiley.com/go/fundamentalsofappliedpathophysiology/instructor4e

Test your prior knowledge

- List three differences between arteries and veins.
- Which has a greater volume of blood – arteries or veins?
- Describe the main differences between the systemic and pulmonary circulation.
- List the physiological factors that affect blood pressure.
- Discuss the common disorders of the vascular system.

Learning outcomes

On completion of this section, the reader will be able to:

- Describe the structures of the arteries, veins and capillaries.

- List some of the differences between an artery and a vein.

- Describe how venous valves function?

- Describe the factors controlling blood vessel diameter.

- Explain the microcirculation of the blood.

Don't forget to visit the companion website for this book (www.wiley.com/go/fundamentalsofappliedpathophysiology/student4e) **where you can find self-assessment tests to check your progress, as well as lots of activities to practise your learning.**

Introduction

Although the heart is the principal organ that pumps blood to the whole body, it is the blood vessels that transport blood throughout the system (Figure 9.1). As the blood flows through the arterial system, it transports nutrients and other substances essential for cellular metabolism and for homeostatic regulation. The waste products of metabolism are transported by the venous system for removal by the kidneys, lungs and skin. This chapter discusses the structure and functions of the blood vessels, factors affecting blood pressure, and vascular disorders and their related care.

Overview of blood vessels

In the human body, there are several kinds of blood vessels. Arteries and arterioles are the vessels that convey blood away from the heart. They transport oxygen-rich (oxygenated) blood, except the pulmonary arteries, which carry oxygen-depleted blood. Veins and venules carry blood towards the heart and transport oxygen-depleted (deoxygenated) blood, except the pulmonary veins, which carry oxygenated blood. Capillaries are the minute blood vessels in between the arterial system and the venous system. They form a delicate network of vessels and are in close proximity to most parts of the body tissues. Blood vessels can dilate, constrict, pulsate and form a closed delivery system for the blood which begins and ends at the heart.

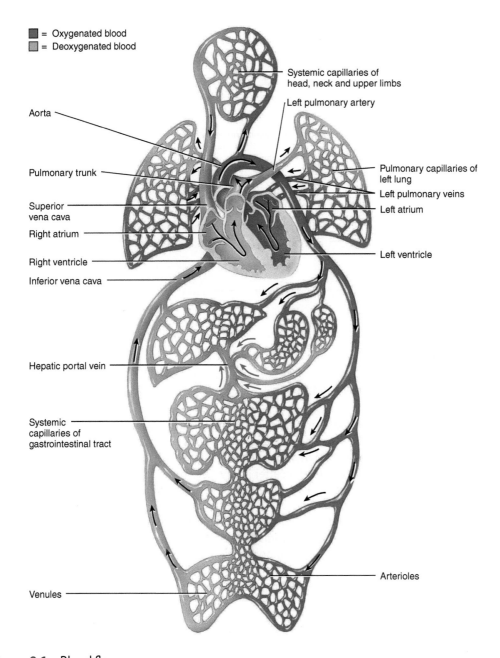

Key:
= Oxygenated blood
= Deoxygenated blood

Systemic capillaries of head, neck and upper limbs

Left pulmonary artery

Aorta

Pulmonary trunk

Pulmonary capillaries of left lung

Left pulmonary veins

Superior vena cava

Left atrium

Right atrium

Right ventricle

Left ventricle

Inferior vena cava

Hepatic portal vein

Systemic capillaries of gastrointestinal tract

Arterioles

Venules

Figure 9.1 Blood flow.

Structure of the blood vessels

Blood vessels, with the exception of the capillaries, are composed of three distinct layers (Marieb and Hoehn, 2019) and a central lumen through which blood flows (Figure 9.2). The outer layer is called the tunica externa, formally known as the tunica adventitia. It is largely composed of collagen fibres that protect and support the blood vessels, and secure them to the surrounding tissues. The tunica externa is supplied with sympathetic nerve fibres and lymphatic vessels; the larger veins are also supplied with elastic fibres (Jenkins and Tortora, 2019).

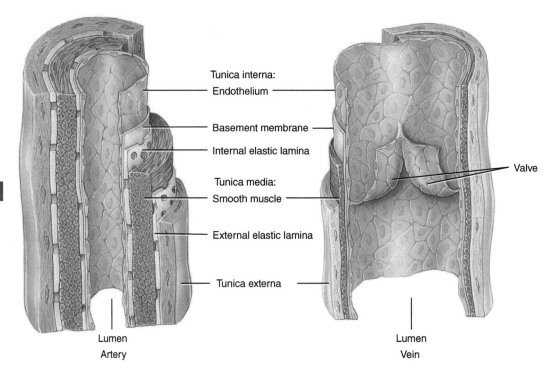

Tunica interna:
Endothelium

Basement membrane

Internal elastic lamina

Tunica media:
Smooth muscle

External elastic lamina

Tunica externa

Valve

Lumen
Artery

Lumen
Vein

Figure 9.2   Structures of an artery and a vein.

The tunica externa is involved in healing after injury, immunity and maintenance of vascular tone. A variety of special cell types are located in this structure to provide these effects. Macrophages, lymphocytes and dendritic cells are involved in immune function. Stem cells and fibroblasts are involved in healing after injury. Cells originating from the tunica externa have been shown to migrate to the tunica media and tunica intima during repair after vessel damage (McCance *et al*., 2018).

The tunica media is the middle layer, and it contains smooth muscle and elastic tissue. The sympathetic nervous system (SNS) also innervates the smooth muscle layer and controls the diameter of the blood vessel. As the blood vessels constrict or dilate, the blood pressure increases or decreases, respectively. The inner layer is called the tunica interna, and it is lined with endothelium. This lining makes the inner surface smooth, thus minimising friction as the blood flows through the vessel.

The endothelium that lines all of the vessels, and makes up the main part of the capillary wall, also has many more dynamic functions. Endothelium is involved in both coagulation and antithrombosis, as well as fibrinolysis, immune function, vasodilation or constriction, tissue growth and wound healing. In particular, the endothelium is involved in a delicate balance between coagulation and anticoagulation as a result of the production of many chemical mediators. Some of these cause vasodilation, such as prostacyclin, NO and endothelium-derived relaxing factor, and some cause vasoconstriction, such as endothelin, angiotensin II and thromboxane. Prostacyclin also reduces platelet adherence, balancing the activity of thromboxane, which increases platelet adherence. The balance between coagulation and anticoagulation relies on the health of the endothelium. A healthy intact endothelium tends towards anticoagulation, but, if damaged, the balance switches in favour of the production of clots. This arrangement generally works well with clots forming where blood vessels are damaged, thus preventing blood loss and enabling the repair process to begin. However, in some conditions where diffuse endothelial damage occurs, such as sepsis, this can lead to the formation of many thrombi, a condition known as disseminated intravascular coagulation (DIC) (McCance *et al.*, 2018).

Although the role of the blood vessels is to transport blood, the tunica externa of the large blood vessels receives its blood supply via a network of blood vessels called the vasa vasorum. Branching from the vessel itself or nearby vessels, it provides nutrients and oxygen, and also removes waste. Vessels with thin walls receive oxygen and nutrients by diffusion from the blood passing through the lumen.

Arteries

Arteries can be subdivided into three groups: elastic arteries, muscular arteries and arterioles. Elastic arteries are thick-walled vessels found near the heart. The aorta is an example of an elastic artery. It is the main artery supplying the systemic circulation from the left ventricle. These vessels contain a high proportion of elastic fibres in the tunica media. Their larger lumen provides low resistance to blood flow. The elastic walls distend when they are filled with blood and then recoil, thus propelling blood onwards (Figure 9.3). This ensures that the blood is moving

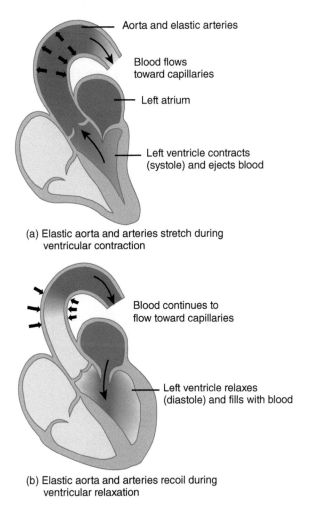

Aorta and elastic arteries

Blood flows
toward capillaries

Left atrium

Left ventricle contracts
(systole) and ejects blood

(a) Elastic aorta and arteries stretch during
ventricular contraction

Blood continues to
flow toward capillaries

Left ventricle relaxes
(diastole) and fills with blood

(b) Elastic aorta and arteries recoil during
ventricular relaxation

Figure 9.3   Elastic recoil of the aorta.

forwards, even though the left ventricle is relaxed. As these arteries conduct blood from the left ventricle to the small arteries, they are sometimes referred to as conducting arteries.

From the elastic arteries, the blood flows into the medium-sized arteries, called the muscular arteries. They contain more smooth muscle and fewer elastic fibres; therefore, they are capable of greater vasoconstriction and vasodilatation. Muscular arteries are also called distributing arteries because they distribute blood to specific organs and parts of the body. Their potential for dilating or constricting allows blood to be distributed to whichever organs are most in need at any given time. They include the axillary, brachial, radial, splenic, femoral, popliteal and tibial arteries.

The muscular arteries then divide into smaller arteries called the arterioles, and these play an important role in determining the amount of blood flowing into organs and tissues. Arterioles branch into smaller arterioles and then into metacapillaries, and direct the flow of blood into the capillaries (Figure 9.4). Larger arterioles have all the three layers, but the tunica media mainly consists of smooth muscle with a few elastic fibres, whilst the metacapillaries near the capillary end are composed of endothelial cells and an incomplete layer of smooth muscle (McCance *et al.*, 2018). Arterioles regulate the blood flow into the capillaries by altering the diameter of the capillaries. When they constrict, blood flow is diverted from the organs or tissue they supply. On the other hand, blood flow increases dramatically when the arterioles dilate.

Capillaries

Capillaries are the smallest network of blood vessels, with walls that are mostly one-cell thick. They connect the arteriole to the venule (see Figure 9.1). The thin walls of the

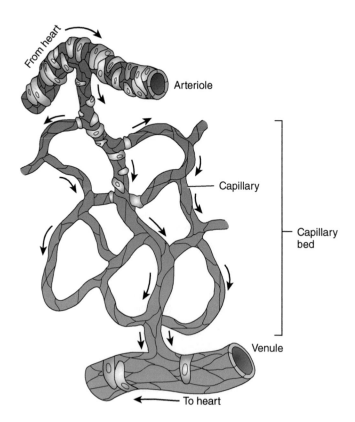

Figure 9.4   Capillaries.

capillaries allow water, nutrients, gases and waste products of metabolism to move in and out of the blood and to nearby cells (Jenkins and Tortora, 2019). Capillaries are composed of a single layer of tunica intima, which is a single layer of endothelial cells attached to the basement membrane. They are found throughout the body, except the epidermis of the skin and the cornea of the eye. Capillaries merge to form venules (see Figure 9.4).

Blood flow into some capillaries can be controlled by tiny circular bands of smooth muscle called precapillary sphincters. There are three main types of capillary: continuous, sinusoid and fenestrated. Sinusoid capillaries are found in the liver and bone marrow. Fenestrated capillaries are responsible for filtration in the glomeruli of the kidneys. Continuous capillaries are found in most tissues and are the most common type (McCance *et al.*, 2018).

Venules

Blood flows from the capillaries to the venules (see Figure 9.4). The smallest venules are mainly composed of endothelium and a few fibroblast cells. The venules are extremely porous and therefore will allow substances such as water, solutes and white blood cells to move in and out of the vessel into the extracellular fluid.

Veins

Venules unite to form veins, and they contain the same three layers as the arteries. The walls of the veins, compared to the arteries, are thinner and contain less elastic and collagenous tissue and smooth muscle. The lumen of the veins is larger compared to the lumen of the arteries. Veins become larger and less branched as they move away from the capillaries and towards the heart. Some veins, most commonly those in the lower extremities, contain paired semilunar bicuspid valves (Figure 9.5) that allow blood flow only towards the heart. Like arteries, veins receive their nourishment from tiny blood vessels called vasa vasorum (McCance *et al.*, 2018).

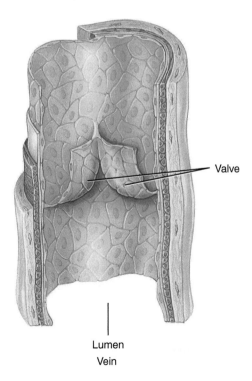

Valve

Lumen

Vein

Figure 9.5   Bicuspid valves of a vein.

Blood pressure

Blood pressure (BP) refers to the force exerted by the circulating blood on the walls of the blood vessel. As the blood moves through the arteries, arterioles, capillaries, venules and veins, the BP drops, and thus BP refers to arterial BP; it is usually measured in the larger arteries. BP fluctuates during the day, and depends on the state of health of the individual. BP is low when the person is sleeping at night and increases as the person wakes in the morning. There are three main factors that regulate BP:

1. Neuronal regulation
2. Hormonal regulation
3. Autoregulation of BP.

Neuronal regulation of BP is achieved via a negative feedback system, which includes baroreceptors and chemoreceptors. The baroreceptors are located in the carotid sinus and the aortic arch, and they are sensitive to arterial BP changes. The chemoreceptors are located in the aortic and carotid bodies. These bodies detect changes in oxygen, carbon dioxide and hydrogen ion concentrations. There are several hormones involved in the regulation of BP, which include the hormones of the renin–angiotensin–aldosterone system, epinephrine (adrenaline) and norepinephrine (noradrenaline), antidiuretic hormone and atrial natriuretic peptide.

Factors that can affect BP

Several factors affect BP:

- Cardiac output, which is a function of heart rate and stroke volume
- Circulating blood volume
- Peripheral resistance, which depends on the degree of constriction of blood vessels
- Blood viscosity, which is most commonly affected by the ratio of red blood cells to plasma.
- Hydrostatic pressure

Other factors that can affect BP include age, gender, stress, hormones and drugs.

Diseases of the blood vessels

On completion of this section, the reader will be able to:

- List some of the common diseases of the blood vessels and the risk factors associated with these diseases.
- Describe the pathophysiological responses associated with specific vascular health problems.
- List the possible investigations.
- Outline the care and management and interventions related to the disorders described.

Snapshot   Leg ulcer

Mrs Carly Symmons is a 66-year-old widow who lives in a first-floor flat. She used to work in the local supermarket as a cashier but is now retired. She suffers from type 2 diabetes, which is controlled by diet and tablets. She is overweight and smokes approximately 30 cigarettes per day but does not drink any alcohol.

Mrs Symmons has a small ulcer on her left ankle, which she cared for herself, but lately has noticed that the ulcer is weeping and she had pains in her left leg. Mrs Symmons made an appointment to see her GP. Her GP, after examining her foot, decided to refer her to the vascular surgeon at the local hospital.

Vital signs

The practice nurse notes and records the following vital signs:

Vital sign	Observation	Normal
Temperature	38.6°C	36.0–37.9°C range
Pulse	98 beats per minute	60–100 beats per minute
Respiration	24 breaths per minute	12–20 breaths per minute
Blood pressure	140/85 mmHg	100–139 mmHg (systolic) range
O$_2$ saturation:	96%	94–98%

A full blood count and urea and electrolytes was performed.

Test	Result	Guideline normal values
White blood cells (WBC)	12×10^9/L	4 to 11×10^9/L
Neutrophils	7.5×10^9/L	2.0 to 7.5×10^9/L
Lymphocytes	4.5×10^9/L	1.3 to 4.0×10^9/L
Red blood cells (RBC)	6.0×10^{12}/L	4.5 to 6.5×10^{12}/L
Haemoglobin (Hb)	158 g/L	130–180 g/L
Platelets	298×10^9/L	150 to 440×10^9/L
C-reactive protein	5.0 mg/L	<5 mg/L
Urea	6.4 mmol/L	2–6.6 mmol/L
Potassium	5.1 mmol/L	3.4–5.6 mmol/L
Sodium	138 mmol/L	135–147 mmol/L

Take some time to reflect on this case and then consider the following:

1. Discuss the possible causes of Mrs Symmons' leg ulcer.
2. Outline the assessments that you will carry out in order to plan her care.
3. Discuss the possible treatment of her leg ulcer.
4. Discuss the health education/promotion advice that you will offer Mrs Symmons before she is discharged from hospital.

Atherosclerosis/arteriosclerosis

Arteriosclerosis is the term describing arterial disorders in which degenerative changes result in decreased blood flow. Atherosclerosis is the most common form of arteriosclerosis, where there is thickening and hardening of the vessel walls due to lipid accumulation. This condition is found mainly in the large- and medium-sized arteries, such as the aorta and its branches, the coronary arteries and the arteries that supply the brain, whereas arteriosclerosis mainly affects arterioles (Nowak and Handford, 2010).

Aetiology

The cause of atherosclerosis is not known, but certain risk factors have been identified:

- Hypertension
- Cigarette smoking (nicotine has a vasoconstricting effect)

- High lipid levels in the blood – most significantly, low-density lipoproteins (LDL) cholesterol
- Familial history
- Obesity. Linked with production of adipokines; hormones produced by adipose tissue (Lelis *et al.* 2019)
- Diabetes mellitus (high serum glucose levels cause vascular damage)
- Lifestyle
- Alcohol
- Gender (men are at a higher risk than women). Oestrogens have a protective effect, reducing LDL cholesterol by increasing the activity of receptors for apolipoprotein B (apoB100), the docking protein on LDLs (McCance *et al.*, 2018).

Investigations

The following investigations may be carried out to confirm diagnosis:

- Full blood chemistry
- Doppler ultrasound
- Electrocardiogram
- Arteriogram.

Clinical investigations

Arteriogram

This is an invasive procedure. The procedure may take approximately 1–2 hours. Special preparations are necessary when patients undergo this procedure. Healthcare professionals must adhere to their local policies in the preparation and in the safe management of patients undergoing the arteriogram, and offer physical and psychological support.

The skin around the groin area is cleansed with antiseptic. A local anaesthetic is injected around the puncture site in the groin. A needle is then inserted into the artery, and a long fine tube (catheter) is placed in position. The special dye (contrast agent) is then injected through the catheter and X-rays taken.

Once the radiologist is satisfied with the X-rays, the catheter will be removed, and the radiologist will press firmly on the skin over the entry site for 10 minutes until the artery stops bleeding. Once the bleeding has stopped, the patient will be asked to lie still for 1 or 2 hours. Once no bleeding is observed, the patient is escorted to the ward.

After the procedure, the nurse must adhere to local policy and procedure in caring and management of patients who have undergone an arteriogram. Regular inspection of the puncture site is important to ensure that there are no complications such as secondary bleeding, excess pain in the groin area and haematoma. Nurses must report to the nurse in charge immediately, if they observe any of these signs, so that prompt action can be taken.

Red flag

Bleeding is one of the risk factors associated with the arteriogram. Every precaution should be taken to ensure that evidence-based practice is carried out following the arteriogram.

Pathophysiology of atherosclerosis

Atherosclerosis is a form of arteriosclerosis where the walls of the arteries are hard, thick and narrow as a result of lipid accumulation within the arterial walls. Lipids (LDL) are deposited on the tunica intima of the damaged blood vessel, where oxidation of LDL takes place. The oxidised LDL then enters the tunica intima of the arterial wall (Jowett and Thompson, 2007), where they are ingested by macrophages. The lipid-filled macrophages then become foam cells.

The oxidised form of LDL cholesterol exerts a variety of effects:

- Causes damage to endothelial cells, which could disrupt the normal balance between procoagulatory and anticoagulatory activity
- Increases proliferation of smooth muscle, which adds to the bulk of the plaque
- Increases the number of adhesion molecules of endothelial cells. These adhesion molecules allow monocytes to bind to the cells and then enter. Once inside, it is these cells that differentiate to form macrophages (McCance *et al.*, 2018).

Once the foam cells accumulate in significant numbers, they form a lesion called a fatty streak, which over time causes a bulge in the lumen of the blood vessel, and this restricts blood flow. The affected blood vessels become hard, lose their elasticity, restrict blood flow and eventually occlude the artery (Figure 9.6). Greater BP is needed to push the blood through these narrow blood vessels, which leads to hypertension. Although atherosclerosis can affect any organ or tissue, the arteries supplying the heart, brain, small intestines,

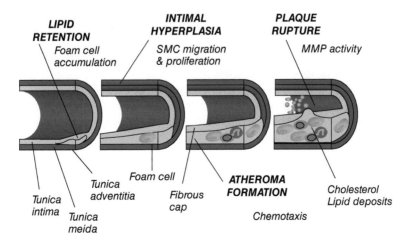

Figure 9.6 Atheroma build-up in an artery.

Table 9.1   Effects of atherosclerosis on different sites.

Site	Effects
Abdominal aorta	Gangrene of toes and feet, aneurysms
Aorto-iliac and femoral arteries	Intermittent claudication gangrene of toes and feet, aneurysms of iliac arteries
Coronary arteries	Angina pectoris, myocardial infarction
Carotid and vertebral arteries	Transient ischaemic attack, cerebrovascular accident
Renal arteries	Hypertension, renal ischaemia
Mesenteric arteries	Intestinal ischaemia

Source: Adapted from Bullock and Henze (2010)

kidneys and lower extremities are mostly affected. Table 9.1 lists the effects at the different affected sites.

The plaques inside the blood vessels are at risk of rupturing. This can be a result of the action of an enzyme complex called matrix metalloproteinases (MMPs). These are normally involved in breakdown of the extracellular matrix as a part of the healing process. If the plaque ruptures, blood will contact the underlying structures, and this will stimulate the production of a thrombus. In some cases, the thrombus could become dislodged to become an embolus.

Signs and symptoms of atherosclerosis

- Diminished or absent pulses
- Skin pallor or cyanosis
- Pain
- Muscle weakness.

Care and management

A full health and care history is essential in order to provide high-quality care for patients with atherosclerosis. The assessment must include the identification of risk factors and symptoms of any cardiovascular disease. The care and management includes the following:

- Health promotion to prevent the disease must include advice on a healthy diet and regulating the lipid levels within a normal range. Regular physical examination by the practice nurse or GP in order to monitor their BP and cholesterol levels should be encouraged.
- Advice on the cessation of smoking and alcohol consumption should be offered, as these are identified risk factors in atherosclerosis.
- Patients should be advised to lose weight if they are obese.
- Encourage the patient to undertake programmed exercise under the supervision of healthcare professionals. This will help in lowering their weight and cholesterol level, and in reducing their BP and stress.

Pharmacological interventions for atherosclerosis

The aim of medications in the treatment of atherosclerosis is to restore blood flow and prevent the disease. The medications include:

- Antihypertensives such as ACE-inhibitors and beta blockers
- Anticoagulant therapy with heparin and warfarin

- Lipid-lowering drugs such as simvastatin
- Antiplatelet drugs such as low dose aspirin and clopidogrel.

In some patients, surgical procedures, such as percutaneous coronary intervention (PCI), may be indicated to improve the blood flow through the vessel.

Medicines management

Statins

Statins are the name given to a group of cholesterol-lowering medicines, which are available on prescription or in low doses over the counter at pharmacies in the UK. Statin therapy is recommended for adults at high risk of cardiovascular disease (heart attack, stroke or peripheral artery disease) and also those who already have a history of cardiovascular disease.

Statins work by inhibiting an enzyme called HMG-CoA reductase. This enzyme is necessary for the synthesis of cholesterol in the liver. This reduces total cholesterol levels in the plasma. The decreased synthesis of cholesterol in the liver also has the effect of upregulating the receptors that many cells have for LDL cholesterol. LDL stands for low-density lipoprotein, and it is one of the specialised carriers used to transport lipids through the blood. Although all cholesterol is essentially the same substance, LDL cholesterol is often termed 'bad cholesterol' because the LDL carrier is the one which is capable of depositing cholesterol and other lipids into the walls of blood vessels to produce atheromatous plaques. The upregulation of the LDL receptors removes more LDL cholesterol from the blood. As a result, statins are particularly good at reducing plasma LDL cholesterol (Ritter *et al.*, 2019).

Some side effects have been documented with this medication including headache, stomach upset, altered liver function and some muscle pain, but these side effects are usually mild, easily recognisable and reversible. It is essential to note that many people will have no side effects at all from this medication.

229

Hypertension

Hypertension refers to sustained elevation in systemic arterial BP (McCance *et al.*, 2018). The elevation may be in either systolic or diastolic pressure, or in both. "Normal" BPs vary widely; generally a BP that is persistently raised over 140/90 mmHg is considered high BP (Royal College of Nursing, 2020). There are many classifications of hypertension, some of which are based on severity, e.g. mild or moderate. Types of hypertension include the following:

- Primary or essential hypertension
- Secondary hypertension where there is an underlying cause, such as renal diseases or tumour of the adrenal medulla
- Malignant hypertension occurs in the younger age groups with renal and collagen diseases
- Isolated systolic hypertension mainly occurs when a combination of factors is seen in the elderly, and is due to increases in cardiac output, increased peripheral resistance and renal vascular resistance. Other possible causes include Paget's disease of the bone and beriberi (McCance *et al.*, 2018).

Note

Blood pressure = cardiac output × peripheral vascular resistance (BP = CO × PVR)

Red flag

Hypertension is the major cause of a stroke and heart attack.
  You can recognise a stroke using the FAST test:

- **F**ACIAL weakness: Can the person smile? Has their mouth or eye drooped?
- **A**RM weakness: Can the person raise both arms?
- **S**PEECH problems: Can the person speak clearly and understand what you say?
- **T**IME to call emergency services.

Aetiology

Although the cause or causes of primary hypertension are unknown, several risk factors have been identified for its development:

- Obesity
- Stress
- Cigarette smoking and alcohol consumption
- Excessive intake of sodium causing fluid retention
- Family history.

Secondary hypertension results from underlying causes such as:

- Renal diseases
- Cushing's syndrome
- Hypo/hyperthyroidism
- Oral contraceptives
- Excessive alcohol consumption
- Coarctation (narrowing) of the aorta.

Investigations

These include:

- Full blood chemistry
- Physical examination
- Electrocardiogram
- Assessment of risk factors.

Common presenting symptoms

Many patients are unaware that they have hypertension and go untreated. They ignore symptoms such as headache, dizziness, nosebleed and fatigue. It is frequently identified through BP screening or as a result of other diseases. Some patients have reported blurred vision and tinnitus, but usually when symptoms of hypertension do occur, the disease is at an advanced stage (Bullock and Henze, 2010).

Pathophysiology

Primary hypertension

Primary hypertension results from a combination of genetic and environmental factors which have an effect on renal and vascular functions; it accounts for 95% of cases.

Primary hypertension may involve dysregulation of the RAAS (renin–angiotensin–aldosterone system). This system is involved in the homeostasis of BP by adjusting the blood volume and the peripheral resistance of blood vessels. If the kidneys are under-perfused, such as would be the case with an excessive drop in blood pressure, juxtaglomerular cells in the kidneys will produce a substance called renin. Renin is classed both as an enzyme and as a hormone. Renin catalyses the conversion of angiotensinogen (a protein circulating in the plasma) to produce angiotensin I. Angiotensin-converting enzyme (ACE), found in many tissues, especially the lungs, converts this to the more active angiotensin II. Angiotensin II causes vasoconstriction and stimulates the adrenal cortex to release aldosterone. Aldosterone increases reuptake of sodium and water from the nephron. These actions have the effect of elevating blood pressure (Tortora and Derricksen, 2017).

231

Secondary hypertension

Secondary hypertension accounts for 5% of cases and is caused by diseases of the organs, resulting in a raised PVR and increased cardiac output. In most cases, the focus is on kidney diseases or excessive levels of hormones such as aldosterone and cortisol. These hormones stimulate the retention of sodium and water, resulting in increased blood volume and BP. Once the underlying cause is treated, such as with the removal of the diseased organ, the BP returns to normal.

Malignant hypertension

This is a rapidly progressive hypertension where the diastolic pressure is in excess of 120 mmHg (Waugh and Grant, 2018), which can result in encephalopathy, cerebral oedema and loss of consciousness. Malignant hypertension does not indicate that there is cellular injury, but because it is life-threatening, it is considered an emergency. If untreated, cerebral oedema and cerebral dysfunction occur, leading to death of the individual. Malignant hypertension can cause a variety of complications, e.g. papilloedema, cardiac failure, cerebrovascular accident and retinopathy. Cerebral oedema will cause increased intracerebral pressure (ICP). This can precipitate seizures, and the pressure increase can cause narrowing of blood vessels, leading to ischaemia (McCance et al., 2018).

Isolated systolic hypertension

This is caused by an increase in cardiac output or PVR and has a higher incidence in the elderly. The rigidity of the vessels is often caused by atherosclerosis. The ageing process leads to hardening of the arteries, increased PVR and decreased baroreceptor sensitivity. In isolated systolic hypertension, the systolic BP is over 140 mmHg, and the diastolic pressure is less than 90 mmHg (Hogan et al., 2014). Isolated systolic hypertension can occur in young and middle-aged people as well as the elderly. It is a major cause of mortality and morbidity. There is a significant increased risk of both coronary artery disease and cerebrovascular disease (Bavishi et al., 2016).

Non-pharmacological interventions

- A single recording of raised BP does not indicate that the patient is suffering from hypertension. At least three recordings of raised BP at different intervals are required to confirm hypertension. Some doctors will monitor the patient's BP using a 24-hour ambulatory monitoring device. This measurement is much more accurate than the BP measurements done in the clinic.
- Advise the patient to restrict sodium intake, as sodium promotes water retention, resulting in increased circulating volume and increased cardiac output, which leads to hypertension.

- Healthcare professionals need to advise the patient on the cessation of cigarette smoking and excessive alcohol consumption. Both are identified as risk factors for hypertension.
- In obese patients, weight reduction through exercise should be encouraged (BMI should be less than 25); this will lower cholesterol levels and help in the control of any underlying problems such as diabetes mellitus (NICE, 2015). Encourage patients to have their weight checked weekly.
- Dietary advice should be offered to the patient. A diet rich in fruit and vegetables and low in saturated fats can help reduce BP. Reduction of salt in cooking should be encouraged, as excessive intake of salt promotes fluid retention, thus increasing circulating volume.
- Encourage patients to reduce their stress levels. Relaxation helps reduce BP by decreasing the workload of the heart. Listening to music, gardening and going for walks have all been identified as helpful in reducing BP.

Orange flag

Due to the asymptomatic nature of hypertension, concordance with medication can be quite poor if the drug that is prescribed produces any unwanted side effects.

Pharmacological interventions

In some patients, non-pharmacological interventions are sufficient to control their BP, while in others combinations of both pharmacological and non-pharmacological methods are used in the treatment of hypertension. The medications include the following:

- Diuretics are prescribed to reduce fluid load, which reduces plasma volume leading to a reduction in BP.
- Medications, e.g. beta blockers, calcium channel blockers and ACE inhibitors, are indicated for the treatment of hypertension (Ritter *et al.*, 2019).

Medicines management

Diuretics

Some of these drugs may decrease the body's levels of the mineral potassium. Symptoms such as weakness, leg cramps or being tired may result. Eating foods containing potassium may help prevent significant potassium loss. If the doctor recommends it, you could prevent potassium loss by taking a liquid or tablet that has potassium along with the diuretic. Diuretics such as amiloride (Midamor), spironolactone (Aldactone) or triamterene (Dyrenium) are called 'potassium sparing' agents. They don't cause the body to lose potassium. They might be prescribed alone, but are usually used with another diuretic. Some of these combinations are Aldactazide, Dyazide, Maxzide or Moduretic.

Some people suffer from attacks of gout after prolonged treatment with diuretics. This side effect is not common and can be managed by other treatments.

People with diabetes may find that diuretic drugs increase their blood sugar level. A change in medication, diet, insulin or oral anti-diabetic dosage corrects this in most cases (Ritter *et al.*, 2019).

Aneurysm

An aneurysm is a permanent dilatation of an artery or a chamber of the heart. Although it can occur in both arteries and veins, the aorta and the arteries at the base of the brain are the vessels most susceptible to aneurysms. It can occur in a localised part of the aorta or all along the vessel (Menzies-Gow, 2020) because it is under constant pressure. The commonest cause of an aneurysm is atherosclerosis, because the fatty deposits erode and weaken the vessel wall. Aneurysms can be classified according to their shape (Figures 9.7a–c) and they include:

- Fusiform – involves the entire circumference of the vessel
- Saccular – appears only on one part or side
- Dissecting – a false aneurysm resulting from a tear in the tunica intima.

233

Red flag

Marfan's syndrome is an inherited condition that affects the genes that control the formation of the body's connective tissue. This includes the connective tissue that makes up some of the walls of larger blood vessels. This is particularly problematic in arteries due to the greater pressure of the blood that they carry. Damage to the structure of the arteries creates weaknesses that can lead to brain aneurysms.

Aetiology

There are several causes of aneurysms, and they include:

- Atherosclerosis – the main cause of an aneurysm affecting the descending aorta
- Infection – mainly due to syphilis affecting the ascending aorta
- Hypertension – due to constant pressure, weakening of the vessel wall can occur in the elderly
- Cystic medial degeneration – it mainly affects the thoracic aorta in a disorder called Marfan's syndrome (see above). It affects the elastic fibres of the tunica media.

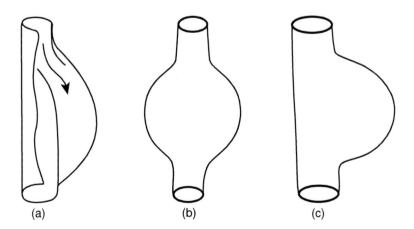

(a)   (b)   (c)

Figure 9.7   (a) A dissecting aneurysm, (b) a fusiform aneurysm, and (c) a saccular aneurysm.

Investigations

These include:

- Full blood chemistry
- Angiography
- Ultrasound
- Chest X-ray.

Symptoms

Most aortic aneurysms are asymptomatic until they start to leak or rupture, and the symptoms vary depending on the affected vessel. Symptoms may include the following:

- Pain in the abdominal region or in the extremities due to compression of neighbouring organs
- Dyspnoea (shortness of breath or difficulty in breathing) due to pressure on internal organs
- Dysphagia (difficulty in swallowing)
- Signs and symptoms of cerebrovascular accident occur if the cerebral arteries are affected.

Care and management

The main treatment for an aneurysm is surgery, and therefore it is vital that a full assessment of the patient is obtained. The surgery may include insertion of a graft (Figure 9.8). It is the healthcare professional's duty in the safe preparation of the patient for theatre to ensure that all the relevant protocols of the individual hospital are adhered to. All care given should be documented in accordance with local policy and procedure and adherence to the Nursing and Midwifery Council Code (2018).

Post-operatively, healthcare professionals should monitor the following:

- ABCDE – airway, breathing, circulation, disability and environment
- Fluid and nutritional management
- Elimination

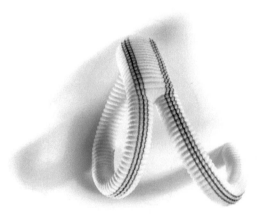

Figure 9.8 Dacron graft for an abdominal aortic aneurysm. Synthetic graft used for surgery. *Source:* Reproduced with permission from Vascutek.

- Pain management
- Wound management
- Detect early signs of postoperative complications of chest infection, deep vein thrombosis and wound infection
- Communication
- Documentation
- Safe preparation of the patient for discharge.

Pharmacological interventions

The following medications may be prescribed for a patient with an aneurysm:

- Antihypertensives
- Anticoagulants
- Antibiotics
- Analgesics.

Snapshot   Intermittent claudication

Mr Ah Peng Lee is a 55-year-old postman. He is married with two children. They live in a council house, and his mother-in-law lives with them. Mr Lee smokes 40 cigarettes per day and drinks two cans of lager every day after work.

Lately his right leg has been aching so much that he has to stop during his delivery rounds to ease the pain and to catch his breath. Over a few weeks the pain has become more severe, so Mr Lee decided to see his GP to find out what is wrong with him and to get some painkillers. His GP examined Mr Lee and decided to refer him to the vascular surgeon at the local hospital.

Vital signs

The following vital signs were noted and recorded by the GP:

Vital sign	Observation	Normal
Temperature	38.8°C	36.0–37.9°C range
Pulse	110 beats per minute	60–100 beats per minute
Respiration	24 breaths per minute	12–20 breaths per minute
Blood pressure	150/80 mmHg	100–139 mmHg (systolic) range
O_2 saturation	95%	94–98 %

A full blood count and urea and electrolytes was performed.

Test	Result	Guideline normal values
White blood cells (WBC)	10×10^9/L	4 to 11×10^9/L
Neutrophils	7.5×10^9/L	2.0 to 7.5×10^9/L
Lymphocytes	3.9×10^9/L	1.3 to 4.0×10^9/L

Test	Result	Guideline normal values
Red blood cells (RBC)	4.8×10^{12}/L	4.5 to 6.5×10^{12}/L
Haemoglobin (Hb)	164 g/L	130–180 g/L
Platelets	298×10^9/L	150 to 440×10^9/L
C-reactive protein	4.2 mg/L	<5 mg/L
Urea	6.0 mmol/L	2–6.6 mmol/L
Potassium	5.1 mmol/L	3.4–5.6 mmol/L
Sodium	138 mmol/L	135–147 mmol/L

Take some time to reflect on this case and then consider the following:

1. What is the possible diagnosis of Mr Lee's condition? Explain your answer.
2. What questions will you ask Mr Lee that will assist diagnosis?
3. Can you explain, in physiological terms, why Mr Lee's aching leg was relieved by rest?
4. Mr Lee states that it is difficult for him to change his lifestyle. What role do you think healthcare professionals can play in helping Mr Lee when he is discharged into the community?

NEWS 2

Ah Peng Lee

Physiological parameter	3	2	1	0	1	2	3
Respiration rate						24	
Oxygen saturation %			95				
Supplemental oxygen				No			
Temperature °C					38.8		
Systolic BP mmHg				150			
Heart rate					110		
Level of consciousness				A			
Score	0	0	1	0	2	2	0
Total		5					

Peripheral vascular disease

Peripheral vascular disease (PVD) is a disease involving reduced blood flow through peripheral blood vessels, leading to ischaemia of the tissues that they supply. It is particularly common in smokers and people with diabetes mellitus. It is likely to cause ischaemia of the lower limbs, and this can result in intermittent claudication, where pain is experienced on movement. If PVD is caused by atheroma, the plaques could result in the formation of a thrombus which occludes the blood vessel. This would be likely to result in the sudden onset of severe pain. Other conditions that can cause PVD include varicose veins and Raynaud's disease (McCance et al., 2018).

Aetiology

The causes of PVD include:

- Cardiovascular disease
- Thrombi
- Pulmonary disease
- Prolonged standing.

Investigations

These include:

- Doppler ultrasound
- Arteriogram/venogram
- Full blood chemistry
- Physical examination
- Electrocardiogram.

Clinical investigations

Doppler ultrasound

The test involves measuring the blood pressure in the ankles and comparing it to the blood pressure in the upper arms. These measurements are taken with a Doppler probe, which uses sound waves to determine the flow of blood in the arteries.

The arterial blood pressure should be about the same in the arms and legs. However, in peripheral arterial disease, the blood pressure in the ankles will be lower than that in the arms.

A full explanation must be provided to the patient and time given to answer any questions that may arise. Ensure that during the procedure the patient is comfortable and dignity is maintained.

Arterial insufficiency

Pathophysiology

If blood flows with reduced pressure, complications can result, such as formation of a thrombus which can occlude the flow of blood through that vessel. The lower limbs are most susceptible to arterial occlusion. The affected limbs are prone to arterial ulcers as a result of tissue hypoxia. A more severe blockage can lead to the development of gangrene, usually in the toe (Toski-Welch and Welch, 2018). Venous insufficiency may occur as the result of an obstruction in the veins by a thrombus or incompetent valves, which can lead to the formation of a venous ulcer as a result of poor circulation. There are distinct differences between arterial and venous insufficiency (Table 9.2).

Signs and symptoms

- Intermittent claudication
- White, pale colour when legs are elevated
- Leg ulcers (Table 9.2)
- Absent pedal pulses
- Numb and cold extremity
- Thickened toe nails.

Table 9.2   Comparison between an arterial and venous insufficiency.

	Arterial	Venous
Pain	Sudden severe pain, rest pain, intermittent claudication	Aching and cramp relieved by elevating the foot
Pulse	Diminished or absent	Present
Ulcer characteristics	Mainly in the toes, feet or other areas of the skin	Mainly over the inner or outer ankle
Skin characteristics	Shiny, cool or cold temperature; mild oedema if present	Thick and tough; skin normal colour; may have oedema, warm to touch
Complications	Gangrene	Poor healing
Blood flow	Doppler pressure readings lower below blockage	Normal pressure reading

Source: Adapted from Hogan *et al.* 2014

Care and management

Pain control is paramount in patients with arterial insufficiency. If pain is caused by exercise, such as walking long distances, then the patient should be advised against it. However, light exercise that can be tolerated should be encouraged as it helps to improve circulation. Patients should be advised to keep themselves warm if they are affected by cold weather, but they should avoid the following:

- Tight fitting clothing as this restricts arterial blood flow.
- Cigarette smoking as it may cause vasoconstriction.
- Very cold temperatures as these may cause vasoconstriction.
- Hot baths or sitting near fires because of the risk of burns with decreased sensation to the limbs.
- Cutting toenails as soft tissue damage may be slow to heal because of poor peripheral circulation. Toenails should be cut by a chiropodist.
- Sitting cross-legged for too long as this will restrict blood flow to the lower limbs.

A well-balanced healthy diet high in fruit, fibre and vegetables and low in saturated fat should be encouraged. Fluid intake of 2.5–3 L should be encouraged as dehydration causes increased blood viscosity and thus increases the risk of clot formation.

Some patients may require bypass surgery to treat the condition, which involves using a vein or Dacron graft (Figure 9.9). It is the healthcare professional's duty to prepare the patient safely for theatre and to monitor their postoperative recovery. Postoperative complications should be reported and treated immediately to prevent undue harm to the patient.

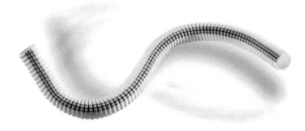

Figure 9.9   Dacron graft for peripheral vascular disease. Synthetic graft used for surgery. *Source:* Reproduced with permission from Vascutek.

Pharmacological interventions

Patients with PVD may be given the following medications:

- Vasodilators
- Anticoagulants
- Antiplatelet drugs.

Medicines management

Aspirin

Aspirin is a medication belonging to the drug class, non-steroidal anti-inflammatory drugs (NSAIDs). Aspirin is available as a generic drug, and is prescribed for treating fever, pain, inflammation, prevention of blood clots, and reduction of the risk of strokes and heart attacks.

Aspirin is an antiplatelet medicine, which means it reduces formation of the platelet plug, leading to reduced likelihood of clots forming in the blood. This reduces the risk of having a stroke or heart attack. Normally, when there is a cut or break in a small blood vessel, a blood clot forms to plug the hole until the blood vessel heals.

Some of the serious side effects include:

- Black, bloody, or tarry stools; due to bleeding into the gut
- Coughing up blood or vomit that looks like coffee grounds
- Severe nausea, vomiting, or stomach pain
- Hyperthermia and increased respiratory rate
- Reye's syndrome
- Salicylism; with tinnitus, vertigo and decreased hearing

(Ritter *et al.*, 2019)

Venous insufficiency/varicose veins

Varicose veins are vessels that have become dilated and tortuous due to incompetent valves, which allow back flow and pooling of blood in the veins. This mainly happens in the saphenous veins of the leg, deep communicating veins and superficial veins (Figure 9.10). One cause of venous distension is prolonged standing, which diminishes the action of the calf-muscle pump (Figure 9.11) (Kuhn-Timby and Smith, 2018). The calf-muscle pump aids venous return to the heart.

People who are susceptible to varicose veins are pregnant women, the obese, those who have to stand for long periods because of the nature of their occupation, e.g. theatre nurses, and the older age group. Several genes have been found to be associated with the development of varicose veins, but the importance of heredity in their development is still unclear. Weight, height, waist and hip circumference have also been found to be important in the development of varicose veins (Shadrina *et al.*, 2019).

Veins affected with varicosity

Any vein in the leg can develop varicosity (Figure 9.12); however, the common veins are the:

- Long saphenous veins
- Short saphenous veins
- Perforating veins.

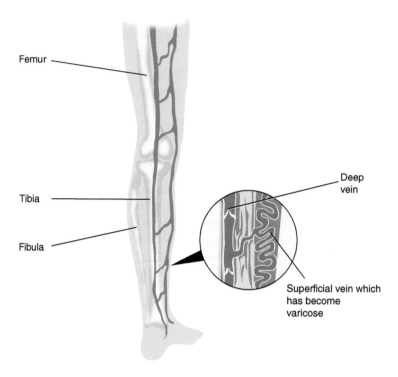

Figure 9.10   Varicose veins.

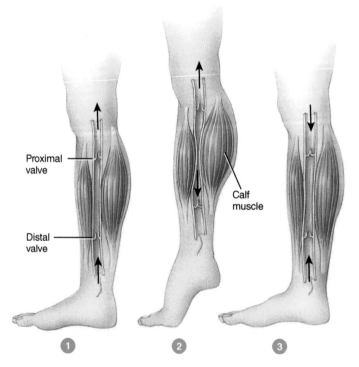

Figure 9.11   Calf-muscle pump.

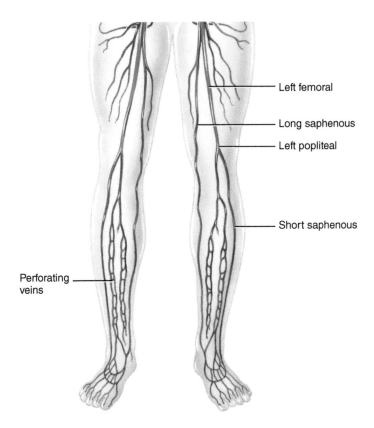

Left femoral

Long saphenous

Left popliteal

Short saphenous

Perforating veins

Figure 9.12   Veins of the leg susceptible to varicosity.

Signs and symptoms

- Swelling of the lower extremities
- Distended and tortuous veins
- Dull aching in the leg
- Ulcers (rare)
- Leg fatigue and heaviness.

Complications

Complications such as venous ulcers, venous eczema, lipodermatosclerosis and skin pigmentation (Figure 9.13a–c) are seen in some patients with varicose veins. Untreated tissue necrosis and infection can occur.

Care and management

In the UK, stripping and ligation of varicose veins are not routinely undertaken in the NHS unless the veins present a health risk; however, varicose veins can be treated privately. After surgery, most patients return to their normal routine within 1–3 weeks. Postoperative care includes applying pressure bandages for about 6 weeks, elevating the foot and gradually increasing ambulation (LeMone *et al.*, 2011). The surgical treatment is successful; however, 20–30% of the patients may require repeat surgery.

Pain should be managed by bed rest and elevation of the feet, which improves venous return. Prolonged standing in one position should be discouraged, and walking (2–3 miles

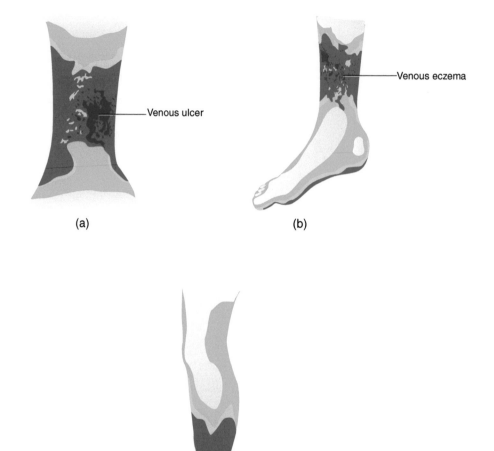

(a)   (b)

(c)

Figure 9.13   (a) Venous ulcer; (b) venous eczema; and (c) lipodermatosclerosis.

per day) should be encouraged to activate the calf-muscle pump, which helps in venous flow (see Figure 9.11) and to reduce oedema and complications such as deep vein thrombosis. Supportive anti-embolism stockings should be worn to reduce swelling in the leg and to provide support to the veins.

- Encourage patients to stop smoking as the nicotine may cause vascular damage.
- Encourage adequate fluid intake of 2–3 L per day and a healthy diet for tissue healing.
- Avoid unnecessary trauma to the feet.
- Inform patients not to cross their leg when seated as this restricts blood return.
- Educate patients in the benefits of regular exercise.
- Encourage all patients to maintain normal weight for their height.

Deep vein thrombosis

Deep vein thrombosis (DVT) is the formation of a thrombus (clot) in the veins when the flow of blood is reduced. It primarily occurs in the veins of the lower extremity (Figure 9.14), such as the femoral, popliteal and the deep veins of the pelvis (Grossman and Porth, 2014).

Aetiology

DVT is associated with the following:

- Stasis of blood in the veins, which can result from immobility after surgery.
- Obstruction to the flow of blood in the veins as a result of trauma.
- Hypercoagulability of blood due to dehydration, hormone replacement therapy and oral contraceptive pills.
- Use of intravenous cannulae may damage the tunica intima, resulting in the formation of clots.

Other factors include age (people over the age of 40 years are at greater risk), obesity, pregnancy, varicose veins and smoking.

Pathophysiology

A thrombus can develop in the superficial or deep veins of the legs. The blood flow is sluggish in the affected vessels, and the clotting cascade takes place. Most clotting factors have a short half-life, and in blood flowing at a normal rate, they would be washed away and diluted before a clot could develop.

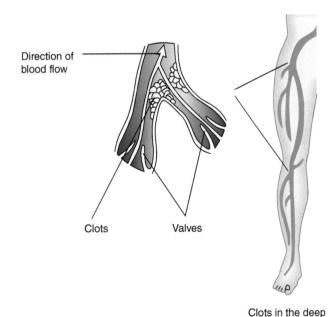

Direction of blood flow

Clots

Valves

Clots in the deep veins of the leg

Figure 9.14 Formation of thrombosis.

Platelets aggregate at the site of injury to the vessel wall or where there is venous stasis (LeMone *et al.*, 2011). Platelet aggregation occurs because platelets are exposed to collagen (a protein in the connective tissue, which is found in the inner surface of the blood vessel). When platelets come into contact with the exposed collagen, they release adenosine diphosphate and thromboxane. These substances make the surface of the platelets sticky and as they adhere to each other, as well as attracting more platelets to the area, and thus a platelet plug is formed (Figure 9.15). This creates a framework around which the fibrin mesh can form. Platelets and blood cells such as red blood cells are trapped in the fibrin mesh (Figure 9.16), and the thrombus grows.

The thrombus triggers the inflammatory response, causing tenderness, swelling and erythema at the affected site. Initially the thrombus stays within the affected area; however, fragments of the thrombus may become loose and travel through the circulation as an embolus, which may lodge in the lungs and cause a pulmonary embolism.

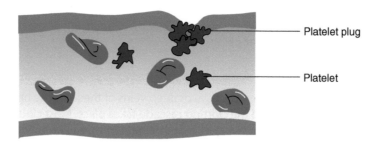

Figure 9.15   Formation of a platelet plug. *Source:* Nair and Peate, 2013.

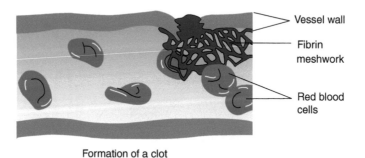

Formation of a clot

Figure 9.16   Formation of a clot. *Source:* Nair and Peate, 2013.

Red flag

A blood clot (thrombus) in the deep venous system of the leg is not dangerous in itself. The situation becomes life-threatening when a piece of the blood clot breaks off (embolus, pleural = emboli), travels downstream through the heart into the pulmonary circulation system, and becomes lodged in the lung. Diagnosis and treatment of a deep venous thrombosis (DVT) is meant to prevent pulmonary embolism.

Signs and symptoms

The signs and symptoms of DVT are as follows:

- Usually asymptomatic
- Dull aching pain in the affected limb, especially when walking
- Oedema of the affected leg
- Cyanosis of the affected leg
- Redness and warmth on the affected part
- Dilatation of the surface vein.

Care and management

- Maintain the patient on bed rest until mobilisation is encouraged.
- Monitor the vital signs (temperature, pulse, respiration and BP) of the patient 1–2 hourly to prevent complications such as pulmonary embolism.
- Observe the calf muscle for swelling. Measure the circumference 10–20 cm above and below the knee. Measurements should be accurately recorded as changes will allow prompt interventions.
- Elevate the foot to promote venous return and to reduce oedema.
- The patient should be advised not to massage the affected calf muscle so as not to dislodge the clot.
- The assessment of pain includes testing for Homan's sign – the patient lies flat with their legs straight and dorsiflexes the foot quickly (Menzies-Gow, 2020). The test is positive if the patient complains of pain in the calf.
- Check every 4 hours if the patient is experiencing any pain or discomfort in the affected leg.
- The patient should be advised to maintain a fluid intake of 2–2.5 L per day to prevent dehydration.
- Check to ensure that compression stockings are fitted correctly.

Pharmacological interventions

The following medications may be prescribed for the patient with DVT:

- Anticoagulants such as low-molecular-weight heparin
- Antiplatelet drugs
- Anti-inflammatory drugs
- Thrombolytic drugs.

Conclusion

The overall aim of this chapter was to provide the reader with an understanding of the vascular system and its related disorders. In order to care for the patient with vascular dysfunction, healthcare professionals need to understand the normal physiology of the vascular system. There are numerous diseases related to the vascular system; however, it is not the remit of this chapter to cover all of them. Some of the main diseases are discussed with their related care and management. The key role of the healthcare professional is to provide comfort, offer advice and prevent complications that could be detrimental to the patient's health. Caring for patients with vascular disorders requires skilled management, which incorporates ongoing assessment, and implementing and evaluating the care.

Test your knowledge

- Describe the process of atherosclerotic occlusion of a vessel.
- List the possible causes of PVD.
- Describe the pathophysiology of hypertension.
- Briefly describe the pathophysiology of an aneurysm.
- Discuss the care and management of the patient with varicose veins.

Activities

Here are some activities and exercises to help test your learning. For the answers to these exercises, as well as further self-testing activities, visit our website at **www.wiley.com/go/fundamentalsofappliedpathophysiology/student4e**

Multiple choice questions

1. In limb ischaemia pain is:
   - (a) Frequently one of the first signs
   - (b) A late sign
   - (c) Only present if there is gangrene
   - (d) In the lower limbs only
2. Acute limb ischaemia is:
   - (a) Seen only in the upper limbs
   - (b) Always bilateral
   - (c) A sudden decrease in limb perfusion that is a threat to the limb's viability
   - (d) A gradual, chronic decrease in limb perfusion that is a threat to the limb's viability
3. Occlusion of a vessel:
   - (a) Leads to an increase in blood flow enhancing oxygen and nutrient delivery to tissues
   - (b) Leads to a reduction in blood flow that compromises oxygen and nutrient delivery to tissues
   - (c) Always causes gangrene
   - (d) Will result in limb ischaemia
4. Ulceration and infection are complications associated with:
   - (a) Low-oxygen state of ischaemic tissues
   - (b) High-oxygen state of ischaemic tissues
   - (c) Hypotension
   - (d) Hypertension
5. Claudication is:
   - (a) Improved after walking, better with limb elevation
   - (b) Worse after walking and worse with limb elevation
   - (c) Improved when heat is applied to the limb and the limb is elevated
   - (d) Worse after walking, better with limb elevation
6. The two most important risk factors for developing acute limb ischaemia are:
   - (a) Hypotension and tachycardia
   - (b) Obesity and hypertension
   - (c) Smoking and diabetes
   - (d) Smoking and excessive alcohol intake

7. Emboli causing limb ischaemia usually originate in the:
   (a) Heart
   (b) Liver
   (c) Spleen
   (d) Kidney

8. Atherosclerosis usually occurs where:
   (a) The walls of the veins and also the arteries are hard, thick and narrow
   (b) The walls of the veins and also the arteries are flaccid, thin and dilated
   (c) The walls of the arteries become infected
   (d) The walls of the arteries are hard, thick and narrow

9. A localised dilatation of a blood vessel due to a weekend arterial wall is known as:
   (a) Arteritis
   (b) Angioplasty
   (c) Arrhythmia
   (d) Aneurysm

10. A group of disorders that results in blood vessel thickening, hardening and losing their elasticity is known as:
    (a) Arthritis
    (b) Arteriosclerosis
    (c) Atherosclerosis
    (d) Sclerosis

11. Of the following, which describes the formation of a blood clot that obstructs blood flow:
    (a) Embolism
    (b) Thrombus
    (c) Fibrillation
    (d) Aneurysm

12. Enlarged, tortuous veins commonly seen in the lower extremities are:
    (a) Thrombocytes
    (b) Phlebitis
    (c) Varicose veins
    (d) Sclerosis

13. Aspirin is a medication belonging to the drug class:
    (a) Anticoagulant
    (b) Non-steroidal anti-inflammatory drugs (NSAIDs)
    (c) Analgesia
    (d) Antidepressant

14. Diagnosis and treatment of a deep venous thrombosis can help to prevent:
    (a) Infection
    (b) Inflammation
    (c) Pulmonary embolism
    (d) Varicose veins

15. Varicose veins mainly occur in:
    (a) The saphenous veins of the leg, deep communicating veins and superficial veins
    (b) The coronary arteries
    (c) The cerebral arteries
    (d) The deep communicating veins and superficial veins in the oesophagus

Conditions

Below is a list of conditions associated with the vascular system. Take some time and write notes about each of the conditions. You may make the notes taken from textbooks or other resources (e.g. people you work with in a clinical area) or you may make the notes based on people you have cared for. If you are making notes about people you have cared for, you must ensure that you adhere to the rules of confidentiality.

Vascular dementia	
Raynaud phenomenon	
Aortic dissection	
Radiculopathy	
Chronic venous insufficiency	

Further resources

Patient

https://patient.info/about-us

This is a comprehensive health information website that GPs and nurses use during consultations. Students should access this website as there is much useful information that can be shared with patients to promote health.

National Institute for Health and Care Excellence (NICE)

Peripheral Arterial Disease: Diagnosis and Management. A clinical guideline that is evidence based regarding the management and diagnosis of peripheral arterial disease.

https://www.nice.org.uk/guidance/cg147/resources/peripheral-arterial-disease-diagnosis-and-management-pdf-35109575873989 last accessed June 2020

National Institute for Health and Care Excellence (NICE)

http://www.nice.org.uk/CG034

This link takes you to the NICE website. This section of the NICE discusses clinical management of primary hypertension. Students accessing this link should bear in mind that every trust will have its own local policies and guidelines.

Department of Health and Social Care (DHSC)

https://www.gov.uk/government/organisations/department-of-health-and-social-care

All healthcare professionals should access this government website. It provides DH publications, including statistical reports, surveys, press releases, circulars and legislation.

British and Irish Hypertension Society

http://www.bhsoc.org/

The British and Irish Hypertension Society provides a medical and scientific research forum to enable the sharing of cutting-edge research into the origin of high blood pressure so as to improve its treatment. This website provides useful information not otherwise found in textbooks.

British Heart Foundation

https://www.bhf.org.uk

This website provides useful information about researches in heart diseases. It also provides healthy living for all ages.

Glossary of terms

Adenosine diphosphate   Found inside cells, it helps to produce ATP during reactions that produce cellular energy and is itself formed from ATP at a later stage. It is this continual synthesis and breaking down of ADP and ATP that produces the energy.

Aneurysm   A localised dilatation of a blood vessel, usually the aorta or the arteries at the base of the brain.

Aorta   First major blood vessel of the arterial circulation. Emerges from the left ventricle of the heart.

Artery   A blood vessel that carries blood away from the heart.

Arteriole   A small artery.

Arteriosclerosis   A condition in which there is thickening, hardening, loss of elasticity of the vessel wall leading to narrowing of the artery.

Baroreceptor   A neuron sensing changes in fluid, air and blood pressures.

Blood pressure   The force exerted by the blood against the walls of the blood vessel due to the contraction of the heart.

Capillary   A small blood vessel where exchanges between blood and tissue cells take place.

Chemoreceptor   A sensory receptor that detects the presence of a specific chemical.

Clotting cascade   A series of steps in the clotting process of the blood.

Collagen fibre   The most abundant of the three fibre types found in the connective tissues.

Endothelium   A single layer of simple squamous cells found in the heart, blood vessels and lymphatic vessels.

Erythema   A superficial redness of the skin.

Extracellular fluid   The fluid that surrounds and bathes the body's cells.

Fibroblast cells   The most common connective tissue cells and only found in the tendons. It is responsible for the production and secretion of extracellular matrix materials.

Hypertension   Raised blood pressure.

Lumen   The inside space of a tubular structure.

Macrophage   A phagocyte produced from monocytes that engulfs and digests cellular debris, microbes and foreign matter.

Oxidation   A chemical reaction where electrons are lost.

Paget's disease   A disorder of the bone. Excessive remodelling of the bone causes enlarged and deformed bones and weakening of the bones, leading to bone pain and fractures.

Papilloedema   A swelling of the optic disc in the eye.

Thromboxane   A compound synthesised in platelets from prostaglandin. It acts to aggregate platelets.

Tunica externa   The membranous outer layer of the blood vessel.

Tunica intima   The inner lining of a blood vessel.

Tunica media   The middle muscle layer of the blood vessel.

Vasoconstriction   A decrease in the diameter of a blood vessel due to the relaxation of smooth muscle in the vessel wall; may occur as a result of hormones or after stimulation of the vasomotor centre leading to increased peripheral resistance.

Vasodilatation   An increase in the diameter of a blood vessel due to relaxation of smooth muscle in the vessel wall; may occur as a result of hormones or after decreased stimulation of the vasomotor centre, leading to decreased peripheral resistance.

Vein   A blood vessel that carries blood to the heart.

Venule   A small vein.

References

Bavishi, C., Goel, S. and Messerli, F. (2016). Isolated systolic hypertension: An update after SPRINT. *The American Journal of Medicine*, 129: 1251–1258.

Bullock, B.A. and Henze, R.L. (2010). *Focus on Pathophysiology*, 4th edn. Philadelphia: Lippincott.

Grossman, S.C. and Porth, C.M. (2014). *Pathophysiology: Concepts of Altered Health States*, 9th edn. Philadelphia: Lippincott Williams & Wilkins.

Hogan, M., Gingrich, M., Hill, K., Scialdo, T. and Wolf, L. (2014). *Pathophysiology: Reviews and Rationales*, 3rd edn. Upper Saddle River, NJ: Pearson Education, Inc.

Jenkins, G.W. and Tortora, G.J. (2019). *Anatomy and Physiology*. Wiley E Books.

Jowett, N.I. and Thompson, D.R. (2007). *Comprehensive Coronary Care*, 4th edn. London: Baillere Tindall.

Kuhn-Timby, B. and Smith, N.E. (2018). Introduction to Medical Surgical Nursing, 12th edn. Philadelphia: Wolters Kluwer Health.

Lelis, de F., de Freitas, F., Machada, S., Crespo, S. and Santos, H.S. (2019). Angiotensin-(1-7), Adipokines and Inflammation. *Metabolism*, 95: P36–45.

LeMone, P., Burke, K. and Bauldoff, G. (2011). *Medical – Surgical Nursing; Critical Thinking in Patient Care*, 5th edn. New Jersey: Pearson.

Marieb, E.N. and Hoehn, K. (2019). *Human Anatomy and Physiology*, Global Edition, 11th edn. London: Pearson.

McCance, K.L., Huether, S.E., Brashers, V.L. and Rote, N.S. (2018). *Pathophysiology: The Biologic Basis for Disease in Adults and Children*, 8th edn. St Louis: Mosby.

Menzies-Gow, E. (2020). Nursing patients with cardiovascular disorders. In: Peate, I. (ed.), *Alexander's Nursing Practice Hospital and Home*, 5th edn. Edinburgh: Churchill Livingstone, Chapter 3, pp. 17–47.

Nair, M. and Peate, I. (2013). *Fundamentals of Applied Pathophysiology: An Essential Guide for Nursing and Healthcare Students*, 2nd edn. Chichester, UK: John Wiley & Sons.

National Institute for Health Care Excellence (2015). *Management of Type 2 Diabetes: Management of Blood Glucose*. (NICE Guideline NG28). Updated August 2019. Available at: https://www.nice.org.uk/guidance/ng28/resources/type-2-diabetes-in-adults-management-pdf-1837338615493. Accessed 8th June 2020.

Nowak, J. and Handford, A.G. (2010). *Essentials of Pathophysiology: Concepts and Applications for Health Care Professionals*, 3rd edn. Boston: McGraw-Hill.

Nursing and Midwifery Council (2018). *The Code. Professional Standards of Practice and Behaviour for Nurses, Midwives and Nursing Associates*. https://www.nmc.org.uk/globalassets/sitedocuments/nmc-publications/nmc-code.pdf Accessed June 2020.

Ritter, J.M., Flower, R.J., Hendersen, G., Loke, H., MacEwan, D. and Rang, H. (2019). *Pharmacology*, 8th edn. Edinburgh: Elsevier, Churchill Livingstone.

Royal College of Nursing (2020). *Blood Pressure*. https://rcni.com/hosted-content/rcn/first-steps/blood-pressure Accessed June 2020.

Shadrina, A., Sharpov, S. and Tsepilov, A. (2019). Varicose veins of the lower extremities: Insights from the first large-scale genetic study. *PLoS Genetics*, Apr.15(4): e10008110.

Tortora, J. and Derrickson, B. (2017). *Principles of Anatomy and Physiology*, 15th edn. New Jersey: John Wiley & Sons.

Toski-Welch, J. and Welch, T.S. (2018). *Limb Ischemia and Gangrene. Emergency Medicine Reports* https://www.reliasmedia.com/articles/143557-limb-ischemia-and-gangrene Accessed June 2020.

Waugh, A. and Grant, A. (2018). *Ross and Wilson Anatomy and Physiology in Health and Illness*. 13th edn. Edinburgh: Elsevier.

Chapter 10

The blood and associated disorders

Barry Hill

Director of Education (Employability), Northumbria University, Newcastle upon Tyne, UK

Contents

Introduction 253	Test your knowledge..........................284
Composition of blood.........................253	Multiple choice questions.................285
Formed elements of blood 257	Conditions..286
Haemostasis 261	Further resources...............................287
Blood groups..263	Glossary of terms................................288
Diseases of the blood.........................264	References...289
Conclusion 284	

Key words

- Erythrocytes
- Platelets
- Haemostasis
- Antigens
- Plasma
- Haemoglobin
- Coagulation
- Agglutination
- White blood cells
- Erythropoietin
- Blood groups
- Haematocrit

Fundamentals of Applied Pathophysiology: An Essential Guide for Nursing and Healthcare Students, Fourth Edition. Edited by Ian Peate.
© 2021 John Wiley & Sons Ltd. Published 2021 by John Wiley & Sons Ltd.
Student companion website: www.wiley.com/go/fundamentalsofappliedpathophysiology/student4e
Instructor companion website: www.wiley.com/go/fundamentalsofappliedpathophysiology/instructor4e

Test your prior knowledge

- What is the composition of blood?
- What is the function of the red blood cell?
- How many types of white blood cells are there? Can you name them?
- Why does arterial blood look bright red?
- What do you understand by the term *blood typing*?

Learning outcomes

On completion of this section, the reader will be able to:

253

- Describe the normal composition of blood.

- List the functions of the red blood cells, white blood cells and platelets.

- Explain the life cycle of the red blood cells and the white blood cells.

- Discuss the factors affecting coagulation.

- Explain the ABO and Rh systems of blood typing.

Don't forget to visit the companion website for this book
(www.wiley.com/go/fundamentalsofappliedpathophysiology/student4e)
where you can find self-assessment tests to check your progress, as well as lots of activities to practise your learning.

Introduction

Blood is a type of connective tissue consisting of cells and cell fragments. It does not connect or give mechanical support. It is called a connective tissue because it develops from mesenchyme and consists of blood cells, which are surrounded by a non-living fluid called plasma. The cells and the cell fragments are formed elements of the blood, and the liquid part is called the plasma. The formed elements are made up of red blood cells (erythrocytes), which account for 45% of the blood. Plasma makes up 55% of the total blood volume (Stanfield, 2013). The remaining 1% consists of white blood cells and platelets (Figure 10.1). The percentage of the formed elements constitutes the haematocrit or packed cell volume. The volume of blood is constant in a healthy person unless the person has physiological problems. This chapter focuses on the composition, structure and functions of various blood cells and their related disorders.

Composition of blood

Blood is composed of plasma, a yellowish liquid containing nutrients, hormones, minerals and various cells, mainly red blood cells, white blood cells and platelets (Figure 10.2). Both the formed elements and the plasma play an important role in homeostasis.

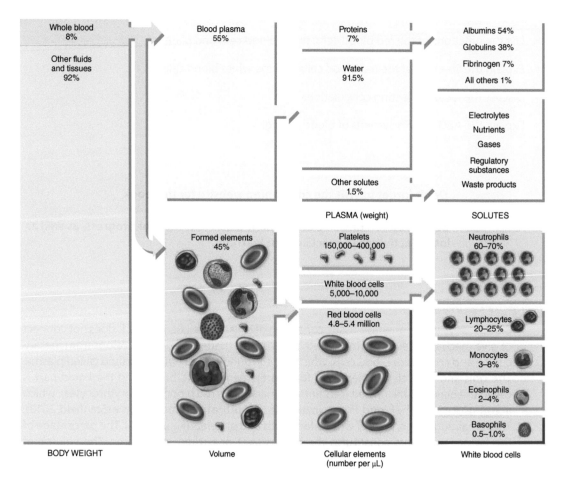

Figure 10.1 Components of clotted blood separated by centrifugation.

Figure 10.2 Cells of the blood.

Properties of blood

In a healthy person, blood forms about 7–9% of total body weight. A man has 5–6 L of blood, while a woman has 4–5 L. Blood is thicker, denser and flows much slower than water due to the red blood cells and proteins, such as albumin and fibrinogen. It has a high viscosity, which offers resistance to blood flow. The red blood cells and proteins contribute to the viscosity of blood, which ranges from 3.5 to 5.5, compared with 1.0 for water. The more red blood cells and plasma proteins there are in blood, the higher the viscosity and the slower the flow of blood. The specific gravity (density) of blood is 1.045–1.065 compared with 1.000 for water, and the pH of blood ranges from 7.35 to 7.45.

Functions of blood

Overall, there are three categories of blood function:

1. Transportation
2. Regulation
3. Protection.

Transportation

Red blood cells in the blood transport oxygen from the lungs to body tissues and waste products of cellular metabolism from the body tissues to the kidneys, liver, lungs and sweat glands for elimination from the body. Blood also transports nutrients, hormones, clotting factors and enzymes throughout the body to maintain homeostasis.

Regulation

Blood regulates blood clotting to stop bleeding; body temperature by increasing or decreasing blood flow to the skin for heat exchange; and acid–base balance to maintain the pH of blood within a normal range (7.35–7.45). It also regulates fluid and electrolyte balance through renal function.

Protection

Blood defends the body against bacteria and viruses (pathogens) in several ways. Some white blood cells, e.g. the neutrophils, engulf and destroy pathogens, while lymphocytes produce and secrete antibodies into blood. Antibodies in the blood play a vital role in the inflammatory and immune response. These responses prevent blood loss after an injury by initiating the clotting mechanisms, without which the person would bleed to death. Clotting involves platelets, the plasma protein fibrinogen and the clotting factors.

Plasma

Plasma is the liquid part of the blood and is composed of water (91%), proteins (8%; albumin, globulin, prothrombin and fibrinogen), and salts (0.9%; sodium chloride, sodium bicarbonate and others) and the remaining 0.1% is made up of organic materials, e.g. fats, glucose, urea, uric acid, cholesterol and amino acids (Mader, 2019). Blood cells are composed of erythrocytes (red blood cells), leucocytes (white blood cells) and thrombocytes (platelets). These substances give plasma greater density and viscosity than water.

Water in plasma

The water in plasma is available to cells, tissues and the extracellular fluid of the body to maintain homeostasis. It is a solvent where chemical reactions between intracellular and extracellular reactions occur. Water contains solutes, e.g. electrolytes, whose concentrations change to meet the body's needs.

Plasma proteins

Plasma contains three principal types of protein:

1. Albumins
2. Globulins
3. Fibrinogen.

Plasma proteins make up 7% of the plasma, and these proteins stay in the blood vessel as they are too large to diffuse through capillaries and are responsible for creating the osmotic pressure of blood. When plasma proteins are lost in patients who suffer from burns, fluid moves into tissues, causing oedema by a process called osmosis.

Albumin

Albumin is the most abundant plasma protein (around 60%). It is synthesised in the liver, and its main function is to maintain plasma osmotic pressure. Albumins also act as carrier molecules for other substances, such as hormones and lipids (Waugh and Grant, 2018).

Globulins

The next most abundant plasma proteins are globulins (around 36%). They are synthesised from the liver and B lymphocytes. They are divided into three groups, based on their structure and function:

1. Alpha globulin
2. Beta globulin
3. Gamma globulin.

The alpha and beta globulins are produced by the liver, and they transport lipids and fat-soluble vitamins. Gamma globulins are immunoglobulins, which are complex proteins produced by lymphocytes, and have a vital role in immunity. They prevent diseases such as measles and tetanus (Waugh and Grant, 2018).

Fibrinogen

Fibrinogen, which is synthesised in the liver, forms approximately 4% of the plasma proteins and is essential for blood clotting. When fibrinogen and several other proteins involved in clotting are removed, the remaining fluid is called serum.

Plasma electrolytes

Electrolytes are inorganic molecules that separate into ions when dissolved in water. They are involved in muscle contraction and transmission of nerve impulses, and play a role in maintaining the pH of blood. The ions are either positively charged (cations) or negatively charged (anions). The principal plasma cation is sodium (Na^+), and the principal anion is chloride (Cl^-).

Gases

Oxygen, carbon dioxide and nitrogen are the principal gases dissolved in plasma. Oxygen is transported by haemoglobin in red blood cells, and some is dissolved in plasma. Most of the carbon dioxide is transported by bicarbonate ions in plasma.

Nutrients and waste products of metabolism

Nutrients such as amino acids, fatty acids and glycerol are obtained from the digestion of food in the gastrointestinal tract. They are vital to cellular function. Waste products of protein metabolism, such as urea, creatinine and uric acid, are transported in the blood to the kidneys for elimination (Mader, 2019).

Formed elements of blood

The formed elements of the blood consist of:

- Red blood cells
- White blood cells
- Platelets.

Red blood cells

Red blood cells are also known as erythrocytes and are small biconcave discs (Figure 10.3). The biconcave shape is maintained by a network of protein called spectrin, which also allows the red blood cells to change shape as they are transported through the blood vessel. There are approximately 4–5.5 million red blood cells in each cubic millimetre of blood (Marieb and Hoehn, 2015). They are a pale buff colour that is lighter in the centre. Young red blood cells contain a nucleus; however, the nucleus is absent in mature red blood cells, as are any organelles such as mitochondria.

The main function of the red blood cell is to transport the respiratory gases oxygen and carbon dioxide (approximately 20%). As red blood cells lack mitochondria to produce energy (adenosine triphosphate), they utilise anaerobic respiration to produce energy and do not use any of the oxygen they are transporting.

Haemoglobin

Haemoglobin is composed of the protein called globin bound to the iron-containing pigment called haem. Each globin molecule has four polypeptide chains consisting of two alpha and two beta chains (Figure 10.4). Each haemoglobin molecule has four atoms of iron, and each atom of iron will transport one molecule of oxygen; therefore, one molecule of

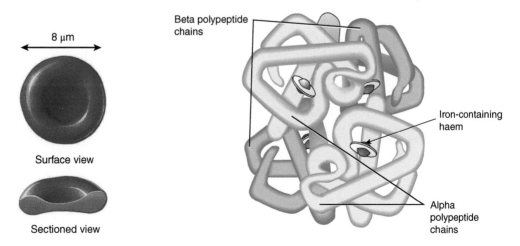

Figure 10.3   Red blood cell.   **Figure 10.4**   Haemoglobin molecule.

haemoglobin will transport four molecules of oxygen. There are approximately 250 million haemoglobin molecules in one red blood cell, and therefore one red blood cell will transport a billion molecules of oxygen.

Formation of red blood cells

Red blood cells are formed from the stem cells in the red bone marrow. In the bone marrow, the multipotent stem cells divide to produce myeloid stem cells, which divide to produce erythroblasts (Figure 10.5). Erythroblasts develop in the red bone marrow to form red blood cells. During maturation, red blood cells lose their nucleus and organelles, and gain more haemoglobin molecules, thus increasing the amount of oxygen they can transport. As mature red blood cells do not have a nucleus, their lifespan is approximately 120 days. It is estimated that approximately 2 million red blood cells are destroyed per second (Mader, 2019); however, these are replaced with an equal number to maintain the balance.

258

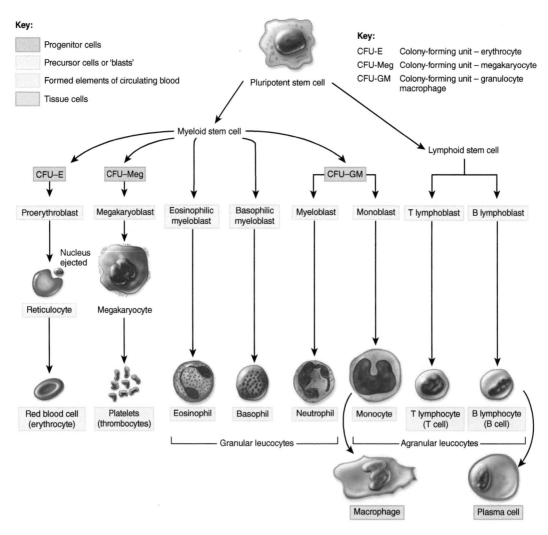

Figure 10.5   Formation of blood cells.

The production of red blood cells is controlled by the hormone erythropoietin (Marieb and Hoehn, 2015), and the essential components for the synthesis of red blood cells are:

- Iron
- Folic acid
- Vitamin B$_{12}$.

Transport of respiratory gases

The major role of red blood cells is to transport oxygen from the lungs to the tissues. The oxygen in the alveoli (air sacs) of the lungs combines with iron molecules in the haemoglobin to form oxyhaemoglobin. This is then transported by the blood to the tissues. As the oxygen level in the red blood cell increases, it becomes bright red, and when the level of oxygen content drops, the colour changes to a dark bluish red (Waugh and Grant, 2018).

In addition to transporting oxygen from the lungs to the body tissues, red blood cells transport carbon dioxide from the tissues to the lungs. Carbon dioxide is transported in three ways:

1. 10% is dissolved in the plasma.
2. 20% combines with the haemoglobin of the red blood cell to form carbaminohaemoglobin.
3. 70% with water to form carbonic acid, which is converted to bicarbonate and hydrogen ions.

$$CO_2 + H_2O \xrightarrow{\text{carbonic anhydrase}} \underset{\text{carbonic acid}}{H_2CO_3} \leftrightarrow \underset{\text{bicarbonate ion}}{HCO_3^-} + \underset{\text{hydrogen ion}}{H^+}$$

The reaction occurs primarily in red blood cells, which contain large amounts of carbonic anhydrase (an enzyme that facilitates the reaction). Once the bicarbonate ions are formed, they move out of the red blood cells into the plasma.

Destruction of red blood cells

Haemolysis (breakdown) is carried out by macrophages in the spleen, liver and bone marrow (Figure 10.6). As red blood cells age, they are susceptible to haemolysis; haem and globin are separated. The globin is broken down into amino acids and used for protein synthesis. Iron is separated from haem and is stored in the muscle and the liver, and reused in the bone marrow to manufacture new red blood cells. Haem is the portion of the haemoglobin that is converted to bilirubin and is transported by plasma albumin to the liver and eventually secreted in bile.

White blood cells

White blood cells are also known as leucocytes. There are approximately 5000–10 000 white blood cells in every cubic millimetre of blood. The number may increase in infections to approximately 25 000 per cubic millimetre of blood. An increase in white blood cells is called leucocytosis, and an abnormally low level of white blood cell is called leucopenia. Unlike red blood cells, white blood cells do have nuclei, and they are able to move across blood vessel

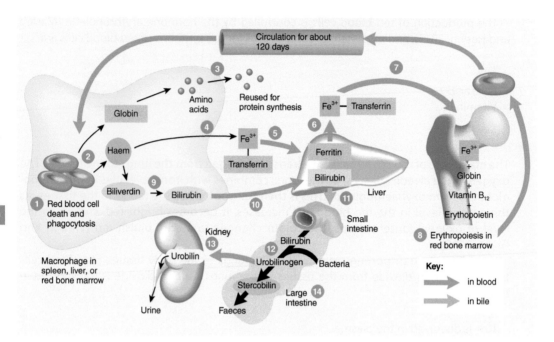

Figure 10.6   Haemolysis of red blood cells and bilirubin metabolism. In point 10: Transport of unconjugated bilirubin to the liver.

walls into the tissues. White blood cells are able to produce a continuous supply of energy, unlike the red blood cells. They are able to synthesise proteins, and thus their lifespan can be from a few days to years. There are two main types of white blood cells:

1. Granulocytes (contain granules in the cytoplasm):
   • Neutrophils
   • Eosinophils
   • Basophils
2. Agranulocytes (despite the name, these contain a few granules in the cytoplasm)
   • Monocytes
   • Lymphocytes.

Neutrophils

Approximately 60–65% of granulocytes are phagocytes. They contain lysozymes, and therefore their main function is to protect the body from any foreign material. They are capable of moving across blood vessel walls by a process called diapedesis and are actively phagocytic. The nuclei of the neutrophils are multi-lobed. The number of neutrophils increases in:

• Pregnancy
• Infection
• Leukaemia
• Metabolic disorder such as acute gout
• Inflammation
• Myocardial infarction.

Eosinophils

These form approximately 2–4% of granulocytes and have B-shaped nuclei. Like neutrophils, they too migrate from blood vessels. They are phagocytes; however, they are not as active as neutrophils. They contain lysosomal enzymes and peroxidase in their granules, which are toxic to parasites, resulting in the destruction of the organisms. Numbers increase in allergy, such as hay fever and asthma, and parasitic infection, e.g. tapeworm infection.

Basophils

Basophils account for approximately 1% of granulocytes and contain elongated lobed nuclei. In inflamed tissue, they become mast cells and secrete granules containing heparin, histamine and other proteins that promote inflammation. Basophils play an important role in providing immunity against parasites.

Monocytes

Monocytes account for 5% of the agranulocytes, and they are circulating leucocytes. Monocytes develop in the bone marrow. Some of them migrate into the tissue, where they develop into macrophages and engulf pathogens or foreign proteins. Macrophages play a vital role in immunity and inflammation by destroying specific antigens.

Lymphocytes

Lymphocytes account for 25% of the leucocytes, and most are found in the lymphatic tissue such as the lymph nodes and the spleen. They get their name from the fluid that transports them – the lymph. They can leave and re-enter the circulatory system. Their lifespan ranges from a few hours to years. The main difference between lymphocytes and other white blood cells is that lymphocytes are not phagocytes. Two types of lymphocytes are identified – T and B lymphocytes. T lymphocytes originate from the thymus gland, while B lymphocytes originate in the bone marrow, hence their names. T lymphocytes mediate the cellular immune response, which is part of the body's own defence. The B lymphocytes, on the other hand, become large plasma cells and produce antibodies which attach to antigens.

Platelets

Platelets are small blood cells consisting of some cytoplasm surrounded by a plasma membrane. They are produced in the bone marrow from megakaryocytes (see Figure 10.5), and fragments of megakaryocytes break off to form platelets. Their lifespan is approximately 5–9 days (Stanfield, 2013). The surface of platelets contains proteins and glycoproteins that allow them to adhere to other proteins such as collagen in the connective tissues. Platelets play a vital role in blood loss by the formation of platelet plugs, which seal the holes in the blood vessels.

Haemostasis

Haemostasis plays an important part in maintaining homeostasis, and it consists of three main components:

1. Vasoconstriction
2. Platelet aggregation
3. Coagulation.

Vasoconstriction

- Results from contraction of the smooth muscle of the vessel wall
- Constriction blocks small blood vessels, thus preventing blood flow through them
- The action of the sympathetic nervous system causes vasoconstriction
- Platelets release thromboxanes.

Platelet aggregation

- Platelets contain contractile proteins called actin and myosin
- Platelet adhesion occurs when platelets are exposed to collagen in the blood vessels
- Platelets release adenosine diphosphate, thromboxane and other chemicals.

Coagulation

If blood vessel damage is so extensive that platelet aggregation and vasoconstriction cannot stop the bleeding, the complicated process of coagulation (blood clotting) will begin. The clotting phase involves several clotting factors (Table 10.1). Most of the clotting factors are synthesised in the liver.

A simplified clotting cascade involves the following stages:

1. Thromboplastinogenase, an enzyme released by the blood platelets, combines with antihaemophilic factor to convert the plasma protein thromboplastinogen into thromboplastin.
2. Thromboplastin combines with calcium ions to convert the inactive plasma protein prothrombin into thrombin.
3. Thrombin acts as a catalyst to convert the soluble plasma protein fibrinogen into the insoluble plasma protein fibrin.
4. The fibrin threads trap blood cells to form a clot.
5. Once the clot is formed, the damaged blood vessel heals, and this restores the integrity of the blood vessel.

Two pathways have been identified in triggering a blood clot: the intrinsic and extrinsic pathways. The extrinsic pathway is a rapid clotting system activated when the blood vessels are ruptured and tissue damage takes place. The intrinsic pathway is slower than the extrinsic pathway and it is activated when the inner walls of the blood vessels are damaged.

Table 10.1   Blood clotting factors.

I	Fibrinogen
II	Prothrombin
III	Thromboplastin
IV	Calcium
V	Proaccelerin, labile factor
VII	Serum prothrombin conversion accelerator
VIII	Antihaemophilic factor
IX	Christmas factor, plasma thromboplastin component
X	Stuart–Power factor
XI	Plasma thromboplastin antecedent
XII	Hageman factor
XIII	Fibrin-stabilising factor

Blood groups

The surface of the red blood cell contains molecules called antigens, and in the plasma there are molecules called antibodies. The antibodies are specific to certain antigens. When an antibody combines with the specific antigen on the red blood cell, they form a link to connect other red blood cells to it. As a result, clumping or agglutination of the red blood cells occurs.

The antigens on the red blood cells have been categorised into blood groups. Although numerous blood groups have been identified, ABO (Figure 10.7) and rhesus (Rh) blood groups are the most important in blood transfusion.

Type A blood group has type A antigen on its surface and anti-B antibody in the plasma; type B blood group has type B antigen on its surface and anti-A antibody in the plasma; type AB blood group has both antigens A and B on its surface but does not contain either antibodies in the plasma; and type O blood group has neither antigens A nor B on its surface but contains both anti-A and anti-B antibodies in the plasma. About 45% of the population in the UK is blood group O, and 55% of the population is either blood group A, B or AB (Waugh and Grant, 2018). People with blood group O are known as universal donors as their red blood cells do not have either A or B antigens on their surface. Conversely, people with blood group AB are known as universal recipients as their red blood cells contain A and B antigens on their surface (Table 10.2).

263

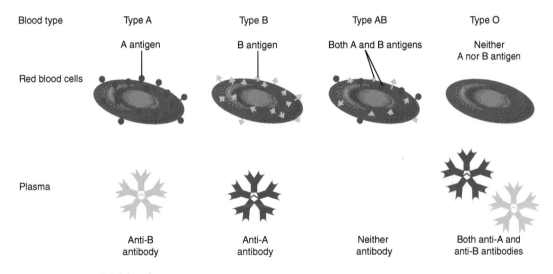

Figure 10.7 ABO blood groups.

Table 10.2 Blood groups.

Blood type	Antigens	Antibodies	Can donate blood to	Can receive blood from
A	Antigen A	Anti-B	A, AB	A, O
B	Antigen B	Anti-A	B, AB	B, O
AB	Antigen A Antigen B	None	AB	A, B, AB, O
O	None	Anti-A	A, B, AB, O	O
		Anti-B		

Red flag

Anaphylaxis is a serious and potentially life-threatening allergic reaction to antibodies or other substances in the blood. In 2013, there were 33 cases of anaphylaxis associated with blood transfusions in the UK, in 2017 there were 442 (Serious Hazards of Transfusion (SHOT), 2017). Participation in UK haemovigilance became more streamlined in March 2017 following the introduction of 'Phase 2' of the unified UK haemovigilance project. This development aimed to link the separate online-reporting systems of the SHOT database (Dendrite), and the Medicines and Healthcare Products Regulatory Agency (MHRA) reporting system, serious adverse blood reactions and events (SABRE). Following successful implementation, there is now a single point of entry to the system via SABRE (https://www.shotuk.org/shot-surveys/).

Nurses need to adhere to the local policy and protocol on the administration and management of a patient on blood transfusion.

Orange flag

Anaphylaxis is a severe and potentially life-threatening allergic reaction. Symptoms can start within seconds or minutes of exposure to the food or substance a person is allergic to and usually will progress quickly. The fact that anaphylaxis can be serious and unpredictable can place a heavy burden on those affected, and on their families. The constant vigilance required and the possibility of being in a life-threatening situation means there is often intense anxiety. It is imperative that the nurse supports the patient and their family by determining if health and well-being needs are being met, ensuring that a holistic approach is being adopted.

Rhesus factor

The rhesus factor (Rh) is another important antigen identified on the surface of red blood cells. The rhesus factor is so called because it was first identified in rhesus monkeys. In the UK, approximately 85% of the population is rhesus positive; i.e. they possess factor D on their red blood cells. The remaining 15% of the population is rhesus negative as their red blood cells do not have factor D. It is important to consider the rhesus factor when cross-matching and transfusing blood to patients to avoid unnecessary complications such as agglutination.

Diseases of the blood
Learning outcomes

On completion of this section, the reader will be able to:

- List some of the common diseases of blood and identify risk factors associated with the diseases.

- Describe the pathophysiological processes related to specific blood disorders.

- Outline the care and management and interventions related to the disorders described.

Snapshot Anaemia

Mr Gerry Oliveira is a 45-year-old man who had a partial gastrectomy 5 years ago due to stomach cancer. Gerry is a second-year student nurse. He is very happy that he can finally achieve something for himself. Gerry is keen to finish his studies and earn some money so that he can help his husband financially. Lately, Gerry has been complaining of tiredness, breathlessness and that his ankles are slightly swollen. He does suffer from gastritis. Gerry does drink alcohol but not excessively. His husband persuaded him to go and see his GP to get some advice and treatment. On arrival to his GP, Gerry was allocated to an advanced nurse practitioner.

265

Vital signs

The practice nurse noted and recorded the following:

Vital sign	Observation	Normal
Temperature	36.8°C	36.0–37.9°C range
Pulse	82 beats per minute	60–100 beats per minute
Respiration	18 breaths per minute	12–20 breaths per minute
Blood pressure	120/62 mmHg	100–139 mmHg (systolic) range
O$_2$ saturation	99%	94–98%

A full blood count and urea and electrolytes was performed.

Test	Result	Guideline normal values
White blood cells (WBC)	9.2×10^9/L	4 to 11×10^9/L
Neutrophils	7.0×10^9/L	2.0 to 7.5×10^9/L
Lymphocytes	3.9×10^9/L	1.3 to 4.0×10^9/L
Red blood cells (RBC)	4.0×10^{12}/L	4.5 to 6.5×10^{12}/L
Haemoglobin	98 g/L	130–180 g/L
Platelets	188×10^9/L	150 to 440×10^9/L
C-reactive protein	5.2 mg/L	<5 mg/L
Urea	6.0 mmol/L	2–6.6 mmol/L
Potassium	5.1 mmol/L	3.4–5.6 mmol/L
Sodium	138 mmol/L	135–147 mmol/L

Take some time to reflect on this case and then consider the following:

1. Which type of anaemia is Gerry suffering from?
2. Discuss the possible investigations that may be carried out to confirm diagnosis.
3. List the medications the advanced nurse practitioner may prescribe to treat his illness.
4. What advice will you give Gerry with regards to his diet and lifestyle?

Anaemia

Anaemia, from the Greek word meaning 'without blood', refers to a reduction in red blood cells and/or haemoglobin. This results in a reduced ability of the blood to transport oxygen to the tissues, causing hypoxia. The normal level of haemoglobin in an adult male is approximately 130–180 g/L of blood, and in an adult female it is approximately 120–160 g/L of blood (Porth, 2014). Anaemia can result from:

- Excessive loss of blood through haemorrhage
- Destruction of red blood cells (haemolysis)
- Deficient red blood cell production due to red bone marrow failure
- Infections such as malaria
- Lack of intake of iron, folic acid and vitamin B_{12}
- Pregnancy.

There are three major types of anaemia:

1. Microcytic anaemia (small red blood cells)
2. Macrocytic anaemia (large blood cells)
3. Normocytic anaemia (normal-sized red blood cells).

Microcytic anaemia

Microcytic anaemia is characterised by small red blood cells. There are several types of microcytic anaemia, of which iron deficiency anaemia is the most common cause of anaemia in the UK. Iron is essential for the production of young red blood cells. As iron is a component of haem, a deficiency of iron leads to decreased haemoglobin synthesis, resulting in impairment of oxygen transport. In iron deficiency anaemia, the red blood cells are small (microcytic) and pale (hypochromic).

Iron deficiency anaemia

Aetiology

Iron deficiency anaemia results from:

- Dietary deficiency of iron
- Loss of iron through haemorrhage
- Poor absorption of iron from the gastrointestinal tract after gastrectomy
- Increased demands, such as growth and pregnancy.

Investigations

The following investigations may be carried out to confirm diagnosis:

- Full blood count (red blood cells, white blood cells, haemoglobin concentration, mean corpuscular volume, haematrocrit)
- Test for levels of ferritin, serum iron, transferring, folate, vitamin B_{12}
- Bone marrow examination
- Physical examination.

Red flag

After a partial or total gastrectomy, the patient may need iron supplement for life.

Orange flag

Care of the surgical patient extends beyond the technical details of a surgical procedure and has to incorporate the psychological needs of the patient. Psychological assessment of the patient includes the search for pre-existing depression and anxiety.

Clinical investigation

Bone marrow sample

Bone marrow samples are usually taken from the top of the pelvic bone. This is the bone that you can easily feel just below each side of your waist. Occasionally, other large bones are used, such as the sternum (breastbone). The patient will be asked to lie on a couch on their stomach or on their side, depending on the exact site the doctor chooses to use. The skin over the bone to be sampled is cleaned with antiseptic.

Some local anaesthetic is then injected into a small area of skin and tissues just over the bone. This stings a little at first, but then makes the skin numb. Some people are given a sedative before the procedure.

To aspirate bone marrow fluid, a needle is pushed through the anaesthetised skin into the bone. A syringe is used to draw out some liquid bone marrow.

In biopsy, a second, thicker, hollow needle is inserted into the bone. This is rotated around as it is pushed slightly forward to force a small sample of bone marrow into the hollow middle of the needle. The needle is then taken out and a pressure bandage applied to prevent bleeding.

After the test, the patient will need to lie on a bed and be observed for an hour to check no serious bleeding takes place.

The patient should be informed that they may have some discomfort and bruising over the test site for a few days. A suitable analgesia will be prescribed to ease the pain.

Pathophysiology

Iron deficiency anaemia is present when the demand for iron in the body exceeds supply; anaemia develops slowly in three stages:

1. The body's iron stores are depleted; however, erythropoiesis continues normally.
2. Iron transportation to bone marrow is diminished, resulting in deficiency in red cell production.
3. The number of microcytic red blood cells increases in the circulation, replacing the normal mature red blood cells.

Iron is constantly used in the production of young red blood cells. Iron is obtained from food sources and absorbed from the gastrointestinal tract. Excess iron is stored in the liver and muscle cells and is readily available for the production of red blood cells.

Some inflammatory disorders such as Crohn's disease will affect the absorption of iron from the gastrointestinal tract, affecting the synthesis of red bloods cells. In some instances, substantial segments of bowel are surgically removed, due to carcinoma of the bowel, again affecting the absorption of iron from the gastrointestinal tract. Inadequate dietary intake also contributes to iron deficiency anaemia in the older adult. Limited access to transportation may make it difficult for the patient to eat a healthy diet rich in meat, fruit and vegetables. Iron deficiency can produce significant gastrointestinal abnormalities such as angular stomatitis and glossitis. Other diseases include peptic ulcer, where the condition produces gastrointestinal bleeding and iron deficiency. The organs affected are the stomach and the duodenum, where there is inflammation and erosion of the membrane.

Signs and symptoms

Patients suffering from iron deficiency anaemia may experience:

- Brittle nails
- Spoon-shaped nails (koilonychias)
- Atrophy of the papillae of the tongue
- Brittle hair
- Cheilosis (cracks at the corners of the mouth)
- Dizziness – due to lack of oxygen supply to the brain
- Hypoxia
- Pica (craving to eat unusual substances such as clay, starch and coal)
- Breathlessness – physiological compensation resulting from the lack of oxygen
- Loss of appetite, which may be due to a sore mouth.

Care and management

The care and management of the patient with iron deficiency anaemia will include a full assessment, including a comprehensive risk assessment to prevent injuries from falls, before planning the appropriate care. The care planned should consider a holistic approach, which includes physical, psychological and social aspects of care.

Patients with iron deficiency anaemia may require blood transfusion. It is the healthcare professional's duty to ensure that the transfusion is administered without complications from transfusion, such as reactions from incompatible blood and hypertension. The patient's vital signs, e.g. temperature, blood pressure, heart rate and respirations, should be monitored every 15 minutes for the first hour as transfusion reactions are likely to occur in the first 15 minutes. Any change in the vital signs should be reported immediately to the nurse in charge and documented in the nursing notes in accordance with local policy and procedure and in alignment with the Nursing and Midwifery Council Code (NMC, 2018).

Patients may be concerned about the risk of contracting HIV or hepatitis C through blood transfusion, and therefore it is the healthcare professional's duty to explain the screening procedures undertaken on donor's blood (Peate, 2020) and the low risk associated with blood transfusion.

Dietary advice on foods rich in iron, such as red meat, liver and vegetables, should be encouraged as iron is an essential component for the production of red blood cells.

Advice on oral hygiene should include the use of a soft-toothed toothbrush, care of dentures and the use of suitable ointments to prevent cracked lips (Renton et al., 2019).

Anaemic patients should be advised not to change position suddenly, e.g. standing up quickly from a sitting position, to avoid falling and injuring themselves as a result of dizziness.

Pharmacological interventions

Patients with iron deficiency anaemia may be prescribed an iron supplement, e.g. ferrous sulphate. Patients should be advised about the side effects, which include constipation, nausea and even diarrhoea. They should be advised to drink 2–3 L of fluid per day to prevent constipation.

Medicine management

Iron tablets

Iron supplements may be taken as capsules, tablets, chewable tablets and liquids. The most common tablet size is 325 mg (ferrous sulphate). Taking more iron than the body needs can cause serious medical problems. Blood counts return to normal after 2 months of iron therapy for most people; however, the patient may continue taking supplements for another 6 to 12 months to build up the body's iron stores in the bone marrow.

Iron is best absorbed on an empty stomach. Yet, iron supplements can cause stomach cramps, nausea and diarrhoea in some people. The patient may need to take iron with a small amount of food to avoid this problem. Milk, calcium and antacids should NOT be taken at the same time as iron supplements. The person should wait at least 2 hours after having these foods before taking the iron supplements.

Constipation and diarrhoea are very common. If constipation becomes a problem, the person should take a stool softener such as docusate sodium (Colace). Nausea and vomiting may occur with higher doses, but they can be controlled by taking the iron in smaller amounts. Black stools are normal when taking iron tablets. In fact, this is felt to be a sign that the tablets are working correctly. Seek medical advice if:

- The stools are tarry-looking as well as black
- If they have red streaks
- Cramps, sharp pains, or soreness in the stomach occur.

Macrocytic anaemia

Macrocytic anaemia is also termed megaloblastic anaemia. It is characterised by defective deoxyribonucleic acid (DNA) synthesis, resulting in the production of unusually large stem cells (macrocytes) in the circulation. In addition to an increase in diameter, the thickness and volume of the cell also increases.

Aetiology

Macrocytic anaemia results from:

- Folate deficiency
- Vitamin B_{12} deficiency.

Both these coenzymes are essential for DNA maturation. Vegans and vegetarians are at risk of developing macrocytic anaemia due to a lack of vitamin B_{12}, which is found in most meat products.

Folate deficiency

Folic acid (folate) is an essential vitamin for the production and maturation of red blood cells. Folate is obtained from the diet and is absorbed from the jejunum and stored in the liver. It is found in leafy vegetables, fruit, cereals and meat; most of it is lost in cooking.

Red flag

Taking folic acid and taking phenytoin (Dilantin) might decrease the effectiveness of phenytoin (Dilantin) and increase the possibility of seizures.

> ## Orange flag
>
> Evidence suggests that folate deficiency may be causatively linked to depressive symptoms (Zhao *et al.*, 2011).

Aetiology
Deficiency in folate can result from:

- Malnutrition
- Malabsorption from the jejunum caused by diseases such as coeliac disease
- Medications that inhibit absorption from the jejunum, e.g. oral contraceptives and anti-convulsants such as phenytoin
- Alcohol abuse – alcohol interferes with folate metabolism in the liver
- Anorexia.

Symptoms
- Fatigue
- Palpitations
- Shortness of breath
- Diarrhoea
- Progressive weakness
- Pallor.

Vitamin B_{12} deficiency
The most common type of megaloblastic anaemia is pernicious anaemia (PA), which results from vitamin B_{12} deficiency. Vitamin B_{12} is essential for the synthesis of DNA, and a deficiency impairs cellular division and maturation, especially in rapidly proliferating red blood cells. The absorption of vitamin B_{12} in the intestine requires the presence of intrinsic factor (IF), which is produced by the gastric mucosa. IF binds to vitamin B_{12} in food, protecting it from gastrointestinal enzymes and facilitating its absorption. Lack of vitamin B_{12} alters the structure and disrupts the function of the peripheral nerves, spinal cord and brain.

Aetiology
Deficiency in vitamin B_{12} can result from:

- Total gastrectomy, partial gastrectomy or gastrojejunostomy
- Gastric lesions
- Carcinoma of the stomach
- Alcohol abuse
- Malabsorption due to inflammatory disease such as Crohn's disease.

Symptoms
- Pallor
- Slight jaundice
- Smooth sore tongue
- Diarrhoea
- Paraesthesias – numbness and tingling in the extremities

- Impaired proprioception (ability to identify one's position in space)
- Problems with balance.

Care and management of people with macrocytic anaemia

Care and management of the patient with macrocytic anaemia is similar to that described earlier for iron deficiency anaemia. A full assessment is essential for planning high-quality care. Most patients with folate deficiency are cared for in the community by their general practice. Patients with folate deficiency anaemia will need dietary advice on which foods contain folic acid and how to avoid destroying it in cooking (Peate, 2020). Advice on folic acid supplements and how to take them should be offered to patients.

Some patients with vitamin B_{12} deficiency may be admitted to hospital for their treatment. The treatment for those patients lacking in IF includes the injection of cyanocobalamin, initially weekly until vitamin B_{12} deficiency is corrected, then monthly. Patients should be advised to eat foods that contain vitamin B_{12} such as eggs, meat and dairy products. PA as a result of vitamin B_{12} deficiency cannot be cured, so the treatment is lifelong. Some patients may need a blood transfusion if they develop complications such as heart failure.

Normocytic anaemia

Normocytic anaemia is characterised by red blood cells that are relatively normal in size and in haemoglobin content, but insufficient in number. It is less common than microcytic and macrocytic anaemias. Normocytic anaemias include:

- Aplastic anaemia
- Haemolytic anaemia
- Sickle cell anaemia.

Aplastic anaemia

Aplastic anaemia (AA) is a serious condition affecting the bone marrow. It is characterised by a reduction of all the blood cells, i.e. the red blood cells, white blood cells and platelets. When all three types of blood cells are low, the condition is termed pancytopenia.

Aetiology

The condition is idiopathic; however, the condition has been associated with:

- Viral diseases, e.g. hepatitis and HIV
- Ionising radiation
- Metastases of the bone
- Cytotoxic drugs
- Chemical compounds, e.g. benzene.

Medicine management

Cytotoxic drugs

Cytotoxic drugs (sometimes known as antineoplastics) describe a group of medicines that contain chemicals which are toxic to cells, preventing their replication or growth, and so are used to treat cancer. They can also be used to treat a number of other disorders such as rheumatoid arthritis and multiple sclerosis. Once inside the body, their action is not generally tightly targeted, and they can produce side effects both in patients and others who become exposed.

Exposure can occur when control measures are inadequate. Exposure may be through skin contact, skin absorption, inhalation of aerosols and drug particles, ingestion and needle stick injuries resulting from the following activities:

- Drug preparation
- Drug administration
- Handling patient waste
- Transport and waste disposal
- Cleaning spills.

Nurses must follow strict protocols to ensure and take preventative measures, to control exposure, such as wearing protective clothing when handling or administering cytotoxic drugs. Procedures must be in place for the safe disposal of waste. Measures to prevent or contain spillages should be used at all times. Any spillages that occur should be dealt with promptly.
Some side effects include:

- Abdominal pain, hair loss, nasal sores, vomiting and liver damage
- Contact dermatitis and local allergic reactions
- Foetal loss in pregnant women and malformations in the children of pregnant women
- Alterations to normal blood cell count
- Abnormal formation of cells and mutagenic activity or mutations forming.

Pathophysiology

AA occurs as a result of reduced bone marrow function, resulting in low numbers of blood cells. Fat cells proliferate to replace stem cells. The formed red blood cells are immature, and the transportation of oxygen is affected. As a result of the shortened lifespan of platelets and white blood cells, patients are prone to infections and bleeding. The most common causes of death are severe haemorrhage, infections and septic shock (Bullock and Henze, 2010). In severe cases, mortality can be high and thus prompt intervention is required.

Symptoms

The initial presenting symptoms include:

- Weakness
- Fatigue
- Pallor caused by anaemia
- Petechiae – small haemorrhages under the skin
- Ecchymoses – bruises on the skin
- Bleeding from mucous membranes of the nose, gums, vagina and gastrointestinal tract may occur as a result of decreased platelet level
- Vulnerability to infections as a result of a low neutrophil count.

Care and management

AA can result in life-threatening complications, such as septic shock, which requires prompt intervention. Specific therapy is determined by the underlying cause of the disorder. The management will include treatment with medications, dietary modifications and blood transfusion if necessary. The healthcare professional's role will include:

- Early detection and treatment of the disease
- Prevention of infections and providing care for septic patients
- Early detection and management of bleeding.

Blood transfusion may be indicated to replace the blood lost, and discontinued as soon as the bone marrow commences the synthesis of blood cells. Healthcare professionals need to be aware of blood transfusion complications such as:

- Hypertension as a result of fluid overload from transfusion
- Transfusion reaction such as rashes and bronchial wheezing
- Electrolyte imbalance
- Incompatibility between a patient's blood and the donor's blood, e.g. back pain, dyspnoea, cyanosis and tachycardia.

As the risk of adverse reaction is high when the blood is transfused, the patient's vital signs must be monitored every 15 minutes for the first hour as many reactions occur within this period (Kozier *et al.*, 2015).

Care and management in the prevention of AA includes teaching good dietary habits, such as having a diet high in iron, folate and vitamin B_{12}, as these are essential in the synthesis of red blood cells. Vegetarians should be encouraged to ingest food rich in vitamin C, as it enhances the absorption of iron from grains and other sources.

Pharmacological interventions

Patients with AA may be prescribed:

- Iron supplement
- Folic acid supplement
- Vitamin B_{12} supplement.

Medicine management

Folic acid

Folate and folic acid are forms of a water-soluble B vitamin. Folate occurs naturally in food, and folic acid is the synthetic form of this vitamin. Folic acid has been added to cold cereals, flour, breads, pasta, bakery items, cookies and crackers as a supplement. Foods that are naturally high in folate include leafy vegetables (such as spinach, broccoli and lettuce), okra, asparagus, fruits (such as bananas, melon, and lemons) beans, yeast, mushrooms, meat (such as beef liver and kidney), orange juice and tomato juice.

Folic acid is used for preventing and treating low blood levels of folate (folate deficiency), as well as its complications, including anaemia and the inability of the bowel to absorb nutrients properly, including ulcerative colitis, liver disease, alcoholism and kidney dialysis.

Side effects include the following:

High doses of folic acid might cause abdominal cramps, diarrhoea, rash, sleep disorders, irritability, confusion, nausea, stomach upset, behavioural changes, skin reactions, seizures, flatus and excitability.

Nurses need to be aware that folic acid can interact with other drugs to increase or decrease its effect. For example, taking folic acid along with methotrexate might decrease the effectiveness of methotrexate, and taking folic acid and phenytoin (Dilantin) might decrease the effectiveness of phenytoin (Dilantin) and increase the possibility of seizures.

Haemolytic anaemia

Haemolytic anaemia results from the premature destruction of red blood cells, leading to the retention of iron and other products of red blood cell destruction. This rare condition is either acquired or inherited. In haemolytic anaemia, the synthesis of red blood cells in the bone marrow is increased to match the number of red blood cells destroyed.

Aetiology

The causes of haemolytic anaemia can be either inherited or acquired and they include:

- Spherocytosis – fragility of the red blood cell membrane
- Haemoglobin defects – thalassaemia and sickle cell anaemia
- Mismatched blood transfusion
- Direct cell injury from drugs, e.g. sodium chlorate
- Disseminated intravascular coagulation
- Haemoglobinopathies – abnormalities in haemoglobin structure.

Red flag

Iron stores increase in haemolysis, and so iron administration is generally contraindicated in haemolytic disorders, particularly those that require chronic transfusion support.

Pathophysiology

The lifespan of red blood cells in haemolytic anaemia is much shorter than the normal lifespan of 120 days. The cell membrane is fragile, resulting in the excessive destruction of the red blood cells; this in turn reduces the number of red blood cells available for the transportation of oxygen, which leads to hypoxia in the tissues. In response to the excessive destruction, the bone marrow becomes hyperactive and produces more red blood cells by erythropoiesis. In haemolytic anaemia, red blood cell destruction can occur in the vascular system or by phagocytosis by the reticuloendothelial system (Porth, 2014). As a result of the increased destruction of the red blood cells, there is an increased level of bilirubin and urobilinogen.

Signs and symptoms

The presence of signs and symptoms depends on the severity of the disease. Some of the clinical manifestations are:

- Jaundice, if red blood cell destruction exceeds the liver's ability to conjugate and excrete bilirubin
- Fatigue
- Hypoxia from impaired oxygen transport
- Dyspnoea
- The spleen may become enlarged in patients with congenital haemolytic disorders.

Care and management

Care and management of the patient with haemolytic anaemia will include advice on diet as for other forms of anaemia, relieving anxiety in patients and their relatives, management of blood transfusion and administration of prescribed medication (see aplastic anaemia). If patients are breathless, they must be nursed upright, supported by pillows and oxygen administered as prescribed.

Sickle cell anaemia

Sickle cell anaemia is a hereditary, chronic haemolytic anaemia characterised by the presence of an abnormal haemoglobin (HbS) molecule (Figure 10.8). This abnormality occurs as a result of a genetic mutation in which one amino acid (valine) replaces another amino acid (glutamic acid). The haemoglobin forms a sickle shape when oxygen is removed from it (Mehta and Hoffbrand, 2014).

In heterozygous twins, if one child inherits the abnormal haemoglobin gene from one parent and a normal haemoglobin (HbA) from the other parent, the child develops the sickle cell trait and is unaware of this until exposed to hypoxic conditions. The trait is passed on to any child. In homozygous twins, the child inherits the abnormal gene from both parents and will suffer from sickle cell anaemia.

275

Pathophysiology

The cause of the sickle shape is the deoxygenation of the haemoglobin. When the haemoglobin is fully saturated with oxygen, the red blood cell has the normal shape, but this changes to the sickle shape as the oxygen content is reduced. Sickled red blood cells are stiff and cannot change shape as normal red blood cells do when they pass through capillaries (Figure 10.9). As a result, the sickled red blood cells obstruct blood flow, causing vascular obstruction, pain and tissue ischaemia.

Sickling is not permanent; most sickled red blood cells regain their normal shape once they are saturated with oxygen. However, repeated sickling causes loss of elasticity of the cell membrane, and over time the cells fail to return to the normal shape when oxygen concentration increases. The weakened red blood cells are haemolysed and removed from the circulation.

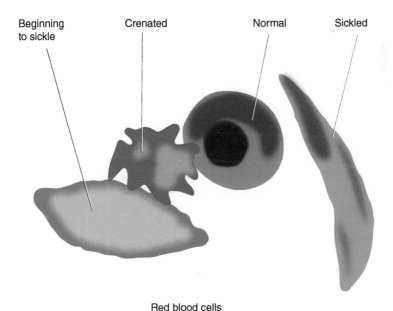

Red blood cells

Figure 10.8   Sickled red blood cell.

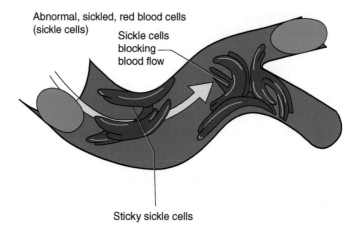

Abnormal, sickled, red blood cells
(sickle cells)
Sickle cells
blocking
blood flow

Sticky sickle cells

Figure 10.9   Sickle cell in microcirculation.

Symptoms

Common presenting symptoms include:

- Pain and swelling caused by occluded blood vessels affecting the hands and feet
- Priapism – persistent painful erection of the penis
- Abdominal pain if the abdominal blood vessels are occluded
- Increased incidence of infection such as osteomyelitis
- Pulmonary hypertension
- Tachycardia
- May present with haematuria (blood in the urine)
- May develop stasis ulcers of the hands, ankles and feet
- White blood cells and platelets are often elevated, thus contributing to vaso-occlusion.

Care and management

There is no known cure for sickle cell anaemia. Care and management of the patient will include alleviation of symptoms and promoting a good quality of life. The care will include:

- Pain management – patients with sickle cell disease may have intensely painful episodes called vaso-occlusive crises. Pain management will require opioid analgesia until the pain has settled. For patients with milder levels of pain, non-steroidal anti-inflammatory drugs such as diclofenac could be the drug of choice. For more severe pain crises, most patients will require admission to hospital for intravenous opioids or patient-controlled analgesia to control their pain level. Treatment for patients experiencing pain crises also includes rest, oxygen therapy, analgesia and hydration.
- Patients will need advice to avoid situations that may trigger a crisis. Risk factors include emotional stress, extreme fatigue and infection.
- Early treatment of infection with antibiotics is important to prevent a crisis occurring. Patients' vital signs should be monitored 2–4 hourly to detect infection in order to commence treatment with antibiotics.
- Blood transfusion is indicated for patients who are breathless as a result of severe hypoxia.
- Genetic counselling should be offered to patients and their families to inform them about the disorder, its inheritance and its consequences.
- During a crisis, fluid therapy is essential to improve blood flow, reduce pain and prevent renal damage and dehydration.

Snapshot   Sickle cell anaemia

Mr David Smith is a 37-year-old man from the Caribbean currently working as an NHS Matron in the UK. He is married to Jess, and they have two children Penny and Alex aged 8 and 13 years. His wife is a self-employed textiles designer who is often busy with her work in her studio. David enjoys socialising, football coaching a local children's team and reading history books.

Over the past 7 days David has been feeling pain in his chest, back and arms, and is pale, breathless, and dizzy. He is worried this may have something to do with his sickle cell anaemia. David visited an emergency nurse practitioner in his hospital ED as after 7 days waiting for the symptoms to resolve; he now thinks this may be serious.

Once the emergency nurse practitioner has completed history taking and physical examination of David's respiratory, cardiac, and muscular skeletal systems in his upper body, she documents his findings and takes his vital signs and his full blood count. After some blood tests and investigations, a provisional diagnosis of sickle cell crisis is made. The consultant decided to admit David for further investigations and treatment.

277

Vital signs

Vital sign	Observation	Normal
Temperature	38°C	36.0–37.9°C range
Pulse	90 beats per minute	60–100 beats per minute
Respiration	26 breaths per minute	12–20 breaths per minute
Blood pressure	130/60 mmHg	100–139 mmHg (systolic) range
O_2 saturation	92%	94–98%

A full blood count and urea and electrolytes was performed.

Test	Result	Guideline normal values
White blood cells (WBC)	3.8×10^9/L	4 to 11×10^9/L
Neutrophils	3.5×10^9/L	2.0 to 7.5×10^9/L
Lymphocytes	1.9×10^9/L	1.3 to 4.0×10^9/L
Red blood cells (RBC)	5.0×10^{12}/L	4.5 to 6.5×10^{12}/L
Haemoglobin (Hb)	70 g/L	130–180 g/L
Platelets	70×10^9/L	150 to 440×10^9/L
C-reactive protein	7.4 mg/L	<5 mg/L
Urea	7.2 mmol/L	2–6.6 mmol/L
Potassium	5.1 mmol/L	3.4–5.6 mmol/L
Sodium	147 mmol/L	135–147 mmol/L

Take some time to reflect on this case and then consider the following:

1. Discuss the possible tests that may be done to confirm diagnosis.
2. What are the risk factors associated with sickle cell crisis?
3. What vital signs and blood results are abnormal, can you identify the correlations between both?
4. What advice would you give David about the treatments for sickle cell crisis?
5. Outline David's care during his stay in hospital.

Leukaemia

Snapshot   Leukaemia

Mr John Tate is a 44-year-old police officer. He is married to Sarah, and they have two sons aged 11 and 13 years. His wife is a teacher who is often busy with her work. Mr Tate enjoys socialising, keeping fit and reading.

Over the past 2–3 months, Mr Tate has been feeling excessively tired. Although he sleeps well at night, he does not feel rested in the morning. Over the past 2 weeks, Mr Tate has been complaining of a sore throat, persistent colds and mouth ulcers. At first he attributed these symptoms to being tired and run down. His wife persuaded him to see his GP. After a thorough physical examination, it was decided that Mr Tate should be seen by a specialist at the hospital.

Mr Tate is seen by the haematology consultant at the local hospital, and after some blood tests and investigations, a provisional diagnosis of acute myeloid leukaemia is made. The consultant decided to admit Mr Tate for further investigations and treatment.

Vital signs

The GP notes and records the following vital signs:

Vital sign	Observation	Normal
Temperature	38.2°C	36.0–37.9°C range
Pulse	84 beats per minute	60–100 beats per minute
Respiration	28 breaths per minute	12–20 breaths per minute
Blood pressure	135/60 mmHg	100–139 mmHg (systolic) range
O_2 saturation	99%	94–98%

A full blood count and urea and electrolytes was performed.

Test	Result	Guideline normal values
White blood cells (WBC)	3.8×10^9/L	4 to 11×10^9/L
Neutrophils	3.5×10^9/L	2.0 to 7.5×10^9/L
Lymphocytes	1.9×10^9/L	1.3 to 4.0×10^9/L
Red blood cells (RBC)	5.0×10^{12}/L	4.5 to 6.5×10^{12}/L
Haemoglobin (Hb)	150 g/L	130–180 g/L
Platelets	290×10^9/L	150 to 440×10^9/L
C-reactive protein	5.4 mg/L	<5 mg/L
Urea	6.2 mmol/L	2–6.6 mmol/L
Potassium	5.1 mmol/L	3.4–5.6 mmol/L
Sodium	138 mmol/L	135–147 mmol/L

Take some time to reflect on this case and then consider the following:

1. Discuss the possible tests that may be done to confirm diagnosis.
2. What are the risk factors associated with acute myeloid leukaemia?
3. What advice would you give Mr Tate if he is to commence chemotherapy?
4. Outline Mr Tate's care during his stay in hospital.

National Early warning Score 2

John Tate

Physiological parameter	3	2	1	0	1	2	3
Respiration rate							28
Oxygen saturation %				99			
Supplemental oxygen				No			
Temperature °C					38.2		
Systolic BP mmHg				135			
Heart rate				84			
Level of consciousness				A			
Score	0	0	0	0	1	0	3
Total	4						

Leukaemia is a malignant disorder where there is an abnormal or excessive proliferation of immature white blood cells. In the UK, leukaemia is the 12th most common cancer in adults, affecting more men than women. There are two principal types – acute and chronic leukaemia. Each of these is further subdivided:

- Acute myeloid leukaemia (AML)
- Acute lymphoblastic leukaemia (ALL)
- Chronic myeloid leukaemia (CML)
- Chronic lymphoblastic leukaemia (CLL).

Red flag

Treatment for ALL is usually urgent and needs to be given within days, and sometimes the same day, as the diagnosis is made. The first phase of treatment, called induction chemotherapy, requires that patients remain in the hospital for approximately four weeks.

Aetiology

The risk factors include:

- Exposure to radiation
- Exposure to benzene (one of the chemicals used in petrol and a solvent used in the rubber and plastic industries)
- Certain genetic conditions such as Down syndrome
- Smoking
- Age – chronic leukaemia is more common over the age of 40 years
- Previous cancer treatments
- Diseases that affect the immune system such as HIV.

Pathophysiology

White blood cells are produced by the bone marrow. They then pass from the bone marrow into the bloodstream and the lymphatic system. White blood cells are involved in various functions of the body's immune system, which protects the body against infections.

Acute leukaemia is more aggressive and develops rapidly. It is more common in the younger age group, and the symptoms develop quickly; if untreated, it becomes life-threatening. Leukaemic cells are immature and poorly differentiated; they proliferate rapidly, have a long lifespan and do not function normally. AML is overproduction of immature myeloid white blood cells, and ALL is the overproduction of immature myeloid lymphocytes, called lymphoblasts. In acute leukaemia, the cells reproduce very quickly and do not become mature enough to carry out their role in the immune system.

CLL is more common in men and occurs most frequently between the ages of 50 and 70 years. In CLL, abnormal lymphocytes proliferate, accumulate in the blood and spread to the lymphatic tissue. Patients affected may live with symptoms for several years. CML has a gradual onset, occurring primarily between the ages 30 and 50 years, and the incidence is slightly higher in men. In CML, there is uncontrolled production of myeloid cells. These cells are abnormal and are not able to carry out the normal functions of white blood cells, such as fighting infections. Their lifespan is long, so over a period of time they replace normal functioning cells (red and white blood cells, and platelets) in the bone marrow. This is a slow process and progressively gets worse over time.

Symptoms

Common presenting symptoms include:

- Tiredness, breathlessness and pale skin (due to anaemia and reduction in red blood cells)
- Abnormal bleeding from the gums and epistaxis
- Bone pain
- Abdominal pain due to an enlarged spleen and/or liver
- Swollen lymph glands in the groin, neck and under the arms
- Weight loss.

Care and management

Patients suffering from leukaemia will need an accurate and full assessment of pain level, activity tolerance, vital signs, nutrition, and signs of bleeding or infection in order to plan high-quality care.

- Advice on preventative measures for bleeding should be offered, i.e. the use of a soft-bristled toothbrush, safety in the use of razors and measures to prevent falls.
- Patients will need advice on measures to maintain hydration and nutrition. Weight is monitored weekly in order to assess weight loss.
- Encourage patients and their relatives to discuss concerns and fears (which may include bone marrow and stem cell transplants).
- Stomatitis (inflammation of the mouth) is a common occurrence, and therefore daily oral hygiene should be encouraged.
- Fatigue as a result of anaemia may be a problem, and therefore patients should be advised to take frequent rest periods and not to overexert themselves.
- Patients should be protected from infections, e.g. washing hands before and after attending to them and discouraging unnecessary visits by others.

Pharmacological and non-pharmacological interventions

Medications and other treatments of leukaemia include:

- Chemotherapy (use of cytotoxic drugs)
- Radiotherapy

- Stem cell and bone marrow transplants
- Monoclonal antibodies
- ATRA (all trans-retinoic acid) is given alongside chemotherapy
- Opioid drugs to control pain.

Thrombocytopenia

Thrombocytopenia is the term for a reduced platelet count. It occurs when platelets are lost from circulation faster than they are produced in the bone marrow. Haemorrhage from trauma or spontaneous bleeding may occur when the platelet count is below 20 000 per cubic millimetre of blood.

Aetiology

Many disease processes can cause thrombocytopenia:

- Anaemia as a result of vitamin B_{12} or folic acid deficiency
- Systemic lupus erythematous
- Sepsis, systemic viral or bacterial infections
- Chemotherapy
- Radiation
- Heparin-induced thrombocytopenia (white clot syndrome)
- HIV.

Pathophysiology

The pathophysiology is related to three basic mechanisms:

1. Accelerated platelet destruction
2. Defective platelet production
3. Disordered platelet distribution.

Three distinct types have been identified:

1. Idiopathic thrombocytopenic purpura (acute and chronic) (ITP)
2. Thrombotic thrombocytopenic purpura (TTP)
3. Haemolytic–uremic syndrome (HUS).

ITP is a disease in which antibodies form and destroy the body's platelets. As the destruction is believed to be caused by the body's immune system, it is classified as an autoimmune disorder. Although the bone marrow increases the synthesis of platelets, it cannot keep up with the demand. Acute ITP is more common in children, while chronic ITP is more common in adults. Platelets become coated with antibodies as a result of the autoimmune response mediated by B lymphocytes. Although the platelets function normally, the spleen identifies them as foreign protein and destroys them.

TTP is a rare disease in which small blood clots form suddenly throughout the body. The numerous blood clots result in a high level of platelet usage in clotting, which reduces their number.

HUS is a rare disorder related to TTP in which the numbers of platelets and red blood cells decrease. HUS can also occur with intestinal infections with *Escherichia coli* and with the use of some drugs such as cyclosporine.

Signs and symptoms

Patients with thrombocytopenia may experience:

- Unexpected bruising
- Petechiae (small red spots under the skin)
- Bleeding from the gastrointestinal tract
- Epistaxis (bleeding from the nose)
- Pain in the joints and muscles
- Heavier than usual menstrual periods in women.

Care and management

As a result of a low level of platelets, the patient is at risk of bleeding, especially from the gums. Early identification of bleeding is important in order to prevent blood loss.

- Monitor vital signs – heart rate, respiratory rate and blood pressure – every 4 hours. Observe for bleeding from other parts of the body, such as in the urine (haematuria), gastrointestinal tract, nasal membrane and vagina.
- Observe the skin for petechiae.
- Advise the patient about the use of safety measures to minimise the risk of bleeding, such as the use of a soft-bristled toothbrush and an electric razor for shaving. Hard bristles may abrade the oral mucosa, causing bleeding, and increase the risk of infection.
- Encourage the patient to rinse the mouth every 2–4 hours to maintain oral hygiene.
- Advise the patient to take 2–2.5 L of fluid over 24 hours to prevent dehydration and infection.
- Advise the patient to avoid medications that interfere with platelet function, such as aspirin.
- A healthy diet high in fibre should be encouraged to prevent constipation. Straining to have a bowel movement could increase the risk of internal bleeding from the gastrointestinal tract.

Pharmacological and non-pharmacological interventions

- Platelet transfusion may be required to treat acute bleeding.
- Oral glucocorticoids such as prednisolone may be prescribed to suppress the autoimmune response.
- Splenectomy may be performed in patients with ITP.

Clinical investigation

Role of history taking and physical examination in thrombocytopenia

Taking a thorough medical history can provide invaluable information and greatly facilitate diagnosis. Aspects of particular relevance that should be investigated include the presence of a family history of thrombocytopenia (a diagnosis of congenital thrombocytopenia is not uncommon in adults); the temporal profile of the thrombocytopenia or of the bleeding manifestations (new onset, chronic, or relapsing); disease history, with particular reference to autoimmune disorders, infections, or malignancies; pregnancy status in premenopausal woman; recent medications and vaccinations;

recent travel (e.g. malaria, rickettsiosis, dengue fever); recent transfusions; recent organ transplantation; ingestion of alcohol and quinine-containing beverages; dietary habits; and risk factors for retroviral infections and viral hepatitis. A history of recurrent, symptomatic thrombocytopenia with platelet counts returning to normal within days, even in the absence of specific treatment, should prompt investigation of a drug-induced thrombocytopenia. The bleeding history does not help in diagnosing the nature of the thrombocytopenia, but gives important clues about its duration and defines its clinical phenotype. Collecting a detailed medical history is not always possible, the typical situation being the unconscious patient with severe thrombocytopenia in the intensive care unit (ICU). However, in such cases, thrombocytopenia is almost always an acute event, and the disease history and exposure to medications (e.g. heparin and antibiotics) immediately preceding the development of thrombocytopenia should be available in the patient's notes.

Physical examination should focus on the location and severity of bleeding risk and other abnormalities that can help in the diagnosis of the thrombocytopenia, such as the presence of organomegaly or skeletal abnormalities. Patients with thrombocytopenia typically experience mucocutaneous bleeding. The presence of joint or extensive soft tissue bleeding suggests the presence of coagulation abnormalities, such as occurs in disseminated intravascular dissemination. The presence of an ischaemic limb or skin necrosis should raise suspicion of heparin-induced thrombocytopenia.

Snapshot   Thrombocytopenia

Mrs LuLu Adebayo is a 67-year-old Nigerian female who has a presenting complaint of non-Hodgkin's lymphoma. Lately, LuLu has been complaining of feeling cold, breathless and a little dizzy when she stands up too quickly. She had chemotherapy 10 days ago but does not want to worry anyone. Eventually she contacts her GP who refers her by telephone immediately to see the cancer team who are already treating her at her local hospital.

Vital signs

The registered nursing associate recorded the following vital signs, and presented the findings to the Registered Nurse for review:

Vital sign	Observation	Normal
Temperature	35.0°C	36.0–37.9°C range
Pulse	96 beats per minute	60–100 beats per minute
Respiration	22 breaths per minute	12–20 breaths per minute
Blood pressure	100/58 mmHg	100–139 mmHg (systolic) range
O₂ saturation	90%	94–98%

A full blood count and urea and electrolytes was performed.

Test	Result	Guideline normal values
White blood cells (WBC)	9.0×10^9/L	4 to 11×10^9/L
Neutrophils	2.0×10^9/L	2.0 to 7.5×10^9/L
Lymphocytes	3.9×10^9/L	1.3 to 4.0×10^9/L
Red blood cells (RBC)	4.0×10^{12}/L	4.5 to 6.5×10^{12}/L
Haemoglobin	g/L	130–180 g/L
Platelets	30×10^9/L	150 to 440×10^9/L
C-reactive protein	5.6 mg/L	<5 mg/L
Urea	6.0 mmol/L	2–6.6 mmol/L
Potassium	5.8 mmol/L	3.4–5.6 mmol/L
Sodium	148 mmol/L	135–147 mmol/L

Take some time to reflect on this case and then consider the following:

1. Which of the blood results were abnormal and why would this be?
2. Discuss the vital signs in relation to these blood results?
3. In relation to LuLu's chemotherapy 10 days ago, do you believe these results to be typical or atypical?
4. What advice will you give LuLu about her breathlessness and dizziness in relation to her vital signs and blood results?
5. What do you know about thrombocytopenia?

Conclusion

This chapter has discussed some of the common disorders of blood that the learner might encounter. Healthcare professionals need to have a good knowledge of the physiology of blood in order to understand the pathophysiology of blood disorders and to provide appropriate care. Patients are often frightened when they are informed that they have a certain blood disorder. It is the healthcare professionals' duty to ensure that the patient receives accurate information relating to their disease and to provide the necessary care.

Test your knowledge

1. List the functions of blood.
2. Explain the clotting process.
3. Explain what would happen if a patient receives mismatched blood.
4. Where is most of the body's blood found?
5. If the blood in the veins is dark red, why does it appear bright red when the vein is cut and bleeding?

Activities

Here are some activities and exercises to help test your learning. For the answers to these exercises, as well as further self-testing activities, visit our website at www.wiley.com/go/fundamentalsofappliedpathophysiology/student4e

Multiple choice questions

1. The formed elements are made up of red blood cells (erythrocytes), which account for what percentage of the blood?
   (a) 25%
   (b) 45%
   (c) 65%

2. Plasma makes up how much of the total blood volume?
   (a) 5%
   (b) 35%
   (c) 55%

3. What percentage do the remaining – white blood cells and platelets – make up?
   (a) 1%
   (b) 16%
   (c) 26%

4. In a healthy person, blood forms about 7–9% of total body weight.
   (a) True
   (b) False

5. Albumin is the most abundant plasma protein.
   (a) True
   (b) False

6. Electrolytes are inorganic molecules that are unable separate into ions when dissolved in water.
   (a) True
   (b) False

7. Vasoconstriction results from contraction of the smooth muscle of the vessel wall.
   (a) True
   (b) False

8. How many red blood cells in each cubic millimetre of blood?
   (a) 3-4.5 million red blood cells
   (b) 4-5.5 million red blood cells
   (c) 5-6.5 million red blood cells

9. The production of red blood cells is controlled by the hormone erythropoietin.
   (a) True
   (b) False

10. White blood cells are also known as leucocytes?
    (a) True
    (b) False

11. How many white blood cells are there in every cubic millimetre of blood?
    (a) 1000 – 2000
    (b) 3000-4900
    (c) 5000–10 000

12. An increase in white blood cells is called leucocytosis.
    (a) True
    (b) False

13. An abnormally low level of white blood cell is called leucopenia.
    (a) True
    (b) False

14. Unlike red blood cells, white blood cells do have nuclei, and they are able to move across blood vessel walls into the tissues.
    (a) True
    (b) False
15. White blood cells can produce a continuous supply of energy, unlike red blood cells.
    (a) True
    (b) False

Conditions

The following is a list of conditions associated with the blood. Take some time, and write notes about each of the conditions. You may make the notes taken from textbooks or other resources (e.g. people you work with in a clinical area), or you may make the notes based on people you have cared for. If you are making notes about people you have cared for, you must ensure that you adhere to the rules of confidentiality.

Septicaemia	
Polycythaemia	
von Willebrand disease	
Disseminated intravascular coagulation	

Myeloma

Further resources

Contact a Family

http://www.cafamily.org.uk/ Accessed 30 March 2020.

Students will find this website a useful source of information on leukaemia. Contact a Family provides support, advice and information for families with disabled children, no matter what their condition or disability. Patients can be referred to this website for support.

National Institute for Health and Care Excellence (NICE) – Treatment for chronic myeloid leukaemia

https://pathways.nice.org.uk/pathways/blood-and-bone-marrow-cancers/myeloid-leukaemia Accessed 30 March 2020.

This link gives access to a NICE pathway and guidance on blood and bone marrow cancers, and recommends treatment for chronic myeloid leukaemia. It is a useful link for your studies of blood disorders.

National Institute for Health and Care Excellence (NICE) – Treatment of anaemia in patients with chronic kidney disease

https://www.nice.org.uk/guidance/ng8/ifp/chapter/Treating-anaemia-in-people-with-chronic-kidney-disease 30 March 2020.

This link gives NICE guidance on how to treat anaemia in people with chronic kidney disease. It is a useful link for your studies of blood disorders.

Health concerns

http://www.lifeextension.com/Protocols/Heart-Circulatory/Blood-Disorders/Page-01 Accessed 30 March 2020.

This is a useful website for students to learn about different blood disorders.

Biomedical Central

http://www.biomedcentral.com/bmcblooddisord/ Accessed 2 August 2016.

BMC Blood Disorders is an open access journal publishing original peer-reviewed research articles in all aspects of the prevention, diagnosis and management of blood disorders, as well as related molecular genetics, pathophysiology and epidemiology. Students may find this website too high powered, but it is nevertheless a useful site for reference.

National Heart, Lung and Blood Institute

https://www.nhs.uk/conditions/stem-cell-transplant/ Accessed 30 March 2020.

This is a good Web link to find out about bone marrow stem cell transplant in patients with blood disorders. This link provides an overview of the type of patients who may need a stem cell transplant and some of the issues before and after the treatment.

Glossary of terms

Adenosine triphosphate (ATP)   A compound of an adenosine molecule with three attached phosphoric acid molecules. Essential for the production of cellular energy.

Agglutination   A process by which red blood cells adhere to one another.

Antibody   A protein in the blood that binds specifically to a particular foreign substance (its antigen). It is a major part of the immune system.

Antigen   A foreign substance (e.g. an infecting microorganism) that can be recognised by the immune system and generates an antibody response.

Bile   An alkaline fluid secreted by the liver that aids digestion of lipids.

Bilirubin   A pigment found in bile resulting from the destruction of red blood cells.

Blood groups   The classification of blood based on the type of antigen found on the surface of the red blood cell.

B lymphocyte   A type of lymphocyte that produces specific antibodies.

Coagulation   The process of transforming a liquid into a solid (especially a blood clot) or the hardening of tissue by physical means.

Coenzyme   A molecule that binds to an enzyme and is essential for its activity, but is not permanently altered by the reaction.

Connective tissue   A primary tissue characterised by cells separated by a matrix; supports and binds other body tissue.

Epistaxis   Bleeding from the nose.

Erythrocyte   Another name for a red blood cell.

Erythropoietin   A hormone produced by the kidneys that regulates the production of red blood cells.

Gastrectomy   Excision of part or the whole of the stomach.

Haematocrit   The percentage of blood volume occupied by erythrocytes.

Haemoglobin   A protein consisting of globin and four haem groups that is found within erythrocytes (red blood cells). Responsible for the transport of oxygen.

Haemostasis   The stoppage of bleeding.

Homeostasis   Maintenance of relatively constant conditions within the body's internal environment despite external environment changes.

Idiopathic   Without a known cause.

Immunity   A protective mechanism that forms antibodies to help protect the body against foreign substances.

Immunoglobulin   Another name for antibody. Antibodies are opsonins that are manufactured by the B lymphocytes and help the phagocytic cells to destroy invading microorganisms in the immune response.

Intrinsic factor   A protein secreted by the parietal cells of the gastric glands and essential for the absorption of vitamin B_{12}.

Lysozyme   A bacteria-destroying enzyme found in lysosomes, sweat, tears, saliva and other bodily secretions.

Mesenchyme   The embryonic mesoderm that develops into connective tissue.

Mitochondria   Cytoplasmic organelles responsible for ATP production.

Molecule   A particle containing two or more atoms joined together by chemical bonds.

Nucleus   A large organelle that contains genetic information and acts as the control centre of the cell.

Organelle   A structural and functional part of a cell that acts like a human organ to fulfil all the needs of the cell so that it can grow, reproduce and carry out its functions.

Osmosis   The passive movement of water through a selectively permeable membrane from an area of high concentration of a chemical to an area of low concentration.

Pathogen   A microorganism that causes problems – is 'infectious'.

Phagocyte   White blood cell that engulfs and destroys microorganisms.

Plasma   The fluid component of the blood.

Platelet   A type of blood cell important in blood clotting.

Polypeptide   A chain of amino acids.

Urobilinogen   A product of bilirubin breakdown.

White blood cell   A leucocyte.

References

Bullock, B.A. and Henze, R.L. (2010). *Focus on Pathophysiology*. Philadelphia: Lippincott.

Kozier, B., Erb, G., Berman, A., Snyder, S.J. and Frandsen, G. (2015). *Fundamentals of Nursing. Concepts, Processes and Practice*, 10th edn. Harlow: Pearson Education.

Mader, S.S. (2019). *Understanding Human Anatomy and Physiology*, 10th edn. Boston: McGraw Hill.

Marieb, E.N. and Hoehn, K. (2015). *Human Anatomy and Physiology*, 10th edn. San Francisco: Pearson Benjamin Cummings.

Mehta, A. and Hoffbrand, V. (2014). *Haematology at a Glance*, 4th edn. Oxford: Blackwell.

Nursing and Midwifery Council (2018). *The Code. Professional Standards of Practice and Behaviour for Nurses and Midwives.* https://www.nmc.org.uk/standards/code/ Accessed March 2020.

Peate, I. (2020). *Alexander's Nursing Practice,* hospital and home, 5th edn. Elsevier.

Porth, C.M. (2014). *Pathophysiology: Concepts of Altered Health States*, 9th edn. Philadelphia: Lippincott Williams & Wilkins.

Renton, S., McGuinness, C. and Strachan, E. (2019). *Clinical Nursing Practice*, 6th edn. Edinburgh: Churchill Livingstone.

SHOT (2017). Annual SHOT report 2017. *MHRA*. Available at: https://b-s-h.org.uk/media/16506/shot-report-2017.pdf Accessed: 31.03.2020

Stanfield, C.L. (2013). *Principles of Human Physiology*, 5th edn. Boston: Benjamin Cummings.

Waugh, A. and Grant, A. (2018). *Ross and Wilson Anatomy and Physiology in Health and Illness*, 13th edn. Edinburgh: Elsevier.

Zhao, G., Ford, E.S., Li, C. *et al.* (2011). Use of folic acid and vitamin supplementation among adults with depression and anxiety: a cross-sectional, population-based survey. *Nutrition Journal*, 10: 102. https://doi.org/10.1186/1475-2891-10-102

Chapter 11

The renal system and associated disorders

Karen Nagalingam

Senior Lecturer, University of Hertfordshire, and Acute Kidney Injury Nurse Specialist Lister Hospital, UK

Contents

Introduction	291
The renal system	291
Disorders of the renal system	300
Conclusion	316
Test your knowledge	317
Multiple choice questions	317
Further resources	319
Glossary of terms	319
References	320

Key words

- Kidneys
- Hilus
- Renal artery
- Nephron
- Ureter
- Renal medulla
- Renal vein
- Glomerulus
- Urethra
- Renal cortex
- Renal pelvis
- Filtration

Fundamentals of Applied Pathophysiology: An Essential Guide for Nursing and Healthcare Students, Fourth Edition. Edited by Ian Peate.
© 2021 John Wiley & Sons Ltd. Published 2021 by John Wiley & Sons Ltd.
Student companion website: www.wiley.com/go/fundamentalsofappliedpathophysiology/student4e
Instructor companion website: www.wiley.com/go/fundamentalsofappliedpathophysiology/instructor4e

- Name four functions of the kidneys.
- Which substances are reabsorbed and which are excreted by the kidneys?
- Describe the structure of the urinary system.
- What is the colour of urine? Think about the destruction of the red blood cells.
- Describe where the kidneys are located in your body.

Learning outcomes

On completion of this section, the reader will be able to:

- Describe the structure and functions of the kidney.

- Describe the microscopic structure of the kidney.

- Explain glomerular filtration.

- To be able to determine if a patient is in Acute Kidney Injury (AKI).

- To understand the difference between AKI and Chronic Kidney Disease (CKD).

Don't forget to visit the companion website for this book
(www.wiley.com/go/fundamentalsofappliedpathophysiology/student4e)
where you can find self-assessment tests to check your progress, as well as lots of activities to practise your learning.

Introduction

The kidneys play an important role in maintaining homeostasis. They remove waste products through the production and excretion of urine, and regulate fluid balance in the body. As part of their function, the kidneys filter essential substances such as sodium and potassium from the blood and selectively reabsorb substances essential to maintain homeostasis. Any substances that are not essential are excreted in the urine. The formation of urine is achieved through the processes of filtration, selective reabsorption and excretion. The kidneys also have an endocrine function, secreting hormones such as renin and erythropoietin. This chapter discusses the structure and functions of the renal system. It also describes some common disorders and their related care, management and treatment.

The renal system

The renal system, also known as the urinary system (Figure 11.1), consists of the:

- Kidneys
- Ureters
- Urinary bladder
- Urethra.

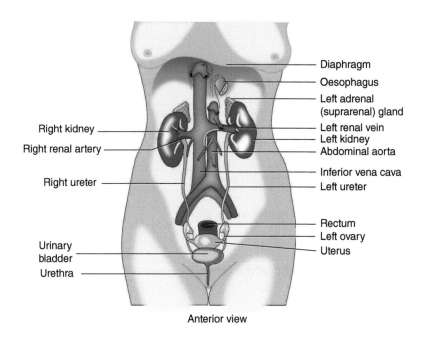

Right kidney

Right renal artery

Right ureter

Urinary
bladder
Urethra

Diaphragm
Oesophagus
Left adrenal
(suprarenal) gland
Left renal vein
Left kidney
Abdominal aorta
Inferior vena cava
Left ureter

Rectum
Left ovary
Uterus

Anterior view

Figure 11.1   Renal system.

The organs of the renal system ensure that a stable internal environment is maintained for the survival of cells and tissues in the body – homeostasis.

Kidneys
External structures

There are two kidneys, one on each side of the spinal column. They are approximately 11 cm long, 5–6 cm wide and 3–4 cm thick (Marieb and Hoehn, 2018). They are bean-shaped organs where the outer border is convex; the inner border is known as the hilum (also known as the hilus), and it is from here that the renal arteries, renal veins, nerves and ureters enter and leave the kidneys. The right kidney is in contact with the liver's large right lobe and hence the right kidney is approximately 2–4 cm lower than the left kidney.

Three layers cover and support the kidneys (Figure 11.2):

1. Renal fascia – outer layer
2. Adipose tissue – middle layer
   Renal capsule – inner layer.

Internal structures

There are three distinct regions inside a kidney (Figure 11.3):

1. Renal cortex
2. Renal medulla
3. Renal pelvis.

The renal cortex is the outermost part of the kidney. It is reddish brown and has a granular appearance, which is due to the capillaries and the structures of the nephron. The medulla is

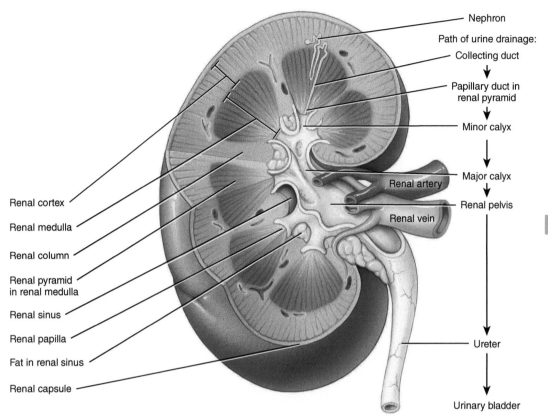

Nephron

Path of urine drainage:

Collecting duct

Papillary duct in
renal pyramid

Minor calyx

Major calyx

Renal artery

Renal pelvis

Renal vein

Renal cortex

Renal medulla

Renal column

Renal pyramid
in renal medulla

Renal sinus

Renal papilla

Fat in renal sinus

Renal capsule

Ureter

Urinary bladder

Figure 11.2   External layers of the kidney. Nephron artificially inserted out of normal proportion.

lighter in colour and has an abundance of blood vessels and tubules of the nephron (Figure 11.3). The medulla consists of approximately 8–12 renal pyramids (Figure 11.3). The renal pelvis is formed from the expanded upper portion of the ureter and is funnel shaped. It collects urine from the calyces (Figure 11.2) and transports it to the urinary bladder.

Nephrons

These are small structures found in the kidney. There are over 1 million nephrons per kidney, and it is in these structures that urine is formed (Figure 11.4). The nephrons:

- Filter blood
- Perform selective reabsorption
- Excrete unwanted waste products from the filtered blood.

The nephron is divided into several Sections and each section performs a different function (Figure 11.4).

Bowman's capsule

Also known as the glomerular capsule, this is the first portion of the nephron (Figure 11.5). It is in this section that the network of capillaries, called the glomerulus (Marieb and Hoehn, 2018), is found. Filtration of blood takes place in this portion of the nephron.

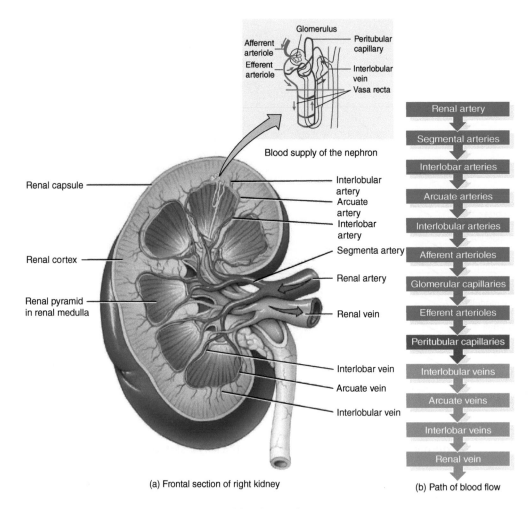

Figure 11.3   Internal structures showing blood vessels.

Proximal convoluted tubule

From the Bowman's capsule, the filtrate drains into the proximal convoluted tubule (Figure 11.4). The cells lining this portion of the tubule actively reabsorb water, nutrients and ions into the peritubular fluid (the interstitial fluid surrounding the renal tubule).

Loop of Henle

The proximal convoluted tubule then bends into the loop of Henle (Figure 11.4). The loop of Henle is divided into the descending and ascending loop. The ascending loop of Henle is much thicker than the descending portion.

Distal convoluted tubule

The thick ascending portion of the loop of Henle leads into the distal convoluted tubule (Figure 11.4). The distal convoluted tubule is an important site for:

- Active secretion of ions and acids
- Selective reabsorption of sodium and calcium ions
- Selective reabsorption of water.

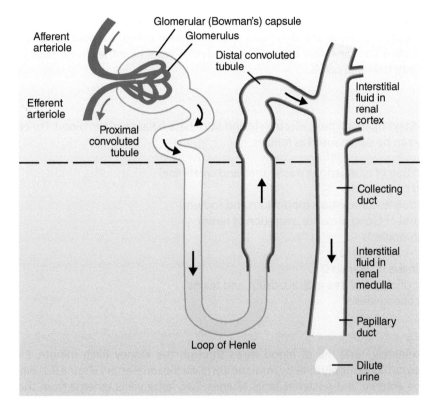

Figure 11.4 Nephron produces dilute urine after the distal tubules and collecting ducts have been passed, which are the site of urine concentration by ADH.

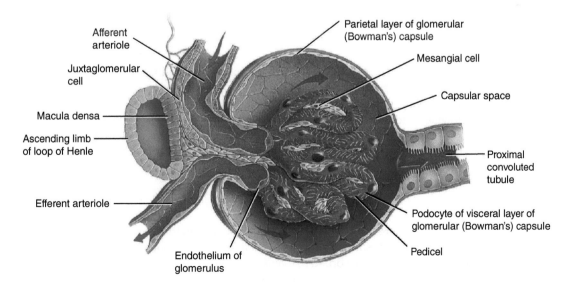

Figure 11.5 Bowman's capsule.

Collecting ducts

The distal convoluted tubule then drains into the collecting ducts (Figure 11.4). Several collecting ducts converge and drain into a larger system called the papillary ducts, which in turn empties into the minor calyx (plural – calyces). From here the filtrate, now called urine, drains into the renal pelvis.

Functions of the kidney

The kidneys maintain fluid, electrolyte and acid–base balance of the blood. Functions of the kidney can be summarised as follows:

- Excretion of nitrogenous waste (urea and creatinine)
- Fluid homeostasis
- Electrolyte homeostasis (potassium and sodium)
- Control of blood pressure (secretion of renin)
- Erythropoiesis
- Acid–base balance
- Synthesis of vitamin D
- Detoxification of free radicals, drugs and toxins
- Gluconeogenesis.

Blood supply

Approximately 1200 mL of blood flows through the kidney each minute. Each kidney receives its blood supply directly from the aorta via the renal artery (Figure 9.2) which divides into the anterior and posterior renal arteries. Two large veins emerge from the hilus and empty into the inferior vena cava.

Urine formation

Three processes are involved in the formation of urine:

1. Filtration
2. Selective reabsorption
3. Secretion.

Filtration

Filtration takes place in the glomerulus, which lies in the Bowman's capsule. The blood for filtration is supplied by the renal artery. In the kidney, the renal artery divides into smaller arterioles. The arteriole entering the Bowman's capsule is called the afferent arteriole, which further subdivides into a cluster of capillaries called the glomerulus. The fluid from the filtered blood is protein free but contains electrolytes such as sodium chloride, potassium chloride and waste products of cellular metabolism, e.g. urea, uric acid and creatinine (McCance and Huether, 2018). The filtered blood then returns to the circulation via the efferent arteriole and finally the renal vein.

Selective reabsorption

Selective reabsorption processes ensure that any substances in the filtrate that are essential for body function are reabsorbed into the plasma. Substances such as sodium, calcium, potassium and chloride are reabsorbed to maintain the fluid and electrolyte balance and the pH of blood. However, if these substances are in excess of body requirements, they are excreted in the urine.

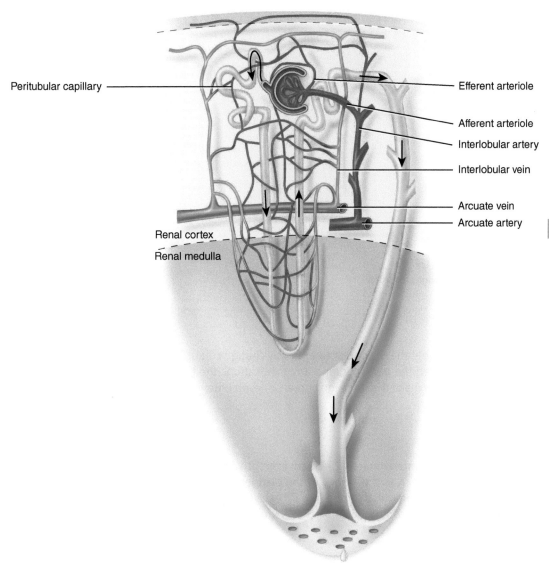

Peritubular capillary

Efferent arteriole

Afferent arteriole

Interlobular artery

Interlobular vein

Arcuate vein

Arcuate artery

Renal cortex

Renal medulla

Figure 11.6 Nephron with capillaries.

Secretion

Any substances not removed through filtration are secreted into the renal tubules from the peritubular capillaries (Figure 11.6) of the nephron (Waugh *et al.*, 2018); these include drugs and hydrogen ions.

Composition of urine

Urine is a sterile and clear fluid containing nitrogenous waste and salts. It is transparent with an amber or light yellow colour. It is slightly acidic, and the pH may range from 4.5 to 8. The pH is affected by an individual's dietary intake. Diet that is high in animal protein tends to make the urine more acidic, while a vegetarian diet may make the urine more alkaline.

Urine is 96% water and approximately 4% solutes. The solutes include organic and inorganic waste products (Table 11.1).

Table 11.1   Summary of the composition of urine.

Composition of urine
Sodium
Potassium
Urea
Creatinine
Uric acid
Chloride
Sulphate
Phosphate
Oxalates
Ammonia
Water (96%)

Source: Adapted from Waugh *et al.,* 2018.

Red flag

It is important to note that urine can temporarily change colour, depending on what has been eaten, how hydrated the person is, and any medications the person is taking. Some medications and foods can make the urine look green, or even blue!

Ureters

The ureters are approximately 25–30 cm in length and 3 mm in diameter (Waugh *et al.,* 2018), and they extend from the kidney to the bladder. The ureters terminate at the bladder and enter obliquely through the muscle wall of the bladder. They pass over the pelvic brim at the bifurcation of the common iliac arteries (Figure 11.7).

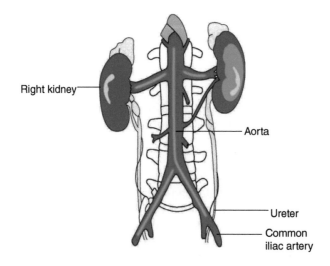

Figure 11.7   Common iliac vessels and ureter.

The ureters have three layers:

1. Transitional epithelial mucosa (inner layer)
2. Smooth muscle layer (middle layer)
3. Fibrous connective tissue (outer layer).

Urine is propelled from the kidney to the bladder by peristaltic contraction of the ureters.

Urinary bladder

The urinary bladder is located in the pelvic cavity posterior to the symphysis pubis. In the male, the bladder lies anterior to the rectum, and in the female, it lies anterior to the vagina and inferior to the uterus (McCance and Huether, 2018); it is a smooth muscular sac which stores urine. As urine accumulates, the bladder expands without a significant rise in the internal pressure of the bladder. The bladder normally distends and holds approximately 350 mL of urine.

The urinary bladder has three layers (Figure 11.8):

1. Transitional epithelial mucosa
2. A thick muscular layer
3. A fibrous outer layer.

Urethra

The urethra is a muscular tube that drains urine from the bladder and conveys it out of the body. The urethra varies in length in both males and females. Sphincters keep the urethra

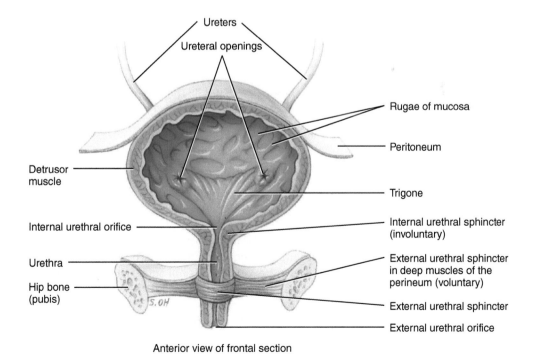

Anterior view of frontal section

Figure 11.8 Layers of the urinary bladder.

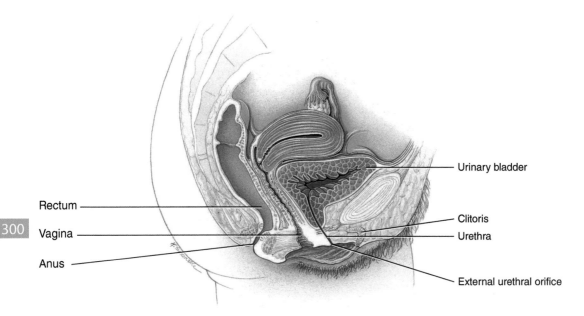

Figure 11.9   Sagittal section pelvis showing the location of the female urethra.

closed when urine is not being passed. The internal urethral sphincter is under involuntary control and lies at the bladder–urethra junction. The external urethral sphincter is under voluntary control.

The male urethra passes through three different regions:

1. Prostatic region – passes through the prostate gland
2. Membranous portion – passes through the pelvic diaphragm
3. Penile region – extends the length of the penis.

The female urethra is bound to the anterior vaginal wall. The external opening of the urethra is anterior to the vagina and posterior to the clitoris (Figure 11.9).

Disorders of the renal system

Case study

Ms Abigail Spears is a 22-year-old with learning disabilities who presents at the local well person clinic with a 48-hour history of needing to urinate frequently, and it hurts when she does. Ms Spears also thinks she may have seen blood in her urine but is not sure. Her mother who has accompanied her says that she has not had a urinary tract infection (UTI) as an adult but had several UTIs as a child. She has some back and loin pain, but no vaginal irritation or discharge. She has an implant for contraception and for regulating her periods, and her mum states it is extremely unlikely that Abigail is pregnant.

Vital signs

The nurse at the clinic notes and records the following:

Vital sign	Observation	Normal
Temperature	38.8°C	36.0–37.9 °C
Pulse	110 beats per minute	60-100 beats per minute
Respiration	18 breaths per minute	12–20 breaths per minute
Blood pressure:	140/75 mmHg	100–139 mmHg (systolic) range
O_2 saturation:	97%	94–98%

A full blood count and urea and electrolytes was performed.

Test	Result	Guideline normal values
White blood cells (WBC)	16×10^9/L	4 to 11×10^9/L
Neutrophils	8.8×10^9/L	2.0 to 7.5×10^9/L
Lymphocytes	5.9×10^9/L	1.3 to 4.0×10^9/L
Red blood cells (RBC)	5.3×10^{12}/L	4.5 to 6.5×10^{12}/L
Haemoglobin (Hb)	158 g/L	130–180 g/L
Platelets	298×10^9/L	150 to 440×10^9/L
C-reactive protein	5.2 mg/L	<5 mg/L
Urea	6.4 mmol/L	2.0–6.6 mmol/L
Potassium	5.1 mmol/L	3.4–5.6 mmol/L
Sodium	138 mmol/L	135–147 mmol/L

Take some time to reflect on this case and then consider the following:

1. What other information about her clinical history would you like to know?
2. You have been asked to do Ms Spears' urinalysis. Explain why you are doing the urinalysis and explain abnormal findings.
3. What advice would you offer Ms Spears to prevent reoccurrence of her UTI?
4. Outline a plan of care for Ms Spears.

Pyelonephritis

Pyelonephritis is inflammation of the renal pelvis and the functional units of the kidney (nephrons). It involves the cortex and the medulla, which is called the parenchyma of the kidney. The incidence is higher in women than in men. There are two main types – acute and chronic pyelonephritis.

Acute pyelonephritis

In acute pyelonephritis, there is sudden or severe infection of the kidney by gram-negative bacteria such as *Escherichia coli* and *Proteus mirabilis*. Gram-negative bacteria are those that do not retain crystal violet dye after an alcohol wash. They may have a red or pink colouration when another dye such as safranin is added to the slide. Gram-positive bacteria will retain the dye and have a purple colouration. They usually ascend from the lower urinary tract (urethra and urinary bladder). In men, prostatitis and prostatic hypertrophy causing urethral obstruction predispose to bacterial infection. Acute pyelonephritis can be caused by blood infection such as septicaemia.

Signs and symptoms

Patients with acute pyelonephritis may present with the following signs and symptoms:

- Sudden onset of fever
- Chills
- Nausea
- Vomiting
- Groin pain
- Haematuria
- Dysuria
- Rigour.

Investigations

The following may be carried out to confirm diagnosis:

- Midstream specimen or catheter specimen of urine to identify causative organism
- Full blood count – raised white blood cells may indicate urine infection
- Ultrasound to identify any obstruction in the urinary tract
- Full nursing and medical history to identify any previous UTI and kidney stones.

Care and management

Patients with acute pyelonephritis may need admitting to hospital if they have signs and symptoms of more serious illness, such as sepsis. Patients who are pregnant, have indwelling catheters, have underlying health issues such as diabetes, genitourinary tract abnormalities or on immunosuppression, are at increased risk of complications (NICE, 2019). It is therefore important to observe for and report signs of pain, agitation and confusion, tachypnoea, low blood pressure and sweating, in order to take prompt action.

Patients may be unable to take oral fluids as a result of nausea and vomiting and can become dehydrated. Therefore, intravenous fluid therapy may be required to support hydration. When able to take oral fluids, the patient should be encouraged to take up to 3 L of fluid per day (Thomas, 2019) to increase urine production and lessen the irritation of urethral mucosa on micturition.

It is important to educate women to wipe front to back after voiding urine or defecating, and it is advised to void urine before and after sexual intercourse in an attempt to flush out bacteria that may have been introduced into the urethra and the bladder.

It is reported that up to 40% of cases of septic shock are as a result of urosepsis (McCance and Huether, 2018). It is therefore important to monitor vital signs and record them using a NEWS2 chart (Royal College of Physicians, 2017). This provides the opportunity to identify trends in observations, which leads to alerts and escalation as required.

Patients with recurrent UTIs will need information on how to recognise the signs and symptoms of urinary tract infection and to take preventative measures.

Pharmacological interventions

The following medications may be prescribed to treat acute pyelonephritis:

- Analgesics for pain management
- Antibiotics to treat the infection
- Anti-emetics for nausea and vomiting
- Antipyretics to treat the pyrexia.

Red flag

Do not perform urine dipstick in adults over the age of 65 years to test for bacteriuria as it is considered unreliable. Up to half of older adults and people with urinary catheters without an infection will have bacteria in their urine tract. These people do not require antibiotics unless they are symptomatic for urinary tract infection.

Orange flag

Elderly patients admitted with new onset confusion need to be investigated for the cause. However, it is important to consider that confusion can occur when there is a urine infection. It is useful to consider this when there is no obvious cause.

Medicines management

Ciprofloxacin

Ciprofloxacin is in a class of antibiotics called fluoroquinolones. Ciprofloxacin is used to treat different types of bacterial infections and is known as a broad-spectrum antibiotic. It is also useful against multi-resistant microorganisms. This antibiotic is useful in fighting infections in the lungs and kidneys.

Nurses need to be aware that special precautions should be taken when administering ciprofloxacin, as detailed below.

Taking ciprofloxacin may worsen muscle weakness in people with myasthenia gravis (a disorder of the nervous system that causes muscle weakness) and cause severe difficulty breathing or death.

Inform the patient not to take ciprofloxacin with dairy products such as milk or yogurt, or with calcium-fortified juice. Patients may eat or drink these products as part of a regular meal, but do not use them alone when taking ciprofloxacin, as they could make the medication less effective.

Chronic pyelonephritis

Chronic pyelonephritis progresses from acute pyelonephritis. The calyces and the renal pelvis of the kidney are affected. Chronic pyelonephritis can begin in childhood. Repeated UTIs can lead to scaring and fibrosis of the kidney then destroys the parenchyma. Over a period of time, the kidneys become small and irregular in shape, resulting in renal failure.

Signs and symptoms

This condition may be asymptomatic in the early stages and until the patient presents with renal failure. The patient may present with:

- Pyrexia
- Abdominal and groin pain
- Hypertension
- Dysuria
- Uraemia
- Proteinuria.

Investigations

The investigations are the same as those for acute pyelonephritis.

Care and management

The care and management of the patient with chronic pyelonephritis is the same as for acute pyelonephritis. However, patients who have recurrence of UTI may require long-term antibiotic therapy. In the event of renal failure as a result of kidney damage, the patient may need renal dialysis. Healthcare professionals should prepare and educate the patient in lifestyle changes resulting from kidney dialysis, such as diet and fluid intake.

Cystitis

Cystitis is the inflammation of the urinary bladder and the inflamed bladder may haemorrhage. Cystitis is the most common form of UTI and affects women more than men (Vecchio et al., 2018). The bacteria responsible for the infection are *E. coli*, which is found in the lower gastrointestinal tract, and *P. mirabilis*. In women, the bacteria gain entry into the urinary bladder through the short female urethra. Cystitis can also result from non-bacterial irritation, such as from clothing that is made from synthetic fibres, hygiene sprays and talcum powder.

Aetiology

There are several causes:

- Bacterial infection
- Sexual intercourse
- Pregnancy
- Rectal intercourse
- Urinary tract obstruction as a result of an enlarged prostate gland
- Chemicals in washing powder
- Nylon underwear
- Talcum powder
- Stress.

Investigations

Midstream specimen urine should be cultured to identify the organism:

- Sometimes a flexible cystoscopy may be carried out to detect abnormalities
- Urine cytology to rule out renal cancer.

Signs and symptoms

The patient may present with the following signs and symptoms:

- Dysuria
- Urgency
- Pyuria
- Haematuria
- Abdominal discomfort
- Nocturia
- Urinary incontinence.

Care and management

The main objective is to identify the cause of cystitis in order to offer the correct treatment; cystitis may not be the result of bacterial contamination. The patient will need reassurance, psychological support and health education. With recurrent urinary tract infection, the patient may need long-term antibiotic therapy. The patient should be advised on the importance of taking the prescribed medication. Information on side effects of antibiotics, such as diarrhoea, vomiting and allergic reactions, should be provided; the role of the nurse and other healthcare professionals is to provide people with information.

Unless contraindicated, the patient should be advised to take 2.5–3 L of fluid per day (Thomas, 2019). This helps produce urine and flush out any bacteria in the renal tract. Measurements of vital signs, e.g. temperature and pulse, should be recorded every 4 hours until symptoms of cystitis subside or as the patient's condition dictates. Health education is the same as for the patient with acute pyelonephritis.

There is much debate regarding the use of cranberry juice in treating UTIs. There are conflicting findings in regard to the benefit of taking cranberry supplements (NICE, 2018). Cranberry and blueberry juices contain benzoic acid, which coats the lining of the bladder wall and prevents bacteria from infiltrating into the bladder wall. Advise the patient to avoid materials or chemicals that may cause bladder irritation, such as underwear made from synthetic material, the use of hygiene sprays or bubble bath.

Acute kidney injury and chronic kidney disease

AKI is a condition in which the kidneys are unable to remove accumulated metabolites from the blood, leading to altered fluid, electrolyte and acid–base balance. The cause may be a primary kidney disorder, or renal failure may be secondary to a systemic disease or other urological defects. AKI may be either acute or acute on chronic.

CKD is a silent disease, developing slowly and insidiously, with few symptoms until the kidneys are severely damaged and unable to meet the excretory needs of the body.

Both forms are characterised by azotemia – increased levels of nitrogenous waste in the blood.

Acute kidney injury

AKI is the acute decline in renal function leading to azotemia (accumulation of nitrogenous waste in the blood), and fluid and electrolyte imbalance. AKI has an abrupt onset and with prompt intervention is often reversible; if left untreated, it leads to permanent renal damage.

Pathophysiology

The causes of AKI can be categorised into prerenal, intrarenal and postrenal (Table 11.2). Prerenal AKI is the most common, with dehydration and infection being the main cause. In prerenal AKI, hypoperfusion leads to AKI without directly affecting the integrity of the

305

Table 11.2   Summary of aetiology of acute kidney injury.

Prerenal	Intrarenal	Postrenal
Fluid loss from: • Haemorrhage • Severe dehydration	Glomerulonephritis	Ureteric calculi/Neoplasm
Cardiac: • Reduced cardiac output: • Heart failure • Myocardial disease	Hypertension	Urethral stricture
Reduced pressure to the kidneys: • Sepsis • Shock • Liver failure	Nephrotoxic drugs/bacterial toxins and chemicals	Prostatic hyperplasia

kidney tissue. Intrinsic (or intrarenal) AKI, due to direct damage to the functional kidney tissue, is responsible for another 40%. Urinary tract obstruction with resulting kidney damage is the precipitating factor for postrenal AKI, the least common form.

Prerenal

Prerenal causes include insufficient blood flow to the kidneys, resulting in reduced cardiac output as a result of heart failure, hypovolaemia resulting from haemorrhage and shock. The kidneys receive 20–25% of cardiac output to maintain glomerular filtration. With a reduction in real or relative renal blood flow, glomerular filtration is affected, and this causes ischaemic changes to the renal tissues.

Intrarenal

Intrarenal causes result from conditions that impair renal function. The renal parenchyma and nephrons are damaged, leading to renal injury. Glomerulonephritis, hypertension, chemicals such as ethyl glycol and drugs, e.g. antibiotics, can all affect renal function.

The nephrons of the kidneys are susceptible to trauma from poor renal blood flow, hypertension and shock. The cell membranes of the nephrons are damaged as a result of the trauma. The renal tubules become blocked with debris, thus increasing tubular pressure, resulting in poor elimination of sodium, water and metabolic waste.

Nephrotoxic drugs such as aminoglycoside antibiotics, non-steroidal anti-inflammatory drugs and toxins from bacteria destroy tubular cells. The damaged tubular cells become permeable to water, sodium and metabolic waste.

Postrenal

Postrenal failure results from obstruction along the ureters, urinary bladder and urethra. Obstruction resulting from stones in the ureters, prostatic hyperplasia and urethral stricture could restrict urine flow, leading to postrenal failure.

Red flag

When a patient presents with AKI, it is essential to think about the cause. Consider if there is a history of acute illness and whether the cause could be related to sepsis or hypovolaemia. Undertaking a urinalysis may help to determine any intrinsic cause. Also consider urinary tract obstruction for the cause of AKI.

Medicines management

Non-steroidal anti-inflammatory drugs such as ibuprofen and aspirin can have adverse effects on the kidneys. Our kidneys require pressure from the vascular system to enable the kidney to filter our blood. These drugs can affect the pressure of blood flow to the kidneys, and this can have a detrimental effect on renal function.

Investigations

The following investigations may be carried out:

- Full blood count may indicate reduced red blood cell count, anaemia.
- Urea and electrolyte studies may indicate an increase in urea level and electrolyte imbalance, such as hyperkalaemia and hyponatraemia.
- Urinalysis may indicate proteinuria, haematuria and increased cell casts.
- Abdominal X-ray may be performed to identify obstructions.
- Ultrasound may be carried out to identify the cause of renal injury.
- Arterial blood gases may indicate metabolic acidosis.

Clinical investigations

Magnetic resonance angiography (MRA)

Magnetic resonance angiography is an MRI examination of the blood vessels. Unlike traditional angiography that involves placing a tube (catheter) into the vessel, MRA is non-invasive. The patient may be asked not to eat or drink anything for 4–6 hours before the scan. The patient is asked to lie on a narrow table, which slides into a large tunnel-shaped scanner. The test may take an hour or more.

Some examinations require a special dye (contrast). Most often, the dye is given before the test through a vein (IV) in the hand or forearm. The dye helps the radiologist to see certain areas more clearly. If the patient has reduced kidney function, it is important to seek advice, as the patient may need additional precautions such as extra fluids or on occasion may require temporary dialysis.

There is no special type of care required after an MRA. The patient may resume their normal diet and activities, unless the doctor advises differently.

Signs and symptoms

AKI is usually secondary to another cause, and therefore it is important to ensure that AKI can be identified as soon as possible. Key signs and symptoms are reduced urine output and a raised urea and creatinine. To work out a patient's urine output, it is important to weigh the patient. A patient should produce a minimum of 0.5 mL/kg/hr of urine an hour.

Stages

AKI progresses through four phases:

1. Initiation
2. Oliguric
3. Diuretic
4. Recovery

Table 11.3   Staging of acute kidney injury.

AKI stage	Serum creatinine changes	Urine output changes
1	≥1.5–1.9 × the baseline	<0.5 mL/kg/hr for 6 hours
2	≥2–2.9× the baseline	<0.5 mL/kg/hr for 12 hours
3	≥3× the baseline	<0.3 mL/kg/hr for 24 hours or anuria

Source: KDIGO, 2013b.

The initiation phase is when the initial diagnosis is made. This can range from several hours to days. During this period, kidney function is suppressed, and the patient may present with oliguria or anuria during this phase. Toxins, electrolytes and drugs can start to accumulate in the blood. It is important that a thorough assessment is undertaken to identify the cause and to ensure that there are no medications that may affect renal function.

During the oliguric phase, which can last from 5 days to 15 days (Dainton, 2019), urine output is minimal. Fluid and electrolyte imbalance occurs during this phase, and serum creatinine and blood urea levels are elevated. Healing of the nephrons occurs with fibrous scar tissue formation. At this point, the patient is susceptible to infection and bleeding.

The diuretic phase is when kidney function starts to return and urine production increases (diuresis). Diuresis can last for 24 hours, and the patient may pass up to 3 L of urine per day. Although a large volume of urine is produced, full renal function is still impaired. Dehydration is a problem as a result of increased fluid loss and the inability of the kidneys to perform selective reabsorption. Therefore, fluid monitoring and monitoring of electrolytes are essential at this point (see Table 11.3).

The recovery phase can last for over a year. Renal function starts to return to normal, and the kidney can respond to the body's needs.

Care and management

A patient with AKI requires supportive treatment and close monitoring of their vital signs. This include regular NEWS2 observations, daily weights, fluid assessment including intake and output, nursing history and assessment of the patient's knowledge of the disease process should all be carried out in order to provide high-quality care.

The Royal College of Physicians (2015) suggests identifying the cause of the AKI and to treat appropriately. To ensure hydration is maintained in the patient and monitored and to stop any nephrotoxic drugs (drugs that harm the kidney).

An accurate fluid intake and output should be maintained to prevent fluid overload in the early stages of the disease and dehydration in the diuretic phase.

A patient's vital signs should be monitored according to recommendations as identified by NEWS2, and these should be escalated as required.

Healthcare professionals should educate the patient on how to avoid AKI in the future, especially if they are at risk of AKI.

It is important to alleviate patient's and relatives' worries and anxieties. Healthcare professionals should give the patient time to ask questions and should respond appropriately. Psychological care is important in the care and management of the patient with AKI.

Pharmacological interventions

The patient may have their medication reviewed to ensure that their kidneys are not being further damaged. Detrimental medications include:

- Certain antibiotics including Gentamycin
- Antihypertensives, such as angiotensin-converting enzyme (ACE) inhibitors, may need to be reviewed temporarily and an alternative medication prescribed.

Snapshot   Patient with Acute Kidney Injury

Barbara Brathwaite is a 71-year-old lady admitted to Accident and Emergency with lethargy and confusion. Her daughter, Pauline, was concerned and rang 111, who advised her to attend the Emergency Department. She lives alone but has a wide social circle and is a regular member of the Women's Institute. She is normally fit and well and only takes Digoxin for her atrial fibrillation, and ibuprofen occasionally for backache.

On admission it is identified that Barbara has had diarrhoea and vomiting for the past 5 days, and this is likely to be infective gastroenteritis. She has struggled to eat or drink much, although she is tolerating small sips of water in the last 24 hours. She is aware that some of her friends have not been well but is not sure if it is the same thing. Jenny's mouth and tongue are dry, and her skin is flaky. She is also complaining of feeling faint.

Her Observations on admission are:

Clinical Observations	On admission
Oxygen saturation	94%
Respiratory rate	28 breaths/minute
Pulse	Irregular; 50 approximately
Blood pressure	102/73
Temperature	36.2° C
AVPU	Alert with confusion
NEWS2 Score	7

Barbara is admitted to the ward, blood chemistry and haematology are taken, and intravenous fluids are commenced. She is started on an input and output chart, as she stated that she has not needed to pass urine for a while. Her blood results are:

Blood results	On admission	Range
Urea	38 mmol/L	3.2–7.0 mmol/L
Creatinine	240 mmol/L	63–111 mmol/L
Potassium	6.2 mmol/L	3.5–5.2 mmol/L
Sodium	143 mmol/L	135–145 mmol/L
pH	7.33	7.35–7.45
AVPU	Alert with confusion	

Barbara is diagnosed with acute kidney injury (AKI), and she is given further IV fluids and medication to lower her potassium.

Take time to reflect and consider:

1. Her NEWS2 score is 7. What does this mean?
2. How would the diagnosis of AKI be determined?
3. What is the link between diarrhoea and vomiting and AKI?

Chronic kidney disease

CKD is defined as the progressive reduction in renal function over months to years. The condition is irreversible and eventually affects all the organs of the body. The parenchyma and the nephrons are destroyed, and the renal function progressively diminishes.

Aetiology

There are many causes for CKD, including:

- Renal disease such as polycystic disease
- Arteriosclerosis
- Chronic glomerulonephritis
- Chronic pyelonephritis
- Diabetes nephropathy
- Hypertension
- Renal calculi
- Prostatic hypertrophy.

Investigations

- Urinalysis to detect abnormalities and specific gravity
- Blood tests are carried out to determine renal function
- Urine culture to identify UTI
- Renal biopsy to detect kidney diseases
- Full blood count to identify the extent of anaemia
- Renal ultrasound to determine the size of the kidney.

Clinical investigations

Estimated glomerular filtration rate (eGFR)

The eGFR is a test that is used to assess how well the kidneys are working. The test estimates the volume of blood that is filtered by the kidneys over a given period of time. The test is called the estimated glomerular filtration rate because the glomeruli are the tiny filters in the kidneys. If these filters do not do their job properly, then the kidney is said to have reduced or impaired kidney function.

The eGFR test involves a blood test which measures a chemical called creatinine. Creatinine is a breakdown product of muscle. Creatinine is normally cleared from the blood by the kidneys. If the kidneys are not working properly, the level of creatinine in the blood goes up. The eGFR is then calculated from the age of the patient, sex and blood creatinine level.

Signs and symptoms

In the early stages of the disease, the patient may be asymptomatic. As the disease progresses, the patient may present with the following symptoms:

- Lethargy
- Headache
- Breathlessness
- Proteinuria
- Haematuria
- Oliguria, anuria
- Symptoms of anaemia
- Hypertension
- Pallor.

Pathophysiology

The pathophysiology of CKD involves the gradual loss of nephrons and reduced renal function. CKD can be relatively asymptomatic and therefore may only be picked up when symptoms begin to appear or when a blood test is taken, as increasing levels of urea accumulate in the blood. CKD is identified if the estimated glomerular filtration rate (eGFR) is persistently low for 3 months.

There are a number of conditions that can lead to CKD, which include hypertension, diabetes as well as a range of autoimmune diseases such as lupus. There are five stages of CKD, and these are classified by KDIGO (2013a); see Table 11.4. When a patient reaches end-stage renal disease, there will be signs and symptoms of uraemia, and renal replacement therapy in the form of dialysis or transplantation will be required.

Care and management

The patient and their relatives will require support to come to terms with the disease. The disease is not curable and can lead to death. The healthcare professional should encourage the patient to express their feelings or concerns and assist the patient with coping strategies. If necessary, the patient should be referred to specialist nurses such as the advanced kidney care team.

CKD has implications for the individual in terms of lifestyle, and this can take time to get used to. It is important to offer advice and support for the individual and their family or friends. Dialysis treatment is the main treatment for a patient with ESRD, and therefore information about what this requires and the impact on lifestyle is required.

A patient may have an arteriovenous fistula or tunnelled line if they are on haemodialysis and a peritoneal catheter if they are having peritoneal dialysis. It is important to note any changes in the wound site and to check for any signs of infection, such as pyrexia, tachycardia and inflammation. Vital signs should be monitored and recorded in line with NEWS2 chart, and any changes reported immediately in order to allow prompt action to be taken. Fluid intake and output should be monitored to prevent fluid depletion or fluid overload.

A renal diet may be required which may be low in potassium and sodium, and advice given for fluid restriction may be necessary.

All care given should be documented in accordance with local policy and procedure and in alignment with the Nursing and Midwifery Council (2018). The effects and side effects of prescribed medications should also be documented

Table 11.4   Chronic kidney disease staging.

GFR	GFR (mL/min/1.73 m^2)	
Stage 1	>90	Normal
Stage 2	60–89	Mildly decreased
Stage 3a	45–59	Mildly to moderately decreased
Stage 3b	30–44	Moderately to severely decreased
Stage 4	15–29	Severely decreased
Stage 5	<15	End-stage renal disease (ESRD)

Source: KDIGO, 2013a.

Orange flag

Patients who are approaching end-stage renal disease (ESRD) may have issues with retaining information, lethargy and generally feeling unwell. This can result in feelings of depression. It is important to return to information given to the patient frequently as high levels of urea can inhibit retention of information. Low haemoglobin and increasing levels of toxins can result in lethargy. Ensuring all medications are taken as prescribed and initiation of renal replacement therapy may help with this.

Red flag

CKD is more common in people of South Asian origin and African or Caribbean people than the general population. The reasons for this include higher rates of diabetes among South Asian people and higher rates of high blood pressure in African or Caribbean people.

Pharmacological interventions

The following medications may be prescribed for CKD:

- Antihypertensives
- Iron, folic acid and erythropoietin for the treatment of anaemia
- Calcium binders and alfacalcidol to manage calcium and phosphate levels

Case study

Mr Lee Hong is a 38-year-old owner of a small restaurant. He lives with his wife and their two children. One day while at work, Mr Hong collapsed with severe pain around his kidney region. His wife, who was at work with him, called for an ambulance, and Mr Hong was rushed to the local hospital. On arrival at the Emergency Department, Mr Hong was still in a lot of pain and asked the student nurse for a urinal to pass some urine. He passed approximately 100 mL of urine and gave it to the student nurse. The student nurse observed that Mr Hong had blood in his urine. Mr Hong was examined by the duty doctor, and a provisional diagnosis of renal colic was made.

Vital signs

On admission to the Emergency Department, the following vital signs were noted and recorded:

Vital sign	Observation	Normal
Temperature	36.8°C	36.0–37.9°C
Pulse	102 beats per minute	60–100 beats per minute
Respiration	22 breaths per minute	12–20 breaths per minute
Blood pressure	92/60 mmHg	100–139 mmHg (systolic) range
O$_2$ saturation	99%	94–98%

A full blood count and urea and electrolytes was performed.

Test	Result	Guideline normal values
White blood cells (WBC)	12×10^9/L	4 to 11×10^9/L
Neutrophils	8.2×10^9/L	2.0 to 7.5×10^9/L
Lymphocytes	4.9×10^9/L	1.3 to 4.0×10^9/L
Red blood cells (RBC)	5.3×10^{12}/L	4.5 to 6.5×10^{12}/L
Haemoglobin (Hb)	132 g/L	130–180 g/L
Platelets	200×10^9/L	150 to 440×10^9/L
C-reactive protein	5.1 mg/L	<5 mg/L
Urea	8.2 mmol/L	2–6.6 mmol/L
Potassium	5.1 mmol/L	3.4–5.6 mmol/L
Sodium	138 mmol/L	135–147 mmol/L

NEWS

Lee Hong

NEWS2 Scoring System

Physiological Parameter	Score						
	3	2	1	0	1	2	3
Respiratory Rate (per minute)	≤8		9-11			21-24	≤25
Sp02 %	≤91	92-93	94-95	≥96			
Air or Oxygen?		Oxygen		Air			
Systolic Blood Pressure (mmHg)	≤90	91-100	101-110	111-219			≥220
Pulse (per minute)	≤40		41-50	51-90	91-110	111-130	≥131
Consciousness				Alert			CVPU
Temperature (°C)	≤35.0		35.1-36.0	36.1-38.0	38.1-39.0	≥39.1	

(Royal College of Physicians, 2017)Take some time to reflect on this case and then consider the following:

1. What is Lee's NEWS2 score and what action should be taken?
2. Discuss the possible medications that may be prescribed for Mr Hong.
3. Explain the role of the drugs you have identified.
4. What advice would you offer Mr Hong regarding his fluid and dietary intake?
5. What advice would you give Mr Hong to prevent a future reoccurrence of his problem?

Renal calculi

Renal calculi are stones in the urinary tract and are the most common cause of upper urinary tract obstruction (Figure 11.10) (Porth, 2015). Men are more at risk than women. Stones may develop and obstruct any part of the urinary tract.

Aetiology

Some of the causes include:

- Dehydration
- Immobility
- Carcinoma of the bone
- Urinary tract infection
- Excessive dietary intake of calcium
- Excessive dietary intake of vitamin D
- Excessive dietary intake of protein
- Gout
- Hyperparathyroidism
- Family history of kidney stones increases the risk of developing kidney stones.

Investigations

- Urinalysis to detect UTI and haematuria
- Abdominal X-ray to identify urinary obstruction
- Ultrasound to determine urinary obstruction
- Intravenous pyelogram to show position of stone
- Full blood count
- Urea and electrolytes to detect electrolyte imbalance
- Cystoscopy (Figure 11.11).

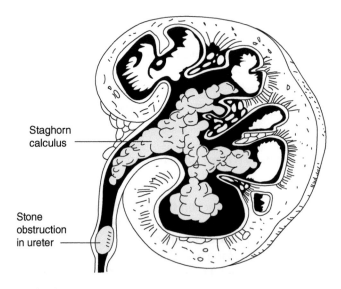

Figure 11.10   Renal calculi.

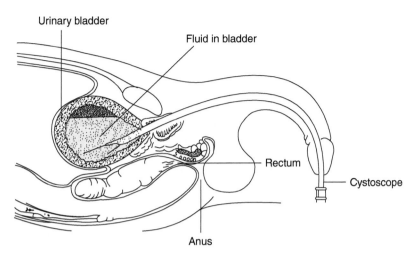

Figure 11.11   Cystoscopy.

Clinical investigations

Intravenous Urogram (IVU) or Intravenous pyelogram (IVP)
The test used to be called an intravenous pyelogram. Intravenous means the injection is given into a vein. Pyelogram refers to the images produced of the internal structure of the kidneys, the collecting systems, and the tubes leading from the kidneys to the bladder, the ureters. With newer techniques, it is possible to get better detail of the whole of the kidney, and the name was changed to urogram. However, both names and both abbreviations are used.

An intravenous pyelogram (IVP) is an X-ray examination of the kidneys, ureters and urinary bladder that uses iodinated contrast material injected into veins. An intravenous pyelogram examination helps the doctors to assess abnormalities in the urinary system, as well as how quickly and efficiently the patient's system is able to handle fluid waste.

There are the usual slight risks associated with ionising radiation, and also from the injection of contrast medium. In particular, female patients who are or might be pregnant must inform a member of staff in advance.

The injection for this test is generally very safe. However, with every injection of the contrast medium, or dye, there is a risk of a reaction. It is not uncommon for people to feel a little warm as the contrast medium flows around the body. Some people may develop a rash, and a few people may get a mild asthma attack. Very, very rarely, someone gets a severe allergic reaction, similar to that with, for example, peanut allergy.

There are no special preparations for an IVP. Nurses need to follow the protocol of the hospital in the safe preparation and care of a patient going for an IVP.

Signs and symptoms

In the early stages, the condition may be asymptomatic. The presenting symptoms depend on the location of the renal stone. Stones forming in the kidney may go undetected for years until identified by routine abdominal X-ray. The patient with stones obstructing the ureters may present with colicky pain, haematuria, nausea and vomiting. Stones in the urinary bladder may not have any symptoms except for a dull pain in the suprapubic region after voiding urine.

Care and management

Full nursing assessment should be carried out to establish the cause of renal calculi. The care, management and treatment will depend on the identified risk factors.

Dietary modification should be encouraged if the renal calculi are the result of excessive intake of calcium, protein, oxalate or vitamin D. Food rich in oxalate includes chocolate, rhubarb and nuts.

The patient should be encouraged to drink 2.5–3 L of fluid per day to flush the kidneys of any bacteria that may cause a UTI and to prevent dehydration. The patient should be taught how to recognise the signs and symptoms of UTI and to take preventative measures.

The patient should be encouraged to undertake exercise, such as walking, swimming or running, to prevent urinary stasis. Exercise improves heart rate and circulation. It also improves blood flow to the kidneys, resulting in good urine output.

The patient should be instructed to take medications as prescribed and educated in the importance of this. The patient should be taught to recognise any side effects of the prescribed medications.

The patient should be taught to test and strain their urine for stones, saving any passed stone for analysis. The patient should be advised to pass all urine into a urinal as small stones can be passed in the urine unobserved by the patient. Kumar and Clark (2017) report that stones less than 0.5 cm in diameter may be passed in the urine without any intervention.

Some patients will require surgery to remove the stones. Approximately one in five stones will not pass spontaneously and may require surgical intervention. If the stone is small, shock-wave lithotripsy may be used to break the stone into smaller pieces; larger stones may be removed using ureteroscopy.

The healthcare professional should provide psychological support to reduce anxiety by actively listening to the patient and relatives and offer information about the prevention of renal calculi.

Pharmacological interventions

The following medications may be prescribed for patients with renal calculi:

- Analgesia for persistent pain
- Antibiotics if the patient presents with UTI.

Conclusion

The renal system consists of the kidneys, ureters, urinary bladder and urethra. This chapter has provided the reader with an overview of the renal system and has discussed some of the disease processes related to the system. It is not the remit of this chapter to discuss all the diseases of the renal system. Healthcare professionals play a vital role in caring for the patient with renal disorders. In order to deliver high-quality care, they need a sound understanding of the anatomy and physiology of the renal system. Apart from the physical aspects, they need to consider the psychosocial aspects of care also.

Patients and their relatives will need advice and support to come to terms with the disease, particularly CKD, which is not curable and can lead to death. Often, nurses are good at providing the physical aspects of care for the patient but fail to include the relatives when planning the patient's care. Chronic renal conditions may lead to lifestyle changes for the patient and their relatives, and healthcare professionals are in the forefront to offer support and guidance to the patient and their relatives.

Test your knowledge

- What happens to the urine output in a patient who is hypovolaemic?
- What happens to urine output if you eat large quantities of salty potato crisps?
- List the functions of the kidney.
- Explain the effect of alcohol on urine production.
- Are males or females more prone to cystitis? Explain.

Activities

Here are some activities and exercises to help test your learning. For the answers to these exercises, as well as further self-testing activities, visit our website at **www.wiley.com/go/fundamentalsofappliedpathophysiology/student4e**

317

Multiple choice questions

1. The renal system is also known as
   - (a) The reproductive system
   - (b) The gastrointestinal system
   - (c) The nervous system
   - (d) The urinary system
2. How many ureters are present in the urinary system?
   - (a) 1
   - (b) 2
   - (c) 3
   - (d) 4
3. The rate at which blood is filtered per minute is known as:
   - (a) The glomerular rate
   - (b) Creatinine clearance
   - (c) Blood urea nitrogen (BUN)
   - (d) Glomerular filtration rate
4. Acute kidney injury was previously known as:
   - (a) Acute renal disease
   - (b) Acute renal failure
   - (c) Chronic kidney disease
   - (d) Chronic kidney failure
5. Acute kidney injury is identified by a rise in what?
   - (a) Creatinine
   - (b) Urea
   - (c) Potassium
   - (d) Sodium
6. How do you determine the minimum amount of urine that a person should pass in an hour?
   - (a) 30 mL/hour
   - (b) 60 mL/hr
   - (c) 0.5 mL/kg/hr
   - (d) 0.3 mL/kg/hr

7. Chronic kidney disease was previously known as what?
   (a) Chronic renal disease
   (b) Chronic renal failure
   (c) Renal failure
   (d) Renal disease

8. Each kidney contains approximately how many nephrons?
   (a) 1 thousand
   (b) 10 thousand
   (c) 1 million
   (d) 10 million

9. One of the main causes of prerenal acute kidney injury is?
   (a) Sepsis
   (b) Diabetes
   (c) High blood pressure
   (d) Renal calculi

10. What are renal calculi?
    (a) They are blockages in the kidney
    (b) Inflammation of the bladder
    (c) Stones within the renal system
    (d) Debris from a urinary tract infection

11. Anuria is a term to describe what?
    (a) No urine output
    (b) Slightly less than normal urine output
    (c) Normal urine output
    (d) Excess urine output

12. Pyelonephritis is what?
    (a) Infection of the kidney
    (b) Infection of the bladder
    (c) Infection of the ureters
    (d) Infection of the stomach

13. What are the main causes of chronic kidney disease (select all that apply)
    (a) Hypertension
    (b) Hypotension
    (c) Diabetes
    (d) Diarrhoea and vomiting

14. Non-steroidal anti-inflammatory drugs are not recommended in patients with renal dysfunction. Identify the reason why.
    (a) Restrict the afferent arteriole going to the nephron
    (b) Restrict the efferent arteriole going to the nephron
    (c) Reduce the absorption of bicarbonate
    (d) Increase the absorption of bicarbonate

15. Acid–base balance is an important function of the kidney what does the kidney do? Select all that apply.
    (a) Reabsorb potassium
    (b) Reabsorb bicarbonate
    (c) Excrete hydrogen
    (d) Excrete potassium

Further resources

Think Kidneys

https://www.thinkkidneys.nhs.uk/
This website provides a range of resources to support patients and professionals with information on kidney disease

National Institute for Health and Care Excellence (NICE)

These links provide guidance on many disorders. See below for specific links for items within this chapter.
Chronic Kidney Disease: https://www.nice.org.uk/guidance/cg182
Acute Kidney Injury: https://www.nice.org.uk/guidance/cg169
Urinary tract infection: https://cks.nice.org.uk/urinary-tract-infection-lower-women
Whether your study is in renal nursing or general field study, this link provides information with regard to treatment and care.

Journal of Kidney Care

https://britishrenal.org/education/journal-of-kidney-care/
This journal will be a valuable resource for students, whether you are a specialist nurse in the renal unit or a nursing student. Here you will find current issues in the care and treatment of renal patients.

Journal of Renal Care

https://onlinelibrary.wiley.com/journal/17556686
This is a valuable journal for students. Here you will find excellence in clinical practice and the journal provides up-to-date accessible, practical and information. From the articles written by experts, you should gain a good knowledge base and learn about evidence-based practice in renal nursing.

The Renal Association

https://renal.org/health-professionals/guidelines/guidelines-commentaries
This link is a valuable source for students who would like to research guidelines for the management of acute kidney injury and chronic kidney disease. Here you will find information on prevention, treatment and management of patients.

Glossary of terms

Anterior   Front.
Anuria   Absence of urine.
Bifurcation   Dividing into two branches.
Calculus   A stone.
Calyces   A small funnel-shaped cavity formed from the renal pelvis.
Diuresis   Excess urine production.
Dysuria   Painful urination.
Erythropoietin   A hormone produced by the kidneys that regulates red blood cell production.
Excretion   The elimination of waste products of metabolism.
Fibrosis   Growth of fibrous connective tissue.
Filtration   A passive transport system.
Glomerulus   A network of capillaries found in the Bowman's capsule.
Haematuria   Blood in the urine.
Hilus   The small indented part of the kidney.
Hyperkalaemia   A high potassium level in the blood.

Hyponatraemia   A low sodium level in the blood.

Involuntary   Cannot be controlled.

Kidney   An organ situated in the posterior wall of the abdominal cavity.

Micturition   The act of voiding urine.

Nephron   The functional unit of the kidney.

Nocturia   Excessive urination at night.

Oliguria   Diminished urine output; deficient secretion of urine; less than 30 mL per hour.

Osmolarity   The osmotic pressure of a fluid.

Parenchyma   The soft tissue of the kidney involving the cortex and the medulla.

Posterior   Behind.

Proteinuria   Protein in the urine.

Pyrexia   Elevated temperature associated with fever.

Pyuria   Presence of white blood cells in the urine.

Renal artery   A blood vessel that takes blood to the kidney.

Renal cortex   The outermost part of the kidney.

Renal medulla   The middle layer of the kidney.

Renal pelvis   The funnel-shaped section of the kidney.

Renal pyramid   A cone-shaped structure of the medulla.

Renal vein   The blood vessel that returns filtered blood into the circulation.

Renin   A renal hormone that alters systemic blood pressure.

Specific gravity   Density.

Sphincter   A ring-like muscle fibre that can constrict.

Ureter   A membranous tube that drains urine from the kidneys to the bladder.

Urethra   A muscular tube that drains urine from the bladder.

Urgency   A feeling of the need to void urine immediately.

Voluntary   Can be controlled.

References

Dainton, M. (2019). Acute Kidney Injury. In: N. Thomas (ed.), *Renal Nursing: Care and Management of People with Kidney Disease*. Newark, United Kingdom: John Wiley & Sons, Incorporated.

KDIGO. (2013a). Clinical practice guideline for the evaluation and management of chronic Kidney disease. *Kidney International*, 3(1). DOI:10.1038/kisup.2012.72

KDIGO. (2013b). *KDIGO clinical practice guideline for acute Kidney injury. Kidney International*, 2.

Kumar, P. and Clark, M. (2017). *Clinical Medicine*, 9th edn. London: Elsevier.

Marieb, E.N. and Hoehn, K. (2018). *Human Anatomy & Physiology, Global Edition*. Harlow, United Kingdom: Pearson Education Limited.

McCance, K.L. and Huether, S.E. (2018). *Pathophysiology - E-Book: The Biologic Basis for Disease in Adults and Children:* Missouri: Mosby.

NICE. (2018). *Urinary Tract Infection (Lower): Antimicrobial Prescribing*. London: NICE. Retrieved from https://www.nice.org.uk/guidance/ng109/resources/urinary-tract-infection-lower-antimicrobial-prescribing-pdf-66141546350533.

NICE. (2019). *Pyelonephritis-Acute: Clinical Knowledge Summaries*. https://cks.nice.org.uk/pyelonephritis-acute#!scenario

Nursing and Midwifery Council. (2018). *The Code: Professional Standards of Practice and Behaviour for Nurses, Midwives and Nursing Associates*. Retrieved from London: https://www.nmc.org.uk/standards/code/

Porth, C.M. (2015). *Essentials of Pathophysiology*, 4th edn. Philadelphia: Wolters Kluwer.

Royal College of Physicians. (2015). *Acute Kidney Injury and Intravenous Fluid Therapy*. Retrieved from London: https://www.rcplondon.ac.uk/guidelines-policy/acute-care-toolkit-12-acute-kidney-injury-and-intravenous-fluid-therapy

Royal College of Physicians. (2017). *National Early Warning Score (NEWS) 2: Standardising the Assessment of Acute-Illness Severity in the NHS*. Retrieved from London: file:///C:/Users/kn12abb/Downloads/NEWS2%20final%20report_0.pdf

Thomas, N. (2019). *Renal Nursing: Care and Management of People with Kidney Disease*. London: Wiley.

Vecchio, M., Iroz, A. and Seksek, I. (2018). Prevention of Cystitis: Travelling between the imaginary and reality. *Annals of Nutrition and Metabolism, 72*(Suppl. 2)(2), 8–10. DOI:10.1159/000488224

Waugh, A., Grant, A., Tibbitts, R., Ross, J.S. and Antbits. (2018). *Ross & Wilson Anatomy and Physiology in Health and Illness*, 13th edn. Edinburgh: Elsevier.

Chapter 12

The respiratory system and associated disorders

Anthony Wheeldon

Senior Lecturer, Department of Adult Health and Primary Care, School of Health and Social Work, University of Hertfordshire, Hatfield, Hertfordshire, UK

Contents

Introduction 323
Anatomy and physiology 324
Disorders of the respiratory system.............331
Conclusion 352
Multiple choice questions...............................353

Conditions...355
Further reading 355
Glossary of terms...356
References..358

Key words

- Carbon dioxide (CO_2)
- External respiration
- Hypoxaemia
- Oxygen (O_2)
- Dyspnoea
- Haemoglobin (Hb)
- Hypercapnia
- Respiration
- Expiration
- Hypoxia
- Inspiration
- Respiratory failure

Fundamentals of Applied Pathophysiology: An Essential Guide for Nursing and Healthcare Students, Fourth Edition. Edited by Ian Peate.
© 2021 John Wiley & Sons Ltd. Published 2021 by John Wiley & Sons Ltd.
Student companion website: www.wiley.com/go/fundamentalsofappliedpathophysiology/student4e
Instructor companion website: www.wiley.com/go/fundamentalsofappliedpathophysiology/instructor4e

- Name five major anatomical structures of the lower respiratory tract.
- List the main functions of the respiratory system.
- Describe the process of gaseous exchange.
- Identify the physiological observations the nurse should use to assess a patient's respiratory status.
- What is the role the healthcare professional in the care of a patient experiencing breathlessness?

Learning outcomes

On completion of this chapter, the reader will be able to:

- List the main anatomical structures of both the upper and the lower respiratory tracts.

- Discuss the four processes of respiration.

- Explain how the body is able to control the rate and depth of breathing.

- Explain the principles of respiratory failure.

- Describe the pathophysiology of a range of respiratory disorders.

- Outline the management of people living with respiratory disease.

Don't forget to visit the companion website for this book
(www.wiley.com/go/fundamentalsofappliedpathophysiology/student4e)
where you can find self-assessment tests to check your progress, as well as lots of activities to practise your learning.

Introduction

All human cells require a continuous supply of oxygen; indeed, cells will only survive for a few minutes without it. Fortunately, around 21% of the air within our atmosphere is oxygen, providing a plentiful supply. As cells use oxygen, the waste gas, carbon dioxide, is produced. If allowed to build up, carbon dioxide can disrupt cellular activity and homeostasis. The principal function of the respiratory system, therefore, is to ensure that the body extracts enough oxygen from the atmosphere whilst disposing of excess carbon dioxide. The collection of oxygen and removal of carbon dioxide is referred to as respiration. Respiration involves four distinct processes – pulmonary ventilation, external respiration, transport of gases and internal respiration. Although all four are examined in this chapter, only pulmonary ventilation and external respiration are the sole responsibility of the respiratory system. As oxygen and carbon dioxide are transported around the body in blood, effective respiration is also reliant upon a fully functioning cardiovascular system.

The respiratory system is divided into the upper and lower respiratory tracts. It is within the lower respiratory tract that external respiration occurs, and the structures involved are microscopic, very fragile and easily damaged by infection. For this reason, both the upper and the lower respiratory tracts are equipped to fight off any invading airborne pathogens.

The air we breathe is contaminated by a wide variety of pollutants (e.g. exhaust fumes, industrial gases, cigarette smoke) and, as a result, respiratory diseases are highly prevalent throughout the world. Respiratory disease accounts for 20% of all deaths in the UK, more than coronary heart disease. The most common respiratory diseases include lung cancer, asthma, chronic obstructive pulmonary disease (COPD), pneumonia and tuberculosis (TB). Respiratory disease places a heavy burden on the NHS, costing an estimated £11 billion a year (British Lung Foundation, 2017).

Anatomy and physiology
The upper respiratory tract

The upper respiratory tract consists of the oral cavity (mouth), the nasal cavity (the nose), the pharynx and the larynx (Figure 12.1). As well as providing smell and speech, the upper respiratory tract ensures that the air entering the lower respiratory tract is warm, damp and clean. First and foremost, the spaces just inside the nostrils are lined with coarse hairs that filter incoming air, ensuring that large dust particles do not enter the airways. The nasal cavity is also lined with a mucous membrane made from pseudostratified ciliated columnar epithelium, which contains a network of capillaries and a plentiful supply of mucus-secreting goblet cells. The blood flowing through the capillaries warms the passing air, while the mucus moistens it and traps any passing dust particles. The mucus-covered dust particles are then propelled by the cilia towards the pharynx where they can be swallowed or expectorated. To add further protection, the upper respiratory tract is lined with irritant receptors,

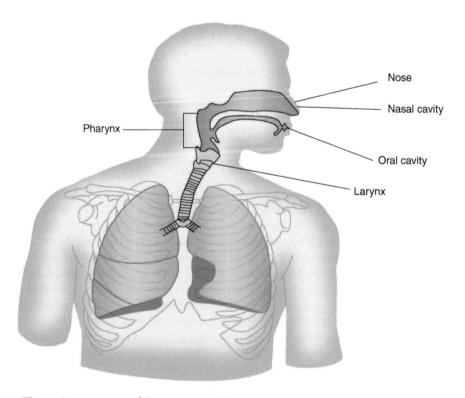

Figure 12.1   The main structures of the upper respiratory tract.

which when stimulated by invading particles (e.g. dust or pollen) force a sneeze, ensuring the offending material is ejected through the nose or mouth.

Unlike the nasal cavity and larynx, the pharynx acts as a passage for food as well as air. The pharynx also contains five tonsils. The two tonsils visible when the mouth is open are the palatine tonsils; behind the tongue lie the lingual tonsils, and the pharyngeal tonsil or adenoid sits on the upper back wall of the pharynx. Tonsils are lymph nodules and part of the body's defence system. The epithelial lining of their surface has deep folds, called crypts. Inhaled bacteria or particles become entangled within the crypts and are then engulfed and destroyed.

The larynx (voice box) also provides a degree of protection, this time from food. The larynx occupies the space between the pharynx and the trachea – the first section of the lower respiratory tract. Also nearby is the oesophagus, which propels food towards the stomach. Attached to the top of the larynx is a leaf-shaped piece of epithelial-covered elastic cartilage, called the epiglottis. On swallowing, the epiglottis blocks entry to the larynx, and food and liquid are diverted towards the oesophagus. Inhalation of solid or liquid substances can block the lower respiratory tract and cut off the body's supply of oxygen – this medical emergency is referred to as aspiration and necessitates the swift removal of the offending substance.

The lower respiratory tract

The lower respiratory tract includes the trachea, the right and left primary bronchi, and the constituents of both lungs (Figure 12.2). The trachea (or windpipe) is a tubular vessel that carries air from the larynx down towards the lungs. The trachea is also lined with pseudostratified ciliated columnar epithelium so that any inhaled debris are trapped and propelled upwards towards the oesophagus and pharynx to be swallowed or expectorated. The trachea and the bronchi also contain irritant receptors, which stimulate coughs that force larger invading particles upwards. The outermost layer of the trachea contains connective

325

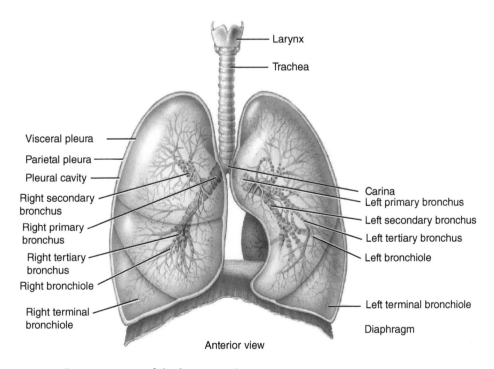

Figure 12.2   Gross anatomy of the lower respiratory tract.

tissue that is reinforced by a series of 16–20 C-shaped cartilage rings. The rings prevent the trachea from collapsing despite the pressure changes that occur during an active breathing cycle. If any obstruction occurs above the larynx, be it a foreign object, inflammation or trauma, a hole or stoma may be created in the trachea and a small tube inserted. This procedure is called a tracheostomy and can ensure that the blocked portion of the upper airway is bypassed, enabling the patient to breathe (Myatt, 2015).

The lungs are two cone-shaped organs that almost fill the thorax. They are protected by a framework of bones, the thoracic cage, which consists of the ribs, sternum (breastbone) and vertebrae (spine). The tip of each lung, the apex, extends just above the clavicle (collar bone), and their wider bases sit just above a concave muscle called the diaphragm. The lungs are divided into distinct regions called lobes. There are three lobes in the right lung and two in the left. The heart along with its major blood vessels sits in a space between the two lungs called the cardiac notch. Each lung is surrounded by two thin protective membranes called the parietal and visceral pleura (Figure 12.2). The parietal pleura lines the walls of the thorax, whereas the visceral pleura lines the lungs themselves. The space between the two pleurae, the pleural space, is minute and contains a thin film of lubricating fluid. This reduces friction between the two pleurae, allowing both layers to slide over one another during breathing. The fluid also helps the visceral and parietal pleura to adhere to one another, in the same way that two pieces of glass stick together when wet.

The airways of the lower respiratory tract divide into branches; for this reason, they are often called the bronchial tree. Within the lungs, the primary bronchi divide into the secondary bronchi, each serving a lobe (three secondary bronchi on the right and two on the left). The secondary bronchi split into tertiary bronchi (Figures 12.2 and 12.3), of which there are 10 in each lung. Tertiary bronchi continue to divide into a network of bronchioles, which eventually lead to a terminal bronchiole. The section of the lung supplied by a terminal bronchiole is referred to as a lobule, and each lobule has its own arterial blood supply and lymph vessels. The bronchial tree continues to subdivide, with the terminal bronchiole leading to a series of respiratory bronchioles, which in turn generate several alveolar ducts. The airways terminate with numerous sphere-like structures called alveoli, which are clustered together to form alveolar sacs (Figure 12.4). There are approximately 490 million alveoli in the lungs (Ochs et al., 2004).

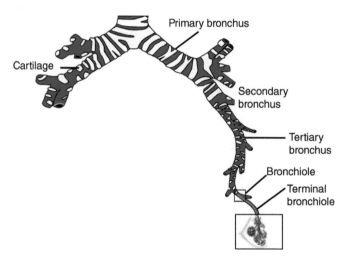

Figure 12.3   The bronchial tree.

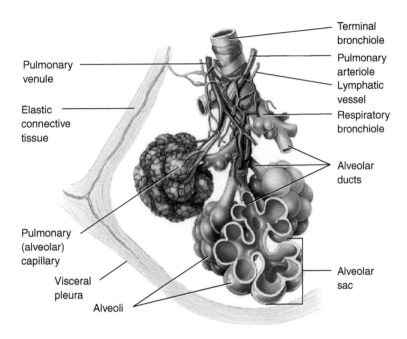

Terminal bronchiole

Pulmonary venule

Pulmonary arteriole

Lymphatic vessel

Elastic connective tissue

Respiratory bronchiole

Alveolar ducts

Pulmonary (alveolar) capillary

Visceral pleura

Alveoli

Alveolar sac

Figure 12.4   Microscopic anatomy of a lobule.

Pulmonary ventilation

Pulmonary ventilation describes the process more commonly known as breathing. The way gases behave helps explain how air flows in and out of the lungs. For instance, gases always flow from an area of high pressure to one of low pressure. All the gases that constitute air collectively exert atmospheric pressure. Air within the lungs also exerts a pressure known as alveolar pressure (Hickin *et al.*, 2015). During inspiration, the thorax expands, and alveolar pressure falls below atmospheric pressure. Because alveolar pressure is now less than atmospheric pressure, air will naturally move into the airways until the pressure difference no longer exists. This phenomenon is explained by Boyle's law, which states that at a constant temperature, the pressure of gas in the lungs is inversely proportional to their size. In other words, as the size of the thorax increases, the pressure inside falls as the gas molecules have more room to circulate (Martini and Nath, 2009).

A range of respiratory muscles are used to achieve thoracic expansion during inspiration (Figure 12.5). The rib cage is pulled outwards and upwards by the external intercostal muscles, whilst the diaphragm contracts downwards, pulling the lungs with it. Expiration is a more passive process. The external intercostal muscles and the diaphragm relax, allowing the natural elastic recoil of the lung tissue to spring it back into shape, forcing air back into the atmosphere (Figure 12.6). Other respiratory muscles can also be utilised. The abdominal wall muscles and internal intercostal muscles, for instance, are utilised to force air out beyond a normal breath, e.g. when playing a musical instrument or blowing out candles on a birthday cake. Muscles such as the sternocleidomastoids, the scalenes and the pectoralis can also be used to produce a deep forceful inspiration. These muscles are referred to as accessory muscles, so called because they are rarely used in normal quiet breathing (Wheeldon, 2016).

External respiration

External respiration occurs only beyond the respiratory bronchioles. For this reason, the end portion of the bronchial tree is called the respiratory zone. The remainder of the bronchial

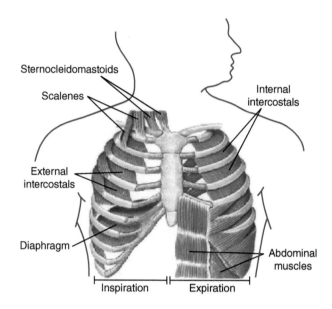

Figure 12.5 Muscles involved in pulmonary ventilation.

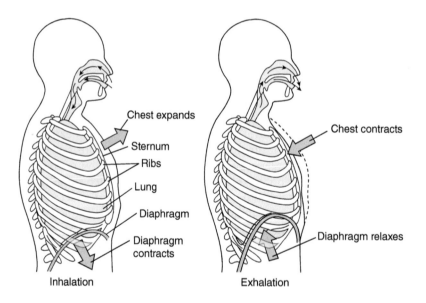

Figure 12.6 Movements of inspiration and expiration.

tree from the trachea down to the terminal bronchioles is the conducting zone. Because the air present in the conducting zone plays no part in supplying the body with oxygen, it is also referred to as the anatomical dead space. External respiration is the diffusion of oxygen from the alveoli into the pulmonary circulation (blood flow through the lungs) and the diffusion of carbon dioxide in the opposite direction. Diffusion occurs because gas molecules always move from areas of high concentration to ones of low concentration. Each lobule of the lung has its own arterial blood supply, which originates from the pulmonary artery, which stems from the right ventricle of the heart. The blood present in the pulmonary artery has been collected from the systemic circulation and is therefore low in oxygen and relatively high in carbon dioxide. The amount (and therefore concentration) of oxygen in the alveoli is far greater than in the passing arterial blood supply. Oxygen therefore moves passively out of the alveoli, into the pulmonary circulation and on towards the left-hand side of the heart. Because there is less carbon dioxide in the alveoli than in pulmonary circulation, carbon dioxide transfers into the alveoli ready to be exhaled (Figure 12.7).

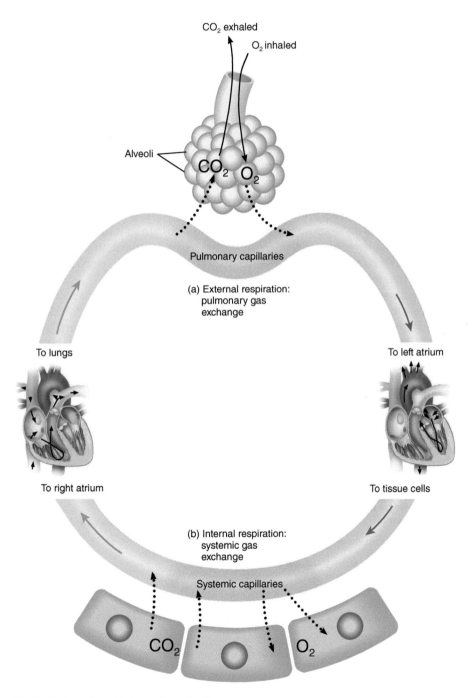

Figure 12.7   External and internal respiration.

Transport of gases and internal respiration

Blood transports oxygen and carbon dioxide between the lungs and all the tissue cells of the body. Cells utilise oxygen when manufacturing their prime energy source, adenosine triphosphate (ATP). In addition to ATP, the cells also produce water and carbon dioxide. Internal respiration describes the exchange of oxygen and carbon dioxide between blood and tissue cells, a phenomenon governed by the same principles as for external respiration. Because cells are continually using oxygen, its concentration within tissue is always lower than within blood. Likewise, the continual use of oxygen ensures that the level of carbon dioxide within tissue is always higher than within blood. As blood flows through the capillaries, oxygen and carbon dioxide follow their concentration gradients and continually diffuse between blood and tissue (Figure 12.7).

Control of breathing

Respiratory centres within the medulla oblongata and pons are responsible for controlling the rate and depth of breathing (Figure 12.8). Within the medulla oblongata, there are chemoreceptors, which continually analyse carbon dioxide levels within the cerebrospinal fluid. As levels of carbon dioxide rise, messages are sent via the phrenic and intercostal nerves to the diaphragm and inter-costal muscles, instructing them to contract. Another set of chemoreceptors found in the aorta and carotid arteries analyses levels of oxygen as well as carbon dioxide. If oxygen falls or carbon dioxide rises, messages are sent to the respiratory centres via the glossopharyngeal nerve and vagus nerve, stimulating further contraction (Figure 12.9). Throughout the day, whether at work, rest or play, the respiration rate changes in order to meet the body's oxygen demands.

Although breathing is essentially a subconscious activity, its rate and depth can be controlled voluntarily or even stopped altogether, e.g. when swimming under water. However, this voluntary control is limited as the respiratory centres have a strong urge to ensure that breathing is continuous. Breathing can also be influenced by the state of mind. The inspiratory area of the respiratory centres (Figure 12.8) can be stimulated by both the limbic system and hypothalamus, two areas of the brain responsible for processing emotions. Fear, anxiety or even the anticipation of stressful activities can cause an involuntary increase in the rate

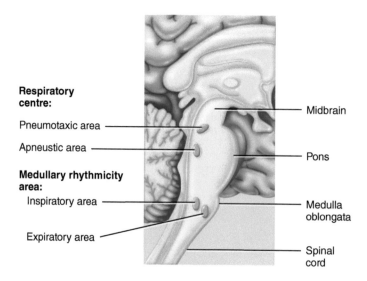

Figure 12.8   The respiratory centres of the brainstem.

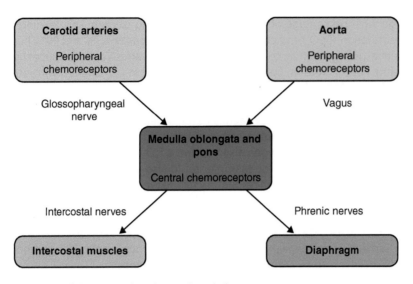

Figure 12.9   Actions of the central and peripheral chemoreceptors.

Table 12.1   Important terminology of breathing.

Term	Definition
Eupnoea	Easy or normal breathing, with a respiration between 12 and 16 breaths per minute
Tachypnoea	Rapid and usually shallow respiration rate, more than 20 breaths per minute
Bradypnoea	Slow respiration rate, less than 10 breaths per minute
Hyperventilation	Increased respiration rate associated with increased ventilation – increased amounts of air entering the alveoli
Hypoventilation	Decreased ventilation – lack of air entering the alveoli
Apnoea	Absence of breathing for more than 15 seconds
Hypopnoea	Shallow breathing with inadequate ventilation
Dyspnoea	Difficult or laboured breathing
Orthopnoea	Difficulty in breathing while lying flat
Cheyne–Stokes breathing	Irregular breathing cycles associated with drug overdose, neurological disturbances and the dying patient

and depth of breathing. Other factors that can affect breathing include pyrexia and pain. Because breathing is largely beyond an individual's control, any changes in respiration rate are clinically significant (Table 12.1).

Disorders of the respiratory system
Respiratory failure

Respiratory failure occurs when respiration is unable to sustain the metabolic needs of the body (Schwartzstein and Parker, 2006). In other words, the lungs are not extracting enough oxygen from the atmosphere. The majority of oxygen (around 98%) is attached to haemoglobin (Hb), which is found in abundance in erythrocytes (red blood cells). A pulse oximeter can gauge what percentage of haemoglobin is carrying oxygen. This reading is called the 'oxygen saturation' (SpO_2). In health, SpO_2 should be between 95% and 99%; however, tremors, anaemia, polycythaemia, cold extremities and nail varnish can all reduce the accuracy of the reading. For this reason, SpO_2 should only be used in conjunction with other observations (Clark *et al.*, 2006). A reduced amount of oxygen in arterial blood is called hypoxaemia. One major symptom of severe hypoxaemia is central cyanosis, a visible bluish hue or tinge visible in the lips and mouth. Hypoxaemia naturally leads to the development of hypoxia, a lack of oxygen in tissue cells. However, hypoxaemia is not the only cause of hypoxia; if you recall, effective transport of oxygen also requires a fully functioning cardiovascular system. Heart failure or haemorrhage, for example, could also result in hypoxia. When a patient is hypoxaemic they are said to be in respiratory failure type 1. Ultimately, the underlying cause should be treated, but oxygen may be prescribed to increase SpO_2.

Around 10% of all carbon dioxide is dissolved in plasma, and the rest diffuses into the erythrocytes. Once inside the erythrocyte, 20% of the carbon dioxide binds to haemoglobin, and the remainder combines with water to form carbonic acid. The carbonic acid then quickly dissociates into bicarbonate ions and hydrogen ions:

$$\underset{\text{Carbon Dioxide}}{CO_2} + \underset{\text{Water}}{H_2O} \leftrightarrow \underset{\text{Carbonic Acid}}{H_2CO_3} \leftrightarrow \underset{\text{Hydrogen ions}}{H^+} + \underset{\text{Bicarbonate ions}}{HCO_3^-}$$

Red flag

Inaccurate pulse oximeter readings

Healthcare professionals need to be aware that there are a number of factors that can lead to inaccurate pulse oximeter readings. Tremors, anaemia, polycythaemia, cold extremities and nail varnish could all lead to inaccurate readings. Always use SpO_2 in conjunction with other nursing observations.

Naturally, the carbon dioxide dissolved in plasma will also generate carbonic acid. However, the reaction that occurs within the erythrocyte is much faster due to the presence of the enzyme carbonic anhydrase. The production of hydrogen and bicarbonate helps to regulate arterial blood pH. A normal arterial blood pH should remain within a very narrow range (7.35–7.45). As levels of hydrogen ion rise and the pH starts to fall below 7.35, more hydrogen ions are combined with bicarbonate to form carbonic acid. As hydrogen ion levels fall and the pH starts to rise, more carbonic acid dissociates. Effective respiration can therefore help regulate hydrogen ion concentration (Clancy and McVicar, 2007).

Respiratory disease often leads to respiratory muscle fatigue, which in turn may lead to a shallower and weaker rate and depth of breathing. Any reduction in ventilation will lead to an accumulation of carbon dioxide, a phenomenon known as hypercapnia. Any patient that is hypoxaemic and hypercapnic is said to be in respiratory failure type 2. Because high carbon dioxide levels lead to a reduction in arterial blood pH, respiratory failure type 2 is also referred to as respiratory acidosis. The only way to reduce carbon dioxide is to 'breathe' it away by improving ventilation. Patients with respiratory failure type 2 may be placed on a mechanical ventilator, which can increase their depth of breathing. One common example of mechanical ventilation used in both hospital and community settings is non-invasive positive pressure ventilation (NIPPV). NIPPV is provided by a special portable machine that delivers breaths via a flexible hose and special facial mask (British Thoracic Society and Intensive Care Society Acute Hypercapnic Respiratory Failure Guideline Development Group, 2016).

Red flag

Non-invasive ventilation and pressure ulcer formation
Healthcare professionals should be aware of that there is a high risk of pressure ulcer formation in patients receiving non-invasive ventilation therapy. The tight-fitting facial masks can cause the breakdown of skin, especially around the nasal bridge where there is less subcutaneous tissue. Pressure ulcers secondary to non-invasive ventilation is reported to occur in up to 70% of cases, and skin lesions can occur within hours of commencing ventilation (Maruccia *et al.*, 2013).

Orange flag

Psychological impact of non-invasive ventilation
Healthcare professionals must acknowledge that being placed on non-invasive ventilation can be a suffocating and claustrophobic experience. While ventilation can help slow and even reverse respiratory failure, wearing the tight-fitting masks can be a frightening experience, especially during the night. Take time to remain with a patient who has recently been commenced on non-invasive ventilation and offer reassurance and take time to answer any questions they may have.

Lower respiratory tract infections

Tuberculosis

TB is a lung infection mainly caused by *Mycobacterium tuberculosis*, an airborne slow-growing bacillus.

The signs and symptoms of TB include:

- Haemoptysis
- Weight loss
- Pyrexia
- Fatigue
- Night sweats.

When the individual is first infected, usually in the upper lobes, lymphocytes and neutrophils congregate at the infection site. The bacilli are then trapped and walled off by fibrous tissue. This phase of TB is referred to as the primary infection, and the infected individual is often asymptomatic and unaware. At some point thereafter, re-exposure to TB or another bacterium causes a secondary infection. The bacilli are then reactivated and start to multiply, after which the patient soon becomes symptomatic and infectious. Bacilli are very resilient and can survive trapped in fibrous tissue for long periods. Individuals can remain unaware that they have TB for many years.

The incidence of TB is growing worldwide, and its rise is attributed to increased international travel, immigration and poverty. TB, however, can be successfully treated on an outpatient basis with a 6-month course of a combination of antibiotics. Because of the recent increases in drug-resistant strains of TB, the major aspects of care are infection control and the maintenance of compliance (NICE, 2016).

Orange flag

Psychological impact of isolation

People with active TB will be asked to isolate themselves at home. Being isolated can have detrimental effects on mental health and well-being. People isolated from others experience loneliness, anxiety, depression and apathy. Anxiety and depression can have a negative influence an individual's appetite and interest in their well-being. Healthcare professionals must prioritise interventions that seek to alleviate anxiety and minimise the impact of social isolation in people living with active TB.

Medicines management

Tuberculosis pharmacological therapy

Tuberculosis is treated with a 6-month combination of four antibiotics, normally rifampicin and isoniazid with pyrazinamide and ethambutol for the first 2 months. In the main, people with TB are cared for in community settings, and the main issue for healthcare professionals is ensuring compliance with the antibiotic regimen to avoid the development of multi-drug-resistant TB (MDR-TB) – TB that is resistant to one or more first-line antibiotics – or extensively drug-resistant TB (XDR-TB) – TB that is resistant to first- and most second-line antibiotics.

While the treatments for TB are generally considered safe, patients will need to be informed of possible side effects. Rifampicin, for example, causes urine to change to an orange red colour and can discolour soft contact lenses. Rifampicin can also reduce the effectiveness of contraceptive pills, and patients should be advised to use alternative methods of contraception while they are taking the drug

Pneumonia

Pneumonia is an infection of the alveoli and small airways. Inflammation and oedema cause the alveoli to fill with debris and exudate. The exudate quickly fills with neutrophils, erythrocytes and fibrin, and a solid mass called consolidation is formed. Consolidation can be patchy and spread throughout both lungs, or concentrated in one mass affecting one or more lobes. Consolidation in the alveoli disturbs external respiration, and less oxygen diffuses from the alveoli into the pulmonary circulation; as a result, the patient becomes hypoxaemic and breathless.

Aetiology

Pneumonia can develop secondary to aspiration or other airway infections (e.g. influenza); however, in the majority of cases, pneumonia is caught from inhaled pathogens. Up to 12% of all GP prescriptions for lower respiratory tract infections are for pneumonia (British Thoracic Society, 2009).

Pneumonia can either be community or hospital acquired. In one-third of cases of community-acquired pneumonia, the cause remains unknown; however, key known pathogens include *Streptococcus pneumoniae*, *Chlamydia pneumoniae* and *Legionella* (Legionnaires' disease). Alcoholism, smoking, drug abuse and chronic heart and lung disease all increase the risk of contracting pneumonia. The immunosuppressed are also vulnerable; however, the invading bacteria in such cases are usually either candida (fungus) or *Pneumocystis jiroveci*, formally known as *Pneumocystis carinii*.

As its name suggests, hospital-acquired pneumonia is contracted during a hospital admission. Inpatients are exposed to a wide variety of risks whilst in hospital. Unconscious patients, for example, require intubation, and postoperative patients may have a suppressed cough, increasing the risk of aspiration. Furthermore, long-term patients are often immunosuppressed and repeatedly exposed to a multitude of pathogens. Hospital-acquired pneumonia is often caused by bacteria such as *Escherichia*, *Klebsiella* or *Pseudomonas* and, regrettably, occurs in 1–5% of all admissions (Hickin *et al.*, 2015).

Signs and symptoms

- Hypoxaemia
- Tachypnoea and dyspnoea
- Tachycardia
- Pyrexia – In response to bacterial infection
- Dehydration – Pyrexia causes fluid loss; also the body loses humidified air on expiration
- Reduced lung expansion – Consolidation makes it hard to expand the lungs and breathing becomes difficult
- Pain – Inflammation can spread to the pleura, causing pleuritic pain (pleurisy)
- Productive cough – The exudate present in the alveoli often produces rust-coloured sputum
- Lethargy.

Investigations

Table 12.2 summarises the investigations used to establish a diagnosis of pneumonia.

Care and management

Pneumonia can develop into a severe infection, and up to 42% of cases will require inpatient care, of which between 5% and 10% of patients will require transfer to intensive care (British Thoracic Society, 2009). The healthcare professional can play an important role in the early detection of deterioration. The main goals of care include:

- Safe administration of prescribed antibiotics.
- Safe administration of prescribed oxygen – To correct hypoxaemia and maintain oxygen saturations above 90%.
- Patient positioning – Placing the patient in an upright position will promote diaphragm and intercostal muscle activity and enhance ventilation.

Table 12.2   The main investigations of pneumonia.

Investigation	Rationale
Full blood count	A white blood cell count above 11×10^9/L indicates inflammation, infection or an immune system response
Urea and electrolytes	Raised urea (>7 mmol/L) is an indicator of severe infection
Blood and sputum cultures	To identify the causative agent and appropriate antibiotic treatment
Liver function test	Acute pneumonia can affect liver function
X-ray	To establish the extent of infected lung tissue

Source: Adapted Hoare and Lim, 2006.

- Establishing and minimising pain levels – To make the patient more comfortable and enhance breathing. An appropriate pain assessment tool should be used (see Chapter 17).
- Temperature management – Safe administration of antipyretic agents, such as aspirin, paracetamol or ibuprofen, electric fans, reducing bed clothes.
- Close monitoring of vital signs – Respiration rate greater than 30 respirations per minute, new hypotension (systolic less than 90 mmHg or diastolic less than 60 mmHg) and new mental confusion could indicate life-threatening pneumonia (NICE, 2014). Vital signs should therefore be recorded hourly until the patient's condition stabilises.
- Fluid balance – As the patient is dehydrated. A minimum of 2.5 L every 24 hours is required. Fluids may be administered intravenously if required (Dunn, 2005).
- Communication – To reduce anxiety and promote comfort.

Snapshot   Pneumonia

Ben is a 32-year-old man who has Down syndrome. Ben has been brought into the urgent care centre by Howard, a care support worker who works at Orange Grove Care Home, where Ben resides. Howard is concerned about Ben as his mood has changed significantly over the past week. Instead of being his happy and cheerful self, Ben is much quieter than normal, is not eating or drinking, and easily becomes angry and agitated.

His vital signs were as follows.

Vital sign	Observation	Normal
Temperature	38°C	36.0–37.9°C range
Pulse	90 beats per minute	60–100 beats per minute
Respiration	22 breaths per minute	12–20 breaths per minute
Blood pressure	119/74 mmHg	100–139 mmHg (systolic) range
O_2 saturation:	97%	94–98 %

NEWS2

Ben Watson

Physiological Parameters	Scores						
	3	2	1	0	1	2	3
Respiration Rate						22	
SpO_2 Scale 1				97			
SpO_2 Scale 2							
Air or oxygen				Air			
Systolic blood pressure				119			
Pulse				90			
Consciousness				A			
Temperature				38			

Note: NEWS score: 2 – Clinical risk Low

When asked, Ben stated that it hurt when he took a deep breath and that he felt very tired. On listening to Ben's chest, the nurse can hear rales, a cracking and bubbling sound, on the right side of his thorax. She sends Ben for a chest X-ray and asks a doctor to review him. The X-ray suggests the development of mild pneumonia, and the doctor prescribes a 5-day course of amoxicillin and paracetamol for pain. The nurse also advises Ben to get plenty of rest and to drink plenty of fluid. Ben is asked to see his GP in 1 week's-time unless he begins to feel worse or sees no improvement after 3 days, in which case he should contact his GP sooner.

After three days of treatment, Howard was pleased to see Ben was much more like his old self, and although Ben stated he still felt a little poorly, he was less agitated and irritable, a little more active and had started to eat a little more. After 1 week, Ben's GP was happy to see that Ben was cheerful and talkative. When she listened to his chest, she could not hear any added breath sounds.

Take some time to reflect on this case and then consider the following:

1. Respiratory disease is the most common cause of death in people with a learning disability. Why do you think this may be?
2. What methods did Howard use to determine the well-being of Ben and why must healthcare professionals take note of a carer's observations?
3. Ben made a good recovery. What were the potential consequences of Ben not receiving such prompt care and attention?

Clinical investigations

Chest X-ray

X-rays are electromagnetic waves which when passed through body produce black-and-white images of internal body structures. Electromagnetic waves are a type of radiation which is absorbed by various organs and structures. The more the radiation absorbed, the whiter they appear on the X-ray image. The calcium in bones, for example, absorbs lots of radiation and therefore bones show up very clearly, enabling clinicians to diagnose bone fractures. Softer tissues and fat absorb less radiation and show up as grey on the X-ray image. Air absorbs the least radiation and appears black on the X-ray. This is useful for clinicians exploring the nature of a patient's breathlessness. On a chest X-ray of a healthy pair of lungs, the ribs, clavicle and spine will be easily identified, as is the heart and some of the larger airways. As the lungs mainly contain air, the X-ray will mainly be black. Inflammation, infection and tumours absorb more radiation than air and will be visible on an X-ray.

Because X-rays use radiation, patients may be anxious about the safety of this investigation. While there is a minor risk of cancer in later years, patients should be advised that this risk very small, estimated to be 1 in 1,000,000 (Public Health England, 2008). However, there is an increased risk to pregnant women, and healthcare professionals should always check to see if their patient is pregnant or thinks they may be pregnant.

Patients should be advised that X-rays are painless. However, they will be asked to remain still for a short period, and this may be difficult if they are in discomfort, breathless or in pain. To ensure safety, the patient will need to be left alone for a very brief period of time while the X-ray is taken. Healthcare professionals will need to assess the potential impact of this on their patient.

Obstructive lung disorders

Obstructive lung disorders involve a degree of obstruction to airflow. In conditions such as asthma and COPD, the obstruction to airflow is associated with narrow airways and increased airflow resistance. If the lumen of an airway is halved, then resistance to airflow will increase

16 times. As resistance increases and more and more gas molecules collide, a noise is generated, accounting for the characteristic wheeze often heard in respiratory patients (Smith and Rushton, 2015). In many patients, airway resistance can be overcome by increasing the work of the respiratory muscles. However, normal passive expiration may not be enough to promote adequate alveoli emptying. Forced expiration generates high intrathoracic pressures that force smaller airways to close, trapping air in the chest.

Investigations

The extent of air trapping can be measured using spirometry, which measures the force and volume of a maximum expiration after a full inspiration. The volume of air that can be forced out is referred to as the forced vital capacity (FVC), and the volume that can be exhaled in the first second of expiration is the forced expiratory volume (FEV_1) (Figure 12.10). By comparing FEV_1 with FVC, the FEV_1:FVC ratio, the severity of airway obstruction can be ascertained. An individual with an FEV_1:FVC ratio of less than 80% has obstructed airways (Sheldon, 2005).

Another important measure of airway resistance is the peak expiratory flow rate (PEFR), or 'peak flow'. PEFR measures the force of expiration in litres per minute. It measures the patient's maximum expiratory flow rate via their mouth. An inability to meet a predicted value based on age, sex and height could indicate airway obstruction. Peak expiratory flow rates provide a quick and simple assessment of the airways; however, regular peak flow measurements are more revealing than single arbitrary readings, and carers should be mindful that peak expiratory flow rates are effort dependent.

Asthma

Asthma is a chronic inflammatory disorder of the lungs. It causes the bronchi and bronchioles to become inflamed and constricted. As a result, airflow becomes obstructed, often resulting in a characteristic wheeze. In the UK, around 8 million people live with a diagnosis of asthma (British Lung Foundation, 2020a).

Asthmatics periodically react to triggers. Triggers are substances or situations that would not normally trouble an asthma-free person's airways. Asthma is said to be either extrinsic or intrinsic. In extrinsic asthma, airway inflammation is a consequence of hypersensitive reactions associated with allergy, i.e. pollen, dust mites or foodstuffs, whereas intrinsic asthma is linked to hyper-responsive reactions to other forms of stimuli, e.g. infection, sudden exposure to cold, exercise, stress or cigarette smoke. Extrinsic asthma is more common in childhood, with many sufferers 'growing out' of it in adolescence; intrinsic asthma usually

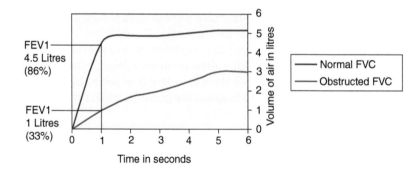

Figure 12.10 Spirometry – a normal forced vital capacity compared to an obstructed forced vital capacity.

develops in adulthood. Many patients, however, have a combination of both types and, irrespective of causative agents, the physiological changes, symptoms and treatments are the same.

Pathophysiology

The pathophysiology of asthma is complicated and intricate. The bronchi and bronchioles contain smooth muscle and are lined with mucous-secreting glands and ciliated cells (Figure 12.11). Close to the airway's blood supply, there are large quantities of mast cells. Once stimulated, mast cells release a number of cytokines (chemical messengers), which cause physiological changes to the lining of the bronchi and bronchioles. Three such cytokines are histamine, kinins and prostaglandins, which cause smooth muscle contraction, increased mucus production and increased capillary permeability. The airways soon narrow and become flooded with mucus and fluid leaking from blood vessels (Figure 12.12). As the airways become obstructed, the patient finds it increasingly hard to breathe and to cough up the mucus. If unresolved, fatigue can occur, and the patient's respiratory effort becomes weak and inadequate, causing hypoxaemia and in severe cases, hypercapnia (Sims, 2006).

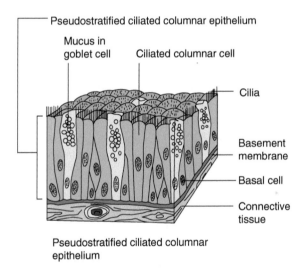

Figure 12.11 Cellular structure of the airways.

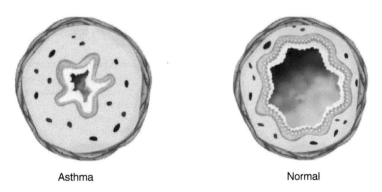

Figure 12.12 Airway pathophysiology, normal compared to status asthmaticus.

Care and management

In the UK, around 1400 people die as a result of their asthma each year. However, asthma is reversible, and it is estimated that two-thirds of asthma deaths are avoidable (Torjesen, 2014). Care should focus, therefore, on close monitoring and health promotion. The main care goals are:

- Continuous monitoring of vital signs until the patient is stabilised.
- Safe administration of prescribed oxygen to maintain oxygen saturation above 92$_{\%}$.
- Safe administration of prescribed bronchodilators and steroids – to alleviate dyspnoea (Tables 12.3 and 12.4).

Table 12.3   Summary of bronchodilator therapies given in asthma and chronic obstructive pulmonary disease.

Type	Actions	Examples	Routes	Care considerations
Beta-2 agonists	Mimics the actions of epinephrine. Beta-2 agonists stimulate beta-2 receptor sites in the airways, promoting rapid bronchodilation within 15 minutes, with a duration of 4–8 hours – depending on dose	Salbutamol Terbutaline Salmeterol	Inhaler Nebuliser Oral Subcutaneous	Patient will need to be advised of the potential for tachycardia and hand tremor
Anticholinergics	Blocks the action of acetylcholine, a neurotransmitter released by the parasympathetic nervous system. Acetylcholine promotes bronchoconstriction and bronchial secretion. Peak bronchodilator effects occur within 1 hour, with a duration similar to beta-2 agonists	Ipratropium bromide	Inhaler Nebuliser	Patient may need frequent mouthwashes, as they have a bitter taste and may cause dry mouth
Methylxanthines	Increases concentration of intracellular cyclic adenosine monophosphate (cAMP). Increased cAMP concentration causes bronchodilation	Theophylline	Oral Intravenous (as aminophylline)	Optimal effects occur when plasma theophylline levels are between 10 and 20 mg/L. Regular blood tests are required

Source: Adapted from Barnes, 2008; and Joint Formulary Committee, 2020.

Table 12.4   Summary of main corticosteroids used in the treatment of respiratory disease.

Indication	Corticosteroids[*]	Route	Care considerations
Prophylaxis and reduction of frequency of exacerbations	Beclomethasone Budesonide Fluticasone	Inhaler	Inhaled corticosteroids can cause hoarseness, loss of voice and candidiasis. Advise patients to rinse their mouths after taking these inhalers
Exacerbation	Prednisolone Hydrocortisone	Oral Intravenous	Patients taking prednisolone and hydrocortisone will need careful monitoring. as can cause the following side effects: • Osteoporosis • Diabetes • Weight gain • Increased body hair • Altered mood

[*] Corticosteroids are potent anti-inflammatory agents. They are used to reduce bronchial hyperactivity in patients with asthma, chronic obstructive pulmonary disease and other respiratory diseases where reversibility is present.
Source: Adapted Barnes, 2008; and Joint Formulary Committee, 2020.

- Communication – as speaking requires a constant flow of air, patients experiencing acute breathlessness are only able to talk for very short periods before the need to breathe interrupts them. The patient's inability to complete a sentence therefore provides a sensitive measure of the extent of a patient's respiratory distress (Higginson and Jones, 2009).
- Regular PEFR measurement – singular or infrequent peak flows will not accurately reflect the patient's status. PEFR should be measured every 15–30 minutes after commencement of treatment and until conditions stabilise. PEFR can also be used to measure the effectiveness of bronchodilator therapy; therefore, PEFR should be measured pre- and post-inhaled or nebulised beta-2 agonists at least four times a day throughout a patient's stay in hospital.
- Comfort and reassurance – Dyspnoea can be a traumatic experience and fear and anxiety also promote hyperventilation. The patient's anxieties should be listened to and continuous explanations provided for the multidisciplinary team's actions.
- Sputum collection – Yellow or green sputum can indicate infection.
- Health promotion – Avoidance of triggers, compliance with prescribed pharmacological therapies, smoking cessation and weight reduction in obese patients may reduce the frequency of asthma attacks.

Red flag

Life-threatening asthma

Healthcare professionals should be vigilant when caring for patients with asthma and be able to detect and determine the signs of acute severe and life-threatening asthma. According to the British Thoracic Society and Scottish Intercollegiate Guidelines Network (2019), if acute severe asthma is suspected, then one or more of the following is present:

- Peak flow 33–50% of predicted or best
- Dyspnoea accompanied by an inability to complete sentences in one breath
- Tachypnoea – respiratory rate 25 breaths per minute or higher
- Tachycardia – heart rate greater than 110 beats per minute.

In addition to the above, if any of the following are also evident, then life-threatening asthma is suspected:

- Peak flow less than 33% of predicted or best
- Oxygen saturation (SpO_2) less than 92%
- Silent chest
- Poor respiratory effort
- Cyanosis
- Hypotension
- Exhaustion
- Arrhythmia
- Altered conscious level
- Arterial oxygen level (PaO_2) less than 8 kPa.

In cases where arterial carbon dioxide ($PaCO_2$) is high (hypercapnia) or doctor's feel mechanical ventilation is required, the patient would be described as having near-fatal asthma.

Snapshot   Asthma

Ayesha is 4 years old and has had a troublesome cough for 4 weeks. At first her mother and father thought she had a common cold, but as the symptoms of the cold abated, the cough remained. Ayesha's father takes her to the GP and explains that the cough is worse at night and stops Ayesha from sleeping. He also states that Ayesha's cough is exacerbated by running and playing with her friends.

The practice nurse listens to Ayesha's chest and asks her to blow into a peak flow meter. The practice nurse concludes that Ayesha has asthma-like symptoms and prescribes a short acting beta2 agonist inhaler and asks that Ayesha comes back to the surgery in two weeks. A practice nurse spends time with Ayesha and her father explaining how to take her inhaler properly, using a device called a spacer to ensure as much of the medication as possible enters Ayesha's airways. The nurse also asks Ayesha's father to monitor the effectiveness of the inhaler.

When Ayesha returns after two weeks her father states that the inhaler makes the cough better, but it still remains, especially at night. In response the practice nurse prescribes an inhaled corticosteroid inhaler to be taken twice a day and for her to be reviewed in 8 weeks.

Take some time to reflect on this case and then consider the following:

1. What do you think is the most likely diagnosis for Ayesha's condition?
2. Why do you think it is challenging for healthcare professionals to make a respiratory diagnosis in children?
3. How does peak expiratory flow rate help healthcare professionals determine the extent of respiratory disease?

Chronic obstructive pulmonary disease

Approximately 600 000 people in the UK have COPD, and it accounts for 5.4% of all male deaths and 4.2% of all female deaths. COPD has been defined as airflow obstruction that is progressive, not fully reversible and does not change markedly over several months. It has one major cause – smoking. COPD is a term now used to describe the traditional diagnosis of chronic bronchitis or emphysema. Chronic asthma sufferers are also at risk of developing fixed airway obstruction as airways become re-modelled over time. Their symptoms may be indistinguishable from COPD, and many COPD patients may also have asthma. Accurate diagnosis therefore is often problematic (Devereux, 2006; NICE, 2018).

Medicines management

Inhaler technique

For patients with asthma and chronic obstructive pulmonary disease, it is very important that their inhaler technique is correct. It is estimated that around a third of patients do not use their inhaler correctly, leading to many people receiving lower doses of their prescribed corticosteroids or bronchodilator therapies. Healthcare professionals need to be aware of the correct techniques for a range of inhalers and be able to advise their patients correctly. Some of the common mistakes made by patients include:

- Not shaking the inhaler before using them – Some inhalers contain a propellant that turns the medication into a spray. Shaking ensures there is an adequate mix of propellant and medication.

- Not waiting between puffs – Waiting 30–60 seconds between puffs allows the medication and propellant to mix together.
- Not breathing out before inhaling – This ensures a deeper and longer inhalation, meaning that more medication enters the airways, increasing its effectiveness.
- Not having a tight lip seal – Having a tight seal around the inhaler will ensure that the maximum amount of medication gets into the airways.
- Not lifting one's chin – An upright chin helps inhalation
- Inhaling too early – Patients often start to inhale before they press their inhaler. This results in too little medication entering the lungs.
- Inhaling too late – It only takes 0.5 of a second for the medication to be delivered, so inhaling too late will result in some of the medication only entering the mouth. Spacers can reduce the chances of this happening.
- Not holding one's breath after inhaling – If patients have been advised to hold their breath after inhaling it is essential, they do so. Holding their breath for 10 seconds after inhaling provides more time for the medication to get into the airways, also increasing its effectiveness.
- Forgetting to use a spacer – Spacers are large plastic tube-like devices which ensure that as much asthma medication as possible is administered. (Asthma UK, 2020)

Signs and symptoms

- Reduced FEV_1 which is less than the predicted value
- Dyspnoea – Due to airway obstruction and air trapping
- Productive cough
- Reduced exercise tolerance
- Respiratory failure types 1 and 2
- Cor pulmonale – Chronic hypoxia causes hypertension within pulmonary circulation. Eventually, the right ventricle becomes enlarged and fails, ultimately leading to peripheral oedema.

Emphysema

Emphysema is defined as the permanent enlargement of airspaces beyond the terminal bronchiole and the destruction of the alveolar wall. The mechanisms behind this degeneration of tissue are thought to relate to the actions of destructive enzymes called proteases, which are released from neutrophils and macrophages in response to infection. In health, lung tissue produces a substance called alpha antitrypsin, which counteracts the destructive action of protease. Smoking, however, is thought to reduce the effect of alpha antitrypsin and increase protease activity, allowing alveolar destruction to continue unabated (Hogg and Senior, 2002). Proteases destroy the elastic fibres essential for elastic recoil, which is much needed during exhalation. As a result, the alveoli become over-inflated as air becomes trapped within the lung (Figure 12.13). The increased volume of air within the thorax pushes the diaphragm downwards, disturbing its natural concave shape and making breathing difficult. Frequent infections can also develop as it becomes increasingly difficult to cough up secretions. The destruction of the alveolar wall and adjacent capillaries will mean that there is less lung tissue available for external respiration, and the patient will be at risk of developing hypoxaemia and hypoxia (Hubert and VanMeter, 2018).

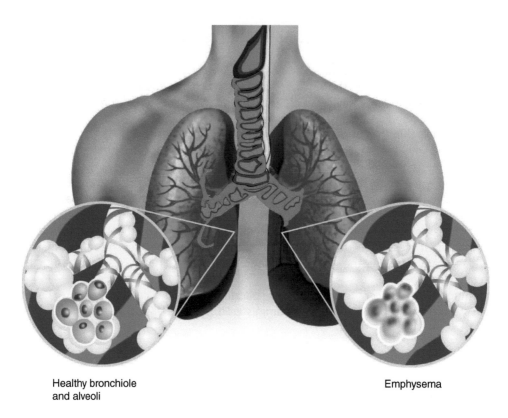

Healthy bronchiole
and alveoli

Emphysema

Figure 12.13   Comparison of a normal bronchiole and alveoli to those in an emphysema sufferer.

Chronic bronchitis

Chronic bronchitis is defined as the presence of a productive cough lasting for three months in each of two consecutive years when other pulmonary and cardiac causes of cough have been ruled out (Braman, 2006). It is characterised by an increase in mucus production and damaged cilia in the bronchi (Figure 12.14). As a result, the bronchi become clogged with mucus, which continues to stimulate the airway's irritant receptors, producing a cough. This chronic irritation causes inflammation and the bronchial wall thickens, causing airway

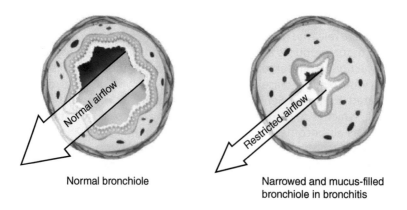

Normal bronchiole

Narrowed and mucus-filled
bronchiole in bronchitis

Figure 12.14   Comparison of a normal bronchiole to that in a chronic bronchitis sufferer.

obstruction. The lack of functioning cilia makes mucus clearance difficult, and as a result, mucus collects and blocks the smaller airways. Secondary infections then occur, causing yet more irritation and inflammation. As more and more airways become blocked, external respiration is reduced and less oxygen is transferred into the bloodstream. The pathophysiological processes behind increased mucus production and cilia dysfunction are thought to involve an inflammatory response to the constant bombardment by cigarette smoke (MacNee, 2006).

Care and management of COPD

The severity of COPD is determined by the FEV_1 (Table 12.5). However, wherever possible, the patient should be managed by the multidisciplinary team in their own home. Factors that may lead to acute exacerbation and necessitate hospital admission for COPD include:

- Inability to cope at home
- Severe breathlessness
- Deterioration
- Poor activity/confined to bed
- Cyanosis
- Worsening peripheral oedema
- Impaired level of consciousness
- Long-term oxygen therapy
- Poor social circumstances
- Confusion or disorientation
- Rapid onset
- Significant co-morbidity, i.e. diabetes, heart disease
- SpO_2 less than 90%
- Chest X-ray changes
- Respiratory failure type 2 (NICE, 2018).

COPD is a diverse and varied condition, and its management requires a holistic approach centred upon self-management and symptom control. The main management goals are:

- Smoking cessation advice
- Education on prescribed oxygen and bronchodilator therapies – to maximise relief of breathlessness
- Immunisation – to minimise the frequency of exacerbations
- Dietary advice – severe weight loss is a feature of both emphysema and chronic bronchitis
- Pulmonary rehabilitation
- Promotion of self-management techniques – COPD is associated with high levels of anxiety and depression.

Table 12.5 FEV_1 as an assessment of airway obstruction (NICE, 2018).

FEV1 post bronchodilator therapy	Severity of airway obstruction
80% or greater	Mild
50–79% predicted	Moderate
30–49% predicted	Severe
Less than 30%	Very severe

Medicines management

Oxygen therapy for patients with COPD

Patients with COPD are at risk of hypercapnia if they receive too much oxygen. Caution should be taken, therefore, when healthcare professionals use oxygen to correct hypoxaemia. It is important to remember that oxygen is a drug and should be prescribed. It should also only be administered or set up by clinicians with the necessary expertise, knowledge and experience.

Oxygen is used to correct hypoxaemia (low levels of oxygen in arterial blood) but not the underlying cause of their breathlessness. The British Thoracic Society stipulates that the minimum amount of oxygen should be given, in order to ensure that oxygen saturations are maintained between 94 and 98%. However, because patients with COPD are at greater risk of retaining carbon dioxide and developing hypercapnia, the target oxygen saturation level should be 88–92%. Healthcare professionals, therefore, must regularly assess oxygen saturation levels to ensure their patient is maintaining a safe oxygen level but also receiving an optimum amount of inhaled oxygen.

Medical oxygen is dry and unlike the moist air we breathe. Entrained oxygen, particularly at high levels, can dry up secretions in the patient's nose or irritate their skin around the oxygen mask. Oxygen can be humidified, passed through sterile water, to soften it and reduce the risk of drying the nose and skin.

Snapshot   Breathlessness

Alison is a 40-year-old single mother of two. Alison rarely drinks alcohol but has smoked 20 cigarettes a day since she was 16 years old. She is currently unemployed and lives in a small council flat on the outskirts of town. She has recently found that she becomes increasingly breathless on exertion, and when she woke up this morning, she could not catch her breath. A concerned friend took her to her local emergency department. On arrival Alison was very distressed and found answering the nurse's questions very difficult as she could not complete a sentence without pausing for breath. The nurses take a set of vital signs, and a doctor takes an arterial blood sample for gas analysis (see below). Alison is prescribed oxygen, salbutamol nebulised and prednisolone orally. Over time Alison's condition stabilises, and later that day she is discharged with salbutamol and beclomethasone inhalers. She is asked to return a few days later for a lung (pulmonary) function test.

Vital signs

On admission to the emergency department, the following vital signs were noted and recorded:

Vital sign	Observation	Normal
Temperature	36.8°C	36.0–37.9°C range
Pulse	120 beats per minute	60–100 beats per minute
Respiration	28 breaths per minute	12–20 breaths per minute
Blood pressure	126/88 mmHg	100–139 mmHg (systolic) range
O_2 saturation	93%	94–98%

NEWS 2   Alison Woodgate

Physiological Parameters	Scores						
	3	2	1	0	1	2	3
Respiration Rate							28
SpO$_2$ Scale 1		93					
SpO$_2$ Scale 2							
Air or oxygen				Air			
Systolic blood pressure				126			
Pulse						120	
Consciousness				A			
Temperature				36.8			

Note: NEWS score: 7 – Clinical risk High, urgent or emergency response required
Source: Royal College of Physicians (2020).

An arterial blood gas was performed:

Test	Result	Guideline normal values
pH	7.36	7.35–7.45
H$^+$	37 nmol/l	35–45 nmol/l
Oxygen (PaO$_2$)	8.1 kPa	11–13 kPa
	60.75 mmHg	75–100 mmHg
Carbon dioxide (PaCO$_2$)	5.9 kPa	4.5–6 kPa
	44 mmHg	34–45 mmHg
Bicarbonate (HCO$_3^-$)	24 mEq/L	22–25 mEq/L
Base excess	–0.9 mmol/l	–2 to +2 mmol/l

Take some time to reflect on this case and then consider the following:

1. Which of Alison's physiological observations do you think are a cause for concern and why?
2. What will the arterial blood gas readings tell the medical team, and how will they influence management decisions?
3. What pharmacological therapies could be used to alleviate Alison's breathlessness?
4. What risk factors may have contributed to Alison's current condition?

Clinical investigations

Lung (pulmonary) function test

A lung function test incorporates a number of investigations that are designed to determine the presence and effect of a number of respiratory diseases. Typically a lung function test will incorporate three specific investigations:

Spirometry: Spirometry measures the force and volume of a maximum expiration after a full inspiration. Two volumes are of particular importance, the total volume of air exhaled or forced vital capacity (FVC) and the volume the patient exhales after 1 second, or FEV_1. A comparison between FEV_1 and FVC, the FEV_1:FVC ratio, determines the severity of airway obstruction. An FEV_1:FVC ratio of less than 80% is indicative of n obstructive airways disease.

Lung Volume: Ascertaining a more accurate measurement of a patient's lung volume will ensure that the spirometry results are more accurate. Spirometry can be performed on wards, in clinics or in GP surgeries. However, for a lung function test, patients are placed in a sealed glass booth, with clips on their noses to prevent air escaping and ensuring a more accurate lung volume measurement.

Gas Transfer: This test measures the effectiveness of gaseous exchange. A harmless dose of carbon monoxide is inhaled, then blood samples are taken, and the level of carbon monoxide present is measured.

It is important that an accurate picture of lung function is ascertained. Therefore, patients may need to abstain from bronchodilator therapy before their test. Analgesia may also affect the results, so patients should tell the medical team if they have taken any pain relief prior to the test.

Patients should be advised to avoid eating large meals before the test, as a full stomach can impede full inhalation. Strenuous exercise and smoking should also be avoided prior to the test. It is advisable that patients wear loose-fitting clothes and avoid wearing jewellery so as to facilitate deep breathing. People who wear dentures should be advised to keep them in to help maintain a seal around the mouthpieces used for inhalation.

Being placed in a glass booth can cause feelings of claustrophobia and anxiety, and patients will need comfort and reassurance that the procedure is harmless and painless.

Bronchiectasis

Bronchiectasis describes an irreversible lung condition caused by recurrent infection and inflammation. The condition is associated with abnormal dilation of the bronchi together with a loss of functioning cilia. Destruction of alveolar walls and fibrosis also occur. It is characterised by a chronic productive cough, in which the patient produces large amounts of purulent sputum. Other symptoms include dyspnoea, pleuritic pain and wheeze. Treatments include chest physiotherapy and antibiotics.

Bronchiectasis is a chronic lung disorder that usually develops secondary to a problem during childhood. Inflammation as a result of severe pneumonia, measles or whooping cough during childhood damages and weakens the bronchial walls. Diseases that cause bronchial obstruction, such as tumours and TB, can also lead to bronchiectasis when infections occur beyond the obstruction. Less common are congenital causes such as cystic fibrosis, in which the overproduction of viscous mucus causes recurrent lung infections, and immunoglobulin deficiencies, which cause recurrent infections (Goeminne and Dupont, 2010).

Restrictive disorders

Patients with restrictive disorders have difficulty in expanding their thorax. Spirometry shows a reduced FVC and FEV_1 but unlike obstructive disorders, the FEV_1:FVC ratio is normal. This is because the airways are not obstructed, but rather chest expansion is restricted. The two main reasons why chest expansion could be impeded are:

1. A condition that directly affects the chest wall, such as kyphosis or scoliosis.
2. A disease that affects lung compliance. Poliomyelitis, amyotrophic lateral sclerosis and botulism, for example, can cause respiratory muscle paralysis, whereas muscular dystrophy causes muscle weakness.

Disorders that restrict lung tissue are in the main chronic conditions caused by the inhalation of industrial or commercial pollutants. The upper respiratory tract is often unable to handle the vast quantities of airborne particles generated by various work practices, e.g. coal dust. Small particles that become lodged within the lungs cause chronic inflammation. Over time, connective tissue within the lungs is eroded, and the lungs become less compliant, making chest expansion difficult. This group of respiratory diseases is called pneumoconioses and the individual diseases are often named after the job or pastime that generated them, e.g. coal worker's lung (Hubert and VanMeter, 2018). Chest expansion can also be restricted by acute problems such as adult respiratory distress syndrome, which occurs after lung trauma or pulmonary oedema.

Lung cancer

Lung cancer has the highest mortality rate of all known cancers in the Western world. In the UK alone, it accounts for around 35 000 deaths a year (British Lung Foundation, 2020b). The most significant risk factor is smoking. Ex-smokers remain at risk, although the likelihood reduces over time. Also susceptible are those exposed to passive smoking, albeit at a much lower probability. Smoking or other irritants (i.e. occupational pollutants) damage the pseudostratified epithelium of lung tissue, rendering it more susceptible to inflammation. Certain chemicals present within cigarette smoke are carcinogenic, and promote the development of tumours within the lung tissue. The vast majority of lung cancers (95%) are bronchial carcinomas, of which there are two major types – non-small cell and small cell. Non-small cell carcinomas account for 70% of all lung cancers and can be subdivided again into squamous cell carcinomas, which tend to develop within the larger bronchi, and adenocarcinomas and large cell carcinomas, which are found in the smaller airways, making them much harder to detect. Small cell carcinomas tend to grow near the large bronchi and are the most aggressive bronchial carcinomas. There are no specific signs of lung cancer, but a diagnosis is usually made in smokers who present with the following symptoms:

- Cough, that does not go away after 2–3 weeks or a long-standing cough that is worsening
- Regular chest infections
- Haemoptysis
- Dyspnoea
- Chest pain when coughing
- Lethargy and tiredness

Snapshot   Pulmonary rehabilitation

Casper is a 77-year-old man living with lung cancer. Recently, Casper had been experiencing increased levels of breathlessness, fatigue and general feelings of being unwell. Casper's daughter made him an appointment with the respiratory nurse as she was increasingly concerned about his well-being, his low mood and his general lack of interest in his garden, which was normally his pride and joy. On examination the nurse noted Casper was experiencing breathlessness on mild exertion and recorded the following vital signs:

Vital sign	Observation	Normal
Temperature	36.2°C	36.0–37.9°C range
Pulse	87 beats per minute	60–1000 beats per minute
Respiration	22 breaths per minute	12–100 breaths per minute
Blood pressure	142/88 mmHg	100–139 mmHg (systolic) range
O_2 saturation	97%	94–98% Or 88–92% in chronic respiratory conditions

349

NEWS 2   Casper Owusu

Physiological Parameters	Scores						
	3	2	1	0	1	2	3
Respiration Rate						22	
SpO$_2$ Scale 1				97			
SpO$_2$ Scale 2							
Air or oxygen				Air			
Systolic blood pressure				142			
Pulse				87			
Consciousness				A			
Temperature				36.2			

Note: NEWS score: 2 – Clinical risk Low
Source: Royal College of Physicians (2020).

The nurse and Casper chatted about the steps he takes to manage his condition, and it was clear that he often felt sad and had lost interest in 'most things'. Casper stated that he felt he had become a burden on his daughter and that he preferred to stay at home rather than visit her and his grandchildren. Based on what she had been told, the respiratory nurse informed Casper that she felt he was depressed.

The respiratory nurse recommended that Casper attend pulmonary rehabilitation sessions as they had been positively evaluated and been shown to effectively reduce depression and anxiety in patients like Casper. There was a local group that met once a week at his local hospital, and she was happy to refer him to the nurse that ran it. Casper agreed to give it a try and attended his first pulmonary rehabilitation session the following week. He was introduced to the service by a physiotherapist, who explained that he would attend eight classes of 2 hours duration, in which he would learn exercises that he could do at home and techniques to help him cope with his breathlessness.

Take some time to reflect on this case and then consider the following:

1. Why do you think people living respiratory disease may be prone to depression?
2. What is pulmonary rehabilitation and why do you think it is beneficial to people like Casper?
3. What impact would depression have on an individual living with a respiratory illness?

Pleural disorders

Only a minute amount of fluid occupies the pleural space (the space between the parietal and visceral pleura). Any condition that causes air or fluid to collect in the pleural space can cause the lung to partially or fully collapse (Figure 12.15). The collapse of a lung results in areas that are under-ventilated, a phenomenon known as atelectasis. The surface area for external respiration is dramatically reduced, and the patient may develop hypoxaemia (West, 2013). The main investigation for pleural disorders is a chest X-ray; the critically ill patient, however, may require a computed tomography (CT) scan.

One fluid that can leak into the pleural space is blood. Trauma, cancer and surgery can all cause bleeding into the pleural space, a phenomenon referred to as haemothorax. Exudate

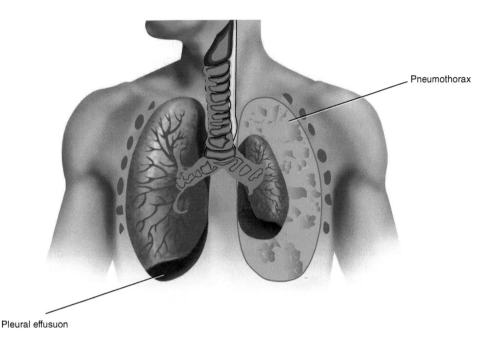

Pneumothorax

351

Pleural effusuon

Figure 12.15   Pleural effusion and a pneumothorax.

and transudate pleural effusions can cause other kinds of fluid to collect in the pleural space. Exudate pleural effusions occur when there is a problem within lung tissue. The fluid that collects in the pleural space is rich in protein and white blood cells because it is generated as a result of inflammation secondary to a tumour or an infection, such as pneumonia or TB. Inflammation increases capillary permeability, allowing fluid to leak out of blood vessels and into the pleural space. Transudate pleural effusions occur as a result of a problem outside of the lungs. A prime example is left ventricular failure, which causes an increase in capillary hydrostatic pressure that forces fluid out of the bloodstream and into the pleural space. A decrease in blood osmotic pressure will also force fluid from blood vessels into the pleural space; causes of reduced blood osmotic pressure include hypoproteinaemia. Some patients may develop an empyema, the formation of pus in the pleural effusion (Dobbin and Howard, 2009). Table 12.6 summarises the signs and symptoms of pleural effusions.

Table 12.6   Signs and symptoms of pleural disorders.

Pleural effusion	Pneumothorax
Dyspnoea	Tachypnoea
Pleuritic pain	Use of accessory muscles
Dry cough	Asymmetrical chest expansion
Cyanosis	Cyanosis
Tachycardia	Tachycardia
	Hypertension or hypotension
	Pulsus paradoxus
	Sweating
	Dry cough
	Restlessness or confusion

The presence of air in the pleural cavity is called a pneumothorax. A pneumothorax can occur as a result of chest trauma, e.g. a stabbing or a broken rib. Patients with chronic respiratory disease are also at risk of developing a pneumothorax. Some individuals have a congenital defect or bleb within the alveolar wall which can rupture spontaneously. Tall young men are at particular risk of this kind of pneumothorax (Ryan, 2005). In certain circumstances, a flap of tissue creates a one-way valve effect and airflow into the pleural space is promoted with each inspiration. As the pneumothorax grows, pressure is exerted on the inferior vena cava, impeding the blood flowing back to the heart (venous return). As a result, the patient becomes hypoxic and breathless. This medical emergency is called a tension pneumothorax (Table 12.6).

Care and management

Chest drains are often used to assist the re-inflation of the affected lung. The monitoring of both the patient and the drain is the responsibility of the healthcare professional, and attention should be paid to the following:

- Patient positioning – Placing the patient in an upright position will encourage drainage and aid expansion of the thorax.
- Position of the chest drain – The drainage bottle must be kept below the patient's chest level to prevent fluid re-entering the pleural space. Coiled and looped tubing should also be avoided as it can impede drainage flow and lead to a tension pneumothorax or surgical emphysema.
- Continuous monitoring of vital signs until the patient's condition stabilises.
- Close monitoring of the chest drain.
- Swinging – The level of the fluid in the underwater seal of the drain should fluctuate between 5 and 10 cm when the patient breathes. Absence of swinging could indicate a kink or blockage in the tubing.
- Bubbling – Bubbles often occur in the water seal bottle without suction when the patient exhales or coughs. Continuous bubbling indicates a problem with the drain or insertion site.
- Administration of prescribed analgesics for pleuritic pain.
- Accurate recording of drainage – The quantity, colour and consistency of the fluid being drained should be noted.
- Infection control – The insertion site should be checked daily for signs of infection, i.e. redness, swelling, heat, pain and discharge (Sullivan, 2008).

Conclusion

This chapter has examined how respiratory disorders can interfere with respiration. Respiration involves four distinct physiological processes: pulmonary ventilation, external respiration, transport of gases and internal respiration. Respiration ensures that the body receives enough oxygen whilst disposing of excess carbon dioxide. In doing so, respiration plays a vital role in the maintenance of homeostasis. Any disease that interferes with pulmonary ventilation or external respiration will disturb homeostasis by reducing oxygen levels and possibly increasing carbon dioxide. The respiratory system has a complex anatomical structure, and so there are a multitude of respiratory diseases. TB and pneumonia, for example, affect the alveoli and neighbouring tissue, whereas COPD and asthma obstruct the airways. Whatever the primary cause of the respiratory disorder, pulmonary ventilation and external respiration will almost always be affected, and hypoxaemia and hypoxia can result. Patients with respiratory disease present with a multitude of symptoms – with dyspnoea, tachypnoea, pleuritic pain, reduced peak expiratory flow rate, low SpO$_2$, cyanosis and an inability to speak in complete sentences being just a few examples.

Activities

Here are some activities and exercises to help test your learning. For the answers to these exercises, as well as further self-testing activities, visit our website at **www.wiley.com/go/fundamentalsofappliedpathophysiology/student4e**

353

Multiple choice questions

1. Which of the following statements is true?
   (a) Cells require a continuous supply of oxygen (O$_2$)
   (b) The organelle lysosome is often referred to as the powerhouse of the cell
   (c) Carbon dioxide is required for the production of adenosine triphosphate (ATP)
   (d) All of the above
2. Which of the following is found in the upper respiratory tract?
   (a) Pharynx
   (b) Alveoli
   (c) Tertiary bronchi
   (d) Trachea
3. How many lobes are there in the left lung?
   (a) 1
   (b) 2
   (c) 3
   (d) 4
4. Which gas law states that the "the pressure of gas in the lungs is inversely proportional to their size."?
   (a) Henry's law
   (b) Dalton's law
   (c) Boyle's law
   (d) Fick's law
5. Which of the following muscles is also known as an accessory muscle?
   (a) Diaphragm
   (b) Sternocleidomastoids
   (c) External intercostals
   (d) Internal intercostals
6. How is the majority of carbon dioxide transported around the human body?
   (a) Dissolved in plasma
   (b) Attached to haemoglobin
   (c) As chloride ions
   (d) As bicarbonate ions

7. Which of the following statements on gaseous exchange is true?
   (a) Arterial pulmonary circulation is low in carbon dioxide
   (b) Venous pulmonary circulation is high in carbon dioxide
   (c) The concentration of oxygen in the alveoli is higher than in lobular circulation
   (d) The concentration of carbon dioxide in lobular circulation is lower than in the alveoli

8. In which of the following structures are the central chemoreceptors located?
   (a) Pneumotaxic and apneustic areas
   (b) Carotid arteries and aorta
   (c) Medulla oblongata and pons
   (d) Inferior and superior vena cava

9. How is the majority of oxygen transported around the body?
   (a) Dissolved in blood plasma (PaO_2)
   (b) Attached to haemoglobin
   (c) Attached to albumin
   (d) As bicarbonate ions

10. Which of the following statements is correct?
    (a) Hypoxaemia and normal carbon dioxide levels suggests Respiratory Failure Type 2
    (b) An arterial blood pH of 7.4 suggests acidosis
    (c) The treatment of respiratory failure type 2 is ventilation
    (d) The correct term for low levels of oxygen in arterial blood is hypercapnia

11. Which of the following is a symptom of tuberculosis?
    (a) Fever
    (b) Haemoptysis
    (c) Night sweats
    (d) All of the above

12. Which of the following best describes forced vital capacity?
    (a) The amount of air left in the lungs after maximal expiration
    (b) The velocity of air expelled in one second
    (c) The proportion of expelled air exhaled in one second
    (d) The maximum amount of air that can be exhaled after maximal inhalation.

13. Which of the following bronchodilator therapies is a beta-2 agonist?
    (a) Theophylline
    (b) Ipratropium
    (c) Aminophylline
    (d) Salbutamol

14. Which of the following statements is true?
    (a) COPD is an umbrella term for chronic tuberculosis, emphysema and chronic pneumonia
    (b) Chronic bronchitis is defined as the permanent enlargement of airspaces beyond the terminal bronchiole and the destruction of the alveolar wall
    (c) The major cause of COPD is smoking
    (d) Emphysema is defined as the presence of a productive cough lasting for 3 months in each of 2 consecutive years when other pulmonary and cardiac causes of cough have been ruled out

15. Which of the following diseases is a restrictive respiratory disorder?
    (a) Asthma
    (b) Pneumoconiosis
    (c) COPD
    (d) Bronchiectasis

Conditions

The following is a list of further conditions that are associated with the respiratory system. Take some time and write notes about each of the conditions. You may make the notes taken from textbooks or other resources (e.g. people you work with in a clinical area), or you may make the notes based on people you have cared for. If you are making notes about people you have cared for, you must ensure that you adhere to the rules of confidentiality.

Fibrosis alveolitis	
Bronchiolitis	
Pneumoconiosis	
Empyema	
Cystic fibrosis	

Further reading

National Institute for Health and Care Excellence

http://www.nice.org.uk/

The National Institute for Health and Care Excellence (NICE) website provides access to the latest guidance on many respiratory conditions. This guidance is based on the best available research and will inform you on how to keep your practice evidence based and up to date.

British Thoracic Society

https://www.brit-thoracic.org.uk/

The British Thoracic Society website provides a range of information and clinical guidance that is based on the best available evidence. Their guidance is essential for all health professionals that wish to provide gold standard care for their respiratory patients. British Thoracic Society guidance will also ensure that your academic work is up to date.

British Lung Foundation

https://www.blf.org.uk/

The British Lung Foundation website provides a wealth of information for patients with respiratory disease. By accessing this site, you can gain insight into the support available for people living with lung disease, which may help you in practice and in your academic studies.

Asthma UK

http://www.asthma.org.uk/

The Asthma UK website provides insight into the support and guidance available to people with asthma. Insight into such guidance can help you to enhance your care.

MacMillan Cancer Support

http://www.macmillan.org.uk

The MacMillan Cancer Support website has an excellent section on managing breathlessness, which you may find useful when caring for respiratory patients.

Respiratory Education UK

http://www.respiratoryeduk.com/

The Respiratory Education UK website has access to a range of courses and information, which you may wish to utilise for your studies. There are also quizzes and exercises, which can test your understanding.

Glossary of terms

Amyotrophic lateral sclerosis A serious neurological disease in which motor neurons gradually deteriorate.

Anaemia Blood lacking in iron. Often used to mean a deficiency in red blood cells (erythrocytes).

Antipyretic agent A drug that can reduce high temperatures (e.g. paracetamol, aspirin, ibuprofen).

Aorta The first major blood vessel of arterial circulation. Emerges from the left ventricle of the heart.

Atelectasis A partial or complete collapse of lung tissue due to a blocked airway.

Bacillus A form of bacteria. Bacilli are rod-shaped, gram-positive and usually have motility.

Botulism A rare but serious bacterial infection which causes muscle weakness and paralysis.

Carcinogen Something capable of causing cancer.

Carotid artery The major artery supplying the brain; stems from the aorta.

Cartilage A type of connective tissue that contains collagen and elastic fibres. This strong tough material on the bone ends helps to distribute the load within the joint; the slippery surface allows smooth movement between the bones. Cartilage can withstand both tension and compression.

Cerebrospinal fluid (CSF) The fluid found within the brain and spinal cord.

Chemoreceptor A sensory receptor that detects the presence of a specific chemical.

Central cyanosis A bluish hue or tinge visible on the lips and mouth that occurs when arterial oxygen levels are abnormally low.

Cilia Hair-like extensions on the outer surface of some cells; used to propel liquids.

Cor pulmonale Right-sided heart failure caused by hypoxia.

Diffusion   The passive movement of molecules or ions from a region of high concentration to one of low concentration until a state of equilibrium is achieved.

Elastic cartilage   Cartilage that contains more elastin fibres, providing strength and stretchability.

Enzyme   A protein that speeds up chemical reactions.

Erythrocyte   Another name for a red blood cell.

Expectorate   To cough up and spit out mucus or sputum.

External intercostal muscle   A muscle that spans the spaces between the ribs. As opposed to the internal intercostal muscles, the external intercostal muscles sit closer to the outside of the thorax.

External respiration   The transfer of oxygen from the alveoli in the lungs to the bloodstream and the transfer of carbon dioxide from the bloodstream into alveoli in the lungs.

Extrinsic asthma   Asthma caused by hypersensitive reactions to an allergy.

Exudate   Escaping fluid that spills from a space; contains cellular debris and pus.

Fibrin   A protein essential for clotting.

Fibrosis   Growth of fibrous connective tissue (scar tissue).

Fibrous   Containing regenerated or scar tissue.

Finger clubbing   Alteration in the angle of finger and toe bases caused by chronic tissue hypoxia.

Goblet cell   A mucus-secreting cell found in epithelial tissue.

Haemoglobin (Hb)   A protein consisting of globin and four haem groups that is found within erythrocytes (red blood cells). Responsible for the transport of oxygen.

Haemoptysis   Coughing up of blood.

Hydrostatic pressure   The pressure exerted by a fluid.

Hypercapnia   Elevated levels of arterial carbon dioxide.

Hypertension   Raised blood pressure.

Hypoproteinaemia   A reduced level of plasma proteins.

Hypotension   Low blood pressure.

Hypoxaemia   Reduced level of oxygen within arterial blood.

Hypoxia   Reduced level of oxygen within the tissues.

Intercostal nerve   A nerve that links the respiratory centres in the brainstem with the intercostal muscles.

Internal intercostal muscle   A muscle that spans the spaces between the ribs. As opposed to the external intercostal muscles, the internal intercostal muscles sit closer to the inside of the thorax.

Internal respiration   The transfer of oxygen from the bloodstream into body cells and the transfer of carbon dioxide from body cells to the bloodstream. This is known as aerobic respiration. Anaerobic respiration does not require oxygen but does require a substance such as nitrate or iron to do the same job as oxygen (accept electrons during the chemical reaction). Only human cells with mitochondria can undertake aerobic respiration.

Intrinsic asthma   Asthma caused by hyper-responsive reactions to non-allergic stimuli.

Intubation   The insertion of a special tube into the pharynx and down into the trachea, in order to maintain a patent airway in an unconscious person.

Kyphosis   Curvature of the thoracic spine.

Lymph node   Part of the lymphatic system, it contains many white cells to destroy bacteria that are trapped within the lymph node.

Lymphocyte   A specialist white blood cell involved in immune responses.

Lymph vessel   A vessel that carries lymphatic fluid. Part of the lymphatic system which forms part of the immune system.

357

Macrophage   A phagocyte produced from monocytes that engulfs and digests cellular debris, microbes and foreign matter.

Mast cell   A cell found in connective tissue that releases histamine during inflammation.

Medulla oblongata   Lowest region of the brainstem; concerned with the control of the internal organs.

Muscular dystrophy   A group of diseases characterised by the progressive loss of muscle fibres. Almost all these diseases are hereditary.

Neutrophil   A type of white blood cell.

Non-invasive positive pressure ventilation (NIPPV)   Respiratory support technique that enhances the person's rate and depth of breathing.

Oedema   The abnormal accumulation of fluid in the interstitial spaces. It may be localised (following an injury = swelling) or it may be generalised (as in heart failure).

Osmotic pressure   The pressure that must be exerted on a solution to prevent the passage of water into it across a semipermeable membrane from a region of higher concentration of solute to a region of lower concentration of solute.

Peak expiratory flow rate   The velocity at which a person can expire their total lung volume.

Phrenic nerve   The nerve that links the diaphragm to the respiratory centre in the brainstem.

Poliomyelitis   An acute viral disease which affects the central nervous system.

Polycythaemia   A condition in which there is an abnormally high number of erythrocytes (red blood cells).

Pons   Upper region of the brainstem. Connects the midbrain to the medulla oblongata.

Pseudostratified ciliated columnar epithelium   Covering or lining of the internal body surface that contains cilia and mucus-secreting goblet cells.

Pulmonary ventilation   Breathing. The inspiration and expiration of air into and out of the lungs.

Pulse oximetry   Non-invasive measurement of the oxygen saturation of the blood (SpO_2).

Pulsus paradoxus   A phenomenon in which the pulse is weaker during inspiration than during expiration.

Pyrexia   Elevated temperature associated with fever.

Respiratory acidosis   A blood pH of less than 7.35 caused by a rise in arterial carbon dioxide.

Scoliosis   A sideways curvature of the thoracic spine.

Spirometry   Diagnostic tool which measures a person's forced vital capacity (FVC) and forced expiratory volume within the first second of expiration (FEV_1).

Surgical emphysema   Air trapped in the tissues, usually as a result of a surgical or invasive procedure.

Systemic circulation   The flow of blood from the left ventricle to all parts of the body.

Tachycardia   A fast heartbeat (usually defined as above 100 beats per minute).

Thorax   The body trunk above the diaphragm and below the neck.

Tracheostomy   A procedure in which an incision is made in the trachea to facilitate breathing.

Transport of gases   The movement of oxygen and carbon dioxide between the lungs and body cells.

References

Asthma UK. (2020) *Common Inhaler Mistakes*. Available at https://www.asthma.org.uk/advice/inhalers-medicines-treatments/inhalers-and-spacers/common-inhaler-mistakes/Accessed 14 June 2020.

Barnes, P.J. (2008). Drugs for airway disease. *Medicine*, 36(4): 181–190.

Braman, S.S. (2006). Chronic cough due to bronchitis: ACCP evidence-based clinical practice. *Chest*, 129: 104S–115S.

British Lung Foundation. (2017). *Estimating the Economic Burden of Lung Illness in the UK*. London: British Lung Foundation.

British Lung Foundation. (2020a). *Asthma Statistics*. Available at https://statistics.blf.org.uk/asthma Accessed 14 June 2020.

British Lung Foundation. (2020b). Lung Cancer Statistics. Available at https://statistics.blf.org.uk/lung-cancer Accessed 14 June 2020.

British Thoracic Society and Intensive Care Society Acute Hypercapnic Respiratory Failure Guideline Development Group (2016). *BTS/ICS Guidelines for the Ventilatory Management of Acute Hypercapnic Respiratory Failure*. London: British Thoracic Society.

British Thoracic Society (BTS) (2009). Guidelines for the management of community acquired pneumonia in adults: Update 2009. *Thorax*, 64(Suppl. III): iii1–iii55.

British Thoracic Society and Scottish Intercollegiate Guidelines Network (2019). *SIGN 158 British Guideline on the Management of Asthma*. Available at: https://www.brit-thoracic.org.uk/quality-improvement/guidelines/asthma/ Accessed 14 June 2020.

Clancy, J. and McVicar, A. (2007). Immediate and long-term regulation of acid-base homeostasis. *British Journal of Nursing*, 16(17): 1076–1079.

Clark, A.P., Giuliano, K. and Chen, H. (2006). Pulse oximetry revisited 'but his O_2 sat was normal!' *Clinical Nurse Specialist*, 20(6): 268–272.

Devereux, G. (2006). ABC of chronic obstructive disease definition, epidemiology and risk factors. *British Medical Journal*, 332: 1142–1144.

Dobbin, K.R. and Howard, V.M. (2009). Understanding empyema. *Nursing*, June: 56cc1–56cc5.

Dunn, L. (2005). Pneumonia: Classification, diagnosis and nursing management. *Nursing Standard*, 19: 50–54.

Goeminne, P. and Dupont, L. (2010). Non-cystic fibrosis bronchiectasis: diagnosis and management in the 21st century. *Postgraduate Medical Journal*, 86: 493–501.

Hickin, S., Renshaw, J., Williams, R. and Horton-Szar, D. (2015). *Respiratory System Crash Course*, 4th edn. London: Mosby.

Higginson, R. and Jones, B. (2009). Respiratory assessment in critically ill patients: airway and breathing. *British Journal of Nursing*, 18(8): 456–461.

Hoare, Z. and Lim, W.S. (2006). Pneumonia: Update on diagnosis and management. *British Medical Journal*, 332: 1077–1079.

Hogg, J.C. and Senior, R.M. (2002). Chronic obstructive pulmonary disease. 2: Pathology and biochemistry of emphysema. *Thorax*, 57: 830–834.

Hubert, R.J. and VanMeter, K.C. (2018). *Gould's Pathophysiology for the Health Professions*, 6th edn. St Louis: Elsevier.

Joint Formulary Committee (2020). *British National Formulary*, 79th edn. London: Pharmaceutical Press.

MacNee, W. (2006). ABC of chronic obstructive pulmonary disease pathology, pathogenesis and pathophysiology. *British Medical Journal*, 332: 1202–1204.

Maruccia, M., Ruggieri, M. and Onesti, M.G. (2013). Facial skin breakdown in patients with non-invasive ventilation devices: report of two cases and indications for treatment and prevention. *International Wound Journal*, 12(4): 451–455.

Martini, F.H. and Nath, J.L. (2009). *Fundamentals of Anatomy and Physiology*, 8th edn. San Francisco: Pearson Benjamin Cummings.

Myatt, R. (2015). Nursing care of patients with a temporary tracheostomy. *Nursing Standard*, 29(26): 42–49.

National Institute for Health and Care Excellence (NICE) (2011). *Clinical Guideline 121. Lung Cancer: Diagnosis and Treatment of Lung Cancer*. London: NICE.

NICE (2013). *Asthma NICE Quality Standard QS25*. London: NICE.

NICE (2014). *Pneumonia in Adults: Diagnosis and Management CG191*. London: NICE.

NICE (2016). *Tuberculosis – NICE Guidance NG33*. NICE, London.

NICE (2018). *Chronic Obstructive Pulmonary Disease in over 16s: Diagnosis and Management*. London: NICE.

Ochs, M., Nyengaard, A.J., Knudsen, L., Voigt, M., Wahlers, T. *et al.* (2004). The number of alveoli in the human lung. *American Journal of Respiratory and Critical Care Medicine*, 169: 120–124.

Public Health England. (2008). *Patient dose information: Guidance*. Available at https://www.gov.uk/government/publications/medical-radiation-patient-doses/patient-dose-information-guidance Accessed 19 June 2020.

Royal College of Physicians. (2020). *National Early Warning Scores (NEWS) 2*. Available at https://www.rcplondon.ac.uk/projects/outputs/national-early-warning-score-news-2 Accessed 18 June 2020.

Ryan, B. (2005). Pneumothorax assessment and diagnostic testing. *Journal of Cardiovascular Nursing*, 20(4): 251–253.

Schwartzstein, R.M. and Parker, M.J. (2006). *Respiratory Physiology: A Clinical Approach*. Philadelphia: Lippincott Williams & Wilkins.

Sheldon, R.L. (2005). Pulmonary function testing. In: Wilkins, R.L., Sheldon, R.L. and Krider, S.J. (eds), *Clinical Assessment in Respiratory Care*, 5th edn. St Louis: Elsevier Mosby.

Sims, J.M. (2006). An overview of asthma. *Dimensions of Critical Care Nursing*, 25(6): 264–268.

Smith, J and Rushton, M. (2015). How to perform a respiratory assessment. *Nursing Standard*, 30(7): 34-236.

Sullivan, B. (2008). Nursing management of patients with a chest drain. *British Journal of Nursing*, 17(6): 388–393

Torjesen, I. (2014). Two-thirds of deaths from asthma are preventable, confidential enquiry finds. *British Medical Journal*, 348: 3108.

West, J.B. (2013). *Pulmonary Pathophysiology: The Essentials*, 8th edn. Philadelphia: Lippincott Williams & Wilkins.

Wheeldon, A. (2016). The respiratory system. In: Peate, I. and Nair, M. (eds), *Fundamental Anatomy and Physiology for Nursing and Healthcare Students*. Chichester: Wiley-Blackwell.

Chapter 13

The gastrointestinal system and associated disorders

Louise McErlean

Lecturer, Department of Nursing, School of Health and Social Work, Ulster University, Northern Ireland, UK

Contents

Introduction 362
The digestive system...363
The upper gastrointestinal tract and its
    accessory organs 364
Accessory organs of digestion.......................373
Disorders of the digestive system 376

Conclusion 392
Multiple choice questions...............................392
Conditions..394
Further resources..394
Glossary of terms..395
References..396

Key words

- Oral cavity
- Duodenum
- Large intestine
- Peristalsis
- Oesophagus
- Jejunum
- Digestion
- Peritoneum
- Stomach
- Small intestine
- Chyme
- Bowel sounds

Test your prior knowledge

- What are the main functions of the digestive system?
- List five functions of the stomach.
- Differentiate between chemical and mechanical digestion.
- Name the accessory organs of digestion.
- Consider the effects of digestive system disorders on the psychosocial well-being of the individual.

Learning outcomes

On completion of this section, the reader will be able to:

- Describe the function of the digestive system.

- List the organs of the digestive system.

- List the accessory organs of the digestive system.

- Outline the pathophysiological changes that can occur within the digestive system.

- Discuss the care of individuals with digestive system disorders.

Don't forget to visit the companion website for this book
(www.wiley.com/go/fundamentalsofappliedpathophysiology/student4e)
where you can find self-assessment tests to check your progress, as well as lots of activities to practise your learning.

Introduction

Human cells require nutrients in order to perform their required function. Conditions of the digestive tract are relatively common, due in some part to its considerable length.

The gastrointestinal system, also known as the digestive system or alimentary canal or tract, is responsible for processing food into the required nutrients. The gastrointestinal system is a continuous tract. It begins at the mouth and ends at the anus, and measures approximately 10 m. The gastrointestinal tract is divided into the upper and lower gastrointestinal tract and the accessory organs. The gastrointestinal system includes the mouth, the pharynx, the oesophagus, the stomach, the small intestine and the large intestine. The accessory organs of digestion are the salivary glands, the liver, the pancreas and the gallbladder (Figure 13.1).

The main function of the gastrointestinal system is to break down the dietary intake into the raw materials required by the cells of the body. The gastrointestinal system does this by digesting the dietary intake, absorbing the nutrients obtained from the process of digestion and eliminating any unwanted material. The products of digestion are processed by the liver.

This chapter discusses the structure and function of the digestive system, and common disorders and their related care and management.

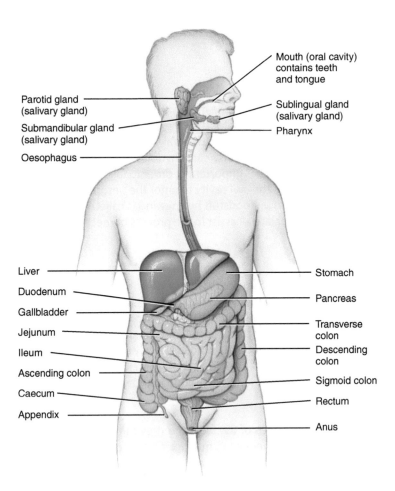

Mouth (oral cavity) contains teeth and tongue

Parotid gland (salivary gland)

Sublingual gland (salivary gland)

Submandibular gland (salivary gland)

Pharynx

Oesophagus

Liver

Stomach

Duodenum

Pancreas

Gallbladder

Transverse colon

Jejunum

Ileum

Descending colon

Ascending colon

Caecum

Sigmoid colon

Appendix

Rectum

Anus

Figure 13.1   The gastrointestinal tract.

The digestive system

Digestion

Food from the diet is broken down throughout the length of the gastrointestinal tract by two types of digestion:

1. Chemical digestion is the chemical breakdown of food. Enzymes are secreted within the digestive tract. The enzymes denature the food, helping to break it down into smaller nutrient molecules. Secretion of the enzymes is dependent upon the action of many hormones.

2. Mechanical digestion is the mechanical breakdown of food. Mechanical breakdown of food begins in the oral cavity with the chewing, grinding and mixing of food. Peristalsis continues to move and churn the ingested food as it moves throughout the length of the digestive system. The smooth muscle contractions of the muscularis layer of the digestive system facilitate the mixing, grinding and denaturing of the ingested food, Mechanical digestion facilitates the breaking down of food into smaller molecules as well as the mixing of the food with the enzymes required for chemical digestion. Smooth muscle contraction occurs as a result of parasympathetic nervous system activity.

The upper gastrointestinal tract and its accessory organs

Oral cavity

The gastrointestinal system begins at the mouth or oral cavity. The mouth receives food and begins the mechanical breakdown of food by the action of chewing and grinding the food. The chemical digestion of food begins in the oral cavity. Food mixes with salivary amylase, which begins the breakdown of dietary carbohydrate (Shier *et al.*, 2018). Mixing the food with saliva adds moisture, which is important in order to taste food and helps form the food into a bolus. The bolus leaves the oral cavity to enter the oesophagus.

The activity of breaking down foodstuff by chewing is called mastication. The lips, gums, teeth, cheeks, tongue and palate all assist in the process of mechanical digestion within the oral cavity (Figure 13.2).

Lips

The lips form the opening into the mouth. They are fleshy folds, which contain skeletal muscles and sensory receptors (Shier *et al.*, 2018). The lips assess the temperature and texture of foods, and direct food into the oral cavity. The ruby red colouring of the lips is attributed to its rich blood supply. Because of their central and usually exposed position, any change in this colouring such as the blue tinge of cyanosis is easily detected. The junction between the upper and the lower lips forms the angle of the mouth. These angles can become sore and dry during periods of ill health and this condition is known as angular cheilitis.

Cheeks

The cheeks form the fleshy sides of the face, and they run from the corner of the mouth to the side of the nose. Subcutaneous fat, muscles and mucous membranes line the cheeks. The cheeks assist in the chewing of food.

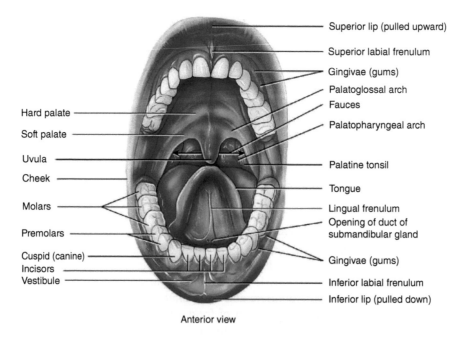

Anterior view

Figure 13.2   The oral cavity.

Palate

The palate is divided into the hard and the soft palates (Figure 13.2); both form the roof of the mouth, whereas the tongue lies at the bottom of the oral cavity and forms the floor of the mouth. The hard and the soft palates are covered by mucous membranes and participate in the mechanical breakdown of food.

Tongue

The tongue is a thick muscular organ composed of skeletal muscles and mucous membranes. The tongue also contains approximately 10 000 taste buds (VanPutte *et al.*, 2016). Taste buds contain sensory gustatory cells that detect different tastes including sweet, bitter, salty, sour and umami. The word *umami* is derived from the Japanese word meaning 'deliciousness' and is a savoury taste.

The tongue is a digestive system accessory organ. In addition to taste, the tongue also has an important role in speech, chewing, directing the food bolus and swallowing.

Teeth

Humans develop two sets of teeth: milk teeth and permanent teeth. There are 20 milk teeth (Figure 13.3), which begin to develop from the age of 6 months. Often one pair of milk teeth grows per month, and they usually fall out between the ages of 6 and 12 years. Once the milk teeth fall out, they are replaced by permanent teeth. There are 32 permanent teeth

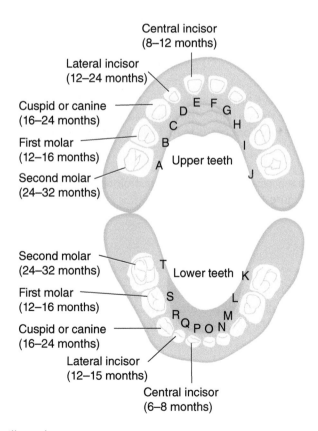

Figure 13.3   The milk teeth.

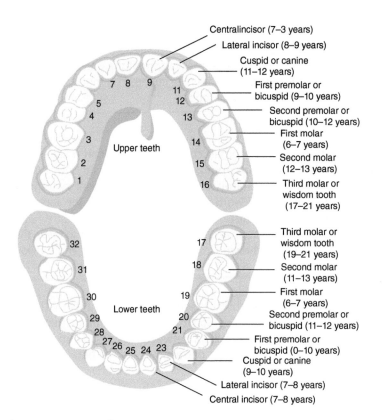

Centralincisor (7–3 years)
Lateral incisor (8–9 years)
Cuspid or canine
(11–12 years)
First premolar or
bicuspid (9–10 years)
Second premolar or
bicuspid (10–12 years)
First molar
(6–7 years)
Second molar
(12–13 years)
Third molar or
wisdom tooth
(17–21 years)

Upper teeth

Third molar or
wisdom tooth
(19–21 years)
Second molar
(11–13 years)
First molar
(6–7 years)
Second premolar or
bicuspid (11–12 years)
First premolar or
bicuspid (0–10 years)
Cuspid or canine
(9–10 years)
Lateral incisor (7–8 years)
Central incisor (7–8 years)

Lower teeth

Figure 13.4   The permanent teeth.

(Figure 13.4), which have the potential to last a lifetime. The first permanent molars appear at the age of 6 years, the second at the age of 12 years and the third may develop after the age of 13 years. The functions of the teeth include cutting, tearing and chewing food.

Salivary glands

Salivary glands are accessory organ of the gastrointestinal system. There are three pairs of salivary glands (Figure 13.5):

1. Parotid
2. Submandibular
3. Sublingual.

The salivary glands are covered by a fibrous capsule and contain secretory cells. The saliva from the secretory cells drains into ducts which lead into the mouth. The salivary glands secrete approximately 1 L of saliva per day (Marieb and Kellar, 2018).
Saliva consists of:

• Water
• Salts
• Salivary amylase
• Mucin (a protein that help form mucus)
• Lysozyme (a bacteriolytic enzyme).

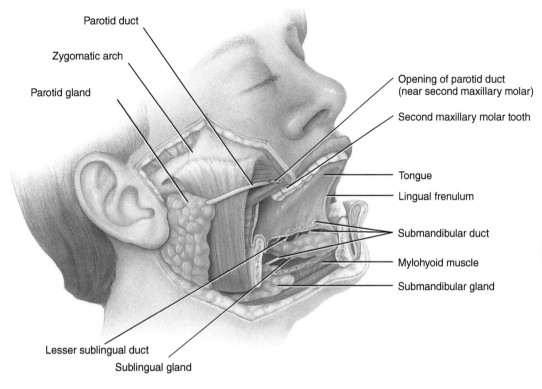

Parotid duct

Zygomatic arch

Parotid gland

Opening of parotid duct
(near second maxillary molar)

Second maxillary molar tooth

Tongue

Lingual frenulum

Submandibular duct

Mylohyoid muscle

Submandibular gland

Lesser sublingual duct

Sublingual gland

Figure 13.5   The salivary glands.

Functions of saliva

The oral cavity is permanently moist due to a continuous coating of saliva. Saliva makes swallowing easier. The action of salivary amylase begins the chemical digestion of carbohydrate. The bactericidal activity of lysozyme present in saliva helps to prevent bacteria that may be present in food from reaching the lower digestive tract. The pH of saliva ranges from 5.8 to 7.4 (Waugh and Grant, 2018).

Pharynx

The pharynx lies behind the nose and mouth. It is divided into three sections – the nasopharynx, oral pharynx and laryngeal pharynx. The pharynx connects with the mouth superiorly and the oesophagus and larynx inferiorly (Longenbaker, 2013). It connects with the two small nasal cavities and two eustachian tubes. When food is swallowed, the soft palate closes the nasal passages, and the epiglottis moves over the glottis to close the larynx and the trachea (Figure 13.6). This allows the foodstuff to move down the oesophagus rather than into the respiratory tract (Figure 13.7).

Oesophagus

The oesophagus is a muscular tube that runs from the pharynx to the stomach. It lies at the back of the trachea and in front of the spinal column (backbone). It is a collapsible muscular tube that channels food into the stomach. The movement of food down the oesophagus occurs as a result of waves of smooth muscle contractions known as peristalsis. It is not possible for a person to swallow and breathe at the same time.

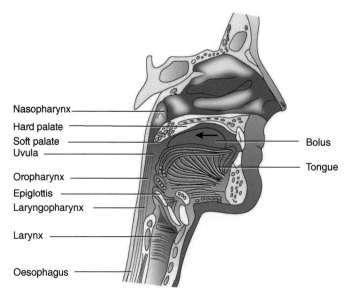

Nasopharynx
Hard palate
Soft palate
Uvula
Oropharynx
Epiglottis
Laryngopharynx
Larynx
Oesophagus
Bolus
Tongue

Position of structures before swallowing

Figure 13.6   The pharynx.

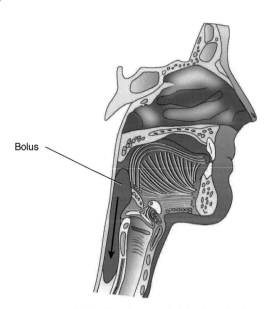

Bolus

During the pharyngeal state of swallowing

Figure 13.7   Swallowing action.

Stomach

The stomach is a J-shaped muscular organ situated below the diaphragm, made up of four regions – an upper portion called the cardiac region, an elevated part called the fundus, a middle section called the body and a pyloric region (Figure 13.8). The layers of the stomach include an outer layer called the visceral peritoneum (also known as the serosa), a muscularis layer, a submucosal layer and a mucosal layer (Figure 13.9).

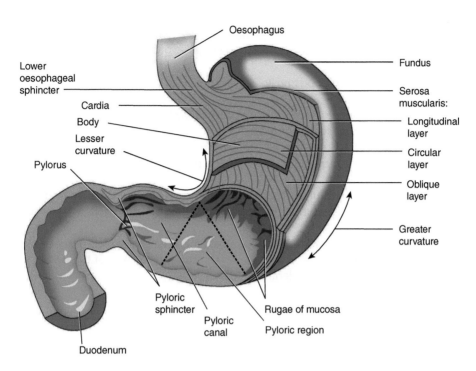

Figure 13.8   The stomach.

369

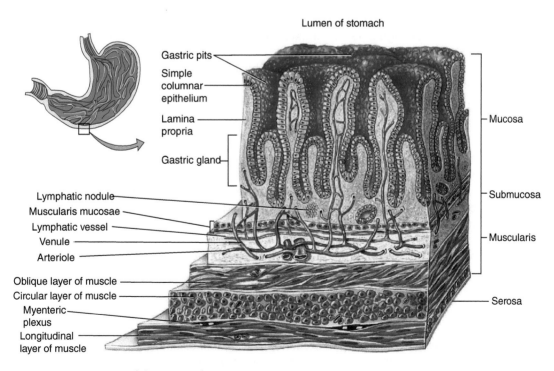

Figure 13.9   Layers of the stomach.

Secretions

The cells of the stomach mucosa secrete numerous enzymes and substances. These are collectively known as gastric juice. Gastric juice contains:

- Mucus, which lubricates food and lines the stomach, protecting it from digestive enzymes and hydrochloric acid.
- Hydrochloric acid, which destroys bacteria that may be present on ingested in food; and is essential for the digestion of proteins.
- Intrinsic factor, which is necessary for the absorption of vitamin B_{12} in the small intestine.
- Pepsinogen, which is required for the chemical digestion of proteins.

Production of gastric juice is dependent upon the hormone gastrin. Gastrin is secreted when food enters the stomach, and secretion stops when the stomach pH drops below 1.5.

The secretions and the ingested food are mixed together into a thick, pasty, semisolid and acidic substance called chyme. Chyme leaves the stomach by way of the pyloric sphincter (Figure 13.8) and enters the duodenum.

Functions

The stomach performs numerous functions:

- It is a temporary reservoir for food until it is ready to be passed into the duodenum.
- Nutrients are liquefied, broken down and mixed with hydrochloric acid to form a semisolid substance called chyme.
- Chemical digestion of proteins begins. Proteins are converted into smaller polypeptides by pepsins.
- Mechanical digestion of food occurs as the three smooth muscle layers of the stomach, the muscularis (Figure 13.8), contract and relax, effectively mixing and churning the stomach contents.
- Milk is curdled, and casein is released from the milk.
- Digestion of fats begins in the stomach.
- Production of intrinsic factor is essential for the absorption of vitamin B_{12}.

Small intestine

Digestion continues in the small intestine and almost all of the absorption of the foods occurs here.

The small intestine is approximately 6 m in length and 3 cm in diameter and is situated in the abdominal cavity. The small intestine is supported by mesenteries (Figure 13.11). The mesenteries convey blood vessels, lymphatic vessels and nerves to the small intestine. The absorptive surface of the small intestine is increased by the presence of microvilli, villi and circular folds (Figure 13.12). The small intestine extends from the pylorus of the stomach to the ileocaecal valve and is divided into three sections: the duodenum, jejunum and ileum (Figure 13.10).

Duodenum

The duodenum is the 'C'-shaped section of the small intestine (Figure 13.10). This is the shortest section. The duodenum commences at the pyloric sphincter and ends at the beginning of the jejunum. The duodenum continues the process of mechanical digestion by the

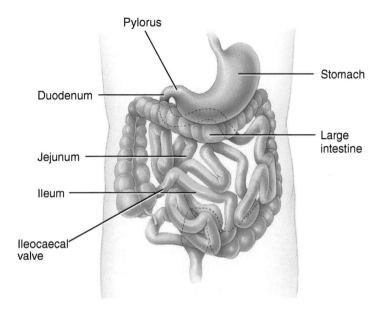

Pylorus

Stomach

Duodenum

Large
intestine

Jejunum

Ileum

Ileocaecal
valve

Figure 13.10   The small intestine.

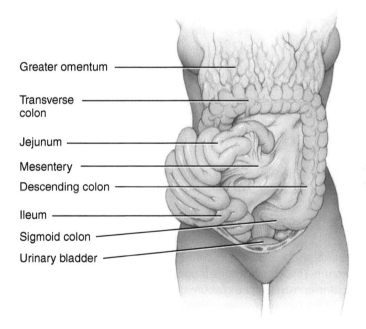

Greater omentum

Transverse
colon

Jejunum

Mesentery

Descending colon

Ileum

Sigmoid colon

Urinary bladder

Figure 13.11   The mesentery of the small intestine.

action of peristalsis. The cells of the intestine produce intestinal juice, which contains some digestive enzymes required for chemical digestion. Pancreatic juice and bile are delivered to the duodenum from the pancreas and gallbladder, respectively. As a result of the many enzymes in intestinal and pancreatic juice, substantial chemical digestion of food occurs in the small intestine. Pancreatic juice is alkaline and therefore neutralises the acidic chyme as it enters the small intestine.

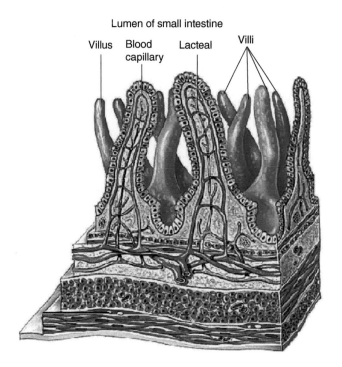

Lumen of small intestine

Villus   Blood   Lacteal   Villi
          capillary

Figure 13.12   Section of the small intestine showing the villi.

Jejunum

The jejunum commences at the end of the duodenum and terminates at the beginning of the ileum. The main function of the jejunum is to further break down the nutrients coming from the duodenum.

Ileum

The ileum commences at the end of the jejunum and terminates at the ileocaecal valve. It is the longest section of small intestine. The main function of the ileum is absorption of nutrients.

Large intestine

The large intestine, also known as the colon, commences at the ileocaecal valve and terminates at the rectum. The large intestine is approximately 2 m in length and 6 cm in diameter. The large intestine consists of the caecum; the ascending, transverse, descending and sigmoid colons; and the rectum and anus (Figure 13.13).

Functions

The functions of the large intestine include:

- Absorption of water, electrolytes and vitamins
- Secretion of mucus for the lubrication of faeces
- Storage of indigestible foodstuff such as cellulose and vegetable fibre
- Production of vitamin K and some B complexes (B_1, B_2 and folic acid)
- Defecation.

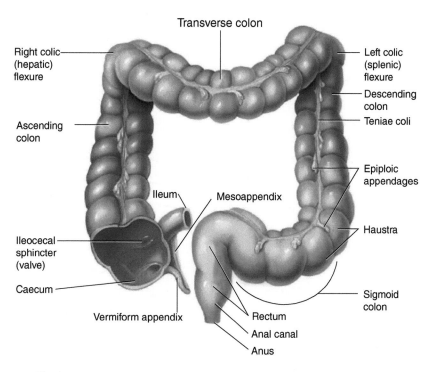

Transverse colon

Right colic (hepatic) flexure

Left colic (splenic) flexure

Ascending colon

Descending colon

Teniae coli

Ileum

Mesoappendix

Epiploic appendages

Ileocecal sphincter (valve)

Haustra

Caecum

Sigmoid colon

Vermiform appendix

Rectum

Anal canal

Anus

Figure 13.13   The large intestine.

Accessory organs of digestion
Liver

The liver is the largest organ in the body. The liver is a wedge-shaped, reddish organ. It is covered by connective tissue and is divided into the right and left lobes (Figure 13.14). It is situated in the upper right quadrant of the abdominal cavity beneath the diaphragm. It is partially protected by the ribs. The right and the left lobes are separated by the falciform ligament, and the liver is covered by a serous membrane called peritoneum.

Blood vessels of the liver

The main blood vessels of the liver include the:

- Hepatic artery – This is a branch of the celiac artery, and it supplies oxygenated blood to the liver.
- The hepatic portal vein – It drains venous blood from the gastrointestinal tract, which contains nutrients absorbed from the small intestine, into the liver.
- The hepatic vein – It drains venous blood from the liver to the inferior vena cava.

Functions

The liver has numerous functions:

- Carbohydrate, protein and fat metabolism
- Modifies waste products and toxic substances, i.e. drugs such as paracetamol, aspirin and alcohol

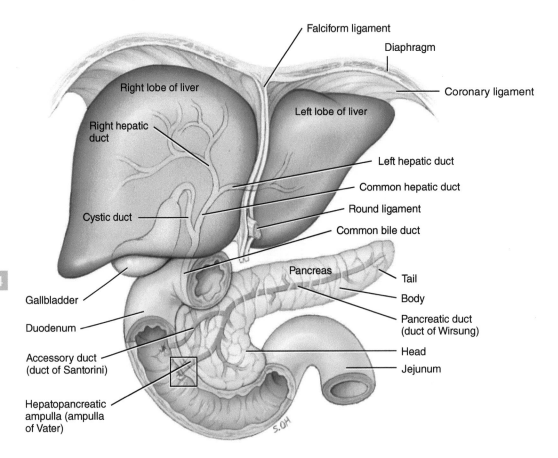

Figure 13.14 The liver.

- Produces and stores glycogen
- Maintains blood glucose levels
- Converts ammonia into urea, which is a waste product
- Forms red blood cells in foetal life
- Plays a part in the destruction of red blood cells
- Stores minerals such as iron and copper
- Stores the fat-soluble vitamins A, D, E and K, and water-soluble vitamin B_{12} [12]
- Manufactures plasma proteins such as prothrombin
- Produces clotting factors
- Produces heat
- Produces bile, which emulsifies fats in the diet for absorption.

Gallbladder

The gallbladder is a pear-shaped muscular sac, which lies beneath the right lobe of the liver (Figure 13.14). The gallbladder's main function is to store and concentrate bile produced in the liver (Figure 13.15). Bile is released from the gallbladder in the presence of the hormone cholecystokinin (CCK). The presence of chyme in the duodenum stimulates the production of CCK. This hormone is transported in the bloodstream to the gallbladder, where it stimulates the smooth muscles of the gallbladder to contract, thus ejecting bile.

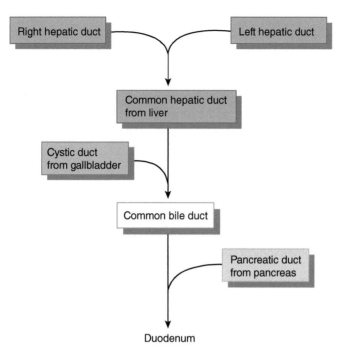

Figure 13.15   Production and storage of bile.

Pancreas

The pancreas is a triangular-shaped organ. It is divided into three sections: head, body and tail (Figure 13.14). It has both an endocrine function and exocrine function.

Exocrine function

The pancreas produces pancreatic juice, which is secreted directly from the pancreas into the duodenum via the pancreatic duct (Figure 13.14). The pancreatic juice contains the following enzymes:

- Pancreatic amylase completes the digestion of carbohydrates
- Trypsin for the digestion of proteins
- Lipase for the digestion of fats.

Approximately 1500 mL of pancreatic juice is produced per day.

Endocrine function

The pancreas also produces hormones that are secreted directly into the bloodstream. The hormones and their functions include:

- Glucagon from pancreatic alpha cells – It increases blood glucose levels
- Insulin from pancreatic beta cells – It lowers blood glucose levels
- Somatostatin from pancreatic delta cells – It regulates both glucagon and insulin levels.

For a more detailed discussion of the endocrine pancreas, see Chapter 15.

Disorders of the digestive system

The digestive system is a large system responsible for processing food and the production of a myriad of enzymes and chemicals; as such it is vulnerable to disorder along its vast length. The remainder of the chapter will examine some of the disorders associated with the digestive system. Professional knowledge is an important area within the NMC Code (NMC, 2018); therefore, reading this chapter and answering some of the associated questions should improve professional knowledge of the digestive system.

Learning outcomes

On completion of this section, the reader will be able to:

- List some of the common disorders of the digestive system.
- Describe the pathophysiology of specific digestive system disorders.
- Discuss the management of digestive system disorders.

Oral Candidiasis

Candidiasis is an infection caused by the yeast Candida. It is also known as oral thrush. *Candida albicans* is the most common of the candidas.

Aetiology

Candida albicans is a commensal microorganism, which can often be found in the digestive system and on the skin. It becomes pathogenic if the conditions are suitable. An excess of sugar such as in diabetes mellitus can lead to an increased risk of developing candidiasis. Treatment with broad-spectrum antibiotics will eradicate the normal flora of microorganisms responsible for keeping Candida at bay and therefore increase the risk of candidiasis. Immunocompromised patients such as cancer patients and patients with neutropenia can be at risk. Asthmatic patients prescribed a steroid inhaler are also at risk, as are the elderly.

Signs and symptoms

These include:

- A sore mouth
- The presence of small creamy white plaques on the tongue or soft palate
- Red and bleeding tissue beneath the white pustules
- Inability to taste food
- The presence of a bad taste in the mouth.

Care and management

Although it can often be diagnosed on visual inspection only, diagnosis can be confirmed by sending a swab taken from the oral cavity for microscopy.

It is important to treat *Candida albicans*, as a painful mouth may stop the patient person from eating and drinking and lead to dehydration and delay the healing process. If left untreated, the infection can spread.

Frequent oral hygiene is required, and an anti-fungal gel, pastille or oral suspension such as nystatin may be prescribed.

Red flag

Oral hygiene is an important part of inpatient care.

Mouth assessment should be carried out and the frequency of oral hygiene established. If candidiasis is present, then dentures should be removed before treatment is given. The nystatin should be administered after mealtimes to allow for as much contact with the affected area as possible. The patient should be encouraged to hold the nystatin in the mouth to increase contact area and time.

Often the medication should be continued as prescribed to ensure the infection has been adequately treated.

Snapshot   Candida albicans

Eliza is 8 weeks old. Eliza's mother Jane is breastfeeding.

Jane has noticed white patches inside Eliza's mouth. The patches rub off when they are wiped, and there are some areas of redness and bleeding. Eliza also has a nappy rash, and she is not feeding as well as she used to. Jane is concerned and calls the midwife.

The midwife explains that this is likely to be oral thrush (*Candida albicans*). As Eliza's immune system is immature, she is more prone to opportunistic infections. The midwife suggests a visit to the GP for some treatment. She also suggests that as *Candida albicans* can be passed to Jane during breastfeeding, Jane should check her breasts for any sign of the infection.

Take some time to reflect on this case and then consider the following:

1. What type of infection is *Candida albicans*?
2. Nystatin is often prescribed to treat oral *Candida albicans* infection. What is the mode of action and side effects associated with this medication?
3. What advice would you give Eliza's mum to prevent the spread of the infection to other members of the household?

Peptic ulcer disease

A peptic ulcer is a break in the lining of the gastrointestinal tract that occurs in the lower part of the oesophagus, the stomach or the duodenum. Duodenal ulcers are the most commonly occurring ulcer. Ulcers can be acute or chronic. Ulcers can be superficial (known as an erosion) or deep, where the ulcer extends through the muscularis mucosae layer. Superficial peptic ulcers usually respond well to drug treatment, but if the ulcer is severe and/or deep, complications can occur, such as perforation of the gastrointestinal wall, haemorrhage and stomach cancer. The prevalence of the disease depends on the ulcer. Gastric ulcers affect those aged 50–70 years. Duodenal ulcers affect those aged from 20–50 years. Women and men are equally affected. Stress ulcers which occur during severe illness are classified as ischaemic or Cushing ulcers.

Figure 13.16 shows the common sites for peptic ulcers.

Risk factors

The following are risk factors for the development of peptic ulcer disease:

- Infection from *Helicobacter pylori* (a gram-negative bacterium)
- Chronic use of non-steroidal anti-inflammatory drugs (NSAIDs) and aspirin derivatives

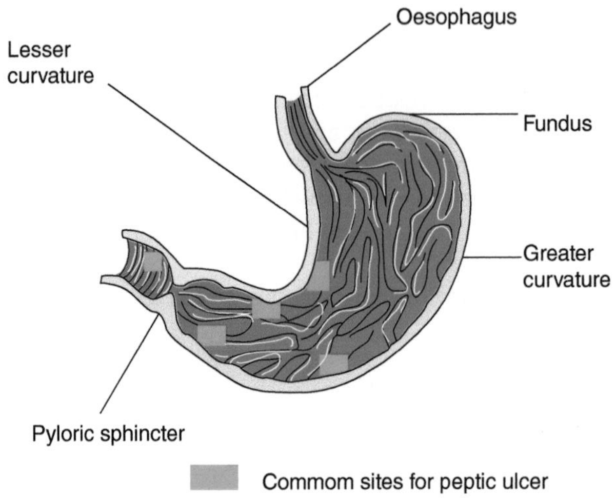

Figure 13.16   Common sites for peptic ulcer (*Source:* Adapted from LeMone *et al.*, 2011).

- Excessive consumption of alcohol
- Cigarette smoking
- Acute pancreatitis
- Cirrhosis
- Chronic obstructive pulmonary disease
- Psychological stress
- Obesity
- Excessive consumption of caffeine
- Genetic predisposition to peptic ulcer disease

Pathophysiology

Mucus lines the digestive tract and acts as a barrier against the acidic gastric secretions. Too little mucus production coupled with too much acid production and exposure to digestive enzymes will leave the digestive tract vulnerable to acid erosion and ulceration. In the duodenum, acid and pepsin (protein-digesting enzyme) breach the mucosal barrier, and this leads to erosions and ulceration. In the stomach, the permeability of the mucosal barrier changes, allowing the mucosa to be more permeable to hydrogen ions. Gastric ulcers form following a period of gastritis. The gastritis prevents the mucosa forming the required protective layer and leaves the mucosa vulnerable. Erosion of the mucosal lining may result in the formation of a fistula. The fistula allows the acidic gastric contents to leak out into the peritoneum, resulting in peritonitis. Stress, caffeine, cigarette smoking and alcohol consumption increase acid production. Medications such as NSAIDs and aspirin inhibit prostaglandins, which protect the mucosal lining (Huether *et al.*, 2019).

H. pylori bacterial infection leads to the destruction of the mucosal epithelial cells of the stomach and duodenum. The bacteria release toxins and enzymes that reduce the efficiency of mucus in protecting the mucosal lining of the gastrointestinal tract. In response to the bacterial infection, the body initiates an inflammatory response, which results in further destruction of the mucosal lining and ulceration.

Stress ulcers can occur in multiple sites in the duodenum and stomach and are associated with physiological stress. Ischaemic ulcers occur following severe burns, multiple trauma, sepsis or heart failure. Cushing ulcers are associated with raised intracranial pressure following brain trauma or surgery. Raised intracranial pressure stimulates the vagus nerve, which leads to increased secretion of gastric acid and a reduction in the blood flow to the mucosa.

Investigations

As well as taking a full health history, the following investigations may be carried out to confirm diagnosis:

- Gastroscopy and biopsy of stomach lining to detect changes as a result of *H. pylori* infection.
- Barium swallow may be performed to detect ulcer formation. This involves swallowing a drink containing barium, which is radio-opaque. The barium coats the lining of the stomach and the duodenum and, if an ulcer is present, this is detected on the X-ray.
- Full blood analysis.

Signs and symptoms

Some patients with peptic ulcer have no symptoms. However, the following symptoms have been reported in patients with peptic ulcer disease:

- Dyspepsia
- Epigastric pain
- Heart burn as a result of the regurgitation of gastric secretion
- Nausea and vomiting
- Haematemesis blood may be present in the vomit if the ulcer bleeds
- Melaena (blood in the stool)
- Loss of weight
- Eructation (belching)

Complications of peptic ulcer disease

- Bleeding – often seen in deeper ulcers and can present as anaemia
- Perforation – can occur as the ulcer erodes through the layers of the gastrointestinal tract and can lead to peritonitis
- Obstruction – can occur due to inflammation and scarring obstructing the lumen of the gastrointestinal tract.

Clinical investigation

Endoscopy is a procedure used to examine an internal organ, structure or tissue. An endoscope is a narrow, long tube with a light and a camera. There are different types of endoscope for different procedures. Gastroscopy is the examination of the oesophagus, stomach and duodenum using an endoscope.

Gastroscopy can be used to diagnose conditions of the upper digestive tract. It can be used to provide treatment, for example, treating small cancerous growths or polyps; for the management of bleeding and for taking biopsies.

Gastroscopy is usually carried out in an outpatient department. Patients are asked to fast before the procedure (6–8 hours for food and 2–3 hours for fluid). The procedure should be explained to the patient and consent gained. Patients are asked to lie on their left-hand side, a local anaesthetic spray is used on the back of the throat and patients are offered some seda-tion. Patients can expect to be awake but drowsy during the procedure.

The endoscope is inserted into the oral cavity, and the patient is asked to swallow to ease the passage of the endoscope through the digestive tract. The images are transmitted to a monitor where the doctor can see and diagnose conditions. Air may be blown into the stomach to enhance the view for the doctor. Small biopsies of tissue can be taken for further laboratory analysis to aid diagnosis.

A diagnostic gastroscopy should last for approximately 15 minutes. If sedation has been admin-istered, recovery may take longer, and a relative or friend is required to escort the patient home.

Gastroscopy is a procedure that is associated with few complications. The complications are associated with the administration of sedation, bleeding or perforation of the GI tract. If treatment is administered during the procedure, this will increase the chance of complications occurring.

Care and management

Once a peptic ulcer has been diagnosed, the healthcare professional should help the person identify any lifestyle factors that may be associated with peptic ulcer disease. Once identi-fied, the person and healthcare professional can discuss ways of reducing the risks. Referral to counselling services, smoking cessation, weight loss group and alcohol awareness may be of benefit.

Dietary advice should be offered to the person. Small regular meals are encouraged – approximately five small meals per day to prevent hunger pain. Spicy food should be avoided as it may irritate the mucosal membrane of the stomach, resulting in inflammation and epi-gastric pain.

Medications such as aspirin and NSAIDs should be avoided, as these drugs may inhibit the action of prostaglandins and may lead to gastrointestinal bleeding.

Complications associated with peptic ulcer disease may require more invasive manage-ment to stop bleeding, treat peritonitis and repair damaged tissue.

Pharmacological interventions

The patient with a peptic ulcer may be prescribed the following medications:

- Antibiotics to treat the *H. pylori* infection
- H$_2$ antagonists inhibit the secretion of acid
- Proton pump inhibitors lead to a reduction in acid production
- Ulcer coating medications prevent the ulcer developing and allow for healing to occur
- Anticholinergic medications to suppress gastric motility.

Snapshot   Acid reflux

Ebele Kanu has been working at the London stock exchange for several years. Four years ago, he was promoted to a very high-powered role with the company he works for. One year later he was diagnosed with depression and has been taking fluoxetine, but he is also increasingly dependent on alcohol with no alcohol-free days in the week. Part of his role involves wining and dining impor-tant clients, and he eats out five days per week. He smokes 20 cigarettes a day. He recently cele-brated his 30th birthday by taking some friends to Ibiza for a week of partying. His lifestyle is now affecting his health. Mr Kanu has gained weight, and his current BMI category is obese. Work has been very stressful of late, and Mr Kanu thought he would benefit from the break. However, on his return, he has severe abdominal pain. He self-refers to the Emergency Department. Mr Kanu describes the pain as burning and gnawing. He tells the doctor he has been having heartburn at night in bed, which is only resolved by taking over-the-counter heartburn remedies and by lying on his left side when in bed to prevent acid reflux. He has also noted a lot more belching of late. This pain is more severe than any he has had before. The doctor suspects that Mr Kanu has peptic ulcer disease. Mr Kanu is assessed and has some blood tests which reveal the following.

Vital signs Gastro-oesophageal reflux disease (GORD)

Vital sign	Observation	Normal
Respiration	16 breaths per minute	12–20 breaths per minute
O_2 saturation (Scale 1)	98% (on room air)	94-98%
Blood pressure	145/76 mmHg	100–139 mmHg (systolic) range
Pulse	102 beats per minute	60–100 beats per minute
Consciousness	Alert	Alert on ACVPU
Temperature	36.8°C	36–37.9°C range

Full blood count and urea and electrolytes

Test	Result	Guideline normal values
White blood cells (WBC)	10×10^9/L	4 to 11×10^9/L
Neutrophils	6.5×10^9/L	2.0 to 7.5×10^9/L
Lymphocytes	3.2×10^9/L	1.3 to 4.0×10^9/L
Red blood cells (RBC)	54.5×10^{12}/L	4.5 to 6.5×10^{12}/L
Haemoglobin (Hb)	128 g/L	130–180 g/L
Platelets	165×10^9/L	150 to 440×10^9/L
C-reactive protein	4.0 mg/L	<5 mg/L
Urea	4.0 mmol/L	2–6.6 mmol/L
Potassium	5.4 mmol/L	3.4–5.6 mmol/L
Sodium	136 mmol/L	135–147 mmol/L

Take some time to reflect on this case and then consider the following:

1. What medication might Mr Kanu be prescribed to treat the acid reflux?
2. Mr Kanu's doctor is concerned that the haemoglobin level is in the lower range of the normal values. What are the signs and symptoms of anaemia that the nurse should look out for?
3. Using your knowledge of the anatomy and physiology of the digestive system, explain why gastric ulcers occur.
4. What lifestyle advice would you offer to Mr Kanu to prevent a recurrence of this condition?
5. Calculate the NEWS2 score, and discuss its implications.
6. Discuss the importance of Mr Kanu's vital signs in relation to haemorrhage as a complication of peptic ulcer disease.
7. The doctor arranges for Mr Kanu to have an endoscopy. What explanation would you give Mr Kanu about what to expect during this procedure?

Chart 1: The NEWS scoring system

Physiological parameter	Score 3	2	1	0	1	2	3
Respiration rate (per minute)	≤8		9–11	12–20		21–24	≥25
SpO$_2$ Scale 1 (%)	≤91	92–93	94–95	≥96			
SpO$_2$ Scale 2 (%)	≤83	84–85	86–87	88–92 ≥93 on air	93–94 on oxygen	95–96 on oxygen	≥97 on oxygen
Air or oxygen?		Oxygen		Air			
Systolic blood pressure (mmHg)	≤90	91–100	101–110	111–219			≥220
Pulse (per minute)	≤40		41–50	51–90	91–110	111–130	≥131
Consciousness				Alert			CVPU
Temperature (°C)	≤35.0		35.1–36.0	36.1–38.0	38.1–39.0	≥39.1	

National Early Warning Score (NEWS) 2: Standardising the assessment of acute-illness severity in the NHS. Updated report of a working party. London: RCP, 2017.

Red flag

Management of obesity

Obesity is often associated with peptic ulcer disease. Obesity can lead to the development of severe or chronic medical conditions. People living with obesity are referred or encouraged to participate in lifestyle weight management programmes. Targets for weight loss can be set, and the first target is often to lose 10% of their current weight. Health benefits include reduction in blood pressure or the prevention of the development of type 2 diabetes mellitus. Additional support may be required to maintain the weight target and the lifestyle change (National Institute for Health and Care Excellence, 2014).

Medicines Management

Proton pump inhibitors (PPIs) reduce the amount of acid in the stomach. Parietal cells produce the acid, and the PPIs block the final step in the production of acid. It does this by the selective inhibition of the H+/K+ ATPase enzyme system responsible for the production of acid. Omeprazole is a PPI that can be prescribed to treat duodenal ulcer. The usual prescribed dose is 20 mg once per day orally. The common side effects associated with omeprazole include the following:

- Abdominal pain
- Constipation

- Diarrhoea
- GI disorders
- Nausea
- Vomiting
- Dizziness
- Headache
- Insomnia
- Skin reactions

Inflammatory bowel disease

Inflammatory bowel disease includes ulcerative colitis and Crohn's disease. Both disorders are characterised by periods of remission and relapse. The aetiology of the conditions is not clear; however, a genetic predisposition, environmental factors and an excessive immune response to gut microflora are thought to contribute to the development of the disorders.

383

Ulcerative colitis

Ulcerative colitis is the chronic inflammation of the mucous membrane of the colon and the rectum. The lining becomes inflamed and ulcerated. Some possible causes of ulcerative colitis include factors such as poor nutrition, stress, bowel infections, genetic factors and auto-immune dysfunction.

Pathophysiology

The inflammatory process occurs in the mucosa and the submucosa of the rectum (proctitis) and spreads along the colon. The inflammation may involve the entire colon up to the junction of the ileocaecal valve. Unlike the lesions in Crohn's disease, the lesions in ulcerative colitis are continuous. The lesions in ulcerative colitis tend to affect the mucosal layer and are not usually transmural as they may be in Crohn's disease.

Inflammation begins in the crypts of Lieberkühn; this leads to the activation of cytokines and macrophages. The epithelial mucosal layer becomes damaged.

The inflammation may be mild, moderate or severe (National Institute for Health and Care Excellence, 2019a).

During mild inflammation, the mucosa may appear hyperaemic and oedematous. The number of stools is usually less than four per day, and there is little evidence of blood in the stool.

During severe inflammation, mucosal destruction leads to swelling, oedema and bleeding, and as the disease progresses, ulceration develops. Mucosal destruction causes an increase in the urge to defecate, with patients having to go to the toilet over six times per day during a period of exacerbation. There will be blood in the stool. This can lead to iron deficiency anaemia. The ulceration spreads through the submucosa, causing necrosis and sloughing of the mucous membrane. In the later stages of the disease, the walls of the colon thicken and become fibrous. This leads to a narrowing of the lumen of the large intestine, which can lead to intestinal obstruction. Loss of normal large intestine function can lead to complications such as dehydration and electrolyte imbalance. Abdominal cramping and pain are associated with these attacks.

Toxic megacolon is a complication of severe inflammation which leads to dilation of the colon (Hubert and Van Meter, 2018)

Long-term complications of ulcerative colitis include an increased risk of developing bowel cancer.

Signs and symptoms

The signs and symptoms will vary depending on the severity of the disease.
In mild disease the symptoms may be minimal.
In severe disease:

- Diarrhoea
- Blood in the stool
- Pus or mucus in the diarrhoea
- Fever
- Anaemia
- Dehydration
- Weight loss
- Poor appetite
- Abdominal pain
- Nausea and vomiting.

384 Crohn's disease

Unlike ulcerative colitis, Crohn's disease can affect the gastrointestinal tract anywhere from the mouth to the anus. The most commonly affected area is the terminal ileum and the ascending colon.

Pathophysiology

In Crohn's disease, the inflammation begins in the submucosa and may extend into the mucosa and serosa. The lesions are not continuous but appear as skip lesions surrounded by normal tissue. The granulomatous lesions have a distinctive cobblestone appearance (Huether *et al.*, 2019). Oedema and continued inflammation can lead to fibrosis, the lumen of the digestive tract may be narrower than usual, and strictures can form. Inflammation can affect transit time through the digestive tract by decreasing it. This, as well as the reduction is surface area available for absorption can lead to symptoms such as weight loss, malnutrition, electrolyte imbalance, vitamin and mineral deficiencies and hypoalbuminaemia.

Anal fissures, anal abscess and fistula between the intestine and the bladder, the intestine and the anus or two loops of intestine may occur.

Complications of Crohn's disease include obstruction.

Signs and symptoms

- Abdominal pain
- Diarrhoea or soft stools
- Anorexia
- Weight loss
- Loss of appetite
- Fatigue
- Anaemia

Investigations for inflammatory bowel disease

The following investigations may be performed to confirm diagnosis:

- Sigmoidoscopy or colonoscopy to examine the mucous membrane of the colon and the rectum. The procedure involves passing a flexible scope via the rectum to examine the lining of the colon.
- A barium enema to identify bowel strictures or ulcerations.
- Stool cultures to rule out any infection.

- Full blood count to exclude anaemia and other complications from ulcerative colitis – a raised white blood cell count indicates infection.
- Plain abdominal X-ray.
- Ultrasound to identify ulcerations.

Clinical Investigation

Calprotectin is a protein released by neutrophils. During inflammation of the gastrointestinal tract, there will be increased neutrophil activity, which increases the amount of calprotectin in the stool. The test is useful in both the diagnosis of inflammatory bowel disease and in the detection of any exacerbation of the condition. The test can help distinguish between non-inflammatory bowel conditions such as irritable bowel disease and inflammatory bowel disease, for example, Crohn's disease (National Institute for Health and Care Excellence, 2013).

Care and management

Orange flag

Psychological support

A diagnosis of inflammatory bowel disease has life-changing implications for people living with this long-term condition. The impact of living with the signs and symptoms such as fatigue and/or frequent visits to the toilet can change future plans and affect lifestyle. Medication effects and side effects can affect mood. There can be issues with intimacy and change of body image following surgery. Debilitating disease can lead to isolation. All of these factors contribute to the development of anxiety and depression. Psychological support is therefore an important part of the care and management of inflammatory bowel disease.

During acute exacerbation

Patient assessment, including vital signs and blood tests, will assist in monitoring the progress of the person living with inflammatory bowel disease during the acute exacerbation.

Dehydration and electrolyte imbalance as a result of the diarrhoea, loss of appetite and poor absorption can occur. It is important to manage fluid intake and output. Administration of intravenous fluid, enteral nutrition or parenteral nutrition may be required to maintain fluid and electrolyte balance.

Anaemia should be treated.

Analgesia and antispasmodic medication should be prescribed for pain management.

A stool chart is a useful indicator of the progression of the illness and success of any treatment.

Dietary intake should be monitored due to the risk of malnutrition.

Perianal skin care should be maintained to prevent skin breakdown due to frequent diarrhoea.

Pharmacological intervention

The following medications may be prescribed in the treatment of inflammatory bowel disease.

- Aminosalicylates (5-ASAs)
- Corticosteroids
- Immunosuppressants
- Biological drugs such as infliximab

These medicines act in a variety of ways to reduce inflammation Where infection is suspected:

- Antibiotics

Other medications that may be required include:

- Antidiarrhoeals
- Antispasmodics
- Analgesia

Medicines management

Infliximab is a biological agent prescribed to treat severe inflammatory bowel disease. In Crohn's disease, it would be prescribed if the disease has not responded to immunosuppressive or corticosteroid treatment or where there is intolerance or contraindications to this treatment (National Institute for Health and Care Excellence, 2019b). In ulcerative colitis, infliximab is only prescribed where there is severely active disease and where ciclosporin is contraindicated (National Institute for Health and Care Excellence, 2015). Tumour necrosis factor – alpha (TNF-α) is a proinflammatory cytokine. Infliximab binds to TNF-α and reduces inflammation. Because the immune response is suppressed, the risk of infection increases, and therefore careful discussion with the patient and consultations must occur before this medication can be prescribed.

Infliximab is given by intravenous infusion. Careful monitoring for allergy is a requirement while the patient is receiving the infusion. Monitoring for the presence of infection before during and for 6 months after administration is essential. People receiving this treatment must carry a hypersensitivity alert card.

Surgical intervention

Ulcerative colitis

In individuals in whom there are few periods of remission, a lack of response to therapy, limited lifestyle, risk of perforation or obstruction, or precancerous changes, then surgical intervention may be required. The surgery will involve the removal of the large intestine and rectum, and the formation of an ileostomy or ileo-anal pouch.

Crohn's disease

Resection of the affected area of intestine may be considered as a form of treatment; however, the benefits and risks, including the risk of a re-occurrence, would have to be discussed in detail. Strictures may be managed with balloon dilation (National Institute for Health and Care Excellence, 2019b).

Snapshot   Ulcerative colitis

Mrs Fiona Brown is a 30-year-old computer analyst. She works part time. She has been married to her husband Ed for 3 years. They have no children but would like to have a family some day. They live close to both sets of parents and siblings.

Mrs Brown was diagnosed with ulcerative colitis when she was 19 years old and has had symptoms and treatment on and off since then. She has been admitted to the surgical ward as her ulcerative colitis has been unremitting for several months now.

Her symptoms include:

- Weight loss of 10 kg in the past 4 months (anorexia)
- Tiredness and lethargy – Mrs Brown has been unable to go to work
- Dry skin and mouth
- Frequent diarrhoea (up to eight visits to the toilet per day)
- Bloody stools (melaena)
- Nausea and vomiting
- Concentrated urine
- Crampy abdominal pain
- Abdominal distension.

Following a consultation with the colorectal surgeon, Mrs Brown has consented to a total colectomy. The doctors are confident that with Mrs Brown's optimistic approach and concordance with prescribed therapy and lifestyle advice, she is a good candidate for the formation if an ileo-anal pouch procedure. This procedure is completed in stages.

On admission to the ward, Mrs Browns observations are recorded as follows:

Vital sign	Observation	Normal
Temperature	38.2°C	36–37.9°C range
Pulse	108 beats per minute	60–100 beats per minute
Respiration	22 breaths per minute	12–20 breaths per minute
Blood pressure	90 mmHg	100–139mmHg (systolic) range
O_2 saturation	95%	94–98%

A full blood count was ordered, and the results return as follows:

Test	Result	Guideline normal values
White blood cells (WBC)	12×10^9/L	4 to 11×10^9/L
Neutrophils	8×10^9/L	2.0 to 7.5×10^9/L
Lymphocytes	3.2×10^9/L	1.3 to 4.0×10^9/L
Red blood cells (RBC)	4.7×10^9/L	4.5 to 6.5×10^9/L
Haemoglobin (Hb)	80 g/L	130–180 g/L
Platelets	160×10^9/l	150 to 440×10^9/l

Take some time to reflect on this case and then consider the following:

1. Discuss how the pathophysiology of ulcerative colitis leads to the signs and symptoms Mrs Brown is experiencing.
2. Calculate the NEWS2 and action required based on the score.
3. Following surgery Mrs Brown returns to the ward. List the postoperative complications that should be watched out for.
4. In relation to the pathophysiology of ulcerative colitis, explain why Mrs Brown's haemoglobin is low.
5. A blood transfusion is prescribed. What checks must be completed before and during the administration of a blood transfusion?
6. Mrs Brown would like to start a family but is worried about the effect of pregnancy on the ileo-anal pouch. What advice would you give Mrs Brown?

Chart 1: The NEWS scoring system

Physiological parameter	Score						
	3	2	1	0	1	2	3
Respiration rate (per minute)	≤8		9–11	12–20		21–24	≥25
SpO₂ Scale 1 (%)	≤91	92–93	94–95	≥96			
SpO₂ Scale 2 (%)	≤83	84–85	86–87	88–92 ≥93 on air	93–94 on oxygen	95–96 on oxygen	≥97 on oxygen
Air or oxygen?		Oxygen		Air			
Systolic blood pressure (mmHg)	≤90	91–100	101–110	111–219			≥220
Pulse (per minute)	≤40		41–50	51–90	91–110	111–130	≥131
Consciousness				Alert			CVPU
Temperature (°C)	≤35.0		35.1–36.0	36.1–38.0	38.1–39.0	≥39.1	

National Early Warning Score (NEWS) 2: Standardising the assessment of acute-illness severity in the NHS. Updated report of a working party. London: RCP, 2017.

Pancreatitis

The pancreas is an accessory organ of the digestive system. Pancreatitis can be acute or chronic. There are many risk factors associated with obstructive biliary tract disease, such as alcoholism, peptic ulcer disease, trauma affecting the abdomen, hyperlipidaemia, some medications and genetic factors. Pancreatitis affects those aged 50–60 years old.

Acute Pancreatitis

Pathophysiology

The pancreas produces pancreatic amylase, lipase and the inactive protein-digesting enzyme precursors, trypsinogen and chymotrypsinogen, which are activated when they reach the small intestine (Marieb and Kellar, 2018). The enzymes reach the small intestine via the pancreatic duct. If there is an obstruction in the bile duct or the pancreatic duct, the enzymes are backed up in the pancreas and become activated. Proteolysis and lipolysis of the cells of the pancreas occurs. Alcohol causes protein plugs to form within the pancreatic ducts. The protein plugs are responsible for obstruction. Gall stones (cholelithiasis) can also lead to obstruction. This process of autodigestion leads to an inflammation. The pancreas becomes oedematous, and pseudocysts containing pancreatic enzymes form. Ischaemia and necrosis may occur. The systemic effects of severe acute pancreatitis can lead to systemic inflammatory response syndrome (SIRS).

If pancreatitis progresses, fibrosis and strictures develop within the pancreas, and duct obstruction continues. This leads to chronic pancreatitis.

Signs and symptoms

- Epigastric or mid abdominal pain that radiate into the back is caused by the presence of oedema in the pancreas.
- Pyrexia is part of the inflammatory response.
- Nausea and vomiting occur due to the presence of paralytic ileus and hypermobility within the digestive tract.
- Abdominal distension due to paralytic ileus and/or the hypermobility of the digestive tract.
- Vital signs in severe acute pancreatitis.
  - Tachypnoea
  - Hypoxaemia
  - Tachycardia
  - Hypotension due to hypovolaemia
  - Renal impairment due to reduced renal blood flow
- Abnormal blood sugar levels as the endocrine function of the pancreas can also be disrupted
- Malabsorption and malnutrition

389

Care and management

Analgesia is required to treat the abdominal pain. Fluid management is required to prevent hypotension and shock. Dietician assessment and enteral nutrition may be required to manage the risk of malabsorption and malnutrition.

Red flag

Severe acute pancreatitis is associated with some serious complications including pseudocysts. Pseudocysts are contained collections of pancreatic enzymes. They can lead to pain, bloating and indigestion. Pseudocysts may need to be surgically drained.

Snapshot   Gallstones

Joseph is 27 years old and has Down syndrome. He has been off-colour and complaining of abdominal pain that is now severe. Two weeks ago, Joseph was diagnosed with gallstones and was waiting for an appointment to have the stones removed. Gallstones are common in people who have Down syndrome due to bile stasis within the bile duct allowing the formation of the stones (Down Syndrome Association, 2018). Joseph's carer has taken him to the GP. The GP suspects that Joseph may have pancreatitis. Joseph will not allow the GP to undertake any physical assessment. The GP is concerned at the amount of pain that Joseph is in and refers to Joseph to the Emergency Department for further investigations and analgesia. The doctor suspects that Joseph has acute pancreatitis.

On admission vital signs and blood tests reveal the following:

Vital sign	Observation	Normal
Temperature	38.2°C	36–37.9°C range
Pulse	112 beats per minute	60–100 beats per minute
Respiration	22 breaths per minute	12–20 breaths per minute
Blood pressure	160 mmHg	100–139 mmHg (systolic) range
O$_2$ saturation	95%	94–98%

A full blood count was ordered, and the results return as follows:

Test	Result	Guideline normal values
White blood cells (WBC)	14×10^9/L	4 to 11×10^9/L
Neutrophils	9×10^9/L	2.0 to 7.5×10^9/L
Lymphocytes	3.6×10^9/L	1.3 to 4.0×10^9/L
Red blood cells (RBC)	4.5×10^9/L	4.5 to 6.5×10^9/L
Haemoglobin (Hb)	135 g/L	130–180 g/L
Platelets	210×10^9/l	150 to 440×10^9/l

Take some time to reflect on this case and then consider the following:

1. Discuss how the cholelithiasis can lead to the development of pancreatitis.
2. Calculate the NEWS2 and action required based on the score.
3. The doctor orders some investigations to assist with the diagnosis. Which two tests should he order and why?
4. Joseph is prescribed codeine phosphate 60 mg intramuscularly for his pain. Discuss the mode of action, choice of route and side effects associated with this medication.
5. An endoscopic retrograde cholangiopancreatography (ERCP) is organised to remove the gallstones. How would you prepare Joseph for this procedure?

Chart 1: The NEWS scoring system

Physiological parameter	Score 3	2	1	0	1	2	3
Respiration rate (per minute)	≤8		9–11	12–20		21–24	≥25
SpO$_2$ Scale 1 (%)	≤91	92–93	94–95	≥96			
SpO$_2$ Scale 2 (%)	≤83	84–85	86–87	88–92 ≥93 on air	93–94 on oxygen	95–96 on oxygen	≥97 on oxygen
Alr or oxygen?		Oxygen		Air			
Systolic blood pressure (mmHg)	≤90	91–100	101–110	111–219			≥220
Pulse (per minute)	≤40		41–50	51–90	91–110	111–130	≥131
Consciousness				Alert			CVPU
Temperature (°C)	≤35.0		35.1–36.0	36.1–38.0	38.1–39.0	≥39.1	

National Early Warning Score (NEWS) 2: Standardising the assessment of acute-illness severity in the NHS. Updated report of a working party. London: RCP, 2017.

Chronic pancreatitis

Chronic pancreatitis occurs secondary to chronic alcohol misuse in the majority of cases; however, it is also associated with smoking, genetic factors, metabolic conditions, pancreatic abnormalities (structural or anatomical) or autoimmune disorders (NICE 2018).

Pathophysiology

Chronic inflammation of the pancreas leads to fibrosis and strictures forming. The islets of Langerhans are destroyed.

Signs and symptoms

- Pain
- Weight loss due to malabsorption
- Steatorrhoea as a result of fat malabsorption
- Diabetes mellitus

Care and management

Lifestyle changes are required to prevent progression of the disease and referral to services to help stop chronic alcohol use. If smoking is a factor, then referral to a smoking cessation service will be required. Dietary advice from a dietician will be needed to manage weight loss and malabsorption. Pancreatic enzyme replacement therapy may be required to prevent malabsorption. A diabetes specialist referral should be made for the management of diabetes mellitus to prevent development of the complications associated with diabetes.

Medicines management

Pancreatic enzyme replacement therapy (PERT) is used to treat pancreatic enzyme insufficiency (PEI). PEI can occur in any condition where the pancreas has been damaged or diseased, for example, chronic pancreatitis. The pancreatic enzymes are responsible for the digestion of fat, protein and carbohydrate. A lack of pancreatic enzymes leads to malabsorption and maldigestion. Pancreatin contains the three digestive enzymes required for the digestion of fat, protein and carbohydrate: lipase, protease and amylase. Pancreatin should be taken with food, and the lowest dose possible should be used to manage the symptoms.

Orange flag

Pancreatitis is a long-term condition. Naylor *et al.* (2016) discuss the lack of integration in managing the psychological effects of long-term illness. Reported issues include reduced life expectancy, poor management of symptoms and lack of support. In order to provide a holistic person-centred approach to care, the psychological impact of chronic pancreatitis should be assessed, and a multidisciplinary approach to minimising the negative effects of this should be implemented.

Conclusion

The gastrointestinal tract, also referred to as the digestive system, provides water, nutrients and electrolytes for bodily functions. Nutrients are extracted from food and transported throughout the body for cellular function. Not only are eating and drinking essential for life and for healing, they are also social activities that contribute to mental and social well-being. Disorders of the digestive tract can therefore have not only a physical impact on people but a psychological impact as well.

This chapter has provided the reader with insight into the normal anatomy and physiology of the gastrointestinal tract and some of the disorders associated with the system. It is not the remit of this chapter to discuss all the related disorders; the reader is advised to read further.

All healthcare professionals work as members of a team assisting or giving advice to patients with gastrointestinal problems. These problems can affect the patient both physically and psychologically and thus may affect the patient's ability to perform the activities of daily living.

Activities

Here are some activities and exercises to help test your learning. For the answers to these exercises, as well as further self-testing activities, visit our website at **www.wiley.com/go/fundamentalsofappliedpathophysiology/student4e**

Multiple choice questions

1. The gastrointestinal system is:
   (a) The body's system of nerves
   (b) The body's food processing system
   (c) The body's lymphatic system
   (d) The body's eliminatory system
2. Where does food pass through between the mouth and the stomach:
   (a) The oesophagus
   (b) The trachea
   (c) The windpipe
   (d) The intestines
3. Which of the following does NOT manufacture digestive juices?
   (a) The liver
   (b) The stomach
   (c) The kidneys
   (d) The pancreas
4. What is the most common type of motility associated with the passage of food from the mouth to the stomach?
   (a) Propulsion
   (b) Segmentation
   (c) Flatus
   (d) Peristalsis

5. Most of the water and electrolytes absorbed across the walls of the gastrointestinal tract is absorbed in this region:
   (a) Mouth
   (b) Stomach
   (c) Small intestine
   (d) Large intestine
6. Which of these best maintains intestinal health?
   (a) Vitamins
   (b) Fibre
   (c) Caffeine
   (d) Fat
7. Which of these can cause heartburn?
   (a) Being overweight
   (b) Lying down soon after eating a large meal
   (c) Drinking excessive alcohol
   (d) All of the above
8. All of the following are substances found in pancreatic juice except
   (a) Trypsin
   (b) Pepsin
   (c) Amylase
   (d) Lipase

9. Bile is produced in the:
   (a) Spleen
   (b) Liver
   (c) Gall bladder
   (d) Stomach
10. The first portion of the large intestine is the
    (a) Jejunum
    (b) Caecum
    (c) Rectum
    (d) Colon
11. Proteins are primarily digested to and absorbed as:
    (a) Amino acids
    (b) Insulin
    (c) Monosaccharides
    (d) Glycerol
12. Proteolysis is the breakdown of:
    (a) Carbohydrates
    (b) Proteins into smaller polypeptides or amino acids
    (c) Blood cells
    (d) None of the above
13. Sigmoidoscopy is used to examine:
    (a) The upper gastrointestinal tract
    (b) Mucous membrane of the duodenum
    (c) Mucous membrane of the rectum
    (d) The stomach
14. *Helicobacter pylori* is:
    (a) A virus
    (b) An infectious disease
    (c) A fungus
    (d) A gram-negative bacterium

15. A pancreatic pseudocyst is:
    (a) A collection of tissue and fluids that forms on the pancreas
    (b) A collection of fluid that forms on the liver
    (c) A collection of fluid that forms on the spleen
    (d) A collection of fluid in the peritoneal cavity

Conditions

Below is a list of conditions that are associated with the digestive system. Take some time and write notes about each of the conditions. You may make the notes taken from text books or other resources (e.g. people you work with in a clinical area) or you may make the notes based on people you have cared for. If you are making notes about people you have cared for, you must ensure that you adhere to the rules of confidentiality.

Hepatitis A	
Portal hypertension	
Diverticular disease	
Gastro-oesophageal reflux disease (GORD)	
Appendicitis	

Further resources

The British Liver Trust

https://britishlivertrust.org.uk/

The British Liver trust are a UK charity who support people living with liver disease and liver cancer, and their carers. They award research grants and provide a wealth of information for patients, carers and healthcare professionals.

The British Society of Gastroenterology

https://www.bsg.org.uk/

This organisation focuses on gastroenterology and hepatology and has a range of resources discussing gastrointestinal conditions and innovation.

Crohn's and Colitis UK

https://www.crohnsandcolitis.org.uk/

Crohn's and Colitis UK is a charity that provides information for patients, carers and healthcare professionals on inflammatory bowel disease. There are some useful resources specifically for healthcare professionals.

Guts UK

https://gutscharity.org.uk/

Guts UK is a charity that was set up to raise money which funds research associated with GI conditions. It also raises awareness of issues around GI health. There are a lot of useful patient resources available via Guts UK about digestive system illnesses and investigations.

The Ileostomy and Internal Pouch Support Group

https://iasupport.org/

The ileostomy and internal pouch support group is a charity set up to support people living with ileostomy or internal pouch, their families and carers. This useful site provides information for people who have had their colon removed. This support group provides a forum for those affected. You can learn more about patient experiences of pregnancy with an ileo-anal pouch.

Glossary of terms

Absorption   The taking of nutrients from the gastrointestinal tract.

Anastomosis   Surgical joining of two parts.

Angular cheilitis   Soreness and dryness in the corners of the mouth.

Barium meal   Examination of the gastrointestinal tract using a contrast medium; under X-ray control.

Bile   An alkaline fluid produced by the liver that aids digestion of lipids.

Calprotectin   A protein released by neutrophils as part of the inflammatory response.

Chyme   A semisolid substance of the stomach.

Digestion   The breakdown of foodstuff.

Duct   A tube.

Dyspepsia   The feeling of epigastric discomfort.

Endocrine gland   A ductless gland that secretes hormones into the bloodstream.

Enzyme   A protein that speeds up chemical reactions.

Eructation   The act of bringing up air from the stomach.

Exocrine gland   A gland that secretes hormones into ducts that carry the secretions to other sites (e.g. the intestine).

Fibrous   Containing regenerated or scar tissue.

Fistula   An abnormal passage from an internal organ to the surface of the skin or between two organs.

Fundus   The upper portion of the stomach.

Gastroscopy   Examination of the gastrointestinal tract using a flexible gastroscope.

Glycogen   A carbohydrate (complex sugar) made from glucose. Excess glucose is stored as glycogen in the liver.

Inflammatory bowel disease   A term used to describe a disorder that involves inflammation within the digestive tract.

Intestine   The small and large bowel.

Large intestine   The colon; large bowel.

Mastication   Chewing, tearing and grinding of food.

Oesophagus   The gullet; food pipe.

Oliguria   Deficient secretion of urine; less than 30 mL per hour.

Oral cavity   The mouth.

Palate   The roof of the mouth.

Pancreatitis   Inflammation of the pancreas that can be acute or chronic.

Paralytic ileus   The absence of peristaltic movement.

Parenteral nutrition   The administration of nutrients other than via the gastrointestinal tract (e.g. intravenously).

Peristalsis   The involuntary movement of the gastrointestinal tract. A wave-like contraction.

Peritoneum   The serous membrane that covers the abdominal cavity.

Pharynx   The throat.

Proctitis   Inflammation of the rectum.

Prostaglandin   Complex unsaturated fatty acid produced by the mast cells and acting as a messenger substance between cells. Intensifies the actions of histamine and kinins. They cause increased vascular permeability, neutrophil chemotaxis, stimulation of smooth muscle (e.g. the uterus) and can induce pain.

Ptyalin   A digestive enzyme; also known as salivary amylase.

Pyloric region   Funnel-shaped portion of the stomach.

Small intestine   The small bowel.

Stomach   The organ that receives food from the oesophagus.

References

Down Syndrome Association (2018). *Gastrointestinal Conditions in Adults*. Middlesex: Down Syndrome Association.

Hubert, R.J. and VanMeter, K.C. (2018). *Gould's Pathophysiology for Health Professionals*, 6th edn. St Louis: Elsevier.

Huether, S.E., McCance, K.L. and Brashers, V.L. (2019). *Understanding Pathophysiology*, 7th edn. St Louis: Elsevier.

LeMone, P., Burke, K. and Bauldoff, G. (2011). *Medical-Surgical Nursing. Critical Thinking in Patient Care*. London: Pearson.

Longenbaker, S.N. (2013). *Mader's Understanding Human Anatomy and Physiology*, 8th edn. London: McGraw Hill.

Marieb, E.N. and Kellar, S.M. (2018). Essentials of Human Anatomy and Physiology, 12th edn. Harlow: Pearson.

National Institute for Health and Care Excellence (2013). *Faecal Calprotectin Diagnostic Tests for Inflammatory Diseases of the Bowel*. Diagnostic guidance [DG11]. https://www.nice.org.uk/guidance/dg11 Accessed 10th June 2020.

National Institute for Health and Care Excellence (2014). *Weight Management: Lifestyle services for Overweight or Obese Adults. Public Health Guideline [PH53]*. London: NICE.

National Institute for Health and Care Excellence (2015). *Infliximab, Adalimumab and Golimumab for Treating Moderately to Severely Active Ulcerative Colitis after the Failure of Conventional Therapy. Technology Appraisal Guidance [TA329]*. https://www.nice.org.uk/guidance/ta329/chapter/1-Guidance Accessed 10th June 2020.

National Institute for Health and Care Excellence (2018). *Pancreatitis. NICE guideline [NG104]*. https://www.nice.org.uk/guidance/ng104 Accessed 10th June 2020.

National Institute for Health and Care Excellence (2019a). *Ulcerative Colitis: Management. NICE guideline [NG130]*. https://www.nice.org.uk/guidance/ng130 Accessed 10th June 2020.

National Institute for Health and Care Excellence (2019b). *Crohn's Disease: Management NICE Guideline [NG129]*.https://www.nice.org.uk/guidance/ng129/chapter/Recommendations#inducing-remission-in-crohns-disease Accessed 10th June 2020.

Naylor, C., Das, P., Ross, S., Honeyman, S., Thompson, J. and Gilburt, H. (2016). *Bringing Together Physical and Mental Health Needs. A New Frontier in Integrated Care*. London: The Kings Fund.

Nursing and Midwifery Council (NMC) (2018). *The Code. Professional Standards of Practice and Behaviour for Nurses, Midwives and Nursing Associates*. London: Nursing and Midwifery Council.

Royal College of Physicians (RCP) (2017). *National Early Warning Score (NEWS) 2. Standardising the Assessment of Acute-Illness Severity in the NHS*. London: RCP.

Shier, D.N, Butler, J.L. and Lewis, R. (2018). *Holes Human Anatomy and Physiology*, 15th edn. London: McGraw Hill Education.

VanPutte, G., Regan, J., Russo, A. and Seeley, R.R. (2016). *Anatomy & Physiology*, 12th edn. London: McGraw Hill.

Waugh, A. and Grant, A. (2018). *Ross and Wilson: Anatomy and Physiology in Health and Illness*, 13th edn. Edinburgh: Elsevier.

Chapter 14

Nutrition and associated disorders

Claire Leader

Senior Lecturer in Adult Nursing, Nursing, Midwifery & Health, Northumbria University, Newcastle upon Tyne, UK

Contents

Introduction 399
Macronutrients...400
Micronutrients...405
Nutritional disorders 410
Conclusion 420
Test your knowledge..420

Multiple choice questions...............................421
Conditions...422
Further resources...423
Glossary of terms...423
References...424

Key words

- Proteins
- Anabolism
- Triglycerides
- Micronutrients
- Vitamins
- Fatty acids
- Glycogen
- Carbohydrates
- Lipids
- Macronutrients

Fundamentals of Applied Pathophysiology: An Essential Guide for Nursing and Healthcare Students, Fourth Edition. Edited by Ian Peate.
© 2021 John Wiley & Sons Ltd. Published 2021 by John Wiley & Sons Ltd.
Student companion website: www.wiley.com/go/fundamentalsofappliedpathophysiology/student4e
Instructor companion website: www.wiley.com/go/fundamentalsofappliedpathophysiology/instructor4e

- What is malnourishment?
- What are micro and macronutrients?
- What is the body's main energy source?
- List the fat-soluble vitamins.

Learning outcomes

On completion of this section, the reader will be able to:

- Discuss the roles of carbohydrates, proteins and fats.

- Discuss the optimum dietary requirements for health.

- Describe the role of micro and macronutrients.

- List some of the nutritional assessment tools.

Don't forget to visit the companion website for this book
(www.wiley.com/go/fundamentalsofappliedpathophysiology/student4e)
where you can find self-assessment tests to check your progress, as well as
lots of activities to practise your learning.

Introduction

Nutrition is vital for human existence. An adequate intake of nutrients is essential for the survival of the body's systems. Nutrients such as the proteins, carbohydrates, lipids and vitamins found in foodstuff are used by the body for energy production, growth and repair. The digestive organs (see Chapter 13) play a vital role in ingestion, absorption, transportation and elimination. When individuals do not receive sufficient nutrients, their body systems do not function efficiently.

This chapter discusses the roles of micro and macronutrients, identifies the different types of food sources and nutritional requirements of the body, and outlines government recommendations with regards to nutritional intake and nutritional disorders, such as obesity and underweight. Nutritional assessment tools and their importance in clinical practice will also be explored.

Healthcare professionals play a vital role in ensuring that the nutritional needs of the patient are met. In a community setting, support will be given to patients to help them make good food choices to optimise health and to effectively manage any chronic disease. In hospital, the key responsibilities of the healthcare professional include nutritional assessment of the patient on admission; managing mealtimes, e.g. providing privacy for the patient; ensuring that they are not disturbed during mealtimes and maintaining an accurate record of the patient's nutritional intake.

Nutrition is a fundamental aspect of maintaining health and preventing disease and yet forms a very small part of educational programmes for healthcare professionals. With diet-related disease soaring and placing a significant disease burden on our society, it is absolutely essential that health professionals are educated about nutrition, not only so that patients receive as clear and consistent a message as possible about what to eat and what to avoid, but also to improve and maintain the health and well-being of the healthcare workforce. This chapter will offer some insight into this important topic.

Let food be thy medicine and medicine be thy food – Hippocrates

Macronutrients

Macronutrients are organic compounds required in relatively large quantities ('macro' means large) for normal physiological functions of the body. Macronutrients include:

- Carbohydrates
- Proteins
- Lipids

Red flag

There is a growing body of evidence indicating that a major imbalance in the relative proportions of macronutrients can increase risk of chronic disease and may adversely affect micronutrient intake.

Carbohydrates

Carbohydrates are organic compounds that contain carbon, hydrogen and oxygen molecules. They make up the body's main source of energy and are required in large quantities. Carbohydrates are found in a variety of whole foods including fruit, vegetables, whole grains (e.g. brown rice, oatmeal, quinoa, whole wheat breads and pasta), legumes (e.g. beans, peas, lentils), seeds and nuts. They are also found in foods less conducive to good health such as white flour, white rice and pasta, confectionary and a myriad of other processed foods. It is here that they gain their bad reputation for contributing to weight gain and ill health.
Carbohydrates are divided into two main groups:

1. Simple carbohydrates (sugars)
   a. Monosaccharides – e.g. glucose (found in fruit, sweet corn and honey) Fructose (fruit sugar), galactose (produced from lactose – sugar in milk),
   b. Disaccharides – e.g. sucrose (glucose and fructose), maltose (glucose) and lactose (glucose and galactose).

More recently, these sugars have been further subdivided; 'free sugars' is the term recommended to describe sugars which are not bound to the food's cellular structure. These may be naturally present, for example, in honey, syrup or unsweetened fruit juices or may be added to food by the cook, manufacturer or consumer, for example, in the form of bread, pastries, confectionary and sweetened beverages. Sugars that are bound to the cellular structure of the food, for example, whole fruits and vegetables, and the lactose contained in milk, fall outside of this definition (Scientific Advisory Committee on Nutrition, 2015, p. 182).

2. Complex carbohydrates
   a. Oligosaccharides, e.g. raffinose, stachyose, verbascose (found in beans, peas, bran and whole grains)
   b. Polysaccharides – e.g. glycogen (stored glucose), starch (e.g. potatoes, squash, rice, pasta), non-starch polysaccharides (dietary fibre).

Current UK guidelines recommend that 50% of the total calorie intake should be from carbohydrates, with no more than 5% from free sugars (BNF, 2019). A recent large-scale meta-analysis of research (Seidelmann *et al.*, 2018) has indicated a U-shaped association between carbohydrate consumption and optimal health. Diets which take less than 47% or more than 70% of calories from carbohydrates are associated with a shorter life expectancy and greater incidence of ill health, with the optimum health benefits conferred at between 50% and 55% carbohydrates. However, the upper level of carbohydrate consumption (greater than 67%) was notably predominant in Asian populations and economically deprived areas, where consumption of higher quantities of carbohydrates from non-whole food sources, e.g. white rice, white bread and other processed foods, is prevalent (Dehghan *et al.*, 2017). Evidence continues to emerge indicating that diets from predominantly whole plant food sources* (complex carbohydrates), are associated with lower rates of all-cause mortality, and this is considered to be in some part attributable to the higher consumption of dietary fibre found with whole food plant-based diets (Kim *et al.*, 2018) in addition to a wider array of micronutrient availability in diets higher in fruit, vegetable and legume intake (Miller *et al.*, 2017).

One gram of carbohydrate provides approximately 4 kcal/g of energy (British Nutrition Foundation (BNF) 2018a). Calories are units of energy found in food and drink. The body burns calories to produce energy, and any excess is stored as fat. In nutrition, values are given for the actual amount of kilocalories in food, but are commonly referred to in calories.

$$1000 \, \text{calories} = 1 \, \text{kcal}$$

Carbohydrates are broken down and converted into glucose by the digestive enzyme amylase found in the saliva and pancreas. Glucose is then oxidised to produce adenosine triphosphate (ATP), providing energy for immediate use by the cells. Glucose that is not required for immediate ATP production is then used for the formation of several amino acids, which are then incorporated into proteins. The remaining glucose may be converted to glycogen, stored in the liver and muscle cells or fat stored in adipose tissue (Tortora and Derrickson, 2017).

The body's capacity to maintain blood glucose levels is achieved by a variety of hormones; the two key hormones are insulin and glucagon. Both these hormones are produced by the pancreas and secreted into the bloodstream. Insulin secretion is increased after a meal has been eaten, and the main function of insulin is to transport glucose into the cells to produce ATP. In the absence of a carbohydrate meal and when the level of blood glucose is low, glucagon stimulates the liver to convert stored glycogen into glucose (a process called glycolysis). Thus, the important role of these hormones is to regulate blood glucose levels. Glucose can be made available by the liver from non-carbohydrate sources, such as proteins and fats, through a process called gluconeogenesis. However, it is important to remember that the body will always demonstrate a preference for taking its energy source directly from carbohydrates converted into glucose (Tortora and Derrickson, 2017).

Glycaemic index (GI) and control

When considering food for optimum health, food structure in addition to food composition is a key component (Wahlqvist, 2016). As discussed, carbohydrates have a significant impact on blood glucose levels, but spikes in these levels depend on how complex the structure of the carbohydrate is. Foods are measured on a scale of 0–100 in relation to their GI. The higher the number, the higher the GI and the quicker and more pronounced is the glucose spike. Simple carbohydrates containing 'free sugars' are quickly absorbed and will cause a sharp rise in blood glucose levels.

---

* A whole food plant-based diet aims to maximise consumption of nutrient-dense plant foods such as fruit, vegetables, whole grains, beans and pulses, and minimise processed foods, oils, meat, fish, dairy and eggs (Tuso *et al.*, 2013).

These are referred to as high-GI foods. Complex carbohydrates take much longer to absorb and will cause a much slower and sustained rise in blood glucose; these foods are low GI.

The rate at which carbohydrates are digested is important for appetite control, for metabolism and for fat burning. Low-GI foods suppress appetite and can keep us feeling fuller for longer, ultimately reducing the amount of food consumed. High-GI foods lead to a slower resting metabolic rate, so fewer calories are burnt in the process of just existing, leading to weight gain. The regular surges in glucose stimulate insulin secretion, necessary for lowering blood glucose levels. Over time these 'spikes' and 'crashes' will take their toll, and cells become increasingly insulin resistant, leading to a gradual onset of type 2 diabetes. Thus, foods that are low GI, are generally unprocessed, whole grain foods high in fibre, and are important for weight control and managing type 2 diabetes (Waugh and Grant, 2018).

Proteins

Proteins are essential for growth and repair. They play a crucial role in virtually all biological processes in the body. All enzymes and many of the hormones are proteins and are vital for the body's function. Muscle contraction, immune protection and the transmission of nerve impulses are all dependent on proteins. Proteins found in the skin and bones provide structural support. The body uses carbohydrate and fat for energy, but when there is excess dietary protein or inadequate dietary fat and carbohydrate, protein is used to produce energy. Excess protein may also be converted to fat and stored in adipose tissue. Approximately 1 g of protein yields 4 kcal/g of energy (BNF, 2018b).

Proteins are highly complex molecules composed of amino acids. Amino acids are simple compounds containing carbon, hydrogen, oxygen, nitrogen, some sulphur and other elements such as phosphorus, iron and cobalt (Tortora and Derrickson, 2017). Amino acids are linked together by peptide bonds to produce new proteins in a process called 'protein anabolism'. There are 20 amino acids in all, and ten of these are known as 'essential amino acids'. These cannot be synthesised by the body and must be obtained from food sources. Different foods contain different proteins, each with their own unique amino acid composition.

Current UK guidance indicates that adults should consume between 10% and 15% of their total calorie intake as protein (with a maximum of 35%) (BNF, 2019). Commonly meat, fish, eggs and dairy products (milk, cheese and yoghurt) have been the major dietary sources of protein. However, with emerging evidence relating to the associations with consumption of these foods and poorer health (e.g. Song *et al.*, 2016), protein from these sources should be limited to within the recommended guideline (Public Health England (PHE), 2016). Seeking protein from a variety of plant-based sources such as quinoa, legumes, soy products, whole grains, leafy greens, etc. is increasingly being recognised as a healthful way to provide adequate amounts of essential amino acids and prevent protein deficiency (Chalvon-Demersay *et al.*, 2017; Richter *et al.*, 2015)

Lipids

Lipid is a term generally used for fat-like substances. They contain carbon, hydrogen and oxygen and make up 18–25% of body mass in lean adults.

Triglycerides are the most plentiful source of natural lipids in the body and diet, accounting for approximately 97% of lipids overall and can be found in solid or liquid form as fat and oils, respectively:

- Saturated fat – A fat that contains mostly saturated fatty acids and becomes solid at room temperature. Occurs mostly in meat (especially red meat) and dairy (milk, cheese and butter) and plant sources such as cocoa butter, coconut oil, palm oil.
- Monounsaturated fat – Oil containing triglycerides consisting mostly of monounsaturated fatty acids. Found in plant foods such as nuts, seeds, olive oil, peanut oil, avocados.

- Polyunsaturated fat – Oil containing polyunsaturated fatty acids, e.g. sunflower oil, soybean oil, oily fish such as salmon, tuna and mackerel.
- Transunsaturated fat (commonly known as trans-fat) – Containing transunsaturated fatty acids, a particular type of polyunsaturated fat that can be made more saturated under high pressure through a process known as hydrogenation, turning the fat into solid form at room temperature. This type of fat is naturally found in small amounts in the gut bacteria of some animals, milk and meat but is more abundant (and harmful) in processed and convenient foods (Baic, 2007).

Lipids are essential for:

- Lubrication of food to facilitate swallowing
- Transportation of fat-soluble vitamins, such as vitamins A, D, E and K
- Synthesis of steroid hormones, such as testosterone and oestrogen
- Transportation of lipid-soluble drugs, such as nicotine and caffeine
- Biological membranes, such as cell and organelle membranes
- Energy production.

403

The simplest lipids are fatty acids. These are used in the synthesis of triglycerides and phospholipids, the major component of the cell membrane. From a nutritional perspective, the essential fatty acids (EFAs) are the most important and, as they cannot be made by the body, they must be included in our diets. The major EFAs are omega-3 and omega-6, which have opposing effects on metabolic functions in the body. Omega-6 is associated with inflammation and platelet aggregation, both essential functions to protect the body against acute infection and injury (Saini and Keum, 2018). However, over-consumption can lead to chronic inflammation and associated diseases including heart disease and cancer (Berquin et al., 2008). Conversely, omega-3 reduces inflammation and has a protective effect against cancer and heart disease (Adkins and Kelly, 2010; Gobbo et al., 2016). Omega-3 can be found in good supply in foods such as flaxseed, walnuts, fish oils and other oils that contain poly-unsaturated fatty acids. Omega-6 is contained in most processed foods, eggs and meat.

Some digestion of fats into free fatty acids begins in the stomach with the aid of the digestive enzyme gastric lipase. The fat is mixed with other nutrients and is passed into the duodenum. Once the contents of the stomach reach the duodenum, the hormone cholecystokinin is released, which stimulates the release of bile from the gallbladder and pancreatic lipase (see Chapter 13). Fats are then further broken down and absorbed from the gastrointestinal tract.

Lipids are insoluble in water ('hydrophobic'), and so most lipids will be combined with proteins from the liver and intestine to be transported as units called lipoproteins (Figure 14.1). There are five types of lipoproteins:

1. Chylomicrons
2. Very low-density lipoproteins
3. Intermediate-density lipoproteins
4. Low-density lipoproteins – 50% cholesterol, 25% protein (often referred to as low-density lipoproteins (LDL) 'bad cholesterol')
5. High-density lipoproteins – 20% cholesterol, 40–45% protein.

Current UK guidance indicates that no more than 35% of calories should be consumed as fat, with a maximum of 11% of these from saturated and trans-fat sources due to their association with ill health (BNF, 2019). There is emerging evidence to support a decrease to the

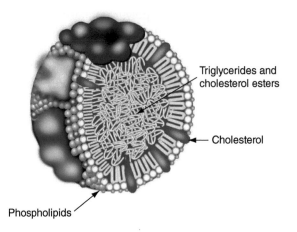

Figure 14.1 A lipoprotein.

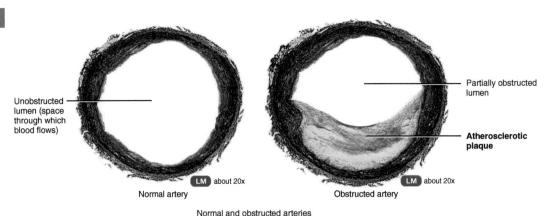

Figure 14.2 An example of plaque.

guidelines for the consumption of saturated and trans-fats further to a maximum of 6–7% of calories in the UK (in line with Japan) to reduce incidences of cardiovascular disease and all-cause mortality (NICE, 2020).

The major health issues associated with the consumption of these fats arise because of increased levels of LDLs. Normally, LDLs transport cholesterol from the liver to aid the body in repair and hormone production. However, where there is an excess, the LDLs accumulate in the artery walls where they interact with substances secreted from the endothelial and smooth muscle cells of the artery, gradually forming a 'plaque' commonly referred to as atherosclerosis, which narrows the path for the blood to flow (see Figure 14.2 for an example of atherosclerosis).

Through a complex interplay involving inflammatory processes and the formation of blood clots (Marzilli, 2012), coronary artery disease develops; the second leading cause of deaths in England and Wales (ONS, 2018). It is thought that these are the same mechanisms that also contribute to many of the other leading causes of death including Alzheimer's and dementia (Roher *et al*., 2011), cancer, stroke as well as chronic conditions such as diabetes and kidney disease, which all contribute to cardiovascular risk (NICE, 2016) and are modifiable through lifestyle changes and a balanced diet that is low in fat.

Red flag

Processed meat and cancer risk
The term 'processed' in relation to meat is defined as 'meat that has undergone treatment through salting, curing, fermentation, smoking or other processes to enhance flavour or improve preservation' (Turesky, 2018, p. 718).

While studies have shown that red and white meat contribute to all-cause mortality, the consumption of processed meat has a particular association with the development of cancer. This has been linked not only to the ingestion of fat and lipids but also cooking at high temperatures, which activates toxins such as nitrates that are present in such foods as link sausages, bacon, ham, cold cuts and hot dogs (Arash et al., 2017). These meats are now categorised along with tobacco in terms of their cancer risk (Bouvard et al., 2015) and ideally should be eliminated from our diets completely to optimise health.

Micronutrients

Micronutrients are organic compounds required in small quantities for the normal physiological functions of the body. They include chemical elements such as hydrogen, nitrogen and carbon, and minerals and vitamins, e.g. vitamins A, B group, C, D, E and K.

Vitamins

Vitamins are organic (carbon-based) substances essential for growth and cellular function. They are required in small quantities and are mainly absorbed from the diet and altered by the body. Some vitamins are synthesised by the body. There are two types of vitamins:

1. Fat-soluble
2. Water-soluble.

Vitamins A, D, E and K are fat-soluble vitamins, and they circulate in the bloodstream; any excess is stored in adipose tissue and used when the levels are low in the bloodstream. As these vitamins can be stored, it is not essential to take vitamins A, E and K daily in the diet.[†] In a healthy individual, fat-soluble vitamin supplements can lead to toxicity. Water-soluble vitamins B group and C circulate freely throughout the body and are not stored (except for vitamins B_{12} and B_6). Excess of these vitamins is excreted in the urine and not stored in the body. Toxicity from these vitamins is less likely and the individual will need a daily intake of these vitamins in the diet. Table 14.1 summarises the vitamins, the food sources containing them and their functions.

Minerals

Minerals form approximately 5% of body weight. Sodium, potassium and calcium form the positive ions (anions), while sulphur and phosphorus form the negative ions (cations).
Minerals are essential for:

- Strong bones and teeth
- Controlling body fluids between intracellular and extracellular fluid compartments
- Turning food into energy.

Table 14.2 summarises the minerals and their functions.

[†] Vitamin D appears to reduce the risk of influenza, and other respiratory tract infections such as COVID-19. Supplementation has been advised in the elderly, diabetic patients and the Black Asian and Minority Ethnic (BAME) community, where vitamin D deficiency is more common, to strengthen immune response, particularly during the winter months in the UK (Grant et al., 2020).

Table 14.1   Summary of vitamins and their functions.

	Food sources	Functions
Fat-soluble vitamins		
Vitamin A	In vegetables as carotenoids: carrots, spinach, kale, sweet potatoes, squash, mangoes In meat as retinol (liver), eggs, milk (including breast milk)	Good vision in dim light. Growth and immunity. Deficiency can lead to dry skin and hair, infections of ear, sinus, respiratory and urinary tract. Slow development of bones and teeth
Vitamin D	Synthesis by ultraviolet rays of the sun Some found in oily fish, eggs, fortified foods such as spreads and cereals	To maintain calcium levels Normal growth, bone and teeth formation. Deficiency can lead to rickets in children and osteomalacia in adults. Also associated with increased risk of respiratory tract infections such as influenza and COVID-19.
Vitamin E	Green vegetables, nuts, whole grains, plant oils, eggs	Antioxidant Maintains immune system
Vitamin K	Brussels sprouts, cabbage, kale, broccoli, spinach, spring onions, kiwi fruit, milk	Important in blood clotting
Water-soluble vitamins		
Vitamin B_1 (thiamine)	Pork, poultry peas, nuts, green beans, soybeans, lentils, rice, yeast, sunflower seeds and whole grains,	Essential for growth and carbohydrate metabolism
Vitamin B_2 (riboflavin)	Asparagus, avocados, beans and peas, mushrooms, sweet potatoes, whole grains, Brussels sprouts, spinach, kale, cabbage, fish, dairy products, eggs and meat	Involved in citric acid cycle
Vitamin B_3 (niacin)	Tuna, chicken and turkey peanuts, quinoa, muesli, yeast extract (marmite/vegemite), wild rice, whole wheat pasta, brown rice, peanuts, mushrooms, nutritional yeast	Involved in glycolysis. Deficiency can cause pellagra causing dermatitis, diarrhoea and psychological disturbances
Vitamin B_6 (pyridoxine)	Chickpeas, potatoes, bananas, turkey, salmon, tuna	Involved in amino acid metabolism, reducing depressive symptoms, anaemia, pre-menstrual syndrome, anxiety, depression, eye health
Biotin	Nuts, legumes, soybeans, green beans, tempeh, avocado, eggs	Synthesis of nucleic acid and fatty acid. Deficiency can lead to muscular pain, depression, dermatitis, fatigue and nausea
Vitamin B_5 (pantothenic acid)	Avocado, squash, mushrooms, baked potato, sweet potato, corn on the cob, mangetout peas, oranges, oatmeal, chestnuts, eggs, lean chicken, fish	Involved in glucose production from lipids and amino acids. Deficiency can cause muscle spasms, fatigue, insomnia and insufficient production of adrenal steroid hormones

(Continued)

Table 14.1 (Continued)

	Food sources	Functions
Fat-soluble vitamins		
Folate (folic acid)	Grain products, broccoli, Brussels sprouts, cabbage spinach and other leafy greens, peas, chick peas, legumes and liver (avoid in pregnancy), eggs.	Synthesis of nucleic acid. Deficiency in pregnant women can lead to higher risk of neural tube defects in infants
Vitamin B$_{12}$	Supplemented in meat, poultry, seafood and eggs. Fortified products such as plant-based milks and nutritional yeast. *Supplement essential in vegan diets*	Production of red blood cells. Deficiency can lead to pernicious anaemia and neuropsychiatric disorders such as memory loss, mood changes
Vitamin C (ascorbic acid)	Citrus fruits, tomatoes, potatoes, green and red peppers, berries, green leafy vegetables	Synthesis of collagen, important component of tendons, blood vessels and bone. Deficiency can lead to scurvy, anaemia, poor wound healing

Source: Adapted from Tortora and Derrickson, 2017.

Table 14.2 Minerals and their functions.

Minerals	Sources	Functions
Calcium (Ca^2)	Broccoli, tempeh, leafy greens, tofu, almonds, beans, lentils, oranges, seeds, dairy, sardines, calcium-fortified foods	For healthy teeth and bone formation, blood clotting, nerve conduction and muscle function
Iron (Fe)	Lentils, chickpeas, beans, tofu, cashew nuts, chia seeds, pumpkin seeds, kale, raisins, quinoa, meat	Production of red blood cells and energy production
Magnesium (Mg)	Nuts, legumes, tofu, seeds, whole grains, leafy greens, bananas, fish	Bone formation, muscle and nerve function
Phosphorus (P)	Poultry, pork, seafood, dairy, sunflower and pumpkin seeds, nuts, whole grains, quinoa, beans and lentils, soy	Teeth and bone formation
Potassium (K)	Bananas, apricots, raisins, dates, leafy greens, sweet potatoes, mushrooms, peas, cucumbers	Muscle and nerve function
Sodium (Na)	Table salt, clams, sunflower seeds, soy sauce, anchovies, (Note: Sodium is added to a range of processed foods, and high sodium is linked to a variety of health issues. Intake to be limited)	Nerve and muscle function; maintains osmotic pressure
Sulphur (S)	Meat and poultry, fish, seafood, eggs, dairy, peaches, apricots, sultanas, asparagus, broccoli, sprouts, red cabbage, leeks, onions, radishes	Components of hormones, vitamins and proteins, required for production of ATP
Zinc (Zn)	Legumes, seeds, nuts, dairy, eggs, whole grains, meat, dark chocolate	Essential for enzyme function, carbon dioxide transport and protein metabolism
Selenium (Se)	Brazil nuts, fish, meat, poultry, cheese, brown rice, beans, mushrooms, oatmeal, spinach, lentils, cashews	Antioxidant properties, required for immune function, synthesis of thyroid hormones, sperm motility. May also prevent certain birth defects, miscarriage and reduce prostate cancer and coronary artery disease

Source: Adapted from Tortora and Derrickson, 2017.

Eating to optimise health

Nutritional requirements vary according to health status, activity pattern and growth. For example, an elderly person's energy requirement is not the same as that of a pregnant woman, a baby or a young adult. During a growth spurt, there is more demand for energy. The energy demand also depends on the activity the individual is engaged in. An athlete who is in training will require more energy than a person who is not undertaking any activity, and a patient recovering from surgery or illness will need more energy during the period of recovery.

Dietary risk factors are ranked second only to tobacco in making a significant impact on the burden of disease in the UK (Steel *et al.*, 2018). As morbidity and mortality continues to escalate, it is becoming increasingly evident that the standard UK diet, high in sugar, salt, saturated and trans-fats, is a major contributory factor. The messages around health and nutrition in the public arena can be conflicting and confusing. Given this, and the availability and convenience of processed and unhealthy foods, it is little wonder that diet-related disease is on the increase.

The WHO recommendations are to 'eat a nutritious diet based on a variety of sources originating mainly from plants, rather than animals' (WHO, 2018), and predominantly plant-based diets have been heralded in the literature as the nutritional equivalent to stopping smoking (Barnard, 2013). A recent large-scale, longitudinal meta-analysis (Zhong *et al.*, 2020), found a significant association with eating processed and unprocessed red meat and poultry and an increased risk of cardiovascular disease and all-cause mortality. Consumption of dairy products including milk, cheese and yoghurt has also been associated with a number of health conditions including prostate cancer (Dagfinn, 2015) and more recently breast cancer (Fraser *et al.*, 2020), with the fats and inflammatory markers present in dairy being thought to contribute to ill health overall.

Aside from the direct links highlighted above, there is a more indirect reason for the over-consumption of processed foods, meat and dairy to be contributing to a poor diet and that is the notable *omission* of the nutrients that are required for the maintenance of good health. Eating processed foods has been associated with a significant increase in salt, sugar and fat intake but also, importantly a significant reduction in the foods required for better health (Rauber *et al.*, 2018). Put more simply, when our plates are crowded with bad food, we do not make room for the good food.

In summary of the evidence around healthful eating, the simplest and best (evidence-based) way to eat is:

- Eat the majority of your calories from predominantly plant-based sources as close to their natural form as possible (whole foods) e.g. vegetables, fruits, nuts, seeds, legumes and whole grains to ensure adequate intake of micro- and macronutrients.
- Avoid added salt, sugar and oil in food and drinks.
- Limit meat intake to a maximum of 70 g per day of lean meat, fish or poultry and avoid completely processed meats (e.g. bacon, sausage, beef cold cuts, ham).
- Incorporate 'meat-free' days into your weekly schedule to further reduce your intake of meat.
- Reduce dairy and egg intake and consume low fat dairy or plant-based alternatives as much as possible.
- Avoid alcohol.

See Figure 14.3 for the Eatwell Guide

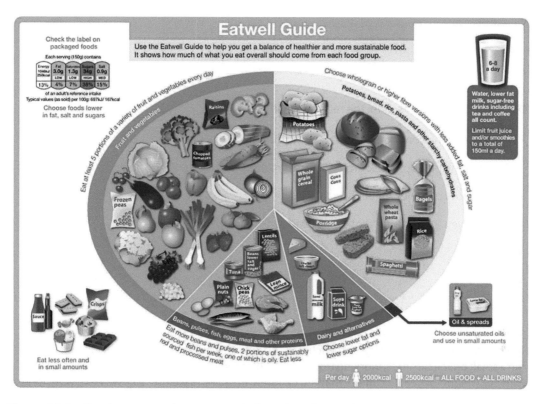

Figure 14.3 Food groups and recommended portions *Source:* PHE, 2016.

Red flag

Alcohol consumption

Moderate alcohol consumption is not *associated with reduced all-cause mortality (Goulden, 2015)*

It has been a generally agreed principle emerging from early evidence (Shaper *et al.*, 1988) that light or moderate alcohol consumption reduces all-cause mortality. Health professionals have based their advice to patients on this guidance, recommending light to moderate alcohol intake as a protection against many health conditions. However, on further scrutiny of many of these studies, it was found that 'ex-drinkers' or 'very light drinkers' were being categorised as 'abstainers'. A significant number of people will reduce or stop alcohol when they experience ill health or take medication. This meant that there was more ill health in the 'abstainer' groups, but when these errors are corrected, there is a direct linear association between alcohol consumption and increased risk of disease (Goulden *et al.*, 2015; Chikritzhs *et al.*, 2015). In short, the more the alcohol consumed, the greater the risks to health, and alcohol consumption should be at a maximum to within government guidance (14 units per week) with maximum health benefits conferred at zero units!

Nutritional disorders

Learning outcomes

On completion of this section, the reader will be able to:

- List some of the common disorders of nutrition.
- Describe the pathophysiological processes related to nutritional disorders.
- List the possible investigations.
- Outline the care and interventions related to the disorders described.

Snapshot   Weight gain

Solomon is a 40-year-old man who lives with his wife Rachel and their two children. Solomon is 172 cm tall and weighs 100 kg, and Rachel is 160 cm tall weighing 88 kg. Solomon and Rachel run a small online business, working from home. Solomon tells you, 'Rachel and I have struggled with our weight for years. I can see that the children are gaining weight, too. We both work long hours sitting at our desks and it is hard to find time to cook. We live mostly on fast food like Chinese and Indian takeaways, kebabs and pizzas'. Solomon went to see his GP because lately he noticed that he had frequent headaches and suffered from dizziness and fatigue. After several tests, his GP informed him that he is hypertensive and that he should consider antihypertensive medication. The GP also informed him that he is overweight and that he should see the practice nurse to get some dietary advice.

Vital signs

The practice nurse noted and recorded the following vital signs were:

Vital sign	Observation	Normal
Temperature	36.2°C	36.0–37.9°C range
Pulse	88 beats per minute	60–100 beats per minute
Respiration	19 breaths per minute	12–20 breaths per minute
Blood pressure	180/115 mmHg	100–139 mmHg (systolic) range
O_2 saturation	98%	94–98%

A full blood count and urea and electrolytes was carried out.

Test	Result	Guideline normal values
White blood cells (WBC)	12×10^9/L	4 to 11×10^9/L
Neutrophils	6.5×10^9/L	2.0 to 7.5×10^9/L
Lymphocytes	2.9×10^9/L	1.3 to 4.0×10^9/L
Red blood cells (RBC)	6.3×10^{12}/L	4.5 to 6.5×10^{12}/L
Haemoglobin (Hb)	160 g/L	130–180 g/L
Platelets	298×10^9/L	150 to 440×10^9/L
C-reactive protein	4.2 mg/L	<5 mg/L
Urea	6.6 mmol/L	2–6.6 mmol/L
Potassium	5.1 mmol/L	3.4–5.6 mmol/L
Sodium	138 mmol/L	135–147 mmol/L

Take some time to reflect on this case and then consider the following:

1. Calculate the body mass index (BMI) for Solomon and Rachel.
2. Discuss the possible complications of obesity.
3. Outline a plan of care for Rachel and Solomon with regard to losing weight.
4. What support systems are available in the community for this family?

Malnutrition

NICE (2012) defines malnutrition as a '... state in which deficiency of nutrients such as energy, protein, vitamins and minerals causes measurable adverse effects on body composition, function or clinical outcome'.

Malnutrition includes undernutrition (wasting, stunting and underweight), inadequate vitamins or mineral intake, overweight and obesity. As discussed above, unhealthy diets and poor nutrition lead to a variety of diet-related non-communicable diseases (e.g. heart attacks, stroke, cancer and diabetes) and contribute to the leading causes of death globally (WHO, 2020). We will now consider how health professionals can effectively care for adults who are suffering because of obesity or being underweight.

Obesity

When we talk about malnutrition we most frequently think of those who are extremely underweight. However, obesity is increasingly being recognised as a disease of malnutrition as although food is consumed in large quantities, the diet may be high in fat and sugar and low in essential vitamins and minerals, causing disease (WHO, 2020).

Obesity is an excessive accumulation of fat cells (adipose tissue) for an individual's height, weight, gender and ethnicity, to such an extent that it can lead to health problems. The fat may settle in the abdominal region (apple-shaped), hips or thighs (pear-shaped). One useful tool for calculating obesity is body mass index (BMI). The formula for BMI is:

$$BMI = \frac{weight(kg)}{height(m)^2}$$

An individual with a BMI between 19 and 24.9 kg/m^2 is of normal weight, of 25–29.9 kg/m^2 is considered overweight and of over 30 kg/m^2 is considered obese. Obesity can reduce life expectancy and lead to complications:

- Heart disease
- Diabetes mellitus
- Vascular disease
- Respiratory disease
- Hypertension
- Bowel cancer
- Deep vein thrombosis
- Varicose veins
- Cerebrovascular accident.

Red flag

The prevalence of obesity and overweight is increasing around the world, but the rates in the UK are among the highest in Europe (OECD, 2017).

Globally, over 4 million people per year die as a result of being obese (Steel *et al.*, 2018), with the UK being in the top 50% of countries with a high BMI with 1 out of every 4 adults classed as obese (NHS, 2019). Public health initiatives raising awareness of the importance of a healthy diet (e.g. PHE, 2016) have had negligible impact, with a notable increase in the prevalence of obesity since 2007 (PHE, 2020). The healthy eating message seems to be slow to translate into a reduction in obesity and sub-optimal nutrition, hitting those living within deprived areas from lower socio-economic backgrounds hardest (PHE, 2020). This places a significant burden on the NHS – direct costs caused by obesity are estimated to be £6.1 billion per year and are forecast to reach £9.7 billion by 2050 (PHE, 2017).

Aetiology

Both hereditary and environmental factors have been associated with obesity, including physiological, psychological and cultural influences. Some of the causes include the following:

Lifestyle factors:

- Diet high in sugar and fat
- Portion size
- Physical inactivity

Social and psychological factors:

- Habits of family and friends
- Low socio-economic status
- Less formal education
- Low self-esteem
- Depression
- Previous psychological trauma (e.g. abuse in childhood)

Physical factors:

- Genetics (may impact how we metabolise food or how we store excess calories)
- Medical conditions (e.g. Polycystic ovary syndrome, hypothyroidism)

- Medications (e.g. beta-blockers, lithium, anti-psychotics, steroids)
- Age (obesity rates increase with advancing age)
- Peri- and menopause

(*Source*: NICE, 2017a)

Orange flag

To increase muscle strength and power beyond the natural limit, some people turn to substances like anabolic-androgenic steroids. Anabolic refers to growth promotion, whereas androgenic refers to the development of male sex characteristics. While steroids' muscle-building capabilities are well documented, they come with several potential side effects. Steroid use has been associated with increased aggression and impulsivity, particularly in male teenagers and adults as well as depression, mood swings and mania.

Signs and symptoms

413

Most practitioners use the BMI assessment tool to identify if a person is overweight or obese:

- BMI between 25 and 29.9 kg/m² is overweight
- BMI between 30 and 39.9 kg/m² is obese
- BMI over 40 kg/m² is extremely obese
- Visible body fat accumulation on hips, waist and thighs
- Increased abdominal girth
- Increased weight
- Waist–hip ratio.

Screening tools for nutritional assessment

The following tools may be used to determine the level of obesity:

- BMI to identify excess adipose tissue, but this needs to be interpreted with caution as it is not a direct measure of adiposity (NICE, 2014).
- Malnutrition Universal Screening Tool (MUST) to determine nutritional status (Malnutrition Advisory Group, 2003).
- Anthropometry measurements to measure skinfold thickness.
- Clinical assessment of the patient.
- Biochemical tests to assess nutrient levels, e.g. protein, HBA1c (to assess for Type 2 diabetes) and lipid profile (NICE, 2014).

Clinical investigations

MUST Tool

The Malnutrition Universal Screening Tool (MUST) was developed by the Malnutrition Advisory Group, a standing committee of British Association for Parenteral and Enteral Nutrition (BAPEN). It has been validated for use in hospitals and the community, and it is the tool recommended by NICE (2014), with its key benefits noted as being quick and easy to use in a variety of care settings. Its use is supported by the British Dietetic Association (BDA), the Royal College of Nursing (RCN) and the Registered Nursing Home Association (RNHA), and it is the most commonly used nutritional screening tool in the UK.

Care and management

In addition to the wide-ranging physical morbidities associated with obesity, patients who are overweight or obese may also suffer from mental health issues such as depression and low self-esteem. These may cause the person to overeat (comfort/emotional eating) or may be as a result of associated social stigma, self-blame or physical constraints such as reduced mobility. Healthcare professionals will need to be sensitive to the patient's feelings when working with these patients and should support the patient to identify the cause of obesity, offering advice on preventative measures, such as dieting and exercise, ensuring that wider determinants such as age, ethnicity and gender are factored in to any package of support.

Advice on diet and healthy eating (Figure 14.2) should be offered as recommended by the Department of Health (PHE, 2016) and outlined in the "Eating to optimise health" section above. The patient should be encouraged to have their weight checked weekly and to keep a record of this.

The patient should be encouraged to take regular exercise for weight reduction unless contraindicated. The British Nutrition Foundation Task Force (2015) recommends 30 minutes of exercise, such as walking, cycling or swimming, at least five times per week, but encouraging the individual to do exercise that they enjoy is more likely to produce positive results. The level of activity should be gradually increased to the level they can tolerate.

Pharmacological interventions

The use of medication has been questioned as an effective weight loss strategy. Studies have shown that weight loss does not generally exceed 4 kg where prescription medications are taken (Haddock *et al.*, 2002) and, given the additional side effects, as well as weight gain as soon as patients discontinue taking them, (Rodríguez and Campbell, 2016), they should be used with caution.

Orlistat is the only drug currently available in the UK that is recommended specifically for the treatment of obesity. It is not recommended for all obese patients and should only be prescribed for those with a BMI greater than 30 kg/m^2 or above after careful assessment of co-morbidities (NICE, 2014).

Medicines management

Orlistat

Orlistat is a lipase inhibitor for obesity management that acts by inhibiting the absorption of dietary fats. Orlistat inhibits dietary fat absorption by approximately 30%. It works by inhibiting pancreatic lipase, an enzyme that breaks down fat in the intestine. Without this enzyme, fat from the diet is excreted undigested, and not absorbed by the body. However, some vitamins are fat soluble, and Orlistat will reduce their absorption. As undigested triglycerides are not absorbed, the resulting caloric deficit may have a positive effect on weight control.

Some common side effects include:

- Bladder pain/discomfort
- Body aches
- Chills
- Cough
- Diarrhoea
- Difficulty with breathing
- Fever

- General feeling of discomfort or illness
- Headache
- Loss of appetite.

Less common side effects include:

- Tightness in the chest
- Tooth or gum problems
- Troubled breathing
- Wheezing.

Surgery

Surgery may be offered to some patients when dieting and exercise have not been success-ful in reducing their weight. Surgical procedures such as gastric bypass (Roux-en-Y connec-tion) may be carried out to limit the quantity of food the individual can eat at any one time (Figure 14.4). A large-scale systematic review of bariatric treatments indicates that gastric bypass may be more effective than other surgeries for weight loss but does carry greater risk of complications (Panagiotou *et al.*, 2018). Many of the benefits of weight loss surgery may be associated with the necessary caloric restriction before and after surgery (Pop *et al.*, 2018), which brings into question whether other means of caloric restriction would be of greater benefit in this group of patients.

Snapshot – weight loss

Miss Fuji Mata is a 79-year-old woman who lives alone. Her neighbour, Afzal, has been visiting Fuji and helping her with shopping. He notices that Fuji has lost quite a bit of weight recently and is looking drawn and pale. She also seems to be confused at times. When he unpacks her shopping, he is throwing away much of what he bought for Fuji previously and is concerned that she is not eating. He speaks to Fuji, who reports a loss of appetite and says she 'cannot be bothered' to cook for herself. Sometimes she will have a bowl of cereal and a few cups of tea in a day, and that is all she wants. Afzal asks Fuji if he can contact her GP and she agrees. Following a telephone consultation with the GP, she asks the community nurse team to visit Fuji at home.

Vital signs

The community nurse records the following vital signs:

Vital sign	Observation	Normal
Temperature	36.8°C	36.0–37.9°C range
Pulse	58 beats per minute (irregular)	60–100 beats per minute
Respiration	18 breaths per minute	12–20 breaths per minute
Blood pressure	90/60 mmHg	100–139 mmHg (systolic) range
O$_2$ saturation	98%	94–98%

A full blood count and urea and electrolytes was performed.

Test	Result	Guideline normal values
White blood cells (WBC)	8.5×10^9/L	4 to 11×10^9/L
Neutrophils	6.6×10^9/L	2.0 to 7.5×10^9/L
Lymphocytes	3.9×10^9/L	1.3 to 4.0×10^9/L
Red blood cells (RBC)	4.5×10^{12}/L	4.5 to 6.5×10^{12}/L
Haemoglobin (Hb)	98 g/L	130–180 g/L
Platelets	198×10^9/L	150 to 440×10^9/L
C-reactive protein	4.8 mg/L	<5 mg/L
Urea	6.5 mmol/L	2–6.6 mmol/L
Potassium	3.5 mmol/L	3.4–5.6 mmol/L
Sodium	138 mmol/L	135–147 mmol/L

Take some time to reflect on this case and then consider the following:

1. Discuss the effects of undernutrition on the systems of the body.
2. Explain what key factors are leading to Fuji's weight loss.
3. Outline a plan of care for Miss Mata's malnutrition.
4. With the aid of a risk assessment tool, what nutritional advice will you offer Miss Mata?

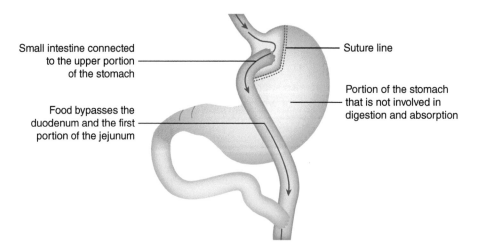

Figure 14.4 Gastric bypass surgery.

Malnutrition and underweight adults

Malnourishment leading to being underweight can be detrimental to health, and if untreated, can result in complications. Malnourishment is most likely to develop in the community setting, and it is reported that malnourished patients visit their GPs more often, when in hospital have longer stays and are more likely to develop complications or infections. Multisystem failure and death can occur from severe weight loss as a result of malnourishment.

Carbohydrates and fats are the main energy source of the body. When dietary intake is not sufficient to meet the energy requirements of the body, stored glycogen, body protein and fats are used to produce energy (Tortora and Derrickson, 2017). In a severe state of malnourishment in underweight people, the body uses its fat reserve and converts it into fatty acid and ketones, which provide energy for the brain. As the disease process progresses, body mass is reduced, and there is a reduction in energy expenditure.

Signs and symptoms
- BMI between 17 and 18.5 kg/m^2 – mild malnourishment
- BMI between 16 and 17 kg/m^2 – moderate malnourishment
- BMI less than 16 kg/m^2 – severe malnutrition
- Severe muscle wasting
- Wrinkled skin in patients with marasmus
- Distended abdomen in patients with kwashiorkor
- Swollen ankles in patients with kwashiorkor.

Aetiology
Causes of malnutrition include:

- Elderly and living on their own
- Eating disorders (e.g. anorexia nervosa, bulimia)
- Medical conditions e.g. cachexia, osteo- and rheumatoid arthritis
- Neuro-degenerative disease e.g. dementia, Alzheimer's
- Socio-economic factors, e.g. poverty, isolation
- Unconscious patients
- Chronic disease such as cardiovascular and renal disease
- Ill-fitting dentures and periodontal disease
- Stomatitis or candida
- Loss of appetite, e.g. as a result of chemotherapy or excessive alcohol consumption or other substance abuse.

Screening tools
- Clinical assessment of the patient
- MUST to determine nutritional status (Malnutrition Advisory Group, 2003)
- BMI
- Anthropometry measurements.

Care and management
Prior to planning care, a full assessment of the patient should be undertaken, including a physical assessment, nutritional assessment, past nursing and medical history, and any problems the patient may present with that could result in undernutrition. Assessment may reveal:

- Changes in dietary habit
- Physiological problems such as swallowing difficulties that may have an effect on nutritional intake
- Poor mental health, e.g. depression, anxiety, dementia
- Socio-economic factors such as lack of finance that may affect purchasing and cooking of food
- Cultural and religious beliefs.

The multidisciplinary team will work with the patient to develop a plan to address the underlying issues and begin to improve and increase their nutritional intake. The plan may include measures such as the completion of a daily food diary and daily weight checking. It is essential that a holistic approach to the care plan is offered, factoring in advice on the best food to purchase that is also in line with patient's preferences, values and religious or cultural requirements.

Where oral supplements (e.g. Ensure Plus) are required, the dietician will be able to give advice on the appropriate supplement for the patient to take in accordance with the NICE (2017b) recommendations and guidelines on nutritional support in adults.

It is also essential that advice is given regarding adequate fluid intake to prevent dehydration, and a fluid balance chart may be commenced to monitor fluid intake and output depending on their condition. The patient should be encouraged to take at least 180 mL of water every hour to prevent dehydration and infection. Any significant changes in fluid balance should be reported immediately to allow prompt action to be taken, e.g. commencement of an intravenous infusion if the patient is dehydrated. Conversely, excessive fluid overload can result in heart or kidney failure.

Any food offered, particularly within a hospital setting, should be as healthy and nutritious as possible and should look appetising. An overview of hospital food standards in 2014 led to a report outlining best practice for the provision of food in hospitals. The report was keen to emphasise an approach whereby the MDT use the term 'eating for health' as a way to describe a diet that is tailored to the individual's therapeutic requirements as 'healthy eating' may be mistaken for calorie restriction (DH, 2014). This includes the consideration of portion size as well as protected mealtimes to ensure patients are given privacy and are appropriately assisted as required. It is the role of the healthcare professional to ensure that the nutritional needs of the patient are met, and this is a key component of the Health and Social Care Act (2008 reg 14: 2014)

Orange flag

Being underweight, whether or not weight is lost intentionally, results from a variety of factors, some psychological, some physiological. A major psychological cause of underweight is depression. Those who experience depression may present with a reduced appetite and rapid weight loss; in these instances, advice from a psychologist or counsellor should be obtained in addition to guidance from a dietician.

Clinical investigations

Malnutrition assessment

Screening should assess BMI and percentage of unintentional weight loss, and consider the timescale of reduced nutritional intake and the likelihood of this continuing in future. Several screening tools exist to aid this assessment, including:

The Malnutrition Universal Screening Tool (MUST), which was developed by the Malnutrition Advisory Group, a standing committee of BAPEN.

The Mini Nutritional Assessment short-form (MNA-SF), which is a practical tool for identification of nutritional status.

Nutritional support should be considered for those:

- With a BMI <18.5.
- With unintentional weight loss of >10% over the previous 3–6 months.

- With a BMI <20 and unintentional weight loss of >5% over the previous 3–6 months.
- Those who have eaten little or nothing for >5 days and who are unlikely not to for the following 5 days or longer.
- For those who have poor absorption, high nutrient losses or increased nutritional needs.

Enteral nutrition

To facilitate enteral nutrition, a tube is inserted directly into the gastrointestinal tract, and the patient is fed a liquid diet through the tube. Enteral feeding is used to supplement oral intake or if the patient is unable to take nutrition orally. Indications include (British Association for Parenteral and Enteral Nutrition (BAPEN), 2018):

- Strokes or other neurological conditions that may impair swallowing
- Surgery of face, neck, gullet or stomach
- Blockages of gullet or stomach
- Radiotherapy of gullet or stomach

419

Types of enteral feeding include:

- Nasogastric (NG) tube feeding involves the insertion of the nasogastric tube via the nasopharynx into the stomach. This procedure is normally carried out by a registered nurse or medical staff.
- Nasojejunal (NJ) tube feeding involves the insertion of a tube via the nasopharynx and the stomach into the jejunum. Insertion of the NJ tube is carried out by medical staff using endoscopy, and it is confirmed to be in place radiologically.
- Percutaneous endoscopic gastrostomy (PEG) or jejunostomy (PEJ) involves the insertion of a tube into the stomach through the abdominal wall. This procedure is carried out surgically by the medical staff.

Care and management of the patient with enteral feeding

Healthcare professionals should support patients with decisions regarding enteral feeding where patients have capacity. Where the patient consents, family members may also be included in discussions and decisions regarding the commencement of enteral feeding (NICE, 2017). Nursing care involves the frequent monitoring for complications, e.g. breathlessness, abdominal distension and recording of vital signs every 2 hours. They should ensure that the enteral feeding tube is correctly positioned before commencing each feed. Local policies, guidelines and the NICE (2017) recommendations in the management and care of the patient with enteral feeding should be adhered to.

Healthcare professionals need to ensure that the patient who is receiving an enteral feed has full care, such as oral and nasal hygiene, washing hands before administering the feed and documenting all the care given as per local policy and procedure and in alignment with the Nursing and Midwifery Council Code (2018).

Red flag

Prior to commencing nasogastric feeding, a range of tests must be performed to confirm that the tube is in the stomach and not the lungs. Local policy and procedure must be adhered to.

Parenteral nutrition

Parenteral nutrition is the direct infusion of a solution into a vein and is used when the patient cannot be nourished with oral or enteral feeding. The solution contains all essential nutritional requirements (micro- and macronutrients) for the body, including fluid replacement. It is a specialised method of feeding which requires specialist care from healthcare professionals. The patient receiving parenteral nutrition in the community will need coordinated support from the district nurse, specialist nutrition nurse, dietician, pharmacist and GP (NICE, 2017b). The patient receiving parenteral nutrition is at risk of developing complications such as infection, fluid overload, heart failure, electrolyte imbalance and respiratory and renal complications. It is not the remit of this chapter to describe this specialist care. Further in-depth discussion regarding the special care of patients receiving parenteral nutrition can be found elsewhere, e.g. Dougherty and Lister (2015).

Conclusion

Nutrition plays a vital role in body function and maintaining homeostasis. Nutrients are classified as micro- and macronutrients. The macronutrients include carbohydrates, proteins and fats, while micronutrients are vitamins and minerals. These nutrients are primarily obtained from the diet and are absorbed from the gastrointestinal tract after digestion. Macronutrients are primarily for energy production, whilst micronutrients promote growth, immunity and development.

Malnutrition leading to obesity and underweight are two major global and national concerns contributing to a significant disease burden and incurring ever-increasing costs to the health and social care sector. The causes of obesity are multi-factorial, associated with lifestyle, social factors as well as physical and mental health disorders. It is a growing issue that is becoming increasingly stigmatised in society. Underweight is becoming increasingly prevalent as the elderly population is increasing. Some elderly people and children are more prone to malnourishment and being underweight as a result of illness or socio-economic factors.

The role of the healthcare professional is varied as regards nutritional care. The responsibilities include preventing malnutrition in patients and offering health education and support relating to obesity and underweight. It is their responsibility to prevent and highlight nutritional problems and to take prompt action to prevent complications, such as heart failure, renal disease, constipation and even death.

Test your knowledge

1. Explain the roles of carbohydrates, protein and fats.
2. Explain the terms micro- and macronutrients.
3. List the fat-soluble vitamins and describe their functions.
4. List the possible causes of obesity and underweight.
5. How are lipids transported in the body?

Activities

Here are some activities and exercises to help test your learning. For the answers to these exercises, as well as further self-testing activities, visit our website at **www.wiley.com/go/fundamentalsofappliedpathophysiology/student4e**

Multiple choice questions

1. Which of the following are simple carbohydrates?
   (a) Oligosaccharides
   (b) Polysaccharides
   (c) Monosaccharides
2. Which of the following foods contain complex carbohydrates?
   (a) Bread
   (b) Cola
   (c) Sweet potatoes
3. What is the current UK recommended intake of total carbohydrates?
   (a) Less than 47%
   (b) 50%–55%
   (c) More than 70%
4. What is the body's preferred energy source?
   (a) Glucose
   (b) Protein
   (c) Ketones
5. What is the process of the production of new proteins called?
   (a) Protein metabolism
   (b) Protein anabolism
   (c) Protein synthesis
6. How many essential amino acids are there?
   (a) 10
   (b) 20
   (c) 40
7. Which of the following foods does *not* contain saturated fat?
   (a) Beef
   (b) Cheese
   (c) Bananas
8. Which of the following foods contain transunsaturated (trans) fat (tick all that apply)?
   (a) Meat
   (b) Milk
   (c) Fish and chip takeaway
9. What does the UK guidance state that the maximum percentage of calories from total fat sources should be?
   (a) 50%
   (b) 35%
   (c) 10%
10. Which of the following vitamins is fat soluble?
    (a) Vitamin C
    (b) Vitamin B
    (c) Vitamin K
11. Which of the following foods contain omega-3 fatty acids?
    (a) Flaxseed
    (b) Lean beef
    (c) Oranges

12. What is the major source of Vitamin D?
    (a) Bananas
    (b) Yellow peppers
    (c) Sunlight
13. Which of the following foods are classed as "legumes" (tick all that apply)?
    (a) Nuts
    (b) Beans
    (c) Lentils
14. How frequently should observations be undertaken on patients receiving enteral nutrition via a nasogastric tube?
    (a) Every 24 hours
    (b) Every 4 hours
    (c) Every 2 hours
15. How many alcohol units is it safest to drink for general health for both men and women?
    (a) 14
    (b) 0
    (c) 28

Conditions

The following is a list of conditions that are associated with nutrition and associated disorders. Take some time and write notes about each of the conditions. You may make the notes taken from textbooks or other resources (e.g. people you work with in a clinical area), or you may make the notes based on people you have cared for. If you are making notes about people you have cared for, you must ensure that you adhere to the rules of confidentiality.

Scurvy	
Hypervitaminosis A	
Rickets	
Constipation	

Anorexia nervosa		

Further resources

Nutrition Facts
https://nutritionfacts.org/ Here you can access a range of evidence-based videos, podcasts and a variety of other resources and peer-reviewed publications all relating to a healthy diet. This is a non-profit, and the founder, Dr Michael Gregor, has written a number of books that are also worth reading including *How Not To Die* and *How Not To Diet*.

Department of Health (DH)
Public Health England (2018). 'Quick Guide to the Government's Healthy Eating Recommendations' can be found here and offer a user-friendly overview of the Eatwell Plate: https://assets.publishing.service.gov.uk/government/uploads/system/uploads/attachment_data/file/742746/A_quick_guide_to_govt_healthy_eating_update.pdf Accessed 14 June 2020.

National Institute for Health and Care Excellence (NICE) – Obesity
http://guidance.nice.org.uk/CG43/Guidance Accessed 3 October 2015.
There is increasing recognition both in the UK and worldwide that there is an 'obesity epidemic'. The issue has received much attention recently from politicians, professionals, the media and the public.
This link gives some insight into a whole range of guidelines from NICE with regards to obesity.

World Health Organization (WHO)
http://www.who.int/topics/nutrition_disorders/en/ Accessed 14th June 2020.
Nutritional disorder is not just a UK problem. It is a worldwide issue. Some of the conditions discussed in this chapter, such as obesity and undernutrition, can lead to other physiological problems, both in adults and in children. WHO provides guidance and recommendations with regards to these health issues. All students should access this website to gain knowledge on these issues.

National Institute for Health and Care Excellence (NICE) – Eating disorders
https://www.nice.org.uk/guidance/ng69 accessed June 2020
In this NICE guidance, you will find information on anorexia nervosa, bulimia nervosa and related eating disorders.

British Medical Journal
http://www.ncbi.nlm.nih.gov/pmc/articles/PMC1118795/ Accessed 3 August 2016.
Students may find this link beneficial as there are numerous articles related to eating disorders and the burden these impose on finance and resources.

Glossary of terms

Anthropometry   Assessment tool used to measure skinfolds.
Body mass index   A number calculated from a person's weight and height.
Buffer   A chemical substance that allows a slight change in pH when acid or base is added to the solution.
Carbohydrate   An organic compound that is composed of carbon, hydrogen and oxygen. Sugars (including glucose) and starch are carbohydrates. They are very important as an energy store.

Coenzyme   A molecule that binds to an enzyme and is essential for its activity, but is not permanently altered by the reaction.

Dysphagia   Difficulty in swallowing.

Enteral   Through the gastrointestinal tract.

Extracellular   Outside the cell.

Fatty acid   Composed of carbon chemically bonded together.

Fistula   An abnormal passage from an internal organ to the surface of the skin or between two organs.

Gastrectomy   Surgical excision of part or the whole of the stomach.

Glucagon   A hormone released by the pancreas, which increase blood sugar levels.

Gluconeogenesis   The production of glucose from non-carbohydrate sources.

Glycogen   A carbohydrate (complex sugar) made from glucose. Excess glucose is stored as glycogen mainly in the liver.

Glycogenolysis   The conversion of glycogen into glucose.

Intracellular   Inside the cell.

Ketone   Product of fat metabolism.

Kwashiorkor   Protein-deficiency malnutrition.

Lipid   An energy-rich organic compound that is soluble in organic substances such as alcohol and benzene.

Lipoprotein   A transport unit for lipids with proteins.

Macronutrient   A nutrient that provides energy.

Marasmus   Protein- and carbohydrate-deficiency malnutrition.

Micronutrient   Vitamins or mineral.

Nutrient   Chemical component of foods.

Obesity   Excess of body fat.

Organelle   A structural and functional part of a cell that acts like a human organ to fulfil all the needs of the cell so that it can grow, reproduce and carry out its functions.

Protein   An organic nitrogenous compound essential as the building material for growth and repair.

Synthesis   Production.

Triglyceride   A major form of lipids in the body.

Undernutrition   Failing health as a result of inadequate nutrient.

Vitamin   An organic compound essential for physiological functions of the body.

References

Adkins, Y. and Kelley, D.S. (2010). Mechanisms underlying the cardioprotective effects of omega-3 poly-unsaturated fatty acids. *Journal of Nutritional Biochemistry*, 21: 781–792.

Arash, E. *et al.* (2017). Mortality from different causes associated with meat, heme iron, nitrates, and nitrites in the NIH-AARP Diet and Health Study: population based cohort study. *BMJ*, 357: j1957. Available at: https://doi.org/10.1136/bmj.j1957 Accessed May 2020.

Baic, S. (2007). Understanding trans fats - theory, evidence, practice. *Practice Nurse*, 33(8): 23–27.

British Association for Parenteral and Enteral Nutrition (BAPEN) (2018). *Enteral and Parenteral Nutrition*. Available at: https://www.bapen.org.uk/nutrition-support/assessment-and-planning/enteral-and-parenteral-nutrition accessed May 2020

Barnard, N.D. (2013). The Physician's role in nutrition-related disorders. From bystander to leader. *Virtual Mentor*, 15(4): 367–372.

Berquin, I.M., Edwards, I.J. and Chen, Y.Q. (2008). Multi-targeted therapy of cancer by omega-3 fatty acids. *Cancer Letters*, 269(2008): 363–377. Available at: 10.1016/j.canlet.2008.03.044.

Bouvard, V. *et al*. (2015). Carcinogenicity of consumption of red and processed meat. *The Lancet Oncology*, 16(16). 15991600. ISSN 1474-5488

British Nutrition Foundation *(BNF) (2018a). Carbohydrate*. Available at: https://www.nutrition.org.uk/nutritionscience/nutrients-food-and-ingredients/carbohydrate.html Accessed May 2020.

British Nutrition Foundation *(BNF) (2018b)*. Protein. Available at: https://www.nutrition.org.uk/nutritionscience/nutrients-food-and-ingredients/protein.html?start=2 Accessed May 2020.

British Nutrition Foundation *(BNF) (2019). Nutrition Requirements*. Available at: https://www.nutrition.org.uk/attachments/article/907/Nutrition%20Requirements_Revised%20August%202019.pdf Accessed May 2020.

British Nutrition Foundation Task Force (2015). *Obesity*. Scotland: British Nutrition Foundation.

Chalvon-Demersay, T. *et al*. (2017). A systematic review of the effects of plant compared with animal protein sources on features of metabolic syndrome. *The Journal of Nutrition*, 147(3): 281–292. https://doi.org/10.3945/jn.116.239574

Chikritzhs, T. *et al*. (2015). Has the leaning tower of presumed health benefits from "moderate" alcohol use finally collapsed? (editorial) *Addiction*, 110(5): 726–727.

Dagfinn, A. (2015). Dairy products, calcium, and prostate cancer risk: A systematic review and meta-analysis of cohort studies. *The American Journal of Clinical Nutrition*, 101(1): 87–117. https://doi.org/10.3945/ajcn.113.067157

Dehghan, M., Mente, A., Zhang, X. *et al*. (2017). Associations of fats and carbohydrate intake with cardiovascular disease and mortality in 18 countries from five continents (PURE): A prospective cohort study. *Lancet*, 390: 2050–2062.

Department of Health *(DH) (2014). The Hospital Food Standards Panel's Report on Standards for Food and Drink in NHS Hospitals*. Available at: https://assets.publishing.service.gov.uk/government/uploads/system/uploads/attachment_data/file/523049/Hospital_Food_Panel_May_2016.pdf Accessed May 2020.

Dougherty, L. and Lister, S. (2015). *The Royal Marsden Hospital Manual of Clinical Nursing Procedures*, 8th edn. Oxford: Blackwell Science.

Fraser, G. et al (2020). Dairy, soy, and risk of breast cancer: those confounded milks, *International Journal of Epidemiology*, dyaa007. https://doi.org/10.1093/ije/dyaa007

Gobbo, F. *et al*. (2016). Cohorts for Heart and Aging Research in Genomic Epidemiology (CHARGE) Fatty Acids and Outcomes Research Consortium (FORCe)ω−3 polyunsaturated fatty acid biomarkers and coronary heart disease: pooling project of 19 cohort studies. *JAMA Internal Medicine*, 176: 1155–1166,

Goulden, R. (2015). Moderate alcohol consumption is not associated with reduced all-cause mortality. *American Journal of Medicine*, 2016; 129(2): 180–186.e4. DOI:10.1016/j.amjmed.10.013

Grant, W. *et al*. (2020). Evidence that Vitamin D supplementation could reduce risk of influenza and COVID-19 infections and deaths. *Nutrients*, 12: 988. DOI: 10.3390/nu12040988 Accessed June 2020.

Haddock, C.K. *et al*. (2002). Pharmacotherapy for obesity: a quantitative analysis of four decades of published randomized clinical trials. *International Journal of Obesity and Related Metabolic Disorders*, 26(2): 262–273.

Health and Social Care Act (2008). Regulations 2014: Regulation 14.

Kim, H., Caulfield, L.E., and Rebholz, C.M. (2018). Healthy plant-based diets are associated with lower risk of all-cause mortality in US adults. *Journal of Nutrition*, 148(4): 624–631. DOI:10.1093/jn/nxy019

Marzilli, M. *et al*. (2012). Obstructive coronary atherosclerosis and ischemic heart disease: An elusive link! *Journal of the American College of Cardiology*, 60(11): 951–956.

Miller, V. *et al*. (2017). Fruit, vegetable, and legume intake, and cardiovascular disease and deaths in 18 countries (PURE): A prospective cohort study. Lancet, 390(10107): 4–10.

NHS. (2019). *The NHS Long Term Plan*. Available: https://www.longtermplan.nhs.uk/ Accessed May 2020.

National Institute for Health and Care Excellence (NICE) (2020). *National Policy on Diet*. Available at: pathways.nice.org.uk/pathways/diet/national-policy-on-diet.pdf Accessed May 2020.

425

Chapter 14 Nutrition and associated disorders

National Institute for Health and Care Excellence (NICE) (2017a). *Obesity What are the Causes and the Risk Factors?* Available at: https://cks.nice.org.uk/obesity#!backgroundSub:1 Accessed March 2020.

National Institute for Health and Care Excellence (NICE) (2017). *Nutrition Support for Adults: Oral Nutrition Support, Enteral Tube Feeding and Parenteral Nutrition*. Available at: https://www.nice.org.uk/guidance/cg32/chapter/1-Guidance Accessed May 2020.

National Institute for Health and Care Excellence (NICE) (2016). *Cardiovascular Disease: Risk Assessment and Reduction, Including Lipid Modification*. Available at: https://www.nice.org.uk/guidance/CG181/chapter/1-Recommendations Accessed: May 2020.

National Institute for Health and Care Excellence (NICE) (2014). *Obesity: Guidance on the Prevention, Identification, Assessment and Management of Overweight and Obesity in Adults and Children*. Available at: https://www.nice.org.uk/guidance/cg189 Accessed May 2020.

National Institute for Health and Care Excellence (*NICE) (2012). Nutrition Support in Adults*. Available at: https://www.nice.org.uk/Guidance/QS24 Accessed May 2020.

Nursing and Midwifery Council (2018). *The Code. Professional Standards of Practice and Behaviour for Nurses, Midwives and Nurse Associates*. Available at: https://www.nmc.org.uk/standards/code/ accessed June 2020

Malnutrition Advisory Group (2003). *The MUST Report. Nutritional Screening of Adults: A Multidisciplinary Responsibility*. London: British Association for Parenteral and Enteral Nutrition.

Office for National Statistics (ONS) (2018). *Deaths Registered in England and Wales (series DR): 2017*. Available at: https://www.ons.gov.uk/peoplepopulationandcommunity/birthsdeathsandmarriages/deaths/bulletins/deathsregisteredinenglandandwalesseriesdr/2017 Accessed June 2020.

Organisation for Economic Cooperation and Development (OECD) (2017). *Obesity Update 2017*. Available: http://www.oecd.org/health/obesity-update.htm

Panagiotou, O.A. *et al*. (2018). Comparative effectiveness and safety of bariatric procedures in Medicare-eligible patients: a systematic review. *JAMA Surgery*, 153(11):e183326.

Pop, L.M., Mari, A., Zhao, T.J. *et al*. (2018). Roux-en-Y gastric bypass compared with equivalent diet restriction: mechanistic insights into diabetes remission. *Diabetes, Obesity and Metabolism*, 20(7): 1710–1721.

Public Health England (2017). *Health Matters: Obesity and the Food Environment*. Available from: https://www.gov.uk/government/publications/health-matters-obesity-and-the-food-environment/healthmatters-obesity-and-the-food-environment–2

Public Health England (2020). *National Diet and Nutrition Survey*. Available at: https://www.gov.uk/government/collections/national-diet-and-nutrition-survey Accessed May 2020.

Public Health England (2016). *The Eatwell Guide*. Available at: https://www.gov.uk/government/publications/the-eatwell-guide Accessed May 2020.

Rauber, R. *et al*. (2018) Ultra-processed food consumption and chronic non-communicable diseases-related dietary nutrient profile in the UK (2008 – 2014). *Nutrients*, 10(5): 587

Rodríguez, J.E. and Campbell, K.M. (2016). Past, present, and future of pharmacologic therapy in obesity. *Prim Care*, 43(1): 61–67.

Roher, A.E. *et al*. (2011). Intracranial atherosclerosis as a contributing factor to Alzheimer's disease dementia. *Alzheimer's & Dementia*, 7(4): 436–444.

Saini, R.K. and Keum, Y.S. (2018). Omega-3 and omega-6 polyunsaturated fatty acids: Dietary sources, metabolism, and significance – A review. *Life Sciences*, 203: 255–267. Available at: https://doi.org/10.1016/j.lfs.2018.04.049 Accessed: May 2020.

Shaper, A.G., Wannamethee, G. and Walker, M. (1988). Alcohol and mortality in British men: Explaining the U-shaped curve. *Lancet*, 11: 1267–1273.

Scientific Advisory Committee on Nutrition (2015). *Carbohydrates and Health*. The Stationary Office. London. Available at: www.tsoshop.co.uk Accessed May 2020.

Seidelmann, S.B. *et al*. (2018) Dietary carbohydrate intake and mortality: A prospective cohort study and meta-analysis. *The Lancet (Public Health)*, 3(9): e419–e428. Available at: https://doi.org/10.1016/S2468-2667(18)30135-X

Song, M., Fung, T.T., Hu, F.B. *et al*. (2016). Association of animal and plant protein intake with all-cause and cause-specific mortality [published correction appears *in JAMA Internal Medicine*, 2016 Nov 1;176(11): 1728]. *JAMA Internal Medicine*, 176(10): 1453–1463. doi:10.1001/jamainternmed.2016.4182

Steel, N. *et al*. (2018). Changes in health in the countries of the UK and 150 English Local Authority areas 1990–2016: A systematic analysis for the Global Burden of Disease Study 2016. *The Lancet*, 392(10158): 1647–1661. Available at: https://doi.org/10.1016/S0140-6736(18)32207-4 Accessed May 2020.

Tortora, G.J. and Derrickson, B.H. (2017) *Tortora's Principles of Anatomy & Physiology*, 15th edn. Singapore: John Wiley & Sons.

Turesky, R. (2018). Mechanistic Evidence for red meat and processed meat intake and cancer risk: A follow-up on the international agency for research on cancer evaluation of 2015. *International Journal of Chemistry*, 72(10): 718–724. Available at: https://doi.org/10.2533/chimia.2018.718 Accessed May 2020

Tuso, P.J., Ismail, M.H., Ha, B.P. and Bartolotto, C. (2013). Nutritional update for physicians: plant-based diets. *The Permanente Journal*, 17(2): 61–66. https://doi.org/10.7812/TPP/12-085

Richter, C.H. *et al*. (2015, November). Plant protein and animal proteins: Do they differentially affect cardiovascular disease risk?. *Advances in Nutrition*, 6(6): 712–728. https://doi.org/10.3945/an.115.009654

Wahlqvist, M. (2016). Food Structure is critical for optimum health. *Food & Function – The Royal Society of Chemistry*, 7: 1245–1250.

Waugh, A. and Grant, A. (2018). *Ross & Wilson Anatomy & Physiology in Health and Illness*, 13th edn. London: Elsevier.

World Health Organization (WHO) regional office for Europe (2018). *Better Food and Nutrition in Europe: A Progress Report Monitoring Policy Implementation in the WHO European Region*. Available at: https://www.euro.who.int/__data/assets/pdf_file/0005/355973/ENP_eng.pdf?ua=1 Accessed: May 2020.

World Health Organization (WHO) (2020). *Malnutrition-Key Facts*. Available: https://www.who.int/news-room/fact-sheets/detail/malnutrition Accessed: May 2020.

Zhong, V.W., Van Horn, L., Greenland, P. *et al*. (2020). Associations of processed meat, unprocessed red meat, poultry, or fish intake with incident cardiovascular disease and all-cause mortality. *JAMA Internal Medicine*, 180(4): 503–512. Available at: doi:10.1001/jamainternmed.2019.6969 Accessed May 2020.

Chapter 15

The endocrine system and associated disorders

Carl Clare

Senior Lecturer, Department of Adult Nursing and Primary Care, School of Health and Social Work, University of Hertfordshire, Hatfield, Hertfordshire, UK

Contents

Introduction 429
Hormones 430
The physiology of the endocrine glands ...433
Disorders of the endocrine system 440
Conclusion 456

Multiple choice questions...............................457
Conditions...458
Further resources...................................459
Glossary of terms...................................460
References...461

Key words

- Hormones
- Homeostasis
- Receptors
- Upregulation
- Downregulation
- Negative feedback
- Hypothalamus
- Calorigenic effect
- Glucagon
- Corticosteroids
- Hyposecretion
- Hypersecretion

Fundamentals of Applied Pathophysiology: An Essential Guide for Nursing and Healthcare Students, Fourth Edition. Edited by Ian Peate.
© 2021 John Wiley & Sons Ltd. Published 2021 by John Wiley & Sons Ltd.
Student companion website: www.wiley.com/go/fundamentalsofappliedpathophysiology/student4e
Instructor companion website: www.wiley.com/go/fundamentalsofappliedpathophysiology/instructor4e

Test your prior knowledge

- Where is the hypothalamus located?
- Name one organ of the endocrine system and one hormone it releases.
- What is the treatment for hypothyroidism?
- Name the two major types of diabetes.

Learning outcomes

On completion of this section, the reader will be able to:

- Name the major endocrine organs.

- Name the hormones that they secrete.

- Describe the principles of the negative feedback control system that affects most endocrine glands.

- Describe the effects of thyroid hormones on the body.

- Discuss the regulation of blood glucose by the pancreas.

Don't forget to visit the companion website for this book (www.wiley.com/go/fundamentalsofappliedpathophysiology/student4e) **where you can find self-assessment tests to check your progress, as well as lots of activities to practise your learning.**

Introduction

The endocrine system is the name given to a collection of small organs that are scattered throughout the body, each of which releases hormones. Hormones are chemical substances that are released into the blood by the endocrine system and exert physiological control over the function of cells or organs other than those that created them (Figure 15.1). The purpose of each hormone varies, but their common primary role is to maintain homeostasis (that is, maintaining a normal physiological balance in the body).

Endocrine-releasing organs can be divided into three main categories:

1. Endocrine glands – These are organs whose sole function is the production and release of hormones. The pituitary, thyroid, parathyroid and adrenal glands are all examples of this category.
2. Organs that are not pure glands but contain relatively large areas of hormone-producing tissue – Examples of these are the pancreas, the hypothalamus and the gonads.
3. Other tissues and organs also produce hormones – Areas of hormone-producing cells are found in the wall of the small intestine, the stomach, the kidneys and the heart.

The organs and their position in the body are shown in Figure 15.2. Each of these organs will typically have a rich vascular (blood vessel) network, and the hormone-producing cells

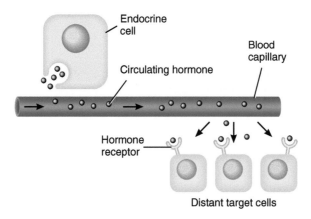

(a) Circulating hormones

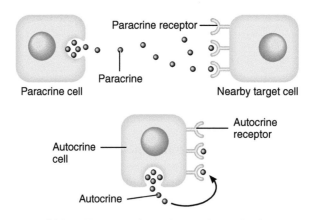

(b) Local hormones (paracrines and autocrines)

Figure 15.1   Hormone release and transport.

within them are arranged into cords and branching networks around this supply. This arrangement of blood vessels and hormone-producing cells ensures that hormones enter the blood rapidly and are then transported throughout the body.

Hormones

There are a great number of hormones produced by the endocrine system, and each has very different effects and affect different cells and organs in the body. The major bodily processes that hormones influence or regulate are reproduction, growth and development, the body's defence mechanisms against stressors, levels of electrolytes, water and nutrients in the body, and cellular metabolism and energy. Hormones are generally made from either amino acids (most) or cholesterol (the steroid hormones). As hormones are released into the bloodstream, they are carried throughout the body, but they do not affect all cells. In order for a hormone to have an effect on a cell, the cell must have receptors for that particular hormone. Cells that have receptors for a particular hormone are known as the target cells for that hormone. Some hormones are very specific, and thus receptors are only found on specific cells (e.g. the adrenocorticotropic hormone), whereas thyroid hormone affects nearly every cell in the body.

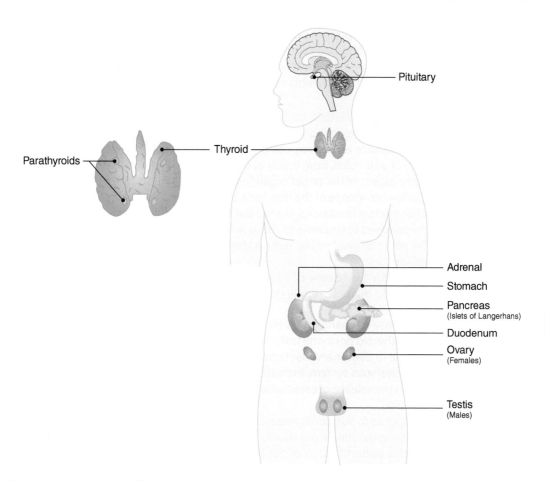

Figure 15.2   Position of the endocrine glands and organs that produce hormones.

431

Receptors for a hormone are proteins that are sited either on the cell wall or inside the cell. The exact location of a receptor depends on the type of hormone that the receptor is for. Amino-acid-based hormones cannot cross the cell membrane, and therefore their receptors are found on the cell wall; activation of these receptors leads to the activation of secondary messenger systems within the cell. One exception is thyroid hormone, which is very small and can diffuse easily across the cell membrane into the cell. The steroid hormones can cross the cell membrane because they are small and lipid soluble, and thus their receptors are found within the cell itself. The activation of a target cell depends on the blood levels of the hormone, the number of receptors on the cell and the affinity of the receptor for the hormone. Changes in all three of these factors can happen relatively quickly in response to a change in stimuli. Changes in the number of receptors are known as upregulation and downregulation.

- Upregulation is the creation of more receptors in response to low circulating levels of a hormone. Thus, the cell becomes more responsive to the presence of the hormone in the blood.
- Downregulation is the reduction in the number of receptors and is often caused by the exposure of a cell to prolonged periods of high circulating levels of a hormone. Thus, the cell becomes less responsive (desensitised) to a hormone, which protects the cell from over-responding to continued high levels of that hormone.

Hormones can have a very powerful effect even at low concentrations, and thus it is essential that the released hormones are disposed of efficiently. Some hormones are rapidly broken down within their target cells; most are inactivated by the liver or the kidneys and then excreted in the urine, but small amounts are excreted in the faeces (Hall and Hall, 2020).

The control of hormone release

The creation and release of most hormones is initiated by an external or internal stimulus; further creation and release is then regulated by a negative feedback system (Figure 15.3). Thus, the influence of a stimulus, from inside or outside the body, leads to hormone release; following this, some aspect of the target organ function then inhibits further reaction to the stimulus and thus further release of the hormone by the organ.

An example of a negative feedback system is the release of insulin by the pancreas. Insulin is released by the pancreas in response to rising levels of glucose, amino acids or fatty acids in the blood. The effect of insulin is to reduce these levels, thus reducing the stimulus for further insulin release.

The initial stimulus for the release of a hormone is usually one of three types, although some organs respond to multiple stimuli (Marieb and Hoehn, 2018):

1. Humoral – A response to changing levels of certain ions and nutrients in the blood, e.g. the release of parathyroid hormone is stimulated by falling blood levels of calcium ions.
2. Neural – A response to direct nervous stimulation. Only a few endocrine organs are directly stimulated by the nervous system. Increased activity in the sympathetic nervous system directly stimulates the release of catecholamines (epinephrine and norepinephrine) from the adrenal medulla.
3. Hormonal – A response to hormones released by other organs. Hormones that are released in response to hormonal stimuli are usually rhythmical in their release (i.e. the levels rise and fall in a specific pattern). Many of the hormones released from the anterior pituitary gland are released in response to releasing and inhibiting hormones from the hypothalamus.

Summary

- Hormones are chemicals that are released into the bloodstream.
- Hormones are released by glands and other organs.
- A hormone's effect on its target cell is through receptors, which are found in the cell wall or contained in the cell itself.

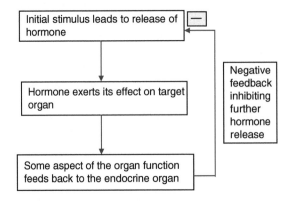

Figure 15.3 Control of hormone release by the negative feedback system.

- The stimulus for a hormone's release can be changing levels of ions or nutrients in the blood, direct stimulation by the nervous system or in response to other hormones.
- Further control of hormone release is regulated by a negative feedback system.

The physiology of the endocrine glands
The hypothalamus and pituitary gland

The pituitary gland is a pure endocrine gland that is located in the brain just below the hypothalamus. It is about the size and shape of a pea on a stalk. The pituitary stalk (infundibulum) connects the pituitary gland to the hypothalamus and contains both nerve fibres and blood vessels (Figure 15.4). The direct link between the hypothalamus and the pituitary gland is essential as it allows direct hypothalamic control of the release of the pituitary hormones.

Anatomically, the pituitary gland is split into two sections (Ritchie and Balasubramanian, 2014). The posterior lobe (the neurohypophysis) is mostly made up of nerve fibres and nerve endings that have their origin in the hypothalamus; it stores two hormones that are created in the hypothalamus and are then transported down the nerve fibres in the stalk (the hypothalamic–hypophyseal tract) and stored in the nerve endings. The anterior pituitary gland (the adenohypophysis) consists of glandular tissues. Whilst the anterior pituitary gland has no direct neural link from the hypothalamus, it does receive its blood supply directly from the hypothalamus through the pituitary portal system. This blood supply is an essential component in the control of the release of hormones from the anterior pituitary gland as it transports inhibiting and releasing hormones created by the hypothalamus to the anterior pituitary gland (Table 15.1).

Growth hormone (somatotropin) stimulates most body cells to increase in size and divide; however, its major targets are the bones and skeletal muscle. Growth hormone also has several other effects, including increasing the cellular uptake of amino acids to be used in the

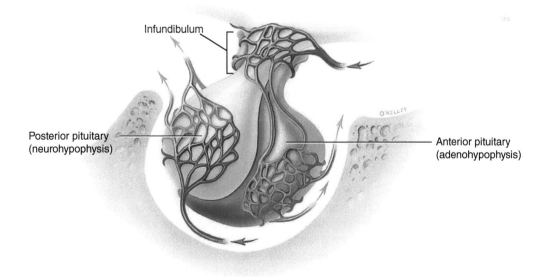

Infundibulum

Posterior pituitary
(neurohypophysis)

Anterior pituitary
(adenohypophysis)

Figure 15.4 The pituitary gland.

Table 15.1 The hormones of the hypothalamus and the anterior pituitary gland.

Hypothalamus	Anterior pituitary gland	Target organ or tissues
Growth hormone releasing factor	Growth hormone	Many
Growth hormone release inhibiting factor	Growth hormone (inhibits release)	Many
Thyroid-releasing hormone	Thyroid-stimulating hormone	Thyroid gland
Corticotropin-releasing hormone	Adrenocorticotropic hormone	Adrenal cortex
Prolactin-releasing hormone	Prolactin	Breasts
Prolactin-inhibiting hormone	Prolactin (inhibits release)	Breasts
Gonadotropin-releasing hormone	Follicle-stimulating hormone	Gonads
	Luteinising hormone	

building of proteins. The secretion of growth hormone is regulated by two hypothalamic hormones: growth hormone-releasing hormone (GHRH) and growth hormone-inhibiting hormone (GHIH). It is usually released in a diurnal cycle (related to the pattern of day and night) and is found at its highest level about an hour after the onset of sleep.

The release of thyroid-stimulating hormone (TSH or thyrotropin) from the anterior pituitary gland is regulated by exposure of the gland to thyroid-releasing hormone (TRH, also known as thyrotropin-releasing hormone) from the hypothalamus and the blood levels of thyroid hormones. The effect of TSH is to stimulate activity in the thyroid gland.

Adrenocorticotropic hormone (ACTH or corticotropin) stimulates the cortex of each adrenal gland to release corticosteroid hormones. The release of ACTH usually follows a diurnal rhythm with the peak being in the morning just after rising (Marieb and Hoehn, 2018). The release of ACTH is stimulated by corticotropin-releasing hormone (CRH) from the hypothalamus; however, other triggers for release include fever, trauma and other stressors (Mihai, 2014).

Gonadotropins is the collective name for follicle-stimulating hormone (FSH) and luteinising hormone (LH). The release of both hormones is regulated by the secretion of gonadotropin-releasing hormone from the hypothalamus. In the adult, FSH stimulates the production of gametes (sperm or egg), and in females it also regulates ovulation in conjunction with LH. LH promotes the production of gonadal hormones in both males and females (Dagklis et al., 2015).

Prolactin stimulates milk production in the breasts and is controlled by releasing and inhibiting hormones produced by the hypothalamus. Prolactin-inhibiting hormone is produced in high levels in men, whereas in women the production of the releasing and inhibiting hormones varies, depending on the amount of oestrogen in the blood.

Two hormones are released from the posterior pituitary gland: oxytocin and antidiuretic hormone (ADH). Oxytocin has an effect on uterine contraction in childbirth and is responsible for the 'let down' response in breastfeeding mothers (the release of milk in response to suckling). In men and non-pregnant women, it plays a role in sexual arousal and orgasm (Borrow and Cameron, 2012).

The primary role of ADH (vasopressin) is to prevent wide fluctuations in the water balance of the body. Osmoreceptors in the hypothalamus monitor the concentration of dissolved ions in the blood (and therefore water levels). An increase in the concentration of dissolved ions leads to an increase in ADH release from the posterior pituitary gland. The main target of ADH is the renal tubules in the kidneys, causing them to increase the reabsorption of water from the urine and back into the blood (thus decreasing urine output and increasing blood volume). A decrease in blood pressure also stimulates ADH release.

The thyroid gland

The thyroid gland is a butterfly-shaped gland located in the front of the neck on the trachea just below the larynx. It is made up of hollow, spherical follicles which contain thyroglobulin molecules with attached iodine molecules; thyroid hormone is created from these. One unique feature of the thyroid gland is its ability to create and store large amounts of hormone; this can be up to 100 days of hormone supply (Hall and Hall, 2020). The thyroid gland releases two forms of thyroid hormone: thyroxine (T_4) and triiodothyronine (T_3), both of which require iodine for their creation. However, T_4 is the primary hormone released by the thyroid gland; this is then converted into T_3 by the target cells (Stathatos, 2012).

Thyroid hormone affects virtually every cell in the body, except the adult brain, spleen, testes, uterus and the thyroid gland itself. In the target cells, thyroid hormone stimulates enzymes that are involved with glucose oxidation. This is the calorigenic effect, and its overall effects are an increase in basal metabolic rate, oxygen consumption and production of body heat. Thyroid hormone also plays an important role in the maintenance of blood pressure, as it stimulates an increase in the number of receptors in the walls of blood vessels (Marieb and Hoehn, 2018).

The control of the release of thyroid hormone is mediated by a negative feedback system which involves the hypothalamus and cascades through the pituitary gland (Figure 15.5).

Increased levels of T_4 (and to a lesser extent T_3) in the blood inhibit the release of TRH from the hypothalamus, thus reducing the stimulation for the release of TSH from the anterior

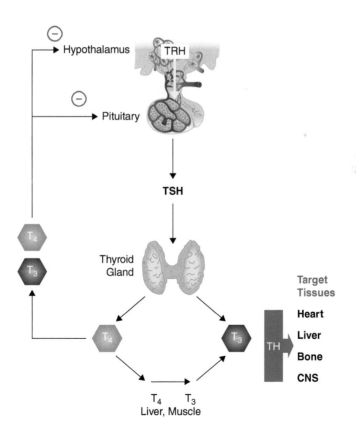

Figure 15.5 The negative feedback control of thyroid hormone production. TSH, thyroid-stimulating hormone; TRH, thyroid-releasing hormone.

pituitary gland. The effect of TSH on the thyroid gland is to promote the release of thyroid hormone into the blood; therefore, a reduction in TSH reduces the release of T_3 and T_4. A reduced level of T_4 in the blood reduces the negative feedback, and thus there is an increase in the release of TRH, which leads to an increase in thyroid gland function. Conditions that increase the energy requirements of the body (such as pregnancy or prolonged cold) also stimulate the release of TRH from the hypothalamus and therefore lead to an increase in blood levels of thyroid hormone. In these situations, the stimulating conditions override the normal negative feedback system (Tortora and Derrickson, 2011).

The parathyroid glands

The parathyroid glands are tiny glands normally located on the back (posterior) of the thyroid gland. There are usually two pairs of glands, but the precise number varies, and some patients have been reported to have up to four pairs (Arrangoiz et al., 2017). The parathyroid glands release parathyroid hormone (PTH), which is the single most important hormone for the control of the calcium balance in the body. Physiologically, calcium is important in the transmission of nerve impulses, is involved in muscle contraction and is required for the production of clotting factors in the blood.

The release of PTH by the glands is controlled by the blood levels of calcium; a reduced calcium level stimulates the release of PTH, and an increased calcium level inhibits its release. PTH increases blood levels of calcium by its action on three target areas in the body (Campbell, 2014):

1. Bones – PTH stimulates the activity of osteoclasts to digest some of the bone and release calcium into the blood.
2. Kidneys – PTH increases reabsorption of calcium.
3. Intestines – PTH increases the absorption of calcium in the intestines by activating vitamin D (which is required for the absorption of calcium in the gut).

The adrenal glands

The adrenal glands are two pyramid-shaped glands that lie on top of each of the kidneys (Ritchie and Balasubramanian, 2014). Each of the adrenal glands is structurally and functionally two glands in one. The inner core of each of the adrenal glands is called the adrenal medulla; this is surrounded by the much larger adrenal cortex (Figure 15.6). Both the medulla and the cortex secrete different hormones and respond to different stimuli.

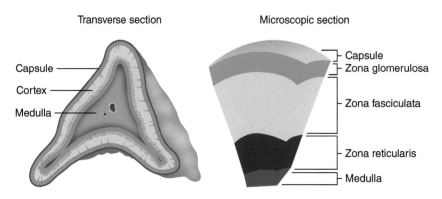

Figure 15.6   Anatomy of an adrenal gland.

The adrenal medulla

The adrenal medulla secretes epinephrine (adrenaline) and (to a lesser extent) norepinephrine (noradrenaline) in response to stimulation by the sympathetic nervous system. Although epinephrine and norepinephrine are essential for normal bodily functioning, the epinephrine and the norepinephrine secreted by the adrenal medulla are not essential and serve only to intensify the effects of sympathetic nervous stimulation (Marieb and Hoehn, 2018).

The adrenal cortex

The adrenal cortex is functionally separated into three different zones (Figure 15.6), each of which produces at least one steroid hormone (hormones made from cholesterol are known collectively as the corticosteroids):

1. Zona glomerulosa – produces the mineralocorticoids
2. Zona fasciculata – produces the glucocorticoids
3. Zona reticularis – involved in the production of glucocorticoids but also produces small amounts of adrenal sex hormones (the gonadocorticoids).

Mineralocorticoids are hormones whose primary function is the regulation of electrolyte concentrations (especially potassium and sodium) in the blood. Several mineralocorticoid hormones are known; however, aldosterone is the most potent and accounts for 95% of all the mineralocorticoid hormones secreted. The effect of aldosterone on the body is to reduce the excretion of sodium in the urine by regulating the reabsorption of sodium from the urine in the distal portion of the renal tubules. Aldosterone also has an effect on the body levels of water and several other ions (including potassium, bicarbonate and chloride) as their regulation is coupled to the regulation of sodium in the body. The stimulus for the release of aldosterone is primarily related to the blood concentrations of sodium (Na^+) and potassium (K^+), blood pressure and blood volume. Increased concentrations of potassium, reduced blood concentrations of sodium and a reduction in blood pressure and/or blood volume all stimulate the release of aldosterone, whilst the opposite inhibits release (Figure 15.7).

There are several mechanisms that regulate the release of aldosterone. The primary control mechanism is the production of angiotensin II by the renin–angiotensin system. However, in response to a severe, non-specific stressor, hypothalamic release of CRH stimulates the increased release of ACTH. This increase in ACTH stimulates a small increase in the release of aldosterone, leading to a slight increase in blood volume and pressure, which will help to ensure the adequate delivery of oxygen and nutrients to the tissues (Marieb and Hoehn, 2018).

The glucocorticoid hormones influence the metabolism of most body cells and are also involved in providing resistance to stressors and promoting the repair of damaged tissues. They also suppress the immune system and inflammatory processes of the body; hence their use in the treatment of inflammatory conditions such as asthma and arthritis. The glucocorticoids include cortisol (hydrocortisone), cortisone and corticosterone; however, only cortisol is secreted in any significant amounts (Mihai, 2014). Cortisol is normally released in a rhythmical pattern, with most being released shortly after the person gets up from sleep and the lowest amount being released just before, and shortly after, sleep commences. Cortisol release is promoted by ACTH from the anterior pituitary gland; increasing levels of cortisol act on both the hypothalamus and the pituitary gland, inhibiting further release of both CRH and ACTH in a negative feedback system. However, this negative feedback system is overridden by acute physiological stress (e.g. trauma, infection or haemorrhage). The increase in sympathetic nervous system activity in response to an acute stress triggers

437

438

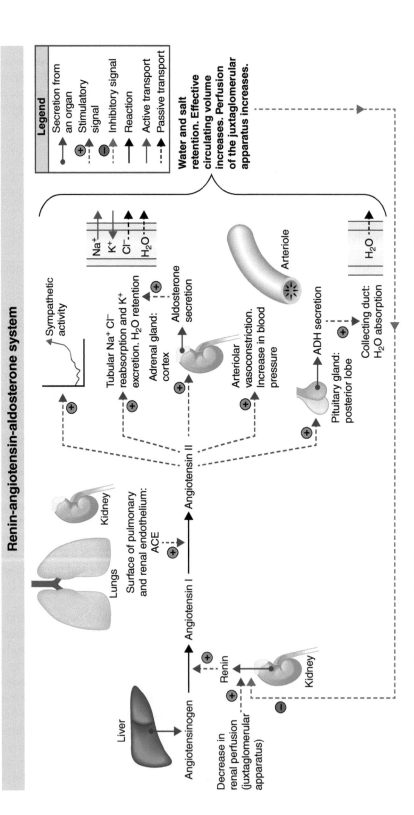

Figure 15.7 Mechanisms for the control of aldosterone secretion. *Source:* By A. Rad (me) – Own work, CC BY-SA 3.0, https://commons.wikimedia. org/w/index.php?curid=549506

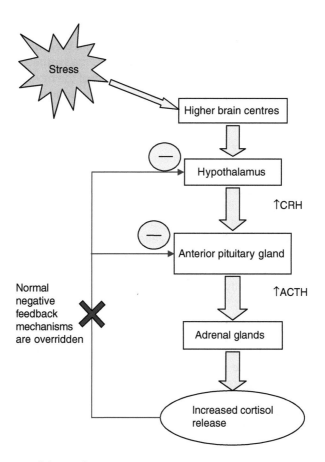

Figure 15.8   Response of the endocrine system to stress.

greater CRH release, and thus there is a significant increase in subsequent cortisol production (Figure 15.8).

The effect of cortisol on the body is to promote gluconeogenesis (the formation of glucose from fats and proteins), the release of fatty acids into the blood and the breakdown of stored proteins to provide amino acids for tissue repair (Mihai, 2014). Cortisol also enhances the vasoconstrictive effect of epinephrine in the control of vascular tone. Thus, cortisol helps to enable the body to respond to stressors of various types.

The pancreas

Located partially behind the stomach, the pancreas is a mixed gland containing both endocrine and exocrine gland cells. The majority of the gland is made up of acinar cells; these cells produce an enzyme-rich fluid that is secreted into the small intestines and aids the digestion of food. Scattered amongst the acinar cells are pancreatic islets, otherwise known as the islets of Langerhans. Each one of these islets is a collection of at least three major endocrine cell types, with each cell type producing a different hormone:

1. Alpha cells produce the hormone glucagon.
2. Beta cells are the most numerous of the cells, and they produce insulin.
3. Delta cells release somatostatin, a hormone that inhibits the release of glucagon and insulin.

Both insulin and glucagon are involved in the control of the blood levels of glucose, but they have directly opposite effects. Glucagon promotes the breakdown of glycogen stored in the liver into glucose (glycogenolysis); it also promotes the synthesis of glucose from fatty acids and amino acids (gluconeogenesis) and the release of the newly created glucose from the liver into the bloodstream. Thus, the major effect of glucagon is to raise glucose levels in the blood. The stimuli for the release of glucagon are decreased blood levels of glucose and increased blood levels of amino acids (e.g. after a protein-rich meal).

Insulin reduces the blood glucose levels and plays a role in the breakdown of protein and in the metabolism of fat. The target cells of insulin are virtually every cell in the body, especially the skeletal muscle cells (but not the brain, the liver and the kidneys). The effect of insulin on these cells is to promote the transport of glucose across the cell membrane into the cell body. Insulin also activates and promotes the enzyme systems within the cell to metabolise glucose to produce adenosine triphosphate (ATP), the basic fuel of body cells. Once the energy needs of the cells are met, insulin promotes the conversion of the remaining glucose into glycogen, and in the adipose tissues it promotes the conversion of glucose into fat molecules and the subsequent storage of these fat molecules in the cells (Bano, 2013). Finally, insulin promotes amino acid uptake by the muscle tissue and the formation of proteins from these amino acids. The release of insulin is stimulated by a rise in glucose levels in the blood, or increased blood levels of amino acids and fatty acids.

As the effect of each of these two hormones leads to the conditions that stimulates the release of the other hormone (e.g. as insulin reduces the blood levels of glucose, so the stimulus for the release of glucagon is increased), insulin and glucagon release is constantly being adjusted. The overall effect is maintenance of homeostasis by preventing large fluctuations in blood glucose.

Disorders of the endocrine system

Learning outcomes

On completion of this section, the reader will be able to:

- Describe the potential impact of hypopituitarism on the endocrine system.

- Describe the symptoms of disorders of the thyroid gland.

- Explain the need for close monitoring and observation of the patient suffering from an adrenal crisis.

- Discuss the role of the healthcare worker in the management of diabetes.

General considerations when caring for patients with an endocrine condition

Regardless of the particular endocrine condition, all patients share a need for psychological support and information, as do their relatives (Department of Health, 2006). Patients will require information on the particular disorders that they are suffering from and the signs and symptoms that they can expect the condition to manifest. Providing the patient with a clear understanding will:

- Reduce anxiety as to what the future may hold.
- Allow the patient to attribute signs and symptoms to their condition rather than enduring them.
- Give the patient control of their health and illness.
- Enable the patient to monitor their own disease and report deviations that may be attributed to a worsening condition or poor control.
- Encourage compliance with treatment regimens.

The pituitary gland

Hypopituitarism

Hypopituitarism is the inability of the pituitary gland to produce enough hormones for normal bodily functioning (Higham *et al.*, 2016). It can be caused by disorders of the pituitary gland itself or the reduction of hypothalamic-releasing hormones due to a disorder of the hypothalamus, thus reducing the stimuli for pituitary gland activity (Figure 15.9).

The most common cause of hypopituitarism is a tumour of either the pituitary gland or the hypothalamus, or a tumour in the same region that is putting pressure on the pituitary gland (Higham *et al.*, 2016). Other causes include genetic causes and, increasingly, the role of trauma to the brain has been recognised (e.g. stroke, trauma or radiation therapy). If a

441

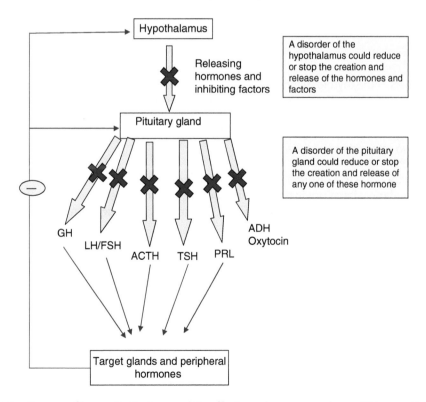

Figure 15.9 Causes of hypopituitarism and its effects on hormone release. GH, growth hormone; LH, luteinising hormone; FSH, follicle-stimulating hormone; ACTH, adrenocorticotropic hormone; TSH, thyroid-stimulating hormone; PRL, prolactin; ADH, antidiuretic hormone.

tumour is identified and surgically removed, then normal pituitary functioning may return; however, if destruction of pituitary gland tissue has occurred, or the cause is not reversible, the condition is chronic and lifelong. The signs and symptoms of hypopituitarism are related to the pituitary hormones that are deficient and their effect on target organs and tissues. In patients who have hypopituitarism caused by a tumour, there may be additional signs and symptoms caused by the tumour pressing on other structures in the same area of the brain, e.g. visual disturbances and headaches.

The treatment for the symptoms of hypopituitarism is to replace the hormones that are not being produced. This can either be a direct replacement of pituitary hormones, such as growth hormone, or replacement of the hormones normally produced by a target organ, e.g. thyroxine replacement therapy if TSH production is reduced. The signs and symptoms that patients may exhibit due to a reduction in the relevant target organ activity are dealt with in the corresponding sections of this chapter.

Diabetes insipidus

Diabetes insipidus is a condition where ADH production and release is reduced (e.g. due to head injury), leading to excessive urine output. A conscious patient can compensate for this increased output by drinking more to replace the fluids passed out as urine. An unconscious patient who may be at risk of diabetes insipidus, e.g. following head injury, requires close monitoring of their urine output. In the event of a reduction in ADH production, the patient will pass large amounts of urine and rapidly dehydrate. The patient should be catheterised and the urine output monitored and recorded at regular intervals. In the event of increased urine output, an unconscious patient cannot replace the excess fluid and will require intravenous fluids, close monitoring of fluid balance and observation for the signs of dehydration.

The thyroid gland

Disorders of the thyroid gland are the most common endocrine disorder encountered in the community setting. These disorders can be classified as either hypersecretion of thyroid hormones (excessive thyroid gland activity – hyperthyroidism) or hyposecretion of thyroid hormones (reduced thyroid gland activity – hypothyroidism). Thyroid disorders can be divided into two categories:

1. Primary – due to a disorder of the thyroid gland itself.
2. Secondary – alterations in thyroid function due to an increase or decrease in the production of either TRH from the hypothalamus or TSH from the pituitary gland.

The diagnosis of a disorder of the thyroid gland is often delayed as the signs and symptoms are vague and diverse, and in the elderly many signs and symptoms may be attributed to age. The introduction of simple laboratory tests for blood levels of the thyroid hormones has now made the diagnosis much easier, but delays in diagnosis are still common. The most useful tests for thyroid disease are the analysis of blood levels of TSH and free T_4. The expected findings of these tests in clinical thyroid disease are detailed in Table 15.2.

Table 15.2 Investigation – common laboratory test findings in the diagnosis of thyroid disease.

	Thyroid-stimulating hormone	Free T_4
Hyperthyroidism	Reduced	Normal or elevated
Hypothyroidism	Elevated	Normal or reduced

Snapshot   Thyroid function

Sarah Thompson is a 14-year-old young woman who has had a prolonged history of struggling though school. During her time at school, she reports she was constantly tired, depressed and 'couldn't be bothered'. She was constantly in trouble for not paying attention, and whenever she has to undertake classwork she found it difficult to concentrate. By the age of 13 years, she had been to the doctors many times. Nothing wrong was found, but she was questioned about her eating habits as she had been gaining weight. Sarah noted that she was constantly cold and even in summer wore a coat to school. Recently her GP had taken blood tests including thyroid function tests (see Table 15.2) and prescribed her tablets to take (levothyroxine), and since then she has been feeling much better. She says that the GP has asked her to go back for blood tests every 2 months.

Take some time to reflect on this case and then consider the following:

1. What are the likely results of Sarah's blood test (thyroid function test) and why are they like this?
2. What is the most likely cause of Sarah's hypothyroidism?
3. Why does the GP wish Sarah to have such regular blood tests?
4. What advice would you give Sarah about her medication?
5. Sarah is worried that there will be long-term consequences to her health from her condition, including dying prematurely. What would you tell Sarah in answer to her concerns?

Orange flag

Though Sarah is of the age of consent for medical treatment, it is highly likely that her parents will be involved in supporting her with managing her newly diagnosed condition. It is important that parents are involved, where appropriate, as they can be useful allies to the child in maintaining healthy behaviours and medication compliance. However, adults have differing learning needs from children and young people, and the information needs of the parents should be assessed as well as the needs of the young person (Nightingale *et al.*, 2015).

Hyperthyroidism

Excessive production of thyroid hormone is commonly due to Graves' disease, an autoimmune disorder where autoimmune antibodies mimic the effect of pituitary TSH, thus stimulating the excessive release of thyroid hormone. Other causes include thyroid cancer, thyroid nodules (usually non-cancerous), viral thyroiditis, postpartum thyroiditis and iodine-containing drugs (such as amiodarone) (Kahaly *et al.*, 2018).

The signs and symptoms of hyperthyroidism are related to the increased levels of thyroid hormone:

- Nervousness, restlessness, fatigue, insomnia
- Tachycardia, palpitations (atrial fibrillation is common in the elderly)
- Shortness of breath
- Weight loss despite an increased appetite, frequency of passing stools, nausea, vomiting
- Muscle weakness, tremors
- Warm, moist flushed skin
- Fine hair

- Staring gaze, exophthalmia
- Goitre
- Heat intolerance.

The long-term effects of hyperthyroidism can include cardiovascular disease (Khan *et al.*, 2020) and osteoporosis. In pregnancy, hyperthyroidism has been linked with higher rates of miscarriage, premature labour, eclampsia and low birth weight of the baby (Pearce, 2015).

Treatments for hyperthyroidism include the following:

- Surgery to remove part or all of the thyroid gland (rarely used except for surgical removal of thyroid tumours).
- Radioactive iodine – This treatment relies on the fact that the most active cells in the thyroid gland will take up the most iodine and thus be destroyed. Radioactive iodine is contraindicated in pregnancy.
- Antithyroid drugs (ATDs) – These reduce thyroid hormone production but do not damage the gland. However, in common with all drugs, ATDs have associated side effects and are poorly tolerated in the long term (Laurberg and Cooper, 2015).
- Symptomatic relief of tachycardia, palpitations, tremors and nervousness can be achieved with beta blockers such as atenolol.

Beyond treatment of the overactive thyroid gland, the management of hyperthyroidism also requires the alleviation of signs and symptoms, the provision of education and support, and monitoring of the patient for any deterioration of the condition:

- Anxiety management is essential, and the use of beta blockers should not be ignored. Psychological support and a calm environment are required to prevent exacerbation of nervousness.
- Provision of a cool, well-ventilated environment and an electric fan will help the patient to remain comfortable.
- Encourage regular fluid intake in patients who are perspiring excessively.
- The patient will be fatigued but will find it difficult to rest. A comfortable environment may aid relaxation and sleep.
- The healthcare worker should be watchful for the potential onset of a thyroid storm (Box 15.1), especially in the newly diagnosed or patients awaiting definitive treatment. Regular monitoring of vital signs and patterns of patient activity/mental state should be carried out.

Hypothyroidism

The causes of hypothyroidism are diverse and include treatment for hyperthyroidism (especially radioactive iodine therapy), radiation therapy of the neck and drugs, such as amiodarone and lithium (Taylor *et al.*, 2018). However, the most common cause of hypothyroidism is Hashimoto's thyroiditis (an autoimmune disorder).

As with hyperthyroidism, the signs and symptoms of hypothyroidism are varied, and it affects virtually every bodily system:

- Confusion, lethargy, memory loss, depression
- Bradycardia, enlarged heart (cardiomegaly), pericardial effusions
- Constipation, weight gain
- Muscle cramps, myalgia (generalised muscle aches), stiffness

Box 15.1   Endocrine emergency – thyroid storm

Thyroid storm is most common in patients with undiagnosed or poorly managed hyperthyroidism; it is due to the effect of high blood levels of thyroid hormone in association with increased sympathetic nervous system activity. There are several known causes of thyroid storm, including emotional or physical trauma and stress (Chiha *et al.*, 2015).

The patient exhibiting thyroid storm will be hyperthermic (temperature over 40°C), tachycardic (commonly atrial fibrillation is found on ECG monitoring), agitated and confused, and may be vomiting or have diarrhoea.

Patients in thyroid storm require close observation and monitoring in a critical care area. The temperature should be reduced by active cooling; intravenous fluids will be required as the patient will rapidly dehydrate, and the tachycardia may require control with beta-blocking drugs (Ferretti and Yee, 2019). Control of thyroid function and the reduction of circulating thyroid hormone are also normally required.

- Dry cool skin
- Brittle nails
- Coarse hair, hair loss
- Oedema of hands and eyelids
- Cold intolerance
- Vacant expression.

However, the development of the symptoms of hypothyroidism is often slow due to the fact that the thyroid gland stores a large amount of thyroid hormone, and this is released despite the inability of the gland to produce more.

In pregnancy, hypothyroidism has been linked to recurrent miscarriages and preterm labour; it is also suspected that untreated maternal hypothyroidism affects the development of the foetus, including the pituitary gland, and this is linked to reduced IQ in the child (Pearce, 2019).

The treatment of hypothyroidism is lifelong thyroxine replacement therapy (Jonklaas, 2016). In the first months of commencing thyroxine therapy, patients will require regular blood tests to ensure that a suitable blood level is achieved, and the dose may need to be altered several times during this period (Jonklaas, 2016). Once a suitable dose has been found, patients will require yearly blood tests to ensure that their needs have not changed; over-replacement of thyroid hormone is one of the leading causes of hyperthyroidism, but can be avoided and is easily rectified. Monitoring of concordance with replacement therapy and the use of strategies to encourage and maintain concordance are essential, as many patients are reluctant to take long-term thyroxine therapy (Eligar *et al.*, 2016). Patients should be counselled as to the possible side effects of thyroid replacement therapy, including temporary hair loss. Patients should be given information regarding what to do in the event of prolonged gastrointestinal disturbance that prevents taking oral medications. Acute illness or trauma may precipitate myxoedemic coma (Box 15.2), and patients must be made aware of the need to seek medical help.

Elderly patients are usually commenced on a lower dose, and their replacement requirements may be lower than those of a younger patient (Biondi and Cooper, 2019). Elderly patients in the community may also require regular health checks to ensure concordance with replacement therapy and monitoring of their symptoms (especially as relatives or carers may attribute symptoms to old age rather than to thyroid disease).

Medicines management

Caution must be exercised in commencing thyroxine therapy in patients with known ischaemic heart disease; these patients are usually commenced on a lower dose, and this is then slowly increased, as giving the patient the full replacement dose may worsen the symptoms of angina or even precipitate a myocardial infarction (Biondi and Cooper, 2019).

Box 15.2   Endocrine emergency – myxoedemic coma

Myxoedemic coma is the end stage of untreated hypothyroidism (Pangtey *et al.*, 2017). This may be due to the previously unrecognised hypothyroidism or the patient stopping replacement therapy; often the crisis is brought on by an underlying illness or trauma. If untreated, it will eventually result in the death of the patient.

The patient in myxoedemic coma will be hypothermic, bradycardic and have a slow, shallow respiratory rate. Blood tests will usually identify low blood levels of sodium and glucose as well as low blood levels of thyroid hormone.

Patients suffering from myxoedemic coma require admission to an intensive care unit for close monitoring, intubation and ventilation, and intravenous replacement of thyroxine, and will require fluid restriction to avoid further diluting the sodium levels in the blood.

The parathyroid glands

Hypoparathyroidism

Prior to the discovery of the parathyroid glands, patients undergoing surgery for removal of the thyroid gland often suffered from hypoparathyroidism as the parathyroid glands were removed along with the thyroid. The patient would subsequently suffer from parasthaesia, tetany and seizures due to the reduced availability of calcium. With the discovery of the parathyroid glands and the reduction of surgery for thyroid disorders, this outcome is now rare. Hypoparathyroidism due to the destruction of the parathyroid gland is now largely due to autoimmune syndromes. These patients require calcium and vitamin D replacement therapy to ensure the availability of calcium for normal muscle functioning.

Hyperparathyroidism

Hyperparathyroidism (excessive production of PTH) is most commonly due to an adenoma (a benign tumour) and is more common in women (Walker, 2016). These patients have raised blood levels of calcium, calcium in the urine and a decreased bone mass; they may also exhibit subtle signs of fatigue and muscle weakness. The current treatment for hyperparathyroidism is the surgical removal of the overactive glands. Traditional opinion has been that many patients will remain asymptomatic as the condition progresses slowly (if at all) and monitoring of parathyroid function is all that is required (Fraser, 2009); however, recent advances in imaging and testing techniques suggest that the effects of asymptomatic hyperparathyroidism are potentially harmful to the patient, and thus surgery may benefit a wider range of patients (Bilezikian *et al.*, 2014).

Red flag

Hypercalcaemia and cardiac arrhythmias

In patients with high calcium levels, for instance, due to hyperparathyroidism, cardiac arrhythmias are common (Walker, 2016). Patients with high calcium levels in the blood should be monitored closely for the onset of arrhythmias through the use of track and trigger systems (such as NEWS). Heart rate should be recorded manually by taking a pulse, as electronic devices often report only heart rate and do not offer information on rhythm and regularity. Abnormalities in vital signs or rhythm should be immediately reported to senior staff.

The adrenal glands

Cushing's disease

Excessive release of the corticosteroids is rare and normally due to a pituitary tumour increasing the release of ACTH; the most common cause of raised blood levels of the glucocorticoids is their therapeutic use in inflammatory conditions (such as asthma and arthritis). Patients with high levels of glucocorticoids in the blood show the signs and symptoms of Cushing's syndrome (Lonser *et al.*, 2017). These patients are commonly obese, with the main distribution of fat being around the face (moon facies), neck (buffalo hump), trunk and abdomen (Figure 15.10). Relative to the central obesity, the patient's arms and legs are often thin and spindly and the patient may report muscle weakness. The patient will often have thin, easily bruised skin and may report slow wound healing or frequent fungal infections; the majority of female patients will report increased hair growth on the face. Osteoporosis is common, and back pain is the most common presenting symptom (Rahaman *et al.*, 2018). The majority of patients with Cushing's syndrome will exhibit some signs of psychological disturbance, e.g. euphoria, mood swings, irritability, poor memory and difficulty in concentrating; disturbance of sleep patterns is common. The long-term effects of persistently high

447

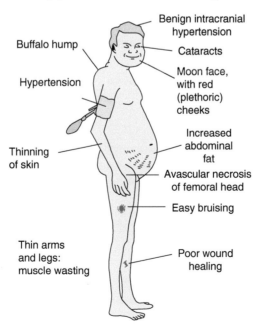

Figure 15.10   Cushing's syndrome (http://www.bmb.leeds.ac.uk/teaching/icu3/lecture/24/index.htm).

levels of glucocorticoids in the blood include hypertension, cardiovascular disease, susceptibility to infection and the development of steroid-induced diabetes.

The treatment of Cushing's disease is to remove or destroy the tumour (Lacroix *et al.*, 2015) or reduction of the doses of glucocorticoid treatment where possible.

Adrenal insufficiency

Adrenal insufficiency (the reduced production and release of corticosteroids from the adrenal glands) is divided into two types:

1. Primary adrenal insufficiency (Addison's disease) due to a disorder of the adrenal glands (Figure 15.11a). The leading cause of Addison's disease in the industrialised world is autoimmune adrenalitis (Hellesen *et al.*, 2018); other causes include tuberculosis, and fungal infection in immunosuppressed patients (such as HIV/AIDS or therapeutic suppression of the immune system).
2. Secondary adrenal insufficiency (Figure 15.11b) is more common and is due to the sudden cessation of glucocorticoid therapy (Paragliola *et al.*, 2017); however, tumours of the hypothalamic–pituitary region and their treatment are also a cause of secondary adrenal insufficiency.

448

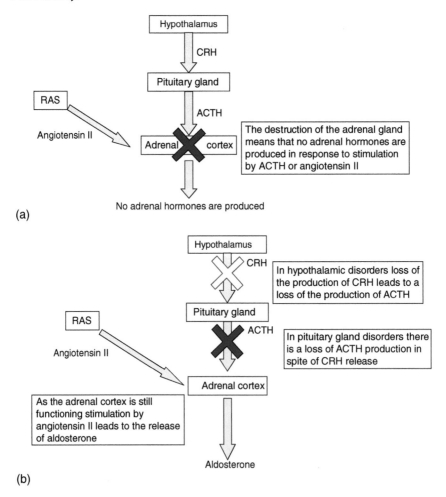

Figure 15.11　(a) Primary adrenal insufficiency and (b) secondary adrenal insufficiency.

The signs and symptoms of primary adrenal insufficiency are related to the lack of both glucocorticoid hormones and mineralocorticoid hormones (in secondary adrenal insufficiency, the release of mineralocorticoid hormones is preserved as it is under the control of the renin–angiotensin system, and thus symptoms related to a lack of aldosterone are not present). In the event of destruction of the adrenal glands (primary adrenal insufficiency), the loss of the adrenal medulla is not associated with clinically important symptoms, as the role of the medullary hormones (epinephrine and norepinephrine) is to magnify the effect of sympathetic nervous system activity, which remains intact.

The signs and symptoms of adrenal insufficiency are vague, and thus the majority of patients will exhibit signs and symptoms for up to a year before diagnosis (Husebye and Lovas, 2009):

- Fatigue, lack of stamina, loss of energy
- Reduced muscle strength
- Increased irritability
- Nausea
- Weight loss
- Muscle and joint pain
- Abdominal pain
- Low blood pressure
- Women may report a reduction in or loss of libido due to the lack of adrenal sex hormones

In addition, in primary adrenal insufficiency only:

- Symptoms related to the loss of aldosterone production, including dehydration, hypovolaemia (with possible postural hypotension), low blood levels of sodium and raised blood levels of potassium.
- Hyperpigmentation of the skin due to the stimulation of skin receptors by increased levels of ACTH. This can show as a darkening of the creases of the skin (e.g. in the palms, knuckles and oral mucosa), vitiligo (pale patches of skin) or an overall darkening of the skin (similar to a sun tan).

However, a proportion of patients will present as an acute adrenal crisis, which is often precipitated by trauma or infection (Box 15.3).

Medicines management

Patients who have been taking high-dose glucocorticoid therapy (such as prednisolone) are at risk of developing temporary adrenal gland atrophy (Paragliola et al., 2017); if the therapy is stopped suddenly, they can present with the signs and symptoms of adrenal insufficiency and even an acute adrenal crisis. Therefore, all patients taking glucocorticoid therapy should never stop their medication suddenly and should carry a 'steroid treatment card' at all times. A reducing dose of glucocorticoids is required to allow for the recovery of the adrenal glands to their full function (British Medical Association/Royal Pharmaceutical Society of Great Britain, 2016).

The treatment of adrenal insufficiency is the replacement of glucocorticoid hormones with oral hydrocortisone in two to three daily doses. In primary adrenal insufficiency, replacement of the mineralocorticoid hormones is also required; this is achieved by the administration of oral fludrocortisone once a day. However, the quality of life of patients with adrenal

449

Box 15.3   Endocrine emergency: adrenal crisis

Adrenal (or Addisonian) crisis is an acute life-threatening event often precipitated by an acute traumatic event, fever or other serious illness. Patients present with severe hypotension resistant to standard therapies such as inotropes, hypovolaemic shock, acute abdominal pain, vomiting, fever, hypoglycaemia, hyponatraemia and hyperkalaemia (Blanshard, 2011).

Treatment of an adrenal crisis requires close monitoring of a patient, including blood pressure monitoring, cardiac monitoring for potential arrhythmias caused by the high potassium levels in the blood, intravenous hydrocortisone to replace the depleted levels of corticosteroids and intravenous fluids to replace volume. Normal saline is the usual fluid used, as it will also replenish the reduced blood levels of sodium. Intravenous glucose may be required and, depending on the levels of potassium in the blood, therapies to reduce these levels may be commenced (e.g. diuretics to promote the excretion of potassium from the kidneys).

insufficiency is often reduced, even with optimum replacement therapy, and patients report fatigue, a lack of energy, depression and anxiety (Erichsen *et al.*, 2009).

Patients with permanent adrenal insufficiency (primary or secondary) will require education on the management of their replacement therapy (Bornstein *et al.*, 2016). Adrenal crises are often the result of a patient not increasing their replacement therapy in response to physical stressors (such as strenuous exercise, trauma, infection or fever). Patients admitted to hospital for a surgical procedure will require either intravenous or intramuscular hydrocortisone prior to surgery to prevent the onset of a crisis. In the event of persistent diarrhoea and vomiting that prevent the patient from taking their normal oral medications, hydrocortisone may be administered by intramuscular injection, and increasingly patients are doing this themselves or with the help of their relatives. Patients are often supplied with an emergency injection kit (hydrocortisone for intramuscular injection, needles and syringes) for the immediate management of an acute traumatic event or illness, and both the patient and their relatives should be trained in its use and their training and knowledge regularly refreshed (Bornstein *et al.*, 2016). It is strongly recommended that all patients with adrenal insufficiency wear a medical alert talisman (typically a bracelet or necklace).

Snapshot   Addison's disease

John Kroll is a 33-year-old gentleman who presents to the ED with a 48-hour history of diarrhoea and vomiting, abdominal pain and extreme dizziness. On questioning he reports a history of lethargy, tiredness, abdominal pain, alternating diarrhoea and constipation and hair loss. The doctor notes that John appears to have darkened skin in his skin creases (such as the creases in the palms, on the knuckles, between the top of the leg and the groin) and at the waistband.

John was diagnosed with an acute adrenal crisis probably due to primary adrenal insufficiency (Addison's disease). He was treated with intravenous hydrocortisone and normal saline infusions (see Box 15.3).

John was discharged a few days later and returned to the day case ward for a rapid ACTH stimulation test. On presentation to the day care unit, John was admitted to a bed, and two separate tubes of blood were taken for baseline cortisol and aldosterone values. Following this, synthetic ACTH was given via intramuscular or intravenous injection. Thirty minutes after these, two further blood tests were taken for cortisol and aldosterone values. Both the post-injection results showed no response to the injection of synthetic ACTH and this confirmed the diagnosis of Addison's disease.

Investigation   Synthetic ACTH as a diagnostic tool

Injection of synthetic ACTH is a commonly used assessment method; the synthetic ACTH stimulates the activity of the adrenal glands, and blood cortisol measures are measured before injection, at 30 minutes post injection and 60 minutes post injection to measure peak cortisol levels as a reflection of adrenal gland function (Saverino and Falorni, 2020).

Red flag

Thyroid function tests in undiagnosed Addison's disease

As the signs and symptoms of Addison's disease can be suggestive of hypothyroidism, the GP will normally request thyroid function tests (TFT) as well as a synthetic ACTH test. It is quite common for the TFT results to be returned before the synthetic ACTH test results. In untreated Addison's disease, the TFT results will show a hypothyroid pattern. It is essential the patient is not commenced on replacement thyroxine until Addison's disease is ruled out, as thyroxine replacement will precipitate a hypo-adrenal crisis in the untreated Addison's patient.

451

Vital signs

On admission to the ward, the following vital signs were noted and recorded:

Vital sign	Observation	Normal
Temperature	37.0°C	36.0–37.9°C range
Pulse	110 beats per minute	60–100 beats per minute
Respiration	26 breaths per minute	12–20 breaths per minute
Blood pressure	85/40 mmHg	100–139 mmHg (systolic) range
Oxygen saturation	96%	94–89%

A full blood count and urea and electrolytes was performed.

Test	Result	Guideline normal values
Potassium	6.2 mmol/L	3.5–5 mmol/L
Sodium	130 mmol/L	135–145 mmol/L
Creatinine	1.4 mg/dL	0.8–1.3 mg/dL
Blood urea nitrogen	23 mg/dL	8–21 mg/dL
Blood glucose	60 mg/dL	65–110 mg/dL

Take some time to reflect on this case, and then consider the following:

1. What do you think is the most likely cause of adrenal crisis?
2. How might you offer physical and psychological support to John?
3. What is the role and function of nurse before, during and after the ACTH stimulation test?

NEWS 2

John Kroll

Physiological parameter	3	2	1	0	1	2	3
Respiration rate							26
Oxygen saturation %				96			
Supplemental oxygen				No			
Temperature °C				37.0			
Systolic BP mmHg	85						
Heart rate					110		
Level of consciousness				A			
Score	3	0	0	0	1	0	3
Total	7						

The pancreas

Hypersecretion of insulin is very rare, and the cause of increased blood levels of insulin in the vast majority of patients is over-administration of insulin in the management of diabetes mellitus (Marieb and Hoehn, 2018).

Diabetes mellitus (diabetes) is a group of disorders characterised by raised blood levels of glucose (WHO, 2006). There are two main types of diabetes: type 1 and type 2 diabetes. However, the signs and symptoms of the two types are similar:

- High blood glucose levels
- Glucose in the urine
- Ketones in the urine
- Frequency in passing urine (including waking at night)
- Thirst
- Increased appetite (usually type 1 only)
- Weight loss (usually type 1 only)
- Fatigue
- Abdominal pain.

Type 2 diabetes can often be asymptomatic and only diagnosed on opportunistic screening or as a chance finding whilst the patient is being investigated or treated for other medical problems.

The signs and symptoms of diabetes are related to the high levels of glucose in the blood and the inability of the cells to utilise glucose due to a lack of insulin production or resistance to the effect of insulin in the body. Glucose is excreted by the renal tubules into the urine, and this leads to increased urine production due to the osmotic effect of the glucose (water is drawn into and retained in the urine by the high levels of glucose). Thus, body levels of water are depleted, and there is subsequent development of chronic thirst. The inability of the cells to use glucose as a primary fuel source leads to the metabolism of fats and amino acids and thus weight loss. Furthermore, the utilisation of fats and amino acids as fuel in the cells leads to the production of ketones (which are strong acids); these are excreted in the urine, and as they are negatively charged they carry sodium and potassium ions with them, leading to electrolyte imbalance, a sign of which is abdominal pain (Marieb and Hoehn, 2018). Eventually, these processes can lead to an acute life-threatening hyperglycaemic event (Box 15.4).

Snapshot   Type 2 diabetes

David Arthur is a 43-year-old factory worker who lives alone following a divorce 10 years ago. He has been admitted to hospital for a routine hernia operation. Routine urinalysis shows a high level of urinary glucose, but he denies having diabetes. Mr Arthur has a long history of psychotic disorders, having first being diagnosed at the age of 20, and he has been taking antipsychotic medication ever since. Talking to Mr Arthur, he reports being frustrated by his weight. Further questioning reveals that he eats a high-fat, high-sugar diet. He has been a smoker since the age of 15 and continues to smoke 20 cigarettes per day. He does no regular exercise as he feels constantly tired and lethargic, which has created problems for him at work. He has read that his medicines may be responsible for his weight and his lethargy, but his GP will only discuss diet and exercise with him, which leaves him frustrated.

Box 15.4   Endocrine emergency: hyperglycaemia

Patients with either type 1 or type 2 diabetes are at risk of developing life-threatening hyperglycaemia (Beltran, 2014).

Hyperosmolar hyperglycaemic state (HHS) is commonly associated with older patients with type 2 diabetes. The onset is usually over days to weeks, and it may be the first indication that a patient is suffering from type 2 diabetes. HHS is characterised by a very high blood glucose (>33.3 mmol/L and often over 50 mol/L), dehydration and confusion, but the absence of significant levels of ketones and therefore no acidaemia (reduced blood pH). Dehydration occurs due to excessive urine output, and low blood levels of sodium and potassium are common.

Diabetic ketoacidosis (DKA) is associated with type 1 diabetes and has a rapid onset (normally less than 24 hours). Patients present with hyperglycaemia (but usually not greater than 40 mmol/L due to the rapid onset of DKA), ketosis (ketones in the blood), acidaemia, dehydration and reduced blood levels of sodium and potassium. The characteristic 'pear drop' or 'acetone' smell to the breath of a patient with DKA is produced by the excess of ketones in the blood.

The management of both HHS and DKA is similar and is aimed at replacing the lost fluid, reducing the blood glucose and correcting electrolyte imbalances. Large amounts of intravenous fluids are given (typically 1–1.5 L in the first hour), and potassium is usually added to subsequent fluids after the initial rapid fluid resuscitation. Low-dose intravenous insulin is commenced to slowly reduce the blood glucose, and the patient is closely monitored, including regular assessment of vital signs, blood glucose and electrolytes (Beltran, 2014).

Take some time to reflect on this case and then consider the following:

1. What risk factors does Mr Arthur have for developing diabetes mellitus?
2. What tests could be carried out to confirm your suspicion that Mr Arthur is suffering from diabetes mellitus?
3. What lifestyle advice would you give Mr Arthur?
4. What is the potential relationship between antipsychotic medicines and diabetes? What advice could you give Mr Arthur? You may wish to read Holt (2019) to help you understand the potential relationship.

Type 1 diabetes

Type 1 diabetes develops most commonly in childhood or early adulthood and comprises about 15% of the total incidence of diabetes in the UK; however, the rate of type 1 diabetes is increasing, particularly in children younger than 5 years of age (Patterson *et al.*, 2019). Type 1 diabetes is normally caused by autoimmune destruction of the beta cells of the pancreas and is therefore associated with a severe reduction in, or complete loss of, insulin production (Kahaly and Hansen, 2016).

The treatment of type 1 diabetes is the replacement of insulin, normally by subcutaneous injection, although alternative methods of administration (including inhaled insulin, nasal administration of insulin and oral insulin) are currently under investigation (Cheung and Senior, 2015). Care must be taken to ensure that the insulin administered is balanced by a sufficient intake of food (particularly carbohydrates, as sugars are quickly used in the body) to avoid low blood sugar levels (hypoglycaemia). Profound hypoglycaemia leads to the patient becoming mentally agitated, possibly aggressive; often the patient will be sweating profusely and will look pale. If the dose of insulin administered is not matched by sufficient intake of food, the patient will eventually become comatose and may die. Conscious patients may be given a sugary snack or drink and some form of carbohydrates; the patient will then require monitoring of their blood glucose until the crisis has passed. Unconscious patients require immediate medical assistance and the administration of an intramuscular injection of glucagon and potentially intravenous glucose (Beltran, 2014).

Orange flag

Diabetes is associated with significant mental health problems in both adults and children. Adults have been shown to suffer from a specialised form of anxiety known as diabetes distress which is related to the stress of the daily management of diabetes. Diabetes distress is associated with increased adverse outcomes in diabetes. In children and young people, diabetes is associated with depression, eating disorders and diabetes distress (Robinson *et al.*, 2018).

Medicines management

When injecting insulin, patients often use the same area (commonly under the umbilicus). However, this repeated use of the same injection areas can lead to the formation of fatty lumps (lipo-hypertrophies or lipos) or atrophy of the site. The absorption of insulin from lipos is known to be slow and erratic, and this can lead to poor glycaemic control. Thus, the user increases their insulin requirements in response to higher blood glucose measurements. Should the patient then choose to inject into a fresh site (with normal blood flow), the increased insulin injected may lead to a hypoglycaemic attack. It is therefore important that patients are educated to rotate injection sites on a daily basis to reduce the formation of lipos.

Type 2 diabetes

This is the most common form of diabetes and is traditionally thought to be a disease of people over the age of 40 years. Overall the number of patients developing type 2 diabetes is increasing, and this increase is occurring across all age ranges, including in adolescents and young adults (Candler *et al.*, 2018). The reasons for this increase are probably related to lifestyle factors, including overeating (particularly sugary foods), a lack of exercise and the increase in the rates of obesity (Candler *et al.*, 2018).

Type 2 diabetes is normally characterised by the development of resistance to the effects of insulin in the tissues, and a reduction in the ability of the beta cells to increase the production of insulin in response to this increased insulin resistance in the body. The resulting high blood levels of glucose lead to damage of the beta cells, thus further reducing the production of insulin. The treatment of type 2 diabetes varies depending on the severity of the condition. In some patients, weight reduction, increased exercise and reduced food intake can resolve the raised blood sugar levels. However, once the beta cell damage has occurred, the need for medications is increased. Current drug therapies for type 2 diabetes (oral hypoglycaemics) target several aspects of the disease, including reducing glucose production by the liver, enhancing insulin output from the pancreas or increasing the sensitivity of the muscle, fat and liver cells to the effects of insulin and thus reducing insulin resistance. Increasingly, a role is being seen for the use of insulin in type 2 diabetes (Ceriello *et al.*, 2020).

Patients with both type 1 and type 2 diabetes will have similar educational needs in terms of their personal control of the diabetes. The aim of disease management is to alleviate the symptoms of diabetes and optimise the control of blood glucose levels, thus preventing long-term complications. Healthcare interventions include the following:

- Advice on appropriate diet – Current advice emphasises the need for a healthy, balanced diet. This includes reducing the amount of sugar and fat that is eaten, increasing the intake of fruit and vegetables, and substituting wholemeal bread and pastas for refined products such as white bread (Diabetes UK, 2011).
- Encouraging regular physical activity – However, strenuous exercise can reduce blood glucose levels, and exercise regimens should be agreed with appropriate healthcare professionals.
- Advice and support for weight loss if required – Weight loss in overweight patients improves the control of diabetes as inactivity and obesity are strongly linked to insulin resistance (Abdelaal *et al.*, 2017).
- Advice and support on stopping smoking – Patients with diabetes have an increased risk of vascular diseases (including heart disease and stroke), and smoking further increases this risk.
- Education on how to monitor blood glucose levels using capillary blood glucose monitoring or urinalysis (as appropriate).
- The use and administration of medications, such as insulin injection techniques and adjusting insulin doses.

Poor control of diabetes often leads to hyperglycaemia and is associated with a range of long-term complications, including blindness or reduced vision, peripheral neuropathy, renal failure, cardiovascular disease, peripheral artery disease and foot ulcers (Box 15.5).

455

Red flag

Mobilising the diabetic patient

Patients under your care who suffer from diabetes must not be mobilised without appropriate footwear to protect the feet from damage. The poor sensation and blood flow in the feet of many diabetic patients mean that any damage to the foot through trauma (such as stubbing a toe, stepping on a sharp item) can lead to the development of foot ulcers. See Box 15.5.

Box 15.5   Focus on diabetic foot ulcers

Excluding accidents, diabetes is the leading cause of lower limb amputations in the UK (Paisey *et al.*, 2018); patients with diabetes have an approximately 15% lifetime risk of developing a foot ulcer (Lebrun *et al.*, 2010).

The causes of diabetic foot ulcers are neuropathic, ischaemic or a mixture of both:

- Neuropathic – The reduced sensation in the feet of patients with peripheral neuropathy means that they are often unaware of the mechanical stresses being placed on their feet due to poorly fitting footwear or trauma (such as standing on a sharp object).
- Ischaemic – The reduced peripheral circulation in patients with long-term complications leads to easily damaged skin with a reduced ability to heal in response to damage.

Not all diabetic foot ulcers become infected, but when they do, the patient's limb, and sometimes life, can be in danger as the wound does not heal rapidly, and infection can spread easily due to the reduction in the delivery of white blood cells to the peripheral tissues.

The treatment of diabetic foot ulcers may require surgical debridement of the wound to remove dead tissue which is a host for bacteria; appropriate wound dressings and antibiotics may also be necessary (Yazdanpanah *et al.*, 2015). Relief of pressure on the ulcer is critical to the success of treatment, and referral to a podiatrist will be required for continued foot care and assessment for pressure-relieving devices (Bus *et al.*, 2016).

Conclusion

This chapter has introduced the physiology of both normal and disordered endocrine functioning and the treatment of the related disorders. The endocrine system has a wide and varied role in the maintenance of normal bodily functioning. Disorders of any of the endocrine organs can produce a variety of signs and symptoms and may even lead to a life-threatening crisis. The healthcare professional has a crucial role in the detection of endocrine conditions, the monitoring of disease progression and treatment effects, and the prevention and treatment of endocrine emergencies. Most patients with an endocrine disorder will take responsibility for the management of their own condition, and it is essential that they are given appropriate advice and support. In order to carry out these roles, the healthcare professional must have a good understanding of the physiology and treatment of endocrine disorders.

Activities

Here are some activities and exercises to help test your learning. For the answers to these exercises, as well as further self-testing activities, visit our website at **www.wiley.com/go/fundamentalsofappliedpathophysiology/student4e**

Multiple choice questions

1. Downregulation is the reduction of:
   (a) Hormone release
   (b) Hormone receptors
   (c) Stimuli for hormone release
   (d) Excretion of hormones.

2. The excretion of the products of hormone breakdown occurs mostly via:
   (a) The faeces
   (b) The urine
   (c) The breath
   (d) The sweat

3. Which hormones are mostly released due to neural stimulation?
   (a) Epinephrine
   (b) Thyroxine
   (c) Insulin
   (d) Luteinising hormone

4. The main type of body cell that are stimulated by growth hormone are:
   (a) Pancreatic
   (b) Brain
   (c) Liver
   (d) Bone

5. The main effect of ADH is to:
   (a) Increase sodium reabsorption
   (b) Decrease sodium reabsorption
   (c) Increase water reabsorption
   (d) Decrease water reabsorption

6. The thyroid gland can store how many days' worth of hormone supply?
   (a) 70 days
   (b) 80 days
   (c) 90 days
   (d) 100 days

7. How many pairs of parathyroid glands do most people normally have?
   (a) 2
   (b) 4
   (c) 6
   (d) 8

8. The role of parathyroid hormone is to help maintain levels of which ion?
   (a) Calcium
   (b) Sodium
   (c) Potassium
   (d) Chloride

9. The main glucocorticoid hormones secreted by the adrenal gland is:
   (a) Corticosteroid
   (b) Cortisol
   (c) Cortisone
   (d) Aldosterone

10. The beta cells of the pancreas secrete what hormone?
    (a) Glucagon
    (b) Insulin
    (c) Somatostatin
    (d) Melatonin
11. The most common cause of thyroid disorders is:
    (a) Autoimmune disorders
    (b) Genetic disorders
    (c) Smoking
    (d) Dietary factors
12. In untreated primary hypoadrenalism, blood tests will show:
    (a) Normal potassium, reduced sodium
    (b) Reduced potassium, reduced sodium
    (c) Raised sodium, reduced potassium
    (d) Reduced sodium, raised potassium
13. Hyperosmolar hyperglycaemic state (HHS) is associated with:
    (a) A serum glucose below 5 mmol/L
    (b) A serum glucose between 5 and 7 mmol/L
    (c) A serum glucose between 20 and 30 mmol/L
    (d) A serum glucose over 33 mmol/l
14. The increase the incidence of type 2 diabetes in children is due to:
    (a) Sugary foods
    (b) Lack of exercise
    (c) Obesity
    (d) All of the above
15. The lifetime risk of developing a foot ulcer for diabetic patients is:
    (a) 10%
    (b) 15%
    (c) 20%
    (d) 25%

Conditions

The following is a list of conditions that are associated with the endocrine system. Take some time and write notes about each of the conditions. You may make the notes taken from text books or other resources (e.g. people you work with in a clinical area), or you may make the notes based on people you have cared for. If you are making notes about people you have cared for, you must ensure that you adhere to the rules of confidentiality.

Hashimoto's disease	
Acromegaly	

Exophthalmia	
Hypopituitarism	
Pheochromocytoma	

Further resources

Addison's Disease Self-Help Group

https://www.addisonsdisease.org.uk/

The website of the only UK-based group specifically for those suffering from Addison's disease (adrenal insufficiency) is not only a good resource for patients diagnosed with Addison's disease, but also contains much information that is useful to the healthcare professional.

Diabetes UK

www.diabetes.org.uk

The website of the largest organisation in the UK for people with diabetes has a large amount of information, including latest news regarding diabetes and guidance ranging from the clinical to the more practical (e.g. recipes for those with diabetes). The two 'Guides to Diabetes' are a useful starting point for anyone wanting to know more about this condition.

EndocrineSurgeon.co.uk

www.endocrinesurgeon.co.uk

The personal website of surgical endocrinologist Mr John Lynn is hugely informative, with detailed sections on endocrine conditions, diagnostic tests and surgical procedures. It is interesting to note that this website is often highly recommended by other websites.

Pituitary Foundation

www.pituitary.org.uk

This website contains many useful resources. There is a comprehensive list of web links, reviews of pituitary-related disorders and proceedings from conferences (which are often hard to find).

The Endocrine Society

www.endo-society.org

This is the website of the world's largest society dedicated to the practice of endocrinology. It is worth viewing regularly as the news section is kept updated, and there is a useful clinical guidelines section, including guidelines on some lesser-known conditions such as Cushing's syndrome.

Glossary of terms

Acidaemia   A state of relative acidity of the blood.

Adenoma   A tumour of glandular tissue (usually benign).

Adenosine triphosphate (ATP)   A compound of an adenosine molecule with three attached phosphoric acid molecules. Essential for the production of cellular energy.

Adrenalitis   Inflammatory condition of the adrenal glands.

Amino acid   The building block of proteins. The type of protein that is produced depends upon the number and types of amino acids that are used to construct it.

Arrhythmia   A disorder of the normal heart beat.

Asymptomatic   Without symptoms.

Atrophy   Wasting away; a diminution in the site of a cell, tissue or organ.

Autoimmune   Immune response to the body's own tissues.

Benign   Causes no problem. In cancer, it means a growth that is not malignant.

Concordance   Current term for the person's adherence to a prescribed treatment.

Debridement   Removal of damaged tissues and cells.

Diuretic   A drug that increases urine output.

Eclampsia   A condition presenting in pregnancy that is characterised by high blood pressure, seizures and even coma.

Electrolyte   A chemical element compound that includes sodium, potassium, calcium, chloride and bicarbonate.

Endocrine gland   A ductless gland that secretes hormones into the bloodstream.

Euphoria   An exaggerated state of well-being; the opposite of dysphoria.

Exocrine gland   A gland that secretes hormones into ducts that carry the secretions to other sites (e.g. the intestine).

Exophthalmos   Excessive protrusion of the eyeballs.

Free T$_4$ Thyroxine in the blood that is not bound to proteins.

Gland   Any organ in the body that secretes substances not related to its own internal functioning.

Glycogen   A carbohydrate (complex sugar) made from glucose. Excess glucose is stored as glycogen, mainly in the liver.

Goitre   Pronounced swelling of the neck.

Homeostasis   Maintenance of relatively constant conditions within the body's internal environment despite external environmental changes.

Hormone   A chemical substance that is released into the blood by the endocrine system, and that exerts physiological control over the function of cells or organs other than those that created it.

Hyperglycaemia   A high blood level of glucose.

Hyperkalaemia   A high blood level of potassium.

Hypersecretion   A high rate of secretion.

Hypertension   Raised blood pressure.

Hyperthermic   High body temperature.

Hypoglycaemia   A low blood level of glucose.

Hyponatraemia   A low blood level of sodium.

Hyposecretion   A low rate of secretion.

Hypotension   Low blood pressure.

Hypothermic   Low body temperature.

Hypovolaemia   Low level of fluid in the circulation.

Inotrope   A drug used to increase the blood pressure in the critically ill.

Insulin resistance   A condition where the usual body reaction to insulin is reduced.

Ion   An atom or group of atoms that carries either a positive or a negative electrical charge.

Ischaemic heart disease   A condition of the heart related to a lack of oxygen reaching the heart muscle.

Ketosis   Ketones in the blood.

Malignant   Invasive, has a tendency to grow and may spread to other parts of the body.

Neuropathy   Inflammation and degeneration of the nerves.

Opportunistic screening   Testing a person for particular diseases or conditions at a point in time they are accessing healthcare for other reasons.

Oral hypoglycaemic   A drugs used in the treatment of diabetes that is taken by mouth and reduces the blood sugar level.

Osmosis   The passive movement of water through a selectively permeable membrane from an area of high concentration of a chemical to an area of low concentration.

Osteoclast   A type of cell that breaks down bone tissue and thus releases the calcium used to create bones.

Osteoporosis   A condition characterised by reduced bone density and an increased risk of fractures.

Palpitations   A feeling of pounding or racing of the heart.

Parasthaesia   Abnormal nerve sensations such as pins and needles, tingling or burning.

Peripheral artery disease   Disease of the arteries of the legs.

Podiatrist   A healthcare professional who specialises in the diagnosis and treatment of disorders of the feet (also known as a chiropodist).

Postural hypotension   Inability of the body to maintain an adequate blood pressure when the person rises from sitting or lying to standing too rapidly. Usually characterised by dizziness or fainting if the person rises too quickly to a standing position.

Tachycardia   Fast heart beat (usually defined as above 100 beats per minute).

Tetany   Prolonged muscular spasms.

Thyroiditis   An inflammatory condition of the thyroid gland.

Thyroid nodule   The growth of thyroid tissue or fluid-filled cyst of the thyroid tissue.

References

Abdelaal, M., le Roux, C.W., & Docherty, N.G. (2017). Morbidity and mortality associated with obesity. *Annals of Translational Medicine*, 5(7): 161.

Arrangoiz, R., Cordera, F., Caba, D., Juárez, M. M., Moreno, E. and Luque, E. (2017). Parathyroid embryology, anatomy, and pathophysiology of primary hyperparathyroidism. *International Journal of Otolaryngology and Head & Neck Surgery*, 6(4): 39–58.

Bano, G. (2013). Glucose homeostasis, obesity and diabetes. *Best Practice & Research Clinical Obstetrics & Gynaecology*, 27(5): 715–726.

Beltran, G. (2014). Diabetic emergencies: New strategies for an old disease. *Emergency Medicine Practice*, 16(6): 1–19.

Bilezikian, J.P., Brandi, M.L., Eastell, R., Silverberg, S.J., Udelsman, R. *et al.* (2014). Guidelines for the management of asymptomatic primary hyperparathyroidism: Summary statement from the Fourth International Workshop. *The Journal of Clinical Endocrinology & Metabolism*. 99(10): 3561–3569.

Biondi, B. and Cooper, D.S. (2019). Thyroid hormone therapy for hypothyroidism. *Endocrine*, 1–9.

Blanshard, H. (2011). Endocrine and metabolic disease. In: Allman, K.G. and Wilson, I.H. (eds), *Oxford Handbook of Anaesthesia*, 3rd edn. Oxford: Oxford University Press, pp. 155–190.

Bornstein, S.R., Allolio, B., Arlt, W., Barthel, A., Don-Wauchope, A. *et al*. (2016). Diagnosis and treatment of primary adrenal insufficiency: an endocrine society clinical practice guideline. *The Journal of Clinical Endocrinology & Metabolism*, 101(2): 364–389.

Borrow, A.P. and Cameron, N.M. (2012). The role of oxytocin in mating and pregnancy. *Hormones and Behavior*, 61(3): 266–276.

British Medical Association/Royal Pharmaceutical Society of Great Britain (2016). *British National Formulary*, 71st edn. London: British Medical Association/Royal Pharmaceutical Society of Great Britain.

Bus, S.A., Armstrong, D.G., Deursen, R.W., Lewis, J.E.A., Caravaggi, C.F. and Cavanagh, P.R. (2016). IWGDF guidance on footwear and offloading interventions to prevent and heal foot ulcers in patients with diabetes. *Diabetes/Metabolism Research and Reviews*, 32(S1): 25–36.

Campbell, I. (2014). Thyroid and parathyroid hormones and calcium homeostasis. *Anaesthesia & Intensive Care Medicine*, 15(10): 481–484.

Candler, T.P., Mahmoud, O., Lynn, R.M., Majbar, A.A., Barrett, T.G. and Shield, J.P.H. (2018). Epidemiology Continuing rise of Type 2 diabetes incidence in children and young people in the UK. *Diabetic Medicine*, 35(6): 737–744.

Ceriello, A., deValk, H.W., Guerci, B., Haak, T., Owens, D., Canobbio, M. *et al*. (2020). The burden of type 2 diabetes in Europe: Current and future aspects of insulin treatment from patient and healthcare spending perspectives. *Diabetes Research and Clinical Practice*, 161: 108053.

Cheung, K.K.T. and Senior, P.A. (2015). Novel and emerging insulin preparations for type 2 diabetes. *Canadian Journal of Diabetes*, 39: S160–S166.

Chiha, M., Samarasinghe, S. and Kabaker, A. (2015). Thyroid storm. An updated review. *Journal of Intensive Care Medicine*, 30(3): 131–140.

Dagklis, T., Ravanos, K., Makedou, K., Kourtis, A. and Rousso, D. (2015). Common features and differences of the hypothalamic–pituitary–gonadal axis in male and female. *Gynecological Endocrinology*, 31(1): 14–17.

Department of Health (2006). *Supporting People with Long-term Conditions to Self Care: A Guide to Developing Local Strategies and Good Practice*. London: Department of Health.

Diabetes UK (2011). *Evidence-based Nutrition Guidelines for the Prevention and Management of Diabetes*. London: Diabetes UK.

Eligar, V., Taylor, P.N., Okosieme, O.E., Leese, G.P. and Dayan, C.M. (2016). Thyroxine Replacement: A clinical endocrinologist's viewpoint. *Annals of Clinical Biochemistry: An International Journal of Biochemistry and Laboratory Medicine*, 53(4): 421–433.

Erichsen, M.M., Lovas, K., Skinningsrud, B. *et al*. (2009). Clinical, immunological, and genetic features of autoimmune primary adrenal insufficiency: Observations from a Norwegian registry. *Journal of Clinical Endocrinology and Metabolism*, 94(12): 4882–4890.

Ferretti, N. and Yee, J. (2019). Thyroid storm. *Journal of Education and Teaching in Emergency Medicine*, 4(3): S1–S24.

Fraser, W.D. (2009). Hyperparathyroidism. *The Lancet*, 374(9684): 145–148.

Hall, J. and Hall, M. (2020). *Guyton and Hall Textbook of Medical Physiology*, 14th edn. Philadelphia: Elsevier Saunders.

Hellesen, A., Bratland, E. and Husebye, E.S. (2018). Autoimmune Addison's disease–An update on pathogenesis. In: *Annales d'endocrinologie* (Vol. 79, No. 3). Elsevier Masson, pp. 157–163.

Higham, C.E., Johannsson, G. and Shalet, S.M. (2016). Hypopituitarism. *The Lancet*, 388(10058): 2403–2415.

Holt, R.I. (2019). Association between antipsychotic medication use and diabetes. *Current Diabetes Reports*, 19(10): 96.

Husebye, E. and Lovas, K. (2009) Pathogenesis of primary adrenal insufficiency. *Best Practice and Research. Clinical Endocrinology and Metabolism*, 23(2): 147–157.

Jonklaas, J. (2016). Update on the treatment of hypothyroidism. *Current Opinion in Oncology*, 28(1): 18.

Kahaly, G.J., Bartalena, L., Hegedüs, L., Leenhardt, L., Poppe, K. and Pearce, S.H. (2018). 2018 European Thyroid Association guideline for the management of Graves' hyperthyroidism. *European Thyroid Journal*, 7(4): 167–186.

Kahaly, G.J. and Hansen, M.P. (2016). Type 1 diabetes associated autoimmunity. *Autoimmunity Reviews*, 15(7): 644–648.

Khan, R., Sikanderkhel, S., Gui, J., Adeniyi, A.R., O'Dell, K. *et al*. (2020). Thyroid and cardiovascular disease: A focused review on the impact of hyperthyroidism in heart failure. *Cardiology Research*, 11(2): 68.

Lacroix, A., Feelders, R.A., Stratakis, C.A. and Nieman, L.K. (2015). Cushing's syndrome. *The Lancet*. 386(9996): 913–927.

Laurberg, P. and Cooper, D.S. (2015). Antithyroid drug therapy in patients with Graves' Disease. In: Bahn, R.S. (ed.), *Graves' Disease*. New York: Springer, pp. 65–82.

Lebrun, E., Tomic Canic, M. and Kirsner, R.S. (2010). The role of surgical debridement in healing of diabetic foot ulcers. *Wound Repair and Regeneration*, 18(5): 433–438.

Lonser, R.R., Nieman, L. and Oldfield, E.H. (2017). Cushing's disease: Pathobiology, diagnosis, and management. *Journal of Neurosurgery*, 126(2): 404–417.

Marieb, E.N. and Hoehn, K. (2018). *Human Anatomy and Physiology*, 11th edn. San Francisco: Pearson Benjamin Cummings.

Mihai, R. (2014). Physiology of the pituitary, thyroid, parathyroid and adrenal glands. *Surgery (Oxford)*, 32(10): 504–512.

Nightingale, R., Friedl, S. and Swallow, V. (2015). Parents' learning needs and preferences when sharing management of their child's long-term/chronic condition: A systematic review. *Patient Education and Counseling*, 98(11): 1329–1338.

Paisey, R.B., Abbott, A., Levenson, R., Harrington, A., Browne, D. *et al*. (2018). Diabetes-related major lower limb amputation incidence is strongly related to diabetic foot service provision and improves with enhancement of services: peer review of the South-West of England. *Diabetic Medicine*, 35(1): 53–62.

Pangtey, G.S., Baruah, U., Baruah, M.P. and Bhagat, S. (2017). Thyroid emergencies: new insight into old problems. *Journal of the Association of Physicians of India*, 65: 68.

Paragliola, R.M., Papi, G., Pontecorvi, A. and Corsello, S.M. (2017). Treatment with synthetic glucocorticoids and the hypothalamus-pituitary-adrenal axis. *International Journal of Molecular Sciences*, 18(10): 2201.

Patterson, C.C., Harjutsalo, V., Rosenbauer, J., Neu, A., Cinek, O. *et al*. (2019). Trends and cyclical variation in the incidence of childhood type 1 diabetes in 26 European centres in the 25 year period 1989–2013: A multicentre prospective registration study. *Diabetologia*, 62(3): 408–417.

Pearce, E.N. (2015). Thyroid disorders during pregnancy and postpartum. *Best Practice & Research Clinical Obstetrics & Gynaecology*, 29(5): 700–706.

Pearce, E.N. (2019). *Hypothyroidism in pregnancy*. In *Thyroid Disease and Reproduction*. Springer, Cham, pp. 101–115.

Rahaman, S.H., Jyotsna, V.P., Kandasamy, D., Shreenivas, V., Gupta, N. and Tandon, N. (2018). Bone health in patients with Cushing's syndrome. *Indian Journal of Endocrinology and Metabolism*, 22(6): 766.

Ritchie, J.E. and Balasubramanian, S.P. (2014). Anatomy of the pituitary, thyroid, parathyroid and adrenal glands. *Surgery (Oxford)*, 32(10): 499–503.

Robinson, D.J., Coons, M., Haensel, H., Vallis, M. and Yale, J.F. (2018). Diabetes and mental health. *Canadian Journal of Diabetes*, 42(Suppl. 1): S130–S141.

Saverino, S. and Falorni, A. (2020). Autoimmune Addison's disease. *Best Practice & Research Clinical Endocrinology & Metabolism*, 34(1): 101379.

Stathatos, N. (2012). Thyroid physiology. *Medical Clinics*, 96(2): 165–173.

Taylor, P.N., Albrecht, D., Scholz, A., Gutierrez-Buey, G., Lazarus, J.H. *et al*. (2018). Global epidemiology of hyperthyroidism and hypothyroidism. *Nature Reviews Endocrinology*, 14(5): 301.

Tortora, G.J. and Derrickson, B. (2011). *Principles of anatomy and physiology, vol. 1: Organisation, Support and Movement, and Control of the Human Body. International Student Version*, 13th edn. Hoboken, NJ: John Wiley & Sons Inc.

Walker, J. (2016). Primary hyperparathyroidism and the role of the nurse. *Nursing Older People*, 28(6): 27–32.

World Health Organization (WHO) (2006). *Fact Sheet No. 312 Diabetes*. Geneva: WHO.

Yazdanpanah, L., Nasiri, M. and Adarvishi, S. (2015). Literature review on the management of diabetic foot ulcer. *World Journal of Diabetes*, 6(1): 37–53.

463

Chapter 16

The reproductive systems and associated disorders

Hazel Ridgers

Freelance Lecturer and Researcher in Nursing and Health, London, UK

Contents

Introduction	465	Male reproductive disorders	486
Reproductive health	465	Conclusion	493
The pelvis	466	Multiple choice questions	494
The female reproductive tract	467	Conditions	496
The menstrual cycle	471	Further resources	496
The female breast	472	Glossary of terms	497
Menstrual disorders	472	References	498
The male reproductive tract	484		

Key words

- Reproduction
- Hormones
- Cancer
- Genitalia
- Ovulation
- Menstruation
- Puberty
- Psychological well-being
- Prostaglandins
- Fertility
- Risk
- Reproductive tracts

Fundamentals of Applied Pathophysiology: An Essential Guide for Nursing and Healthcare Students, Fourth Edition. Edited by Ian Peate.
© 2021 John Wiley & Sons Ltd. Published 2021 by John Wiley & Sons Ltd.
Student companion website: www.wiley.com/go/fundamentalsofappliedpathophysiology/student4e
Instructor companion website: www.wiley.com/go/fundamentalsofappliedpathophysiology/instructor4e

1. Describe the changes occurring during the menstrual cycle.
2. Outline the role and functions of the prostate gland.
3. Discuss how disorders of the reproductive tract may impact an individual's psychological well-being.
4. Describe how reproductive and sexual health are interlinked.
5. Define the multifaceted role of the health professional in caring for people experiencing disease of the reproductive tract.

Learning outcomes

On completion of this chapter, the reader will be able to:

- List the internal and external organs and structures of the female and male reproductive tracts.

- Describe the key functions of the male and female reproductive tracts.

- Explain the normal and abnormal pathophysiological changes that may occur in the male and female reproductive tracts.

- Outline the care and management required for a range of reproductive tract disorders.

Don't forget to visit the companion website for this book (www.wiley.com/go/fundamentalsofappliedpathophysiology/student4e) **where you can find self-assessment tests to check your progress, as well as lots of activities to practise your learning.**

Introduction

Reproduction is a complex activity requiring a series of integrated anatomical and physiological events. The physiological and anatomical aspects of the reproductive tract are primarily associated with procreation. However, the psychological and social aspects of reproduction can be equally important, as is the pleasure that is usually provided by the reproductive organs. Reproductive pathophysiology may be acute or chronic, cause physical and psychological distress, and may result in loss of life.

This chapter offers an outline of the male and female reproductive tracts. Several reproductive health conditions are discussed alongside the care these conditions may require.

Reproductive health

Reproductive health is a human right and a fundamental component of overall health throughout the lifespan regardless of the way a person chooses to express their sexuality. It is an essential feature of human development and is defined by the United Nations (1994) as:

A state of physical, mental and social well-being in all matters relating to the reproductive system at all stages of life. Reproductive health implies that people are able to have a satisfying and safe sex life and that they have the capability to reproduce and the freedom to decide if, when and how often to do so.

This enduring definition emphasises that individuals have rights to reproductive and sexual health; these rights are enshrined in international and UK law. The Human Rights Act 1998: Article 8 provides people with a right to respect for their private and family life. The right to reproductive and sexual health falls within this article.

Reproductive health includes the reproductive processes and functions necessary to have children. As such, reproductive health encompasses the notion that people may have a responsible, enjoyable sex life, the ability to have children and to decide if, when and how frequently to do so.

Reproductive health is inherently interlinked with sexual health and personal relationships (World Health Organisation, 2020). Sexual activity is an important part of sexual expression for most adults. One element of sexual expression is sexual behaviour, some of which may result in an increased risk of reproductive and sexual ill health, for example, as a result of a sexually transmitted infection.

The way a person chooses to express themselves sexually is not just a fundamental aspect of human health; sexual health and freedom of sexual expression are human rights. Healthcare professionals must respect and uphold these rights. Additional expectations are placed on healthcare professionals regarding professional standards of practice and behaviour. For example, nurses and nursing associates are expected to avoid assumptions, recognise diversity and individual choice and challenge discriminatory attitudes and behaviours. This is enshrined in The Code (Nursing and Midwifery Council, 2018). These expectations are also written into organisational policies.

There have been several pioneering developments and the introduction of new technologies over the years that are associated with reproduction; it could be suggested that these innovations have been in response to the national and global incidence of subfertility. For some people, having children and bringing up a family are important aspects of their lives, and for those who experience problems with their fertility, this can be devastating, denying them their opportunity to realise their aspirations and hopes.

The role of the healthcare professional in reproductive health is therefore multifaceted, acting as a health educator, promoting good reproductive and sexual health, preventing ill health and supporting people whose reproductive pathophysiology may have a fundamental impact on both physical and psychological well-being. It is vital therefore that health professionals working in reproductive health provide patient-centred, compassionate and non-judgemental care.

In order to care for those who have reproductive health issues, and to be able to assess and plan care in a safe and effective manner, the healthcare professional must be familiar with the anatomy and physiology of the reproductive tract.

The pelvis

The male and female pelve (singular pelvis) differ, with the female pelvis being wider and shallower than the male pelvis, so that the baby at birth can pass through it (Figure 16.1). The thickness of the bones of the pelvis also differs in the male and female. The female pelvic bones are thinner and more delicate than in the male.

Generally, the pelvis is a ring of bone that supports the weight of the upper body. It can be described as a basin-shaped cavity. The bones of the pelvis are:

- The innominate bones
- The sacrum
- The coccyx.

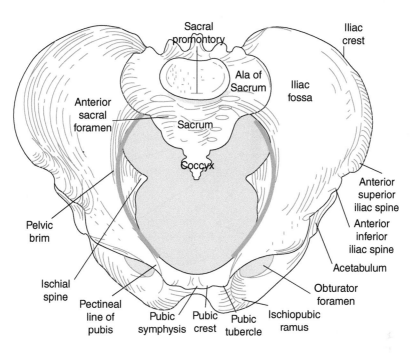

Figure 16.1   The female pelvis.

There are two innominate bones, and both are made up of:

• The ilium
• The pubic bone
• The ischium.

Towards the front of the pelvis (anteriorly), the bones join at the symphysis pubis. The sacrum and the coccyx come together at a joint that is moveable (inferiorly): the sacrococcygeal joint. Strong connective tissues (ligaments) join the pelvis to the sacrum at the base of the spine. Large nerves and muscle pass through the pelvis, and there are several digestive and reproductive organs within it.

The female reproductive tract
Female external genitalia

The external genitalia, i.e. external to the vagina, are also known as the accessory structures of the female reproductive tract. Collectively, they are known as the vulva or pudendum and consist of the (Figure 16.2):

• Mons pubis
• Prepuce
• Clitoris
• Labia majora
• Labia minora
• Urethral orifice
• Vagina
• Bartholin's glands.

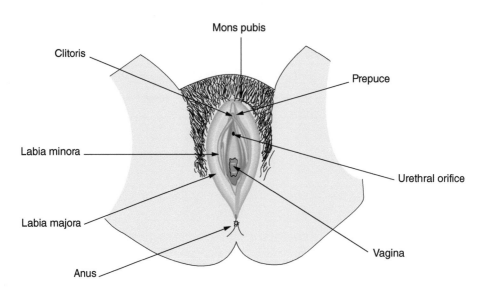

Figure 16.2   The female external genitalia (also known as the pudendum or vulva).

There is a soft mound of fatty tissue covering the symphysis pubis at the front of the vulva – the mons pubis; post puberty, this area is covered with pubic hair. The labia majora extend to both sides of the vulva and are covered with pubic hair – these are two longitudinal prominent folds of tissue. The outer surface of the labia majora is covered by a thin layer of skin containing hair follicles, sweat and sebaceous glands, and the inner surface is smoother, without pubic hair and contains a larger number of sebaceous follicles. Both the labia majora and minora are protective structures, protecting the inner structures of the vulva. Two soft folds of skin make up the labia minora within the labia majora and are situated either side of the opening of the vagina. The labia minora join close to the prepuce; these then cover the clitoris (the vulval vestibule) and extend backwards, enclosing the urethral and vaginal orifices. Connective, fatty and elastic tissues are what chiefly comprise the labia minora; there are no sweat glands or hair follicles as seen in the labia majora, but there are sebaceous glands present. The size and colour of the labia minora will change in response to sexual stimulation.

The clitoris (a sexual organ) is situated where the labia meet near the anterior folds of the labia minora; it is situated above the urethral and vaginal orifices. The clitoris is composed of erectile tissue; it is a small rounded area enclosed in fibrous membranes in layers. It is homologous to the penis and originates embryologically from the same tissue that forms the penis.

The clitoris becomes enlarged, erect and sensitive during sexual stimulation; it initiates and elevates sexual tension levels, and functions solely to bring about sexual pleasure. It is possible for female orgasm to occur when the clitoris is stimulated.

The Bartholin's glands are situated slightly below and to the left and right of the opening of the vagina (Marieb and Keller, 2017). As the female becomes sexually aroused, these glands secrete lubrication in the form of mucus; it is suggested that this can facilitate intercourse and allows for sexual stimulation, but the exact purpose is not fully understood. The secretions are known to contain pheromones; these are chemicals that can trigger a natural behavioural response in another person. Usually, the Bartholin's glands cannot be felt (palpated); however, in the event of obstruction, cyst formation can occur, and the cysts may become infected, resulting in abscess formation. It must be noted that not all Bartholin's cysts are the result of an infection.

Female internal genitalia

The four organs of the female reproductive tract are the:

1. Fallopian tubes
2. Ovaries
3. Vagina
4. Uterus.

The uterus is a dense, muscular, pear-shaped hollow organ and is approximately 7.5 cm long. It is situated deep in the pelvic cavity between the urinary bladder and the rectum; it also touches the sigmoid colon and the small intestines. The uterus has three main parts:

1. The fundus – the thick muscular region that is situated above the insertion of the fallopian tubes.
2. The body (sometimes called the corpus) – the main aspect of the uterus joined to the cervix by an isthmus of tissue.
3. The cervix – this is the narrower lower segment of the uterus, with an external os extending into the vagina.

The cavity of the uterus is continuous (laterally) with the lumen of the fallopian tubes and narrows as it reaches the cervix, creating a triangular, pear shape. The size of the uterus varies amongst women, and during pregnancy, changes size, shape, structure and position. Postpartum, it usually returns to its normal shape and size within 6–8 weeks. The uterus has three layers (Figure 16.3):

1. The perimetrium – This layer is the peritoneum and fascial outer layer. It supports the uterus within the pelvis. Sometimes it is called the parietal peritoneum.
2. The myometrium – This layer is the middle layer and is composed of smooth muscle. The muscles in the myometrium stretch during pregnancy to allow for the growing foetus, and contract during labour. After delivery, the myometrium contracts further to expel the placenta and control blood loss.

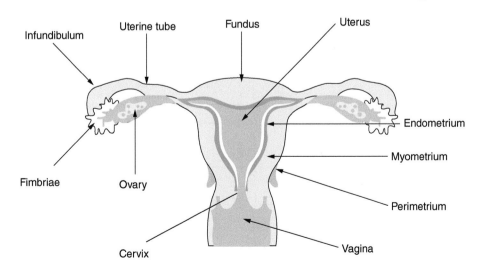

Figure 16.3   The uterus and associated structures.

3. The endometrium – This is the inner lining of the uterus and has a mucous lining. The surface is continuous with the vagina and the uterine tubes. During menstruation the layers of the endometrium slough away from the inner layer. During the menstrual cycle, the endometrium thickens and becomes rich with blood vessels and glandular tissue.

A direct route exists from the vagina through the cervix, uterus and the fallopian tubes to the peritoneum, as there is an opening of the uterus near the fundus into the lumen of the fallopian tubes.

The cervix (a Latin word for neck) is the lower constricted segment of the uterus; it is conical in shape and is a little wider in the middle than it is at the lower or upper ends; it joins to form the upper aspect of the vagina (Figure 16.4).

The ectocervix is the aspect of the cervix that projects into the vagina and has an epithelial surface. The opening of the cervix is known as the external os, and it opens to the endocervical canal; the canal terminates at the internal os. The cervix provides a channel for discharge of the menstrual fluid; it secretes secretions to assist in the transport of semen; during labour, it dilates to allow the passage of the foetus.

The fallopian tubes (also known as the salpinges) are two fine tubes that lead from the ovaries to the uterus; they range from 8 to 14 cm in length (Marieb and Keller, 2017). Collectively, the fallopian tubes, ovaries and support tissues are known as the adnexa. The key functions of the fallopian tubes are to provide a site for fertilisation and transport of the ovum to the uterus; this allows sperm and ova to meet for fertilisation in the tube. The ova are transported along the tube by the action of cilia and peristalsis. The fallopian tubes terminate at or near one ovary, becoming a structure called the fimbria (Figure 16.3).

The egg-producing organs are called the ovaries; they are the size and shape of a large almond, and the two of them are situated on either side of the uterus. As well as being the reproductive organs, they are also endocrine glands. The ovaries are homologous to the testes in the male.

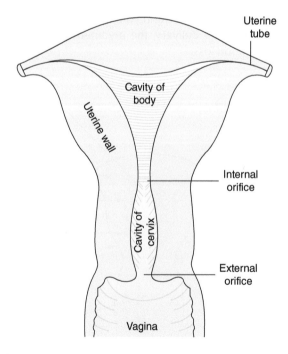

Figure 16.4   The cervix.

When a girl is born, each ovary will contain approximately 200 000–400 000 follicles – these are all the eggs that she will ever possess; the follicles are the shells of each egg. As the girl reaches puberty, the number of follicles will gradually decline, i.e. at puberty the number is between 100 000 and 200 000, and as the woman ages the number of follicles continues to decline.

The menstrual cycle

As a girl reaches puberty, she begins to ovulate – her first menstruation is termed the menarche. Ovulation is the release of a ripe, mature egg from one of the ovaries every month until the menopause, a term used to describe the cessation of the menstrual cycle. Ovulation occurs as the body prepares the woman to become pregnant. If pregnancy does not occur, the woman has a menstrual period, and the cycle begins again. The cycle is complex and is under the control of the reproductive hormonal system.

The cycle begins when a gland in the brain (the pituitary gland) releases a hormone called follicle-stimulating hormone (FSH); this hormone causes approximately 20 eggs to begin to grow and mature in the ovaries. The eggs grow within the follicle (its own shell), and FSH causes the follicle to produce oestrogen. As the levels of oestrogen (another hormone) increase, FSH production is stopped. Only one egg in the follicle will continue to grow and mature; the others die (Grossman and Porth, 2014).The next stage in the cycle occurs when the egg becomes mature; at this stage the pituitary gland produces another hormone called luteinising hormone (LH), and this causes the follicle to burst and the egg is released from the ovary. The follicle is now empty and becomes known as the corpus luteum; oestrogen continues to be produced by the corpus luteum, and it then begins to produce another hormone called progesterone (Thibodeau and Patton, 2013). The role of progesterone at this stage is to begin to prepare the uterus to receive a fertilised egg.

The lining of the uterus (the endometrium) responds to the effects of oestrogen and progesterone and starts to thicken, resulting in a soft, nourishing environment for the fertilised egg. Implantation occurs as a result of the two hormones, and the egg attaching itself to the endometrium. When implantation is successful, the egg then begins to divide by meiosis, forming cells and tissues that will eventually become a human being. Figure 16.5 provides a diagrammatic representation of the ovarian menstrual cycle.

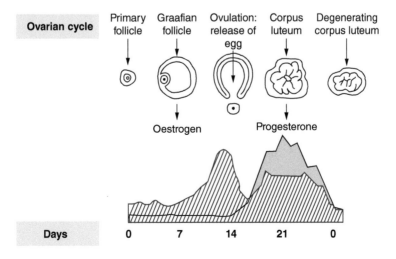

Figure 16.5 The menstrual cycle (ovarian).

If fertilisation fails to occur (and there are many reasons why), then the egg will pass into the uterus and dissolve. When the hormone production slows down, the endometrial lining begins to break down and sloughs off; this then passes through the cervix and vagina and is known as menstruation. The menstrual cycle is said to begin from the first day of one menstrual period until the start of another one and is on an average from 22 to 45 days (Kenny *et al.*, 2017).

The female breast

The female breasts are usually considered as accessory organs of reproduction and play a key role in feeding the young by producing milk. Structurally, the male breast is identical to the female breast but less prominent; male and female breasts develop embryologically from the same tissue (Marieb and Keller, 2017). Figure 16.6 shows a cross-section of the female breast.

The breast is composed of lobes. The lobes contain glandular tissue and fat; breasts are modified sweat glands that produce milk (lactation). The hormone prolactin is produced by the pituitary gland at the end of pregnancy and stimulates the glandular tissue to lactate (Marieb and Keller, 2017). The glandular tissue is further stimulated when the infant suckles at the breast, resulting in contraction, and milk is transported via the ducts to the nipple. The breasts are covered with skin, and each breast contains a nipple surrounded by a pink to dark brown tissue called the areola. The areola contains several sebaceous glands. Marieb and Hoehn (2018) suggest that the role of sebum produced by the sebaceous glands is to reduce chapping and cracking of the skin of the nipple.

During the menstrual cycle, some women may experience changes in their breasts. In the premenstrual period, in response to the increasing levels of oestrogen and progesterone, the breasts may enlarge and become tender or nodular. After menstruation, this growth reverts.

Menstrual disorders

Some women may experience problems with their menstrual cycle, and these include:

- Irregular periods
- Excessive pain
- Excessive bleeding.

This section addresses some of these problems.

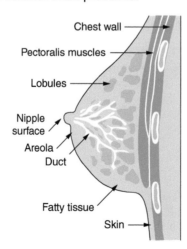

Figure 16.6   A cross-section of the female breast.

Snapshot   Dysmenorrhoea

Carrie Adams is a 24-year-old charity volunteer. She presents for an annual learning disability health check with her GP with a history of increasing lower abdominal pain associated with her menses. Carrie has autistic spectrum disorder (ASD) and a learning disability. She is accompanied by a learning disability support worker whose support Carrie wants her during the consultation. With encouragement from her support worker, Carrie tells the doctor that the pain starts a few days before the first day of her period and lasts about 5 days. Carrie's support worker says that Carrie's behaviour suggests that she is also experiencing lower back pain, and headaches. The support worker advises that Carrie's partner says Carrie is sometimes nauseous and eating less than usual. Carrie explains that her symptoms seem to be worsening. Carrie's medical notes show that menarche occurred at the age of 13 years. Carrie reports that bleeding happens every month for a few days; she cannot give further details on the length of her cycle or length of bleeding. Healthcare appointments and physical examinations make Carrie feel very anxious, and she initially does not give consent for examination. Following sensitive, careful explanation and in line with Carrie's wishes, Carrie's support worker acts as a chaperone, and a physical and pelvic examination is performed. This reveals no abnormalities. Carrie is not on the contraceptive pill, and she explains she does not like taking pills; Carrie's partner uses condoms. Carrie says that she has recently been finding sexual intercourse painful. Carrie's medical notes also show that her mother had a hysterectomy when she was aged 28 years.

473

Vital signs

The following vital signs were noted and recorded on the National Early Warning Score (NEWS2) system:

Vital sign	Observation	Normal
Temperature	36.9°C	36.0–37.9°C range
Pulse	78 beats per minute	60–100 beats per minute
Respiration	14 breaths per minute	12–20 breaths per minute
Blood pressure	138/70 mmHg	100–139 mmHg (systolic) range
O₂ saturation (Scale 1)	100%	94–98%

Physiological parameter (Score)	3	2	1	0	1	2	3
Respiration rate				14			
Oxygen saturation % (Scale 1)				100			
Supplemental oxygen				No			
Temperature °C				36.9			
Systolic BP mmHg				132			
Heart rate				78			
Level of consciousness				Alert			
Total				0			

A full blood count is performed, with the following results:

Test	Result	Guideline normal values
White blood cells (WBC)	5×10^9/L	4 to 11×10^9/L
Neutrophils	6.2×10^9/L	2.0 to 7.5×10^9/L
Lymphocytes	3.2×10^9/L	1.3 to 4.0×10^9/L
Red blood cells (RBC)	4.7×10^9/L	4.5 to 6.5×10^9/L
Haemoglobin (Hb)	130 g/L	130–180 g/L
Platelets	320×10^9/L	150 to 440×10^9/L

Reflect on this case and consider the following:

1. What might be the most likely diagnosis?
2. Provide a list of further tests and investigations that may be required.
3. What treatment options might be available? Consider which may be most suitable.
4. Do you need any other information from Ms Adams in order to ensure that you are able to offer her a safe, patient-centred treatment plan?
5. How would you demonstrate a patient-centred approach in the context of Ms Adams's diagnosis of ASD with a learning disability and her anxiety regarding healthcare appointments and examinations in particular?
6. What guidelines are available to you regarding the use of chaperones for people with learning disabilities?

Clinical investigations

Ultrasound

Ultrasound imaging is also called ultrasound scanning, or sonography, and involves the use of a small transducer (a probe) and ultrasound gel placed directly on the person's skin.

The healthcare professional provides the person with information prior to the test, which should supplement the information offered to the patient by the person who is to perform the investigation. Information should be provided in such a way that the person understands why the test is being carried out and is able to make an informed decision. Provide time for any questions, and if the person is unable to respond to the questions, a registered healthcare professional should be called.

Local policy may dictate that the person needs to remove all clothing and jewellery in the area to be examined. A gown may need to be worn during the procedure. The healthcare professional must assist with the preservation of dignity, exposing only the aspect of the body that is being examined.

Preparation for the procedure depends on the type of examination; for some scans the person may not be allowed to eat or drink for as many as 12 hours prior to the investigation. For others they may be asked to drink up to six glasses of water 2 hours before the exam and to avoid urinating so that the bladder is full when the scan begins.

Explain to the person that they will need to lie prone on the examination table. The healthcare professional may need to assist the person into the optimum position. At all times attention to the person's safety is paramount.

A warm water-based gel is applied to the area of the body being studied; this helps the transducer make secure contact with the body and eliminate air pockets between the transducer and the skin that can block the sound waves from passing into the body. The transducer is placed on the body and moved back and forth until the desired images are captured.

Usually there is no discomfort from pressure as the transducer is pressed against the area being examined.

After imaging is complete, the gel is wiped off the skin. The healthcare professional should reassure the person that the gel does not stain or discolour clothing.

If needed, assist the person with redressing, providing comfort and safety as the person gets down from the examination table.

Document the activity undertaken according to local policy.

Red flag

Use of chaperones

All patients should have the right, if they so wish, to have a chaperone present during an examination, procedure, treatment or any as aspect of care, regardless of organisational constraints or settings in which this is delivered.

The healthcare professional can act as advocate for the patient, helping to explain what will happen during the examination or procedure as well as the reasons why. They can assess the patient's understanding of what has been told to them, and the chaperone will also be a reassuring presence whilst the person is having the examination or procedure, safeguarding against any unnecessary discomfort, pain, humiliation or intimidation. For patients with learning disabilities for whom examinations may be challenging, guidelines suggest that the person chaperoning be someone with whom they are familiar (National Health Service Wales, 2013).

Dysmenorrhoea

Dysmenorrhoea is defined as pain that occurs shortly before or during menstruation (National Institute for Health and Care Excellence (NICE), 2018). During the menstrual cycle, the woman may experience pain in the abdomen, and the pain can be so severe that it can impact her ability to perform the activities of living, such as going to work; often it is because the woman is unable to carry out these activities that she seeks help.

Prior to the beginning of the menstrual period, the breasts can feel larger and they may ache or feel tender. Some pain during the menstrual period is normal; however, extreme pain is not. Women can experience pain prior to and during the menstrual period, and it usually decreases towards the end of the period. The pain can be sharp, intermittent or a dull ache, and is mostly felt in the pelvic region/lower abdomen; it may also be experienced in the back and thighs and is described as 'dragging'. The abdomen may become distended and can be tender to touch, and the woman may have constipation. The woman can experience significant blood loss and can become incapacitated.

There are two types of dysmenorrhoea:

1. Primary dysmenorrhoea
2. Secondary dysmenorrhoea.

Table 16.1 outlines the differences between primary and secondary dysmenorrhoea.

Table 16.1 Primary and secondary dysmenorrhoea – distinctions.

	Primary dysmenorrhoea	Secondary dysmenorrhoea
Age at symptom onset	Adolescence	Symptoms start after a few years of pain-free menstruation
Pain at other times of menstrual cycle	First 2–3 days of period	Exacerbated by menstruation but may occur intermittently or persistently throughout the menstrual cycle
Other types of pain?	No	Dyspareunia

Source: Adapted from Mazza, 2011.

Primary dysmenorrhoea

This refers to menstrual pain that is a result of the physiological activities of menstruation accompanied by muscle contraction. This type of pain exists in women who are otherwise healthy (NICE, 2018).

Secondary dysmenorrhoea

In contrast to primary dysmenorrhoea, secondary dysmenorrhoea is attributed to some form of organic pelvic disease (underlying pelvic pathology). In secondary dysmenorrhoea, there is evidence of an underlying disease process or some type of structural abnormality within or outside of the uterus. Secondary dysmenorrhoea is uncommon in women before the age of 25 years (Kenny *et al.*, 2017). The most common cause is endometriosis, when the endometrial lining of the womb grows outside the uterine cavity.

Risk factors

Increased risk of primary dysmenorrhoea is associated with those who are in the younger age group. There is conflicting evidence linking dysmenorrhoea and modifiable risk factors such as smoking, diet, obesity and depression (NICE, 2018), but evidence suggests there is an increased risk if a woman has a past medical history that includes:

- Early age of menarche
- Nulliparous
- Heavy menstrual flow
- Family history of dysmenorrhoea

In secondary dysmenorrhoea, risk factors depend upon the underlying causative pathology. Secondary causes include:

- Endometriosis
- Adenomyosis (when the endometrium grows into the myometrium of the uterus)
- Fibroids
- Pelvic inflammatory disease
- Cervical cancer
- Ovarian cancer
- Intrauterine device

Pathophysiology

Prostaglandins are released by the uterus during menstruation due to the breakdown of the endometrial cells and the release of their contents. Excessive levels of prostaglandin are closely related to dysmenorrhoea. The increased production of prostaglandins by the uterus results in intense uterine contractions (uterine hypercontractility); the uterus can go into spasm, and the muscle becomes ischaemic, producing uterine pain that is similar to the pain experienced in angina (see Chapter 8). The excessive amount of prostaglandin can also cause the woman to experience:

- Nausea
- Vomiting
- Diarrhoea
- Faintness
- Headache
- Lower backache.

The reason why some women produce excessive prostaglandin is unknown (Linhart, 2007); prostaglandin levels have been found to be much higher in those women with excessive menstrual pain as opposed to those who feel moderate to no pain.

Diagnosis

Diagnosis is made by obtaining a full health and medical history from the woman. The healthcare professional should pay attention to the type of pain that the woman describes, the duration and what (if any) remedies she uses to alleviate the pain as well as the impact on her quality of life and emotional well-being.

To confirm diagnosis of primary or secondary dysmenorrhoea, the following investigations may be required:

- Ultrasound (abdominal/transvaginal)
- Laparoscopy
- Laparotomy.

Care and management

Controlling the pain associated with dysmenorrhoea is a key care intervention. Medications including non-steroidal anti-inflammatory drugs (NSAIDs), for example, ibuprofen, mefenamic acid and naproxen are very effective in the treatment of the pain. NSAIDs can inhibit the synthesis of prostaglandin (Kenny *et al.*, 2017).

In rare cases, surgical intervention may be required for some women. Hysterectomy can be a success in terms of relieving women of their presenting symptoms. This procedure should be performed once childbearing is complete.

There are several non-pharmacological treatments that may help women with dysmenorrhoea. Transcutaneous electrical nerve stimulation (TENS) can help with or without pharmacological analgesics (Wang *et al.*, 2009). Khan *et al.* (2012) suggest that that there is a lack of good-quality evidence to support the use of interventions such as acupuncture or herbal remedies in reducing abdominal pain. Some women may find relief in the use of heat therapy, for example, the use of a hot-water bottle. Exercise can have the effects of releasing endogenous endorphins – the body's own analgesic.

Referral to a specialist gynaecology service should be considered for a woman with suspected or confirmed dysmenorrhoea secondary to endometriosis (NICE, 2018).

Oral contraceptives

The oral contraceptive pill is an effective alternative first-line agent for the treatment of pain in primary dysmenorrhoea where the women does not wish to conceive (NICE, 2018). Oral contraceptives can block ovulation and reduce blood flow to the uterus and may also be used to manage pain in the context of secondary dysmenorrhoea as a result of endometriosis.

Red flag

NSAIDs

The healthcare professional must be aware that there are some patients who are unable to take NSAIDs as they can cause:

- Gastrointestinal bleeding
- Nephrotoxicity
- Nausea
- Vomiting
- Dyspepsia
- Headache.

It must also be remembered that these drugs are contraindicated in those who have:

- Aspirin-induced asthma
- Peptic ulcer
- Renal disease
- Clotting disorders.

Medicines management

NSAIDs

NSAIDs in the context of primary dysmenorrhoea are used to prevent pain rather than acting as an analgesic, and the woman should be informed that she should take the NSAID as soon as she knows that the period is imminent or as soon as the bleeding begins; the medication should be taken on a regular basis for the first 1–3 days of the period as it prevents pain. Paracetamol can be used as an alternative or in addition to NSAIDs where the effect of NSAIDs alone is insufficient.

In secondary dysmenorrhoea, pain management depends upon the underlying causative pathology. For example, a short trial of NSAIDs may be considered as first-line management of pain associated with endometriosis (NICE, 2018).

A woman's preferences, priorities regarding conception and personal circumstances should always be considered regarding the choice of treatment offered. Adherence to the method of pain control, i.e. the woman's ability to take the appropriate dose at correctly time intervals, should be assessed to ensure that this component of her treatment plan is safe and achievable.

Amenorrhoea

Amenorrhoea is the absence or cessation of menses and can occur:

- Prior to the menarche
- After the menopause
- During pregnancy
- Postoperatively
- Post treatment.

Primary amenorrhoea refers to a failure of menstruation by the age of 16 years in the presence of normal sexual characteristics. Secondary amenorrhoea is the absence of menstruation for at least 6 consecutive months in women who have had regular periods of for three consecutive cycles in women with irregular periods (Royal College of Obstetricians and Gynaecologists, 2020).

The most common cause of primary amenorrhoea is gonadal dysgenesis, a condition in which ovary development is incomplete or defective, resulting in total or partial dysfunction. Whilst the most common cause of secondary amenorrhoea is pregnancy, other causes according to the Royal College of Obstetricians and Gynaecologists (2014) include:

- Polycystic ovary syndrome
- Hypothalamic causes – due to excessive weight loss (anorexia) or excessive exercise
- Hyperprolactinaemia – an elevated level of prolactin in the blood; in women this may be caused by a prolactinoma
- Contraception – the contraceptive pill and depot injection.

Diagnosis

The healthcare professional must undertake a full health, medical and menstrual history, including:

- Sexual history in order to rule out pregnancy
- Family history to determine if there are any genetic abnormalities
- The presence of any associated illness, for example, hypothyroidism or diabetes mellitus
- Emotional upsets
- Changes in body weight
- Increase in exercise
- Drug history, e.g. contraceptive pill/injection, chemotherapy
- Previous surgery.

In all women who present with amenorrhoea, it is advisable to perform a pregnancy test (Royal College of Obstetricians and Gynaecologists, 2020), to rule out pregnancy. In secondary amenorrhoea, several blood tests may be carried out in order to assess levels of hormones, such as FSH and LH, as well assessment of thyroid function. Prolactin levels will also need to be assessed to determine if there is any evidence of hyperprolactinaemia. A pelvic ultrasound can demonstrate the presence of polycystic ovaries (enlarged ovaries), and magnetic resonance imaging (MRI) or computer tomography (CT) scans can identify a pituitary tumour; a hysteroscopy may be required.

Care and management

The role and function of the healthcare professional is to provide the woman with emotional as well as physical support, and information that she can understand in order to make informed decisions about her treatment options. Healthcare professionals are ideally placed to discuss lifestyle issues with women, such as smoking and alcohol consumption, and stress-reducing activities, and to provide information about diet and weight gain (if needed), and the balance between excessive and therapeutic levels of exercise. The woman may need support in relation to the perceived threat to her self-esteem and with concerns associated with fertility as a result of amenorrhoea. Explanations should be provided about the type of investigations that may be required and the reason why they are being performed. The treatment required will depend on the cause. Surgical intervention or hormone replacement therapy may be needed.

Snapshot   Heavy menstrual bleeding (HMB)

Benita Rodriguez is a 48-year-old woman. She visits her local primary healthcare centre with a 7-month history of heavy periods. Mrs Rodriguez has a history of depression, for which she takes an antidepressant. She works as an administrator in a busy office. Mrs Rodriguez becomes very tearful when she describes that during menstruation, she feels worried and anxious about managing her level of blood loss. There have been several situations at work where she was not able to manage with her normal sanitary products. She feels embarrassed that others may have noticed menstrual blood had leaked onto her clothes. She is now taking time off work and declines all social invitations when menstruating, preferring to be at home with easier access to a bathroom. This is having a negative impact on her relationship with her employer, her husband, grown-up children and her friends, in part because Mrs Rodriguez is not comfortable disclosing the reasons for her changed behaviour. She says that her sexual relationship with her husband has been impacted too and where they used to enjoy regular sex together, this is no longer the case. As a result, she reports feeling anxious, lonely and says that she feels her depression is worsening and her antidepressants no longer satisfactorily managing her depressive symptoms. She reports no other symptoms. Heavy menstrual bleeding is suspected.

Vital signs

The following observations are noted and recorded using the National Early Warning Score (NEWS2) system.

Vital sign	Observation	Normal
Temperature	36.8°C	36.0–37.9°C range
Pulse	71 beats per minute	60–100 beats per minute
Respiration	17 breaths per minute	12–20 breaths per minute
Blood pressure	124/70 mmHg	100–139 mmHg (systolic) range
O_2 saturation	98%	94–98%

Physiological parameter	3	2	1	0	1	2	3
Respiration rate				17			
Oxygen saturation %				98			
Supplemental oxygen				No			
Temperature °C				36.8			
Systolic BP mmHg				124			
Heart rate				71			
Level of consciousness				Alert			
Total				0			

A full blood count (FBC) is drawn, with the following results:

Test	Result	Guideline normal values
White blood cells (WBC)	5×10^9/L	4 to 11×10^9/L
Neutrophils	6.2×10^9/L	2.0 to 7.5×10^9/L
Lymphocytes	3.2×10^9/L	1.3 to 4.0×10^9/L
Red blood cells (RBC)	4.7×10^9/L	4.5 to 6.5×10^9/L
Haemoglobin (Hb)	120 g/L	130–180 g/L
Platelets	320×10^9/L	150–440×10^9/L

Take some time to reflect on this case and then consider the following:

1. What do you consider to be the priorities for Mrs Rodriguez's care?
2. How would you describe the impact of HMB on Mrs Rodriguez's quality of life?
3. Consider what services are available in your own healthcare setting to support women's mental health in the context of reproductive pathophysiology.
4. Are you concerned about Mrs Rodriguez's haemoglobin? How might this be managed?

Heavy menstrual bleeding (menorrhagia)

Heavy menstrual bleeding (HMB) is sometimes referred to as menorrhagia. It is defined as excessive menstrual blood loss that occurs over several consecutive cycles. It can significantly impact a woman's physical, emotional, social and material quality of life (NICE, 2020). Normal levels of menstrual blood loss are difficult to define. However, the evidence suggests that rapid changes in blood chemistry occur at two levels of menstrual blood loss: 60 mL and 120 mL (NICE, 2007).

Diagnosis

A detailed healthcare and menstrual history will need to be undertaken in order to offer the woman appropriate and effective treatment. Issues to be explored should include the following:

- The nature of the bleeding, for example, how long periods last, how much bleeding occurs (for example, how often sanitary napkins, tampons or menstrual cups need to be changed) and whether blood clots are present?
- Any other related symptoms, such as bleeding after sex or bleeding between periods?
- Any previous treatment for HMB or co-morbidities?
- What is the impact on the woman's quality of life?

There is natural variation in the amount of blood loss women experience during menses. Blood volume loss may also be impacted by issues such as approaching menopause, and many women will experience an increased volume of blood loss towards the end of peri-menopause. The National Institute for Health and Care Excellence (2020) emphasise that the aim of any intervention for HMB should be to improve the woman's quality of life.

A physical examination is not always required, but may be offered depending on the patient's history, for example, if related symptoms such as persistent intermenstrual bleeding, pelvic pain and/or pressure are reported. Examinations may include an internal and external abdominal examination (palpation). The person carrying out the examination may then identify, for example, if there are any indications of fibroids.

A FBC should be ordered for all women reporting HMB (NICE, 2020) to identify whether the woman is anaemic. There are a variety of tests and investigations that may be undertaken in order to help determine why a woman is experiencing HMB; these should only be ordered on the basis of a woman's medical history. For example, a coagulation screen should be reserved for women whose history indicates HMB since menarche alongside a personal or familial history of coagulation disorders, and other laboratory testing such as endocrine screening should not be ordered routinely (NICE, 2020).

An ultrasound scan may be needed to determine if there are any structural abnormalities. In some instances, a biopsy may be needed to exclude any potential disorders, e.g. endometrial cancer. If the ultrasound demonstrates that there are abnormalities (or it is inconclusive), then hysteroscopy can be performed to aid diagnosis or to determine the exact location of the fibroid.

Care and management

Pharmacological approaches to treatment may be commenced immediately if the woman's history and/or examination suggests a low risk of structural or endometrial pathologies (NICE, 2020). Table 16.2 outlines the different pharmacological interventions that may be used in the treatment of HMB. The woman must be provided with all the information she requires to make an informed decision; however, for some women hormonal contraception as a form of treatment may be unacceptable, e.g. religious reasons or the desire to conceive. The woman may need to be treated with hormone replacement therapy; she may also require other interventions such as a referral to counselling services to help manage the psychological impacts of HMB.

Medicines management

Contraceptive implant
A contraceptive implant is a small flexible tube approximately 40 mm in length that is inserted under the skin of the inner side of the upper arm. The implant steadily releases a hormone into the bloodstream. The implant can only be inserted by a trained registered healthcare professional.

An injection of local anaesthetic is used to anaesthetise the skin. A special needle is used to place the implant under the skin. A dressing is applied; the area around the implant may bruise and can be sore, tender and swollen for a day or two.

An implant can be left in place for three years or taken out sooner if the woman decides to stop using it. A trained registered healthcare professional must take it out. The nurse or doctor palpates the arm to locate the implant and then injects a local anaesthetic into the area where the implant is. A small incision is made in the skin and the implant is gently pulled out. A dressing is applied and is kept in place for a few days.

It usually only takes a few minutes to remove the implant, and it should not be difficult to remove. If an implant is difficult to feel under the skin, it may prove difficult to remove. If this happens, referral is made to remove the implant with ultrasound guidance.

When the pharmacological approach fails or is unacceptable, surgical intervention may be recommended after the woman has been given the opportunity to review and agree any treatment decision. Ensure that sufficient time has been provided and appropriate support given to the women during the decision-making process. There are several interventions that need consideration (Table 16.3).

Table 16.2 Drugs that may be used in the treatment of HMB.

Drug	What it is	How it works	Possible side effects	Comments
Levonorgestrel – a hormone	A small plastic device placed in the uterus, slowly releasing progestogen	The hormone prevents the lining of the uterus from growing too quickly	Irregular bleeding. Breast tenderness. Acne. Headaches. Amenorrhoea	This is also a contraceptive. First-line treatment
Tranexamic acid	Tablet format. The medication is taken from the start of the menstrual period for up to 4 days	Promotes clot formation within the uterus; reducing the amount of bleeding	Indigestion. Headaches. Diarrhoea	If symptoms do not improve within 3 months, treatment should be stopped. Considered as second-line treatment
Non-steroidal anti-inflammatory drugs (NSAIDs)	Tablet format. Medication to be taken from the start of the menstrual period or just before and until heavy bleeding stops	Reduction in prostaglandin production	Indigestion. Diarrhoea	If symptoms do not improve within 3 months, treatment should be stopped
Combined oral contraceptives	Pill format that contains the hormones progestogen and oestrogen. One pill is taken for 21 days, then stopped for 7 days, and the cycle is repeated	Prevents the menstrual cycle from occurring	Mood change. Headache. Nausea. Fluid retention. Breast tenderness	This is also a contraceptive. Considered as second-line treatment
Oral progesterone (norethisterone)	Tablets taken 2–3 times per day from the 5th to 26th day of the menstrual cycle	Prevents the lining of the uterus from growing too quickly	Weight gain. Bloating. Breast tenderness. Headache. Acne	This is also a contraceptive. Considered as third-line treatment
Injected or implanted progesterone	Progestogen is injected or implanted. The implant releases the hormone slowly for 3 years	Prevents the lining of the uterus from growing too quickly	Weight gain. Bloating. Breast tenderness. Headache. Acne. Irregular bleeding. Amenorrhoea. Bone density loss can occur	This is also a contraceptive. Considered as third-line treatment
Gonadotropin-releasing hormone analogue	An injection preventing the production of oestrogen and progesterone	Prevents the menstrual cycle from occurring	Menopause-like symptoms (hot flushes, increased sweating, vaginal dryness)	Considered as third-line treatment

Source: Adapted from NICE, 2007.

483

If surgical intervention is required, the woman (and her family) will need support; this can be physical and psychological as well as socio-economic support. It is important to organise service provision with the women need's as the central focus and a coordinated multidisciplinary/multiagency approach is advocated.

The information provided to the woman must be offered in a format she understands, and it must also be relevant to her circumstances; this may mean that the information may need to be translated into her preferred language. Information must point out the risks as well as

Table 16.3   Potential surgical treatments for women with heavy periods.

Proposed surgical intervention	What it is	Possible side effects	Comments
Endometrial ablation: Thermal balloon endometrial ablation (TBEA). Impedance-controlled bipolar radiofrequency ablation. Microwave endometrial ablation (MEA). Free fluid thermal ablation	A device is inserted in all techniques through the vagina and cervix into the uterus When the device is *in situ*, several methods can be used to heat the device, e.g. by using radio energy microwaves. The purpose is to destroy the lining of the uterus	Vaginal discharge. Increased pain during the menstrual period. Infection	In some women, the procedure may need to be repeated as the lining of the uterus can grow back. This procedure is not suitable if the woman wishes to become pregnant
Uterine artery embolisation (UAE)	The aim is to block the blood supply to the uterus. Small particles are injected into the blood vessels that take blood to the uterus, blocking any blood supply to fibroids in the expectation that they shrink	Vaginal discharge. Pain. Nausea. Vomiting	There may be need for further surgery. Women undertaking this procedure may be able to become pregnant
Myomectomy	Surgical removal of a fibroid can be performed either through an abdominal incision or via the vagina. The vaginal route necessitates the use of a hysteroscope	Adhesions and as a result a possibility of pain and impaired fertility. Infection Perforation of the uterus	Those undergoing this procedure may be able to become pregnant
Hysterectomy	There are two main methods of performing a hysterectomy: vaginally or abdominally. In total hysterectomy, the uterus and cervix are removed, whereas in subtotal hysterectomy, only the uterus is removed	Haemorrhage during or after surgery. Infection. Damage to adjacent organs, e.g. bowel or urinary tract. Urinary/faecal dysfunction	Women wishing to have a hysterectomy will not be able to become pregnant. Removal of the uterus means the women will no longer have a menstrual period

the benefits of the various treatments and procedures being offered, and an opportunity must be provided for the woman to ask questions. It must be emphasised that she can change her mind at any stage should she wish, and she is entitled to a second opinion should this be required.

The male reproductive tract

The male reproductive tract is designed to produce spermatozoa and deposit these inside the female vagina; this contributes to reproduction. The spermatozoa are responsible for the fertilisation of the female egg. Unlike the female genitalia, male genitalia are found outside of the body (Figure 16.7).

Male genitalia

The penis and scrotum comprise the male external genitalia. Within the scrotal sac, a loose bag-like sac of skin, suspended by the spermatic cord, in between the thighs, are the testes.

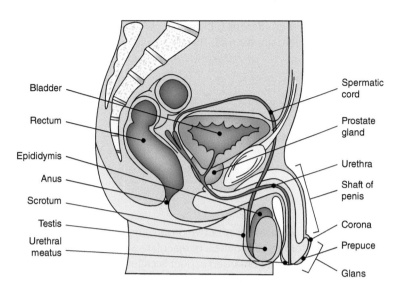

Figure 16.7   The male reproductive system.

They are approximately 4.5 cm in length, 2.5 cm in breadth and 3 cm in diameter; they feel smooth and move freely within the scrotal sac (Thibodeau and Patton, 2013). The testes are found outside of the abdominal cavity in the scrotum; however, they begin their development in the abdominal cavity and normally descend into the scrotal sac during the last 2 months of foetal development. The testes traverse the inguinal canal and inguinal rings and move into the scrotum where they are suspended.

It is normal for one testis to hang lower than the other. As the cremasteric muscle contracts, the spermatic cord (to which it is attached) shortens, and the testes moves up towards the abdomen; the result of this is that it provides the testes with more warmth. For effective development of sperm, the testes must be at a lower temperature than the rest of the body; this is the reason why the testes are situated outside of the body. The testes have two functions – to secrete the hormone testosterone, which is responsible for the development of the male secondary sex characteristics (deep voice, beard growth, body hair), as well as the function of the male reproductive system in the production of spermatozoa (Tortora, 2017). The testes are the essential male organs of reproduction.

The composition of the testes, contained under a membranous shell, is glandular tissue that is made up of several lobules differing in size according to their location. The lobule consists of approximately 660–1200 seminiferous tubules that are small convoluted structures, responsible for the production of sperm. The spermatozoa develop in different stages in different parts of the tubules. The tubules form sperm continuously; in a young man, sperm is produced at the rate of 120 million per day. The sperm travel from the seminiferous tubules to the rete testis, to the efferent ducts onwards to the epididymis, where spermatogenesis takes place and newly created mature sperm cells are formed. Spermatogenesis is complex and can be divided into three phases:

1. Mitotic proliferation to produce a large number of cells
2. Meiotic division to produce genetic diversity
3. Maturation, preparing sperm for transit and penetration of the oocyte in the female tract.

The sperm cells are then moved on to the vas deferens and expelled through the urethra as a result of rhythmic contractions.

Situated between the seminiferous tubules are cells called the Leydig cells, where testosterone and other androgens are formed. The physical changes in the male related to testosterone are:

- Increase in penile size
- Enlargement of the scrotum
- Growth in the size of the testes
- Enlargement of the larynx and deepening of the voice
- Increase in muscle mass
- Increase in basal metabolic rate
- Increase in sebaceous glands
- Thickening of the bones.

The penis is an external male reproductive organ, and within the penis is the urethra. The penis provides a route for the elimination of ejaculate and urine via the urethral orifice situated at the tip of the penis; the enlarged aspect is called the glans penis. The glans penis is homologous with the female clitoris.

The penis is made up of three columns of erectile tissue:

- Two corpora cavernosa
- One corpus spongiosum.

The end of the corpus spongiosum is the bulbous glans penis; the glans is covered with a thin layer of skin that allows for erection and, in uncircumcised males, the skin at the glans folds over on itself to form the prepuce or foreskin; the area where the foreskin is attached, underneath the penis, is called the frenulum, which is homologous with the female clitoral hood. The urethra, the terminal end of the urinary tract, lies on the tip of the glans and is known as the urethral meatus. Erection requires complex vascular activity – dilation of the arteries supplying blood to the penis and sympathetic nervous system activity.

The prostate gland is approximately 2.5 cm and lies at the base of the urinary bladder surrounded by the upper part of the urethra (Marieb and Hoehn, 2018). The function of the prostate gland is not fully understood. The gland is described as chestnut-shaped, made up of 20–30 compound tubular–alveolar glands; these glands are embedded in a mass of smooth muscle and dense connective tissue. A thin milky fluid is secreted, adding bulk to semen on ejaculation. Prostatic fluid accounts for approximately one-third of semen volume. During orgasm, sperm cells are transmitted from the urethra via the ejaculatory ducts situated in the prostate gland; smooth muscle within the prostate gland contracts during ejaculation and this helps to expel semen.

Male reproductive disorders

This section discusses four common male reproductive tract disorders:

1. Phimosis
2. Paraphimosis
3. Hydrocele
4. Benign and malignant prostate enlargement.

It is not possible in a chapter of this size to outline in depth all the detail associated with these disorders. The reader is advised to delve deeper into the subject in order to gain more comprehensive insight into the care and management of men with reproductive tract disorders.

Snapshot   Testicular torsion

Anil Gupta is 16 years of age and was playing football in the park with friends and family. The ball hit Anil in his groin with some force. This caused him to double up and gasp for breath. Anil recovered and played the rest of the game. Following the game Anil began to complain of nausea and vomited twice. With considerable prompting from his mother, Anil eventually disclosed that the pain in his groin was severe and was worsening. Anil's parents took him to the local emergency department. A full history was taken and on examination Anil's right testicle was found to be swollen and extremely painful. He was hesitant to let anyone near him and reluctant to take any deep breaths. Based on Anil's history and presentation testicular torsion is diagnosed. Anil's vital signs were recorded. Anil was given intravenous pain relief, and his family were instructed that he must remain nil by mouth, and he and his family were prepared for emergency surgery.

Vital signs

The following vital signs were noted and recorded using the NEWS2:

Vital sign	Observation	Normal values
Temperature	37.2°C	36.0–37.9°C range
Pulse	90 beats per minute	60–100 beats per minute
Respiration	18 breaths per minute	12–20 breaths per minute
Blood pressure	126/60 mmHg	100–139 mmHg (systolic) range
O$_2$ saturation (Scale 1)	98%	94–98 %

Physiological parameter	3	2	1	0	1	2	3
Respiration rate				13			
Oxygen saturation % (Scale 1)				98			
Supplemental oxygen				No			
Temperature °C				36.4			
Systolic BP mmHg				116			
Heart rate				80			
Level of consciousness				Alert			
Total				0			

Take some time to reflect on this case, and then consider the following questions:

1. Why is testicular torsion treated as a medical emergency?
2. What type of surgery may be performed on Anil?
3. Other than trauma, what other causes may lead to testicular torsion?
4. Why do you think Anil was reluctant to report testicular pain to his mother?
5. How might you communicate with a teenager undergoing and recovering from testicular surgery who may be embarrassed by talk about parts of the body he considers to be 'private'?

Phimosis

Phimosis in adults occurs when the opening of the foreskin (or prepuce) is unable to be retracted behind the glans penis; the foreskin is too tight for retraction. It is important to note that almost all baby boys have a non-retractable foreskin at birth. The ability to retract the foreskin happens spontaneously in most boys by around 10 years of age (British Association of Paediatric Urologists, 2006).

Phimosis can be congenital, or it can occur as result of infection, inflammation or trauma; it is most frequently due to a condition known as balanitis xerotica obliterans (BXO), the aetiology of which is unknown (British Association of Paediatric Urologists, 2006). BXO (sometimes referred to as lichen sclerosus) is a fibrosing condition resulting in thick (sclerosing) scarring of the skin of the penis, because of which the skin becomes discoloured.

Orange flag

Phimosis and skin changes
Phimosis can cause changes in the cosmetic appearance of the skin of the penis, resulting in psychological distress and may impact confidence, self-esteem and can have a negative impact on intimate relationships (Shasi et al., 2010).

Diagnosis

As the foreskin cannot be retracted, this may result in poor hygiene and the man with phimosis may present with balanoposthitis. The glans penis becomes infected (balanitis) as does the foreskin (posthitis); the man may complain of itching and irritation, pain, discomfort, bleeding on sexual intercourse or masturbation, white discharge (smegma) and there may be dysuria and retention of urine due to restriction of the foreskin. Urethral stenosis and inflammation can also occur.

Care and management

A holistic assessment of individual needs is required along with appropriate health promotion activity by teaching the patient how to ensure, and reinforcing the need for, good personal hygiene. Emphasis should be placed on daily washing of the penis and the avoidance of soap or bathing products that may be irritant. If an infection is present, depending on the cause of the infection, antibiotic therapy, antifungal or topical steroid preparations may be necessary (National Health Service, 2020); analgesia may also be required. The healthcare professional must ascertain if the man is sexually active; if this is the case, his partner may also require treatment. If a barrier method of contraception is not being used, then the use of a condom for sexual intercourse should be advocated to prevent transmission of infection.

In severe cases of foreskin restriction, e.g. when urinary retention occurs, an emergency circumcision may be required. Post-circumcision, wound healing must be promoted; a non-adherent dressing and patient education focusing on ways to reduce inflammation are required. The man should be taught how to perform personal hygiene associated with the genitalia and given a supply of non-adherent dressings to protect the wound whilst it heals. Patient education regarding the signs of infection is key to reducing the risks of complications. The man should be informed that if excessive bleeding occurs, then he will need to contact his general practice or emergency department. Sexual intercourse and masturbation should cease until after the wound has healed.

Paraphimosis

Conversely, paraphimosis occurs when the foreskin is retracted over the glans penis and forms a constriction near the base of the glans. The cause is usually related to failure of the foreskin to return to its usual position covering the glans penis after manipulation has occurred. The band of foreskin that is retracted remains behind the glans penis leading to vascular engorgement, oedema of the glans and pain. Acute paraphimosis needs rapid evaluation and should be considered a medical emergency (The Royal College of Surgeons, 2016) to prevent lasting damage to, or loss of, the glans.

It may be possible to manually manipulate the foreskin back over the glans penis. Oral and/or topical analgesia and a small amount of lubricant can be used to help with manipulation. The use of ice packs rather than a manual technique to reduce swelling is considered controversial on the basis that it may further compromise distal arterial inflow (Bradley *et al.*, 2020). If manipulation fails, then a dorsal slit may be made in the foreskin, and circumcision advised at a later date due to the risks of recurrence.

Medicines management

Topical preparations

Topically applied medicines can include creams, ointments, lotions, scalp applications and skin patches. They are used for the administration of a number of medicines, for example, anaesthetics, antibiotics or steroids.

The manufacture's guidelines should be followed in conjunction with the prescription. Use local policy concerning the administration of medications.

When applying a topical medication, the area should be gently washed to remove previously applied medication and any debris. Assess the site where topical medications are to be applied and check for irritation and skin breakdown.

Because topical medications are absorbed by the skin, wear gloves when applying them to protect yourself against exposure. If the patient's skin is intact, clean technique is acceptable. However, if the skin is not intact, you must use an aseptic non-touch technique to reduce the risk of introducing a pathogenic organism into the wound.

The dose of medication to be used (e.g. steroidal preparations) is measured in terms of the length of cream or ointment squeezed out of the tube. This is measured in a fingertip unit. One fingertip unit is the distance from the tip of an adult index finger to the first crease of that finger.

After the application of any topical preparation, local policy will need to be adhered to, and this includes the documentation of procedure.

When assisting those men who are unable to carry out the activities of living independently, for example, when assisting them with their personal hygiene or performing catheter care, ensure that the foreskin (in uncircumcised men) is fully retracted to cover the glans penis.

Hydrocele

A hydrocele occurs when there is collection of fluid in the membranous sac that surrounds the testes; it is usual for a hydrocele to appear unilaterally. A hydrocele may occur spontaneously, and the cause may be unknown, or it can be the result of inflammatory conditions such as epididymitis or orchitis – inflammation of the epididymis or testes respectively; trauma may also cause hydrocele. In some cases, the cause may be a testicular tumour.

Diagnosis

A detailed healthcare and medical history will need to be taken, asking the patient about any recent injury or trauma, other medical conditions and a sexual history is required. The scrotum can swell to a considerable size and usually it is painless (asymptomatic), but the excessive swelling can cause discomfort. It becomes painful when the fluid that surrounds the testes becomes infected. The patient may seek help because the size of the swelling can prevent him from enjoying and taking part in social activities such as swimming, running, walking and sexual activity. The swelling can progress and cause the blood supply to the testes to become compromised.

Examination of the contents of the scrotal sac reveals a dullness when the sac is percussed; the swelling feels smooth and is usually located in front of the testes. A hydrocele and tumour can be differentiated using illumination, i.e. a light source (transillumination): a hydrocele allows the light to pass through, whereas a tumour is dense and prevents this from occurring (Bryson, 2017). Ultrasound may be required to determine if there is any underlying cause, e.g. testicular cancer.

Care and management

Where underlying pathology is excluded, intervention to treat a hydrocele is not usually required. Elevation of the scrotum by the wearing of a scrotal support may reduce the swelling. Hydrocelectomy (also known as hydrocele repair) is a surgical procedure used to correct a hydrocele; this can be performed with the patient attending the hospital as a day case. Postoperatively, the patient will be observed for any signs of haemorrhage, and there is also a risk of infection; however, this is rare. There is also a risk of damage to the spermatic vessels, but again this is rare.

In cases where the hydrocele is large, causing discomfort or infected, surgery may be offered as first-line treatment. As an alternative for men unable to undergo surgery and for whom fertility is not a priority, fluid can be aspirated with a cannula or needle and a sclerosing fluid such as tetracycline or alcohol injected to reduce the likelihood of recurrence (Kogan & Erdem, 2020). Aspiration of the fluid carries with it the risk of infection. If the fluid is infected, the man will need to be prescribed antibiotics.

Benign and malignant prostate enlargement

As a man ages, his prostate gland becomes larger, and as ageing progresses the gland atrophies and connective tissue accumulates. Tumours of the prostate gland (benign and malignant) usually grow slowly and as such the symptoms may occur over many years. The accumulation of connective tissue and atrophy is not usually due to cancer and is known as benign prostate hyperplasia (BPH) or benign prostatic enlargement (BPE). BPH is the most common neoplastic growth in men; over 50% of men aged 60 years will have BPH, and not all men will have symptoms (they may be classed as asymptomatic). BPH does not appear to be a risk factor for malignant prostate cancer.

Certain factors increase the risk of prostate cancer:

1. Increasing age
2. A family history of prostate cancer
3. Being black African or black Caribbean

Diagnosis

When symptoms are present, they are the same for BPH and malignant prostate cancer and include:

- Dysuria
- Frequency of micturition
- Urgency

- Nocturia
- Hesitancy.

There may be a history of recurrent urinary tract infection, and increasing urinary obstruction can cause back pressure, leading to renal impairment. Acute urinary retention can occur if the prostate gland becomes enlarged, and this is further complicated if the gland is also infected (prostatitis). Pathological changes as a result of abnormal enlargement of the prostate gland or cell multiplication in either benign or malignant prostate tumours can occur; the key change is pressure caused by the enlarged gland on the prostatic urethra, which can lead to impeded urinary outflow. Over time, urinary retention can impair urinary function, and prostatic obstruction can result in:

- Obstruction of the urethra
- Diverticulum of the bladder
- Hydroureter
- Hydronephrosis
- Infection
- Renal failure.

After a detailed medical history has been undertaken, diagnosis may be confirmed by digital rectal examination (DRE), transrectal ultrasound (TRUS), assessment of prostate-specific antigen (PSA) and other blood tests, such as measurement of serum acid phosphatase. Biopsy of the prostate gland may be undertaken whilst the TRUS is happening. A general physical examination is usually undertaken; the abdomen is palpated along with examination of the lymph glands.

491

The malignant cancer cells of the prostate gland can spread to other parts of the body (metastasise), to the bones as well as the lymph glands and lungs.

Care and management

The care and management of the man with prostate cancer is complex and will depend on the individual. There are several factors that must be given consideration, and a key element of the healthcare professional's role is to provide the man with the information that he requires and in a format that he understands for him to make an informed decision. The staging of the cancer will reveal its size and how far it has spread. The treatment options for a cancer that is small and has not spread far will be different from those for a cancer that is large and has spread widely. The cells of the cancer are examined under the microscope, which then allows it to be graded. The more abnormal the cells, the higher the grade is likely to be; low-grade cancers usually spread more slowly. Other factors that need to be considered include the man's preferences and the results of the PSA, DRE and TRUS.

The following treatment options are available, requiring discussion between the man and the urology team. Treatment depends on the wishes of the individual man and whether the cancer has spread (NICE, 2014):

- Surveillance
- Surgery
- Laser therapy
- Transurethral ablation
- Transurethral microwave therapy
- External beam radiotherapy
- Brachytherapy.

Chemotherapy, radiotherapy and hormone therapy can also be considered, again depending on the individual case.

Surgical intervention may be required to remove the whole gland or the part of the gland that is causing the obstruction. The most common surgical procedure used for BPH is transurethral resection of the prostate gland (TURP). When TURP is performed, a cystoscope is passed into the urinary bladder to visualise the interior of the urinary bladder; a rectoscope is then passed, and resection begins by chipping away small sections of the gland tissue that is compressing the urethra and the neck of the bladder.

Postoperatively, a three-way urethral catheter will be *in situ*, and the urinary bladder is continuously flushed out with a non-electrolyte solution to prevent blood clots from forming.

There are potential complications that can arise in association with surgery on the prostate gland:

- Haemorrhage
- Infection
- Clot retention
- Deep vein thrombosis
- Urethral stricture
- Incontinence
- Erectile dysfunction
- Retrograde ejaculation/ejaculatory volume loss

Snapshot   TURP

Winston Clarke is a 70-year-old small business owner who recently retired. He underwent a TURP procedure 48 hours ago. He has recovered well and following a plan for discharge made during the morning's ward round, is preparing to go home. He would like to discuss resuming sexual activity with his husband and has asked to speak to one of the healthcare team about this before he leaves the ward.

Reflect on Mr Clarke's case and consider:

1. How would you approach this conversation to facilitate an open, patient-centred discussion about sexual well-being and sexual activity?
2. What information will be important to share with Mr Clarke in regard to safely resuming sexual activity following TURP surgery?
3. List the services, including psychosexual support, that are available in your own healthcare setting for patients who may experience an impact on sexual function following surgery to the reproductive tract.

Red flag

Sexual health history language

The healthcare professional must give serious consideration to the use of sexually explicit language within the sexual history consultation and use language that is clear, understandable and with which both clinician and patient are comfortable.

One issue that concerns healthcare professionals is whether to bring vernacular terms into the discussion because of their emotional charge, and some use only medical terms. Often patients are also embarrassed about using colloquialisms in case they cause offence, and some try to express their problem in medical terms but in doing so may misunderstand each other. Such misunderstandings may lead to difficulties in obtaining an accurate history and inappropriate care being provided, so careful judgement must be used in deciding if it would be more appropriate to use colloquial rather than medical terms.

Clinical investigations

PSA testing

PSA is a protein produced by both healthy and cancerous epithelial cells in the prostate gland. It is normal for men to have a small amount of PSA in the blood: the normal range for a PSA test is 3 ng/mL or less. Slightly higher levels may be normal in some older men.

Whilst PSA testing is useful in the management of patients with confirmed prostate gland malignancy, the result of PSA testing alone is not considered an accurate indicator of the presence of malignant prostate disease. This is because PSA levels increase for a variety of reasons, such as increasing age, prostate enlargement, prostatitis (inflammation of the prostate gland) or urinary tract infection. Activities such as anal sex may also increase PSA levels; as can any activity that stimulates the prostate gland, including the DRE. Rarely, PSA test results may be in the normal range in patients with prostate cancer.

The National Institute for Health and Care Excellence (2015) recommend consideration of a PSA test alongside a DRE to assess for prostate cancer in all men who present with lower urinary tract symptoms, erectile dysfunction or visible haematuria (the presence of frank blood in the urine). It is important that the health professional advises patients to refrain from activities that may temporarily increase PSA levels prior to PSA blood testing as well as providing accurate information about the benefits and limitations of this test.

493

Orange flag

TURP and sexual function

Research analysing the impact of TURP on sexual function is unclear. Some research suggests that whilst TURP is commonly associated with retrograde ejaculation, the surgery is unlikely to adversely impact the man's physical sensation of orgasm, libido or erectile function (Mishriki *et al.*, 2011). Health professionals should nevertheless be aware that there may be a perception amongst patients (and their partners) that TURP can lead to erectile dysfunction. Such a perception may have a significant impact on the man's psychology and self-confidence when resuming sexual activity following surgery. The adrenaline released in response to the anxiety of not achieving a firm erection may result in a vicious cycle culminating in erection loss. Patient-centred discussions about the variety of factors that may influence sexual function following surgery are an important element of preparation for this procedure. Men should also be encouraged to report ongoing concerns about sexual function following TURP and should be made aware that support is available if problems occur. Whilst pharmacological interventions such as sildenafil may be appropriate, it is important to also consider the value of psychosexual counselling.

The healthcare professional is required to ensure that the patient is kept pain free postoperatively. It is vital that a strict fluid balance is maintained, and that catheter care is ensured, making every effort to prevent infection. The patient should be encouraged to mobilise as soon as possible as his condition permits. If the patient is to be discharged home with his catheter *in situ*, he will need to be taught how to care for this, and referral will need to be made to the community nurse.

Conclusion

Reproduction of the human species is complex, with the key function of the male and female reproductive tracts being associated with procreation. Whilst the physiological functions associated with reproduction are important, it is also essential to remember that there is pleasure associated with the reproductive tract and that this component is also important for many people.

This chapter has provided insight into the normal and abnormal anatomy and physiology, as well as providing discussion on several pathological changes that may occur in the male and female reproductive tracts. Emphasis has been placed on providing evidence-based information for patients and service users in a format that the person understands, in order to help them make complex decisions about their treatment options and care pathways.

Activities

Here are some activities and exercises to help test your learning. For the answers to these exercises, as well as further self-testing activities, visit our website at **www.wiley.com/go/fundamentalsofappliedpathophysiology/student4e**

Multiple choice questions

1. The United Nation's (1994) definition of reproductive health refers to a state of physical, mental and social well-being in all matters related to the reproductive system during which stages of life?
   (a) During puberty
   (b) During adulthood, including older age
   (c) At all stages of life
   (d) During episodes of disease
2. Demonstrating an understanding of which of the statements below is important to the practice of health professionals caring for those with disease of the reproductive tract?
   (a) Sexual health is a human right
   (b) Freedom of sexual expression is a human right
   (c) The ability to understand and integrate both statements into their practice is fundamental
3. Which of the following is a commonly reported side effect following a transurethral resection of the prostate (TURP)?
   (a) Retrograde ejaculation
   (b) Permanent loss of sexual desire
   (c) Permanent loss of sexual pleasure
4. Name the three layers of the uterus in order, starting with the innermost layer
   (a) Perimetrium, myometrium, endometrium
   (b) Endometrium, myometrium, perimetrium
   (c) Myometrium, perimetrium, endometrium
5. Which of the following problems are reported in association with menses?
   (a) Irregular menstruation
   (b) Excessive pain
   (c) Excessive bleeding
   (d) All of the above.
6. In dysmenorrhoea, which of the lists below most accurately describe the areas of the body where women may report experiencing pain/ discomfort?
   (a) Lower abdomen, pelvic region, back and thighs
   (b) Abdomen and lower back
   (c) Abdomen and thighs.

7. In relation to heavy menstrual bleeding (HMB) at which points are changes in blood chemistry most commonly seen?
   (a) 60 mL
   (b) 120 mL
   (c) Both of the above.

8. Why is a full blood count (FBC) advised for women with heavy menstrual bleeding (HMB)?
   (a) To check for cancer
   (b) To check for anaemia
   (c) To check for hormonal changes

9. What is a contraceptive implant?
   (a) An intrauterine device
   (b) A contraceptive device inserted into the subcutaneous tissue of the arm
   (c) A long-acting intramuscular injection of the hormone progesterone

10. Which of the following correctly list the symptoms of both benign and malignant prostate disease?
    (a) Dysuria, frequency, urgency, hesitancy, nocturia
    (b) Dysuria and frequency
    (c) Nocturia and hesitancy

11. What does the contraction of the cremasteric muscle do?
    (a) Contraction shortens the spermatic chord bringing the testes closer to the body, facilitating temperature regulation
    (b) Contraction helps expel semen during ejaculation
    (c) Contraction enables the uterus to shed endometrium during menstruation

12. Which of the following statements apply to acute paraphimosis?
    (a) Acute paraphimosis is considered a medical emergency
    (b) Reduction should only be attempted once oedema has resolved
    (c) Catheterisation usually resolves the problem

13. How does transillumination help to differentiate a hydrocele from a testicular tumour?
    (a) Light passes through a hydrocele; it does not pass through a tumour
    (b) Light passes through a tumour; it does not pass through a hydrocele
    (c) Transillumination is not recommended to enable differentiation between a hydrocele and a testicular tumour

14. According to current guidelines, what are the limitations of a PSA test in assessing a man for malignancy of the prostate gland?
    (a) Any level of PSA in the blood indicates the presence of malignancy
    (b) There are no limitations, PSA on its own is an accurate way of diagnosing prostate malignancy
    (c) PSA is a protein produced by both healthy and cancerous epithelial cells in the prostate gland. As a result, using currently available PSA testing alone to diagnose cancer is not reliable

15. When taking a sexual history, the health professional should do the following:
    (a) Always use the patient's choices of words to describe sexual organs in order to make the patient feel comfortable
    (b) Carefully consider use of terminology to ensure an accurate, reliable sexual history is taken in a way that does not make either patient or clinician feel uncomfortable
    (c) Always ask the patient to use a pro forma to avoid any embarrassment being caused by discussion

Conditions

Below is a list of conditions that are associated with the reproductive systems. Take some time and write notes about each of the conditions. You may make the notes taken from textbooks or other resources (e.g. clinical colleagues you work with) or you may make the notes based on people you have cared for. Please ensure that you adhere to the rules of confidentiality.

Endometriosis	
Cervical cancer	
Chlamydia	
Penile cancer	
Balanitis	

Further resources

National Institute for Health and Care Excellence (NICE)

http://www.nice.org.uk/

NICE provides guidance, sets quality standards and manages a national database to improve people's health and prevent and treat ill health. There are many excellent resources on this website that can help guide and inform practice.

Men's Health Forum

http://www.menshealthforum.org.uk/

This is a charity that provides an independent and authoritative voice for male health in England and Wales, and tackles the issues and inequalities affecting the health and well-being of men and boys. The site is packed with data and a numerous links to other sites and resources

Sexual Advice Association

http://sexualadviceassociation.co.uk

This is the website of a charitable organisation with the aim of helping to improve the sexual health and well-being of men and women and to raise awareness of the extent to which sexual conditions affect the general population. It also has a helpline that can be used to discuss concerns that people feel they cannot discuss with their doctor.

Verity

http://www.verity-pcos.org.uk/home

A self-help group for women with polycystic ovary syndrome. Verity organises conferences and conducts research.

Caring for people with a learning disability. Resources from the Royal College of Nursing

https://www.rcn.org.uk/library/subject-guides/learning-disability-nursing

The Royal College of Nursing offers a variety of resources to support standards of care for people with a learning disability.

Prostate Cancer UK

www.prostatecanceruk.org

The first National organisation for prostate cancer in the UK. Prostate Cancer UK supports the care and well-being of men with prostate cancer in the UK, increase investment in prostate cancer research and raise the profile of prostate cancer with the public. They offer a free online learning module for health professionals on discussing sex with people with and affected by prostate cancer.

Women's Health Forum Royal College of Nursing

https://www.rcn.org.uk/get-involved/forums/womens-health-forum

This forum provides nurses and others with up-to-date information and news associated with women's health. The forum organises a number of events, conferences and meetings. The site has a variety of useful links and other resources.

Glossary of terms

Ablation   To destroy (e.g. endometrial ablation means to destroy the layer of the cells that lines the uterus).

Asymptomatic   Without symptoms.

Atrophy   Wasting away; a diminution in the size of a cell, tissue or organ.

Bartholin's glands   Two small round structures on either side of the vaginal opening. Secretions from these glands provide vaginal lubrication. The exact purpose of the fluid secreted is not fully understood.

Benign   Causes no problem. In cancer, it means a growth that is not malignant.

Brachytherapy   In prostate cancer, implantation of tiny radioactive seeds under anaesthetic directly into the prostate gland.

Cilia   Small hair-like structures on the outer surface of some cells; used to propel liquids.

Clitoris   A small body of tissue that is highly sexually sensitive; it is protected by the prepuce. Becomes enlarged and erect during sexual stimulation.

Cystoscope   A thin tube with a light and eyepiece attached to it, allowing the user to see the inside of the urinary bladder.

Diverticulum   A pouch or sac opening from a tubular or saccular organ (e.g. the urinary bladder).

Dorsal   Pertaining to the back; the rear aspect.

Dyspareunia   Pain with intercourse.

Fibroid   A non-cancerous growth in the uterus.

Hydronephrosis   An abnormal enlargement of the kidney that may be due to ureteral obstruction.

Hydroureter   Distension of the ureter with urine as a result of blockage.

Hysterosalpingogram   X-ray examination of the uterus and uterine tubes after radio-opaque dye has been injected.

Ischaemia   A low oxygen state in a part of the body. Usually the result of an obstruction to the blood supply to tissues.

Labia majora   The inner layers of the vulva – thinner than the labia minora; protects the urethra, vagina and clitoris.

Labia minora   The outer layers of the vulva, covered with pubic hair and containing sweat and sebaceous glands. Situated on either side of the vagina.

Laparoscopy   The passage of a laparoscope into the abdominal cavity via the abdominal wall to allow the cavity to be viewed.

Laparotomy   A surgical procedure that requires an incision to be made into the abdomen.

Lumen   The inside space of a tubular structure.

Malignant   Invasive, has a tendency to grow and may spread to other parts of the body.

Mons pubis   Also known as the mons Veneris (Latin for the Hill of Venus, the Roman Goddess of love). Fatty tissue covering the symphysis pubis.

Nulliparous   Never having given birth to a viable infant.

Os   Mouth; a term applied to an opening in a hollow organ such as the cervix.

Peristalsis   A wave-like contraction.

Prepuce   A loose fold of skin covering the glans penis and glans clitoris.

Prolactin   A hormone primarily associated with lactation. Secreted by the anterior pituitary gland.

Prolactinoma   A prolactin-producing tumour of the anterior pituitary gland; a slow-growing benign swelling.

Prostaglandin   Complex unsaturated fatty acid produced by the mast cells and acting as a messenger substance between cells. Intensifies the actions of histamine and kinins. They cause increased vascular permeability, neutrophil chemotaxis, stimulation of smooth muscle (e.g. the uterus) and can induce pain.

Slough   Dead tissue that has separated from the living structure.

Trocar   A sharp-pointed surgical instrument that fits inside a tube (cannula).

Unilateral   Affecting only one side; as opposed to bilateral, affecting both sides.

References

Bradley, N. Bragg, S. and Leslie, W (2020) *Paraphimosis*. Florida: StatPearls. https://www.ncbi.nlm.nih.gov/books/NBK459233 Accessed June 2020.

British Association of Paediatric Urologists (2006) *Foreskin Conditions*. https://www.baps.org.uk/resources/management-foreskin-conditions/ Accessed June 2020.

Bryson, D. (2017). *Transillumination of Testicular Hydrocele*. Clin Med Image Library. https://clinmedjournals.org/articles/cmil/cmil-3-075.php?jid=cmil. Accessed June 2020.

Grossman, S. and Porth, C.M. (2014). *Porth's Pathophysiology: Concepts of Altered Health States*, 9th edn. Philadelphia: Lippincott.

Kenny, L., Bickerstaff, H. and Myers, J. (2017). *Gynaecology by Ten Teachers*, 19th edn. London: Hodder.

Khan, K.S., Champeneria, R. and Latthe, P.M. (2012) How effective are non-drug, non surgical treatments for primary dysmenorrhoea? *British Medical Journal*, 344: e3011.

Kogan, B.A. and Erdem, E. (2020). Hydrocele. *Best Practice: British Medical Journal*. http://newbp.bmj. com/topics/en-gb/1104. Accessed June 2020.

Linhart, J. (2007). *Female Reproductive Problems*. In: Monahan, F.D., Sand, J.K.,

Neighbors, M., Marek, J.F. and Green, C.J. (eds), *Phipps' Medical Surgical Nursing: Health and Illness Human Anatomy and Physiology Perspectives*, 8th edn. St Louis: Mosby, pp. 1685–1720.

Marieb, E.N and Keller. S.M (2017). *Essentials of Human Anatomy and Physiology*, 12th edn. San Francisco Park: Pearson.

Marieb, E.N. and Hoehn, K. (2018). *Human Anatomy and Physiology*, 11th edn. New Jersey: Pearson.

Mazza, D. (2011). *Women's Health in General Practice*. Edinburgh: Elsevier.

National Health Service (2020). *Phimosis and Paraphimosis*. https://www.nhs.uk/conditions/phimosis/ Accessed June 2020.

National Health Service Wales (2013). *Guidelines for Chaperoning or Escorting*. NHS Wales: Aneurin Bevan Health Board.

National Institute for Health and Care Excellence (2007). *Treatment and Care for Women with Heavy Periods*. London: NICE.

National Institute for Health and Care Excellence (2014). *Prostate Cancer: Diagnosis and Treatment*. London: NICE. https://www.nice.org.uk/guidance/cg175 Accessed June 2020.

National Institute for Health and Care Excellence (2015). *Lower Urinary Tract Symptoms: Management. Guidance; CG97*. London: NICE.

Nursing and Midwifery Council (2018). *The Code: Professional Standards of Practice for Nurses, Midwives and Nursing Associates.* https://www.nmc.org.uk/globalassets/sitedocuments/nmc-publications/ nmc-code.pdf Accessed June 2020.

Royal College of Obstetricians and Gynaecologists (RCOG) (2013). *Chronic Pelvic Pain, Initial Management: Green Top Guideline Number 41*. London: RCOG.

Royal College of Obstetricians and Gynaecologists (RCOG) (2014). *Long-term Consequences of Polycystic Ovary Syndrome: Green TopGuideline Number 33*. London: RCOG.

Royal College of Obstetricians and Gynaecologists (RCOG) (2020). *Evaluation of Amenorrhoea*. London: RCOG. https://elearning.rcog.org.uk//causes-and-management-amenorrhoea/evaluation-amenorrhoea Accessed June 2020.

Royal College Surgeons (2016). *Management of Paediatric Testicular Torsion*. London: RCS.

Shasi, P., Chapman, H. and Evans, D. (2010). Psychological and psychiatric morbidity in lichen sclerosus in a cohort recruited from a genitourinary medicine clinic. *International Journal of STD and Aids*, 21. 1: 17–18.

Thibodeau, G.A. and Patton, K.T. (2013). *The Human Body in Health and Disease*, 6th edn. St Louis: Elsevier.

Tortora, G.J. (2017). *Principles of Anatomy and Physiology*, 15th edn. New York: Wiley.

United Nations (1994). *International Conference on Population and Development*. Report of the International Conference on Population and Development: Cairo, New York: United Nations.

Wang, S-F., Lee, J.P. and Hwa, H-L. (2009). Effect of transcutaneous electrical nerve stimulation on primary dysmenorrhea. *Neuromodulation*, 12(4): 302–309.

World Health Organisation (2020). Sexual and reproductive health: definition. World Health Organisation: Europe. https://www.euro.who.int/en/health-topics/Life-stages/sexual-and-reproductive-health/ news/news/2011/06/sexual-health-throughout-life/definition Accessed June 2020.

Chapter 17

Pain and pain management

Anthony Wheeldon

Senior Lecturer, Department of Adult Nursing and Primary Care, School of Health and Social Work, University of Hertfordshire, Hatfield, Hertfordshire, UK

Contents

Introduction 501
The physiology of pain 502
Pain classification 507
The pain experience 509
Pain theories..510
Pain pathophysiology and management..511

Conclusion 530
Multiple choice questions...........................531
Conditions...532
Further resources...533
Glossary of terms...534
References..536

Key words

- Acute pain
- Chronic pain
- Neuropathy
- Opioid
- Ascending pain pathway
- Descending pain pathway
- Nociceptors
- Somatic pain
- Analgesia
- Gate control theory
- Non-opioid
- Visceral pain

Fundamentals of Applied Pathophysiology: An Essential Guide for Nursing and Healthcare Students, Fourth Edition. Edited by Ian Peate.
© 2021 John Wiley & Sons Ltd. Published 2021 by John Wiley & Sons Ltd.
Student companion website: www.wiley.com/go/fundamentalsofappliedpathophysiology/student4e
Instructor companion website: www.wiley.com/go/fundamentalsofappliedpathophysiology/instructor4e

Test your prior knowledge

- What is the difference between acute and chronic pain?
- How would you assess a patient's pain?
- Discuss the pain pathway.
- Explain the difference between opioid and non-opioid medications.
- List five non-pharmacological methods of pain control.

Learning outcomes

On completion of this chapter, the reader will be able to:

- Describe the physiology of pain transmission and sensation.

- Explain the difference between acute and chronic pain.

- Explain the principles of the gate control theory of pain.

- Discuss the pathophysiology of a range of pain disorders.

- Discuss the impact of pain on an individual's well-being.

- Identify an effective range of pain assessment strategies.

501

Don't forget to visit the companion website for this book (www.wiley.com/go/fundamentalsofappliedpathophysiology/student4e) **where you can find self-assessment tests to check your progress, as well as lots of activities to practise your learning.**

Introduction

Pain is an integral part of life. Everyone experiences it at various times throughout their lifetime; indeed, pain is the most common reason for an individual to seek medical advice. Yet, despite its prevalence, it remains difficult to define. One common definition states that "Pain is whatever the experiencing person says it is, existing when he says it does" (McCaffery, 1979, p. 11). Pain is not only an unpleasant or uncomfortable sensation that occurs as a result of injury, strain or disease, it can also be an emotional experience unrelated to tissue damage. For example, pain is a term used to describe feelings relating to loss, grief and even unrequited love. Pain is also an individual and personal experience. The way someone expresses and deals with their pain will be determined by their culture, life experiences and personality.

Unresolved pain can have an adverse effect on the cardiovascular, respiratory, gastrointestinal, neuroendocrine and musculoskeletal systems. It can also promote anxiety and sleeplessness (MacIntyre and Schug, 2015). The management of pain is often associated with the administration of analgesia; however, there are a wide range of non-pharmacological methods of pain control available. Because it is an emotional as well as physiological phenomenon, the successful assessment and control of pain is reliant upon an individualised holistic plan of care, which utilises both pharmacological and non-pharmacological treatments.

The physiology of pain

The physiology of pain is complex and in some instances not fully understood. However, the generation of pain follows a basic three-step process (Figure 17.1):

1. An irritation or injury, such as a cut or burn, is detected in the peripheral nervous system by special nerve cells called nociceptors.
2. A nerve impulse is then generated, sending a pain impulse towards the central nervous system.
3. This message is received by the brain where the extent and significance of the irritation or injury is interpreted and pain is sensed.

Nociceptors

Nociceptors are free nerve endings present in every tissue in the body, except for the brain. They are activated by noxious stimuli, of which there are three broad types: thermal, mechanical and chemical. As the name suggests, thermal stimuli are sensations of severe heat or cold. Mechanical stimuli, on the other hand, are produced by tissue damage caused by trauma or disease, including:

- Damage to tissue due to trauma or minor injury
- Lack of blood flow and oxygen, i.e. ischaemia and hypoxia

502

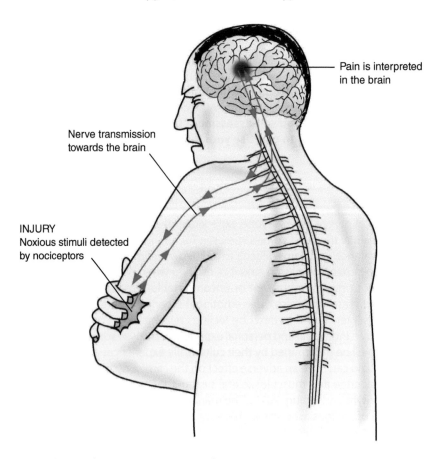

Figure 17.1   Pathway of pain transmission and interpretation.

- Ulceration
- Infection
- Nerve damage
- Inflammation.

Chemical stimuli detect the presence of chemicals such as histamine, kinins and prostaglandins, which are released as a result of tissue damage and inflammation.

The actions of nociceptors are not clear; however, two types have been identified – polymodal nociceptors, which detect mechanical, thermal and chemical stimuli, and mechanoceptors, which sense intense mechanical stimuli only.

The ascending pain pathway

Nociceptor stimulation leads directly to the transmission of a pain impulse along special sensory fibres towards the thalamus and somatosensory cortex within the brain, where the severity and meaning of the pain is analysed. This line of communication is called the ascending pain pathway. It consists of three linked neurons called first-, second- and third-order neurons, depending on their place in the pathway. The first-order neurons travel from the nociceptors to the spine; second-order neurons travel upwards through the spinal cord towards the thalamus in the brain; and third-order neurons run from the thalamus through the brain towards the somatosensory area of the cerebral cortex

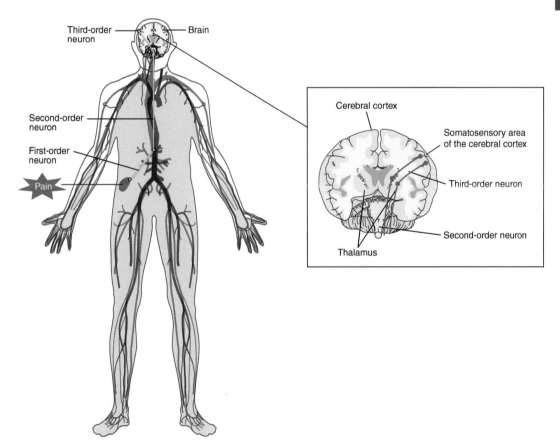

Figure 17.2   The ascending pain pathway.

(Figure 17.2). The line of communication between the first-, second- and third-order neurons is maintained by a number of neurotransmitters, such as substance P and serotonin (MacLellan, 2006).

The two first-order neurons responsible for the transmission of the pain impulse between the nociceptors and the spinal cord are A-delta (Aδ) fibres and C fibres. The speed of this transmission depends upon the diameter of the fibre and whether or not the fibre is myelinated. The axons of myelinated fibres are surrounded by a sheath of myelin, which electrically insulates them and increases the speed of nerve conduction (Figure 17.3). Aδ fibres are thicker and are myelinated, and therefore transmit pain impulses faster than C fibres, which are thinner and non-myelinated (Table 17.1).

Pain is often described as having two phases, referred to as first and second pain. First pain is described as a sharp or pricking pain, whereas second pain is the dull, burning or aching pain that follows. Aδ fibres are thought to receive input from mechanoceptors and also generate the first pain sensation. C fibres, on the other hand, are thought to receive input from polymodal nociceptors and are more likely to produce second pain. Pain impulses follow the same pathway as touch and mild heat and cold. The sensory fibres responsible for these sensations are A-beta (Aβ) fibres. Aβ fibres are myelinated and are thicker than both Aδ fibres and C fibres and therefore can transmit signals much faster. Stimulation of Aβ fibres, by rubbing a mild injury, for example, can alleviate the pain.

504

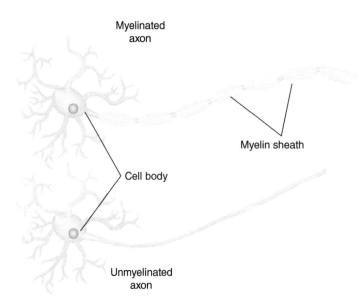

Figure 17.3   Basic structure of myelinated and unmyelinated nerve fibres.

Table 17.1   Size and speed of first-order sensory fibres.

Sensory fibre	Diameter (μm)	Myelinated	Speed of conduction (m/s)
A-beta (Aβ) fibres	6–12	Yes	35–75
A-delta (Aδ) fibres	1–5	Yes	5–35
C fibres	0.2–1.5	No	0.5–2

The first-order neurons enter the spinal cord at a location called the dorsal horn (Figure 17.4). Here they synapse (connect) with second-order neurons, of which there are two types: nociceptive-specific (NS) and wide dynamic range (WDR) neurons. Both respond to noxious stimuli; however, WDR neurons also react to non-noxious input, such as those transmitted by Aβ fibres, i.e. touch, heat and cold. Both NS and WDR neurons cross over the spinal cord into white matter, where they continue to rise up the spinal cord towards the thalamus along a pathway called the spinothalamic tract (Figure 17.5).

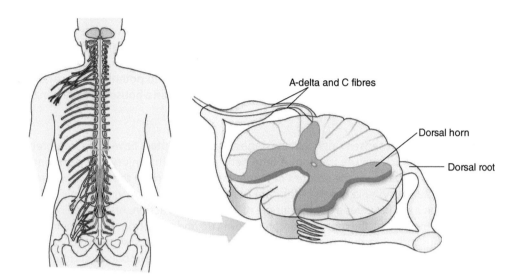

Figure 17.4 Cross-section of the spinal cord. Note that both sides are identical.

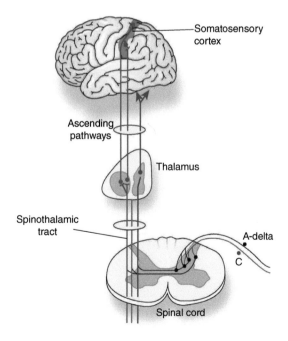

Figure 17.5 The spinothalamic tract.

Pain interpretation

The spinothalamic tract ends at the thalamus, where second-order neurons meet third-order neurons. Third-order neurons travel through the brain towards the somatosensory cortex, a part of the brain that allows the individual to locate pain and describe it. As well as locating the pain, the brain will also generate an emotional response, be it anger or distress or mild irritation. The area of the brain thought to influence this emotional response is the limbic system (Figure 17.6). Often referred to as the 'emotional brain', the limbic system deals with feelings of pain, pleasure, affection and anger. An individual's response is not predictable as it is dependent upon their personality, life history and culture. The limbic system also evaluates the seriousness of the pain and helps the individual to remember why the pain occurred. Over time people learn to avoid painful stimuli, such as sharp objects and broken glass, and thus protect themselves from injury (Godfrey, 2005a). However, this protective element has its limits; e.g. individuals may deliberately expose themselves to potential injury and pain if it means rescuing a loved one from a perilous situation, i.e. from a house fire (Johnson, 2005).

Reflex arcs

Because pain is not sensed until pain messages from nociceptors have been interpreted by the brain, there is a minute fraction of time between the initial injury and pain sensation. Reflex arcs aim to reduce the amount of tissue damage by forcing the body away from the source of the injury quickly and before the brain processes the inevitable pain messages. Stepping on a pin provides a good example of a reflex arc in action. After stepping on a pin, reflex arcs ensure that the foot involuntarily moves up and away from the pin before pain is sensed, thus reducing the amount of tissue damage. Reflex arcs work by collecting pain impulses from first-order neurons and then immediately sending impulses, via interneurons, along motor nerves back towards skeletal muscle (Figure 17.7).

Descending pain pathways

Descending pain pathways seek to inhibit the sensation of pain. They involve the release of special neuropeptides that have analgesic properties. They bind with opiate receptors, which are present throughout the central nervous system, and block the action of the neurotransmitter, substance P.

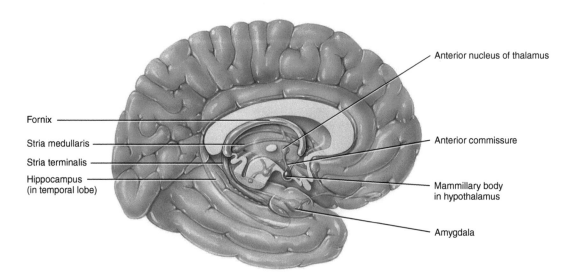

Figure 17.6   The limbic system.

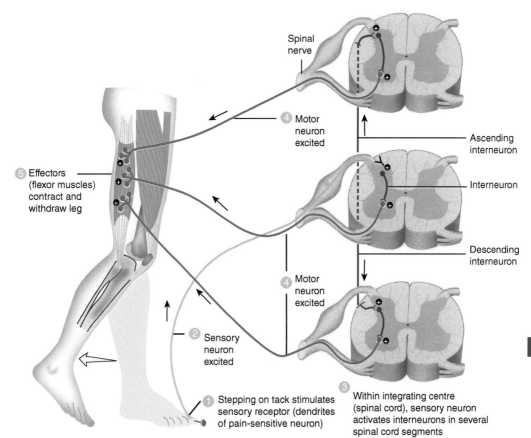

Spinal nerve

④ Motor neuron excited

Ascending interneuron

⑤ Effectors (flexor muscles) contract and withdraw leg

Interneuron

Descending interneuron

④ Motor neuron excited

② Sensory neuron excited

① Stepping on tack stimulates sensory receptor (dendrites of pain-sensitive neuron)

③ Within integrating centre (spinal cord), sensory neuron activates interneurons in several spinal cord segments

Figure 17.7   Example of a reflex arc working in response to pain.

Because of their analgesic effect, these neuropeptides are often referred to as endogenous or natural opiates. There are three groups of endogenous opiate – endorphins, encephalins and dynorphins – and there are four major categories of opiate receptor: mu (μ), kappa (κ), sigma (σ) and delta (δ). Levels of endorphins, encephalins and dynorphins increase during periods of stress and pain. However, stimulation of opiate receptors also promotes feelings of euphoria and well-being, and it is endogenous opiates such as endorphins that are associated with the pleasant sensations experienced during excitement, sexual activity and even exercise.

Pain classification
Transient, acute and chronic pain

Pain is classified according to its duration. A short episode of pain, as a consequence of a stubbed toe or a cut finger, for example, is classified as transient pain. The injured individual, despite perhaps becoming momentarily upset, will consider the pain to be of no consequence and not seek medical attention.

Acute pain is associated with a severe sudden onset; however, unlike transient pain, it is prolonged and continues until healing begins. Acute pain is intense and can be an intolerable experience; in response, areas of the brain seek to restore homeostasis by initiating an autonomic response. The thalamus, hypothalamus and reticular formation (Figure 17.8), for example, promote diaphoresis, tachycardia, hypertension and tachypnoea in response to acute pain.

507

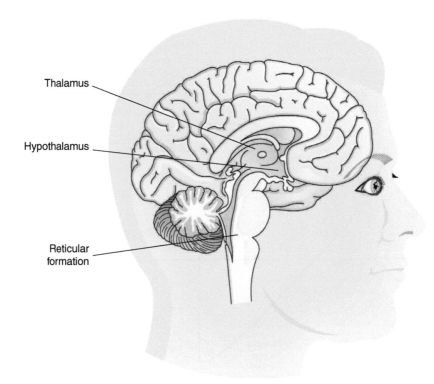

Figure 17.8   Location of the thalamus, hypothalamus and reticular formation.

The term *chronic pain* is used to describe pain that continues even though healing is complete. Although the pain may remain as intense as acute pain, there is little or no autonomic response. Acute pain is a symptom of an associated medical condition or injury. Chronic pain, on the other hand, exists after the injury or disease has ceased. For this reason, chronic pain is often considered to be a syndrome – a medical condition in its own right (Melzack and Wall, 1988).

Red flag

Absence of symptoms may not indicate a lack of pain – pain is what the patient says it is.
   Chronic pain may not generate some of the classic visible symptoms that are often present in acute pain, for example:

- Tachycardia
- Hypertension
- Diaphoresis
- Grimace
- Guarding

However, the intensity of their pain may be as severe as an episode of acute pain. Therefore, individuals with chronic pain will require the same level of comfort, reassurance and analgesia as individuals in acute pain. Remember, 'pain is what the patient says it is'.

Superficial and deep pain

Pain is categorised according to location and is often called deep or superficial. Superficial pain occurs due to nociceptor stimulation in the skin. Because there are large numbers of nociceptors in skin, pain can be easily located. Acute superficial pain is often described as a sharp, pricking sensation. Deep pain, on the other hand, is dull and prolonged. Deep pain can be either somatic or visceral. Somatic pain emanates from structures such as bones, muscles, joints and tendons. Visceral pain is produced when nociceptors in organs such as the kidneys, stomach, gallbladder and intestines are stimulated. Unlike the skin, these organs and others like them have far fewer nociceptors, and therefore it is often difficult for an individual to describe the exact location of their pain (MacLellan, 2006).

The pain experience

The term *pain threshold* is often used to describe an individual's response to pain; e.g. a patient may be said to have a high or low pain threshold. Pain threshold is the point at which an individual will report pain. It is generally accepted that all humans have a similar pain threshold. People nevertheless express pain in a variety of ways. This is because the expression of pain is influenced by emotional state, personality, past experience, culture and social status, rather than a personal pain threshold.

The limbic system, which processes emotional responses to pain, interacts closely with the frontal lobes, which are responsible for cognitive thought. This explains why people in acute pain may at times behave irrationally. Conversely, people can often control their emotions if pain occurs when it is socially unacceptable to cry out or complain (Marieb and Hoehn, 2018). The person's state of mind also influences pain intensity. Anxiety and depression, for example, have been shown to increase pain levels (Carr *et al.*, 2005), whereas reducing anxiety levels through education can reduce pain (Lin and Wang, 2005).

An individual's attitude towards pain can also affect its intensity. Attitudes towards pain are often influenced by the meaning of the pain experience. For example, patients having undergone elective surgery report less pain than patients involved in sudden traumatic accidents. This may be because postsurgical pain may be viewed as a symptom of surgery and healing, and therefore as something positive. The meaning of pain can change and alter pain perception. For instance, mild abdominal pain may become severe when the individual learns that it may be something serious (Melzack and Wall, 1988). Past experiences are also a contributing factor. Patients who have been exposed to severe pain during a prior medical procedure may become anxious about future treatments and ultimately sense greater levels of pain. People also learn how to express and react to pain by observing those around them. A person's attitude towards their pain may be influenced by the experiences of family members or their ethnicity and culture (Briggs, 2010).

Orange flag

Pain is a personal experience

Pain is a personal experience and unique to the sufferer. If holistic and effective care is to occur, healthcare professionals must shelve their own pain experiences and focus on the experience of the individual in pain. The way they react may be different from how you would react. 'Pain is what the patient says it is', and therefore healthcare professionals must take an objective and person-centred approach. Inadequate care and attention to the individual's feelings could lead to psychological harm.

Pain theories

Most pain theories acknowledge that the pain experience is both emotional and psychological. The specificity theory hypothesises that pain is experienced when specific nerve endings are stimulated. Information is then carried to a pain centre in the brain. It is the characteristics of the stimulus rather than the brain that determine the intensity of the pain. Pattern theory, on the other hand, suggests that no separate system for pain sensation exists. Rather pain is interpreted by the brain when intense peripheral nerve stimulation occurs. Such theories do not explain why pain can occur as a result of a gentle stimulus, i.e. neuralgia, or when no tissue damage exists. Neither do they explain why two people with the same injury may experience different levels of pain. For this reason, Melzack and Wall's gate control theory is more widely accepted as the most important pain theory.

Gate control theory of pain

The gate control theory of pain proposes that pain impulses must pass through a theoretical 'gate' at the dorsal horn of the spinal cord before ascending towards the brain (Figure 17.9).

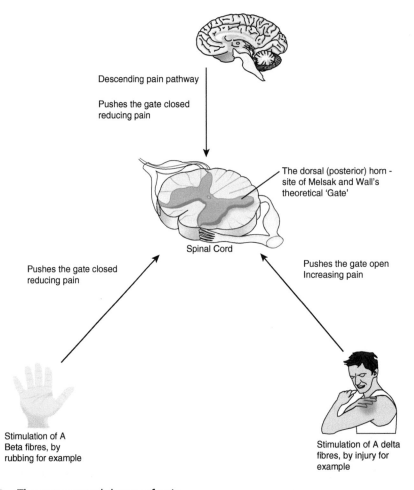

Descending pain pathway

Pushes the gate closed reducing pain

The dorsal (posterior) horn - site of Melsak and Wall's theoretical 'Gate'

Spinal Cord

Pushes the gate closed reducing pain

Pushes the gate open Increasing pain

Stimulation of A Beta fibres, by rubbing for example

Stimulation of A delta fibres, by injury for example

Figure 17.9   The gate control theory of pain.

Pain messages from Aδ and C fibres will push open the gate. However, the actions of Aβ fibres and the descending pain pathway will push the gate closed. The intensity of an individual's pain, therefore, is determined by a balance between noxious stimuli and Aβ fibre or descending brain activity. The wider the gate opens, the more intense the pain; if the gate closes, the pain ceases (McCaffery *et al.*, 2003).

Stimulation of the larger Aβ fibres with touch or heat can inhibit pain transmission via Aδ and C fibres. This helps explain how rubbing mild injuries, acupuncture and transcutaneous electrical nerve stimulation (TENS) may reduce pain levels. Increased activity in the descending pain pathway also seeks to close the gate to pain. This may explain why a person's emotional state, personality and culture may determine how pain is expressed. For example, increased levels of endogenous opiates can push the gate closed. The gate control theory also proposes that pain intensity is influenced by the action of transmission cells and substantia gelatinosa cells, which are found within the dorsal horn of the spinal cord. Transmission (T) cells transmit pain messages towards the brain. Substantia gelatinosa (SG) cells, on the other hand, inhibit T-cell activity and thus push the gate to pain closed. The activity of both T cells and SG cells are enhanced by the descending pain pathway and therefore the individual's state of mind. In depressive and anxious states, T-cell activity is enhanced, pushing the gate open and increasing pain intensity. However, in relaxed and contented states, SG cell action is increased, pushing the gate closed and decreasing pain levels (Melzack and Wall, 1988; Figure 17.10).

511

Orange flag

Depression and its influence on pain
Depression and low mood can enhance the intensity of pain. Long-term and unresolved pain can lead to depression and anxiety. Often people living with chronic pain get locked into a vicious cycle of depression and exacerbation of pain that can be difficult to break out of. Healthcare professionals must ensure that they account for psychological status when assessing a patient in pain and planning their care.

Pain pathophysiology and management
Pathophysiology
Referred and phantom limb pain

Referred pain occurs when tissue damage in one area of the body leads to pain elsewhere, e.g. pain as a result of angina. Although the tissue damage arises in the coronary arteries, pain is also felt radiating down the left arm. Despite sensing intense pain, the tissue there remains healthy. Referred pain happens because the damaged or inflamed organ and the area where pain is felt are served by nerves from the same segment of the spinal cord. Other examples include pain due to liver or gallbladder inflammation being sensed in the right shoulder. Figure 17.11 highlights the main instances of referred pain (Tortora and Derrickson, 2017).

The term *phantom limb pain* describes the pain sensed by amputees where the removed limb once was. The pain is often described as burning, cramps, tingling, electric shocks,

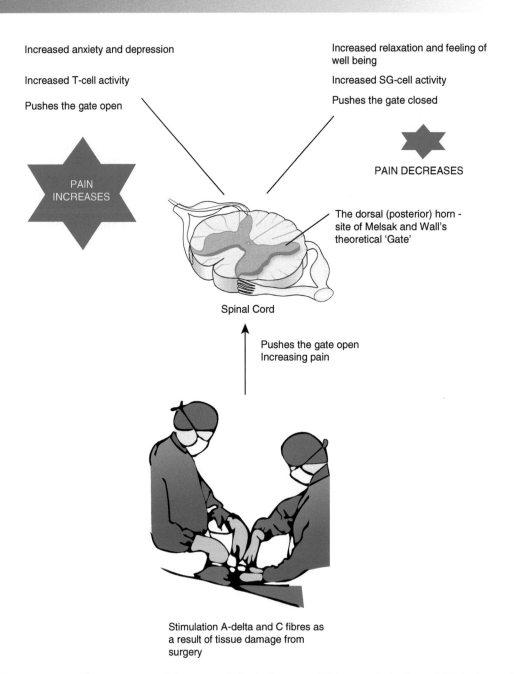

Increased anxiety and depression

Increased T-cell activity

Pushes the gate open

PAIN INCREASES

Increased relaxation and feeling of well being

Increased SG-cell activity

Pushes the gate closed

PAIN DECREASES

The dorsal (posterior) horn - site of Melsak and Wall's theoretical 'Gate'

Spinal Cord

Pushes the gate open
Increasing pain

Stimulation A-delta and C fibres as a result of tissue damage from surgery

Figure 17.10   The gate control theory and the influence of T (transmission), and SG (substantia gelatinosa)-cell activity.

itching or pins and needles, and it has been reported by the majority of trauma and surgical amputees (Colquhoun *et al.*, 2019). The precise pathophysiology is unknown. However, a number of possible explanations have been hypothesised. One suggests that the brain continues to receive 'signals' from the amputated limb. Another proposes that painful limbs create 'pain memories' before amputation, while another common assumption is that tissue damage leads to increased sensitivity in nociceptors stimulating neighbouring nerves not originally involved in the initial injury (Virani *et al.*, 2014).

512

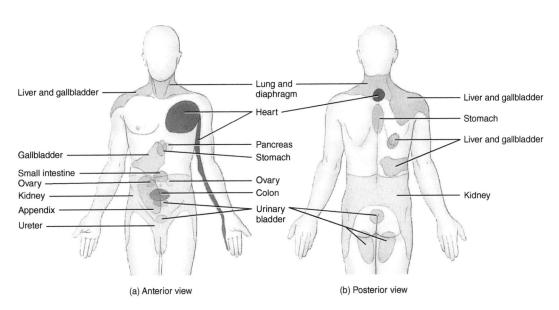

Figure 17.11   Examples of referred pain and the origin of the tissue damage.

Neuropathy

513

Neuropathic pain occurs when the nociceptors and neurons are damaged. There are many conditions that lead to the development of neuropathic pain:

- Entrapment (trapped nerves)
- Causalgia (sensory nerve damage)
- Scar tissue
- Thoracotomy
- Amputation
- Diabetes
- Herpes
- Ischaemia.

Neuropathies produce pain that is described as a burning, electric or tingling, and the pain can be continuous or spasmodic. The nervous tissue in the ascending pain pathways is said to be plastic, meaning it can change in response to psychological and physical stimuli. This includes changes to the sensitivity of nociceptors, which can begin to generate pain impulses in response to ordinary feelings of touch. The patient may complain of pain when slight pressure is exerted on the site of injury, a phenomenon called allodynia. Damaged neural tissue also leads to increased sensitivity to painful stimuli, and the individual will feel pain that is out of proportion to the level of tissue damage. This increase in pain sensitivity is referred to as hyperalgesia (Scadding, 2003).

Postoperative pain

Up to 90% of patients experience pain after surgery, with up to 30% reporting severe pain (Ingadottir *et al*, 2017). A significant contributory factor to postoperative pain is anxiety, which can increase pain intensity. Anxiety and apprehension prior to surgery lead to high levels of pain postoperatively (Theunissen *et al.*, 2012). In order to reduce postoperative pain, carers should invest in preoperative care strategies that minimise preoperative anxiety, such as patient education (Alanazi, 2014). Carers are also ideally placed to minimise postoperative pain as they are responsible for the administration and evaluation of prescribed analgesics.

Unresolved pain leads to a complicated postsurgical recovery. Pain in the chest or abdomen, for example, can affect respiration. People in pain tend to breathe shallowly and avoid coughing. Painful movement can also render patients reluctant to mobilise. Pain also slows down gastric emptying and reduces intestinal motility, probably due to the activation of a reflex arc. Prolonged pain also increases levels of anxiety. Indeed, pain and anxiety are intertwined problems, as during the postoperative period one inevitably leads to the other. The effects of unresolved anxiety can have a severe detrimental effect on the patient's postoperative recovery. Prolonged anxiety will lead to a stress response as the body attempts to maintain homeostasis. During stress, the neuroendocrine system releases numerous hormones that increase blood pressure, pulse and metabolism. Epinephrine (adrenaline), for example, increases heart rate, and aldosterone increases blood pressure. Cortisol and glucagon, on the other hand, liberate more glucose for the production of energy. Cortisol also decreases immune function (MacIntyre and Schug, 2015). The combination of unresolved pain and anxiety affects many major body systems, which can lead to chest infection, impaired wound healing and deep vein thrombosis among other complications (Table 17.2).

Cancer pain

There is a high prevalence of pain in patients with cancer. Indeed, in some studies, up to 96% of patients with cancer experience pain, more than those with HIV (80%), heart disease (77%), renal disease (77%) and chronic obstructive pulmonary disease (50%) (Solano *et al.*, 2006).

Table 17.2   Effects of pain and stress on four major body systems.

Respiratory system	Hypoventilation	Hypoxaemia	Gastrointestinal system	Delayed gastric emptying	Nausea and vomiting
	Decreased cough	Hypoxia		Intestinal motility	Reduced nutrition
	Tachypnoea	Retained sputum			Poor wound healing
		Chest infection			
Cardiovascular system	Tachycardia	Elevated heart workload	Renal system	Increased retention of sodium and water	Lower urine output
	Hypertension	Deep vein thrombosis			
	Reduced venous return	Pulmonary embolism			
	Coronary vasoconstrictive				
Musculoskeletal system	Reduced mobility	Prolonged postoperative recovery	Pancreas	Increased glucagon	Increased blood sugar levels
	Muscle atrophy	Deep vein thrombosis		Decreased insulin	
		Pulmonary embolism			

Source: Adapted from Cousins and Power, 2003; MacIntyre and Schug, 2015.

Table 17.3   Types of cancer pain, their source, causes and descriptions.

Type of pain	Structures affected	Causes	Patient description
Somatic nociceptor	Muscle and bone	Bone metastases. Surgical incisions	Aching, sharp, gnawing or dull. Easily located
Neuropathic	Nerves	Chemotherapy. Tumour	Burning, itching, numbness, tingling, shooting
Visceral nociceptor	Organs of the abdomen, pelvis and thorax	Tumour	Crampy, colicky, aching, deep, squeezing, dull
			Less easily located

Source: Adapted from Kochhar, 2002.
Note: Listed in order of prevalence. Most patients have a combination of somatic and visceral nociceptor pain.

The causes of cancer pain are wide and varied, but the most common cancer pain is that caused by bone metastases. Cancer pain can be classified as being either nociceptive or neuropathic. Table 17.3 lists the common causes and descriptions of cancer pain.

The aim of palliative care is to minimise pain and its associated distressing symptoms (WHO, 2008). Cancer pain is therefore classified according to when it occurs or if it becomes more intense and unmanageable. There are three classifications of cancer pain:

1. Breakthrough pain – pain that is more intense than normal.
2. Incident pain – pain caused by specific activities, i.e. walking, lifting, etc.
3. End-of-dose failure pain – occurs if effects of analgesia subside before the next dose is due.

Breakthrough and incident pain are common, even in patients whose pain is well controlled. End-of-dose pain, however, is an indicator that the patient's current pain control may need reviewing (Hayden, 2006).

Snapshot   Appendicitis

Chloe Anderson is a 34-year-old teacher. She was brought into the emergency department by her husband after complaining of severe abdominal pain for the past 2 hours. On examination she is cold and clammy to touch, and she is guarding her abdomen. Chloe tells the nurse that the pain started in the middle of her tummy but has now moved to the lower right-hand side of her abdomen. She states that on a scale of 1 to 10, where 10 is the worst pain imaginable, her pain scores 9, and that the pain is constant and intense. Chloe feels nauseous but has not vomited; she last opened her bowels yesterday. The nurse records a set of vital signs (below) and orders an abdominal ultrasound.

Vital signs

On admission to the emergency department the following vital signs were noted and recorded:

Vital sign	Observation	Normal
Temperature	39.1°C	36.0–37.9°C range
Pulse	100 beats per minute	60–100 beats per minute
Respiration	16 breaths per minute	12–20 breaths per minute
Blood pressure	155/110 mmHg	100–139 mmHg (systolic) range
O_2 saturation	98%	94–98 %

A full blood count was performed.

Test	Result	Guideline normal values
White blood cells (WBC)	12.3×10^9/L	4 to 11×10^9/L
Neutrophils	8.1×10^9/L	2.0 to 7.5×10^9/L
Lymphocytes	4.9×10^9/L	1.3 to 4.0×10^9/L
Red blood cells (RBC)	4.08×10^{12}/L	3.8 to 5×10^{12}/L
Haemoglobin (Hb)	136 g/L	130–180 g/L
Platelets	278×10^9/L	150 to 440×10^9/L
C-reactive protein	2 mg/L	<5 mg/L

NEWS 2   Chloe Anderson

Physiological Parameters	Scores						
	3	2	1	0	1	2	3
Respiration Rate				16			
SpO$_2$ Scale 1				98			
SpO$_2$ Scale 2							
Air or oxygen				Air			
Systolic blood pressure				155			
Pulse						120	
Consciousness				A			
Temperature						39.1	

Note: NEWS Score: 4 – Low risk
Source: Royal College of Physicians (2020)

Take some time to reflect on this case and then consider the following:
1. What type of pain is Chloe suffering from, and how would you classify and categorise this kind of pain?
2. Chloe is going for surgery. How do you think she will feel prior to the surgery and how might her level of pain impact on postoperative pain?
3. Which analgesia may be prescribed for Chloe and what are their major side effects?

Clinical investigations

Abdominal ultrasound

Ultrasound uses sound waves to produce images of internal organs. This can be a very useful diagnostic tool for healthcare professionals trying to establish the cause of abdominal pain. The abdomen contains all the organs of digestion, the kidneys, spleen and abdominal aorta, and it can be difficult to discern the source of a patient's discomfort or the extent of any tissue damage. Abdominal ultrasounds can aid diagnosis by detecting organ enlargement, kidney stones, gallstones, aortic aneurysm. Doppler ultrasounds can also establish disruption of blood flow, clots, narrowing of blood vessels or tumours.

Ultrasounds are a painless and non-invasive procedure, but patients with abdominal pain may find the procedure uncomfortable. Care should be taken therefore to provide reassurance, and time should be taken to explain the procedure to the patient and provide a rationale for this investigation. Although the investigation only takes 10–20 minutes, the patient must expose their abdomen, and this may involve the removal of clothes. Healthcare professionals must, therefore, ensure that privacy and dignity are maintained.

Pain assessment

Effective pain assessment allows the practitioner to best select appropriate pharmacological and non-pharmacological interventions. However, pain is a complex multifaceted phenomenon, and its assessment can be challenging. Pain is a holistic experience, which is influenced by biological, psychological and physical stimuli (Ford, 2019). Any health assessment must pay attention to physiological, psychological, emotional and social aspects of pain if effective holistic care is to occur. Furthermore, pain is a subjective experience, and the healthcare professional must rely on the patient's own description of the pain. However, many patients are often unable to verbalise or describe their pain. For this reason, non-verbal cues are of particular importance.

A description of pain is rarely enough to determine appropriate treatment. Further information on the location, duration and onset of pain can aid healthcare professionals in managing the patient's pain. Every pain assessment must also include the following:

517

- Location of pain – where is the pain, does it radiate anywhere?
- Duration of pain – how long has the patient had the pain?
- Onset – when did the pain start and what was the patient doing at the time?
- Frequency – how often does the pain occur?
- Intensity – how painful is it; does the level of pain change?
- Aggravating factors – what makes the pain worse?
- Relieving factors – what makes the pain feel better?
- Other symptoms – does the patient feel dizzy, nauseous, sweaty or short of breath?
- Sleep patterns – does the pain keep the patient awake? (Godfrey, 2005b; MacLellan, 2006).

Further information on the patient's psychological and emotional response to their pain should also be gathered. For example:

- The patient's expectations of any potential treatments
- The patient's concerns regarding the cause of their pain
- Any personal or spiritual beliefs
- Acceptable pain levels
- Pain levels that will allow the patient to return to work
- Feelings of stress and anxiety
- Any coping mechanisms
- The patient's preferences regarding treatment options (MacLellan, 2006).

Acute pain also produces an autonomic response, and often patients will present with hypertension, tachycardia and changes in respiratory rate. Pain assessment should therefore include measurement of blood pressure, pulse, temperature and respiration rate. However, chronic pain may not have an adverse effect on these vital signs; therefore, the patient's description of the pain should remain the principal indicator of pain intensity.

Red Flag

Pain assessment – beware of misconceptions and stereotypes

There are a number of popular misconceptions regarding pain perception that are often based on stereotypes and assumptions. Healthcare professionals must provide individualised and holistic care and avoid such preconceived views. Popular pain myths include the following:

- You can teach people to tolerate pain.
- Over time people become used to pain.
- Healthcare professionals are an authority on pain and the nature of pain.
- People often lie about pain to acquire analgesia or exaggerate its intensity to avoid work.
- Visible symptoms of pain can be used to determine its severity.
- Analgesia should not be administered/prescribed until a cause for pain has been determined.

A more accurate representation of the above popular pain myths would be:

- Tolerance of pain is different for each individual.
- People with prolonged pain are more likely to become more sensitive to pain stimuli.
- Healthcare professionals are not an authority on pain; only the patient knows how their pain affects their life and well-being.
- Very few people lie about the existence of pain, and exaggeration of its intensity is rare.
- The absence of pain expression does not imply lack of pain, as often people living with chronic pain have the ability to carry on as usual.
- People have a right to have their pain accepted, assessed and acted upon and should be treated and cared for, even if there is no immediate discernible cause.

(McGann, 2007)

Formal structured pain assessment tools can facilitate pain assessment. There is a variety of pain assessment tools at the carer's disposal, ranging from simple single-dimension scales to comprehensive pain questionnaires. The most common single-dimension scales are the verbal rating scale, the visual analogue rating scale and the numerical rating scale. Verbal rating scales ask the patient to select which adjective from a list best describes their pain (Figure 17.12), and with a numerical scale the patient assigns a number to match the pain intensity (Figure 17.13). The visual analogue scale is much simpler. The patient is shown a

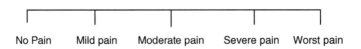

No Pain   Mild pain   Moderate pain   Severe pain   Worst pain

Figure 17.12   An example of a verbal rating scale.

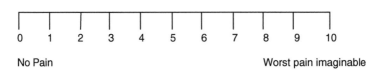

0   1   2   3   4   5   6   7   8   9   10

No Pain   Worst pain imaginable

Figure 17.13   An example of a numerical rating scale.

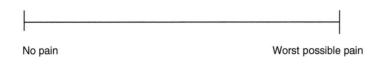

No pain	Worst possible pain

Figure 17.14   An example of a visual analogue scale.

basic continuum running from no pain to worst pain possible. The patient can point or state whereabouts on the continuum their pain is (Figure 17.14). The main advantage of simple rating scales is their ease of use. They can be utilised swiftly and do not overburden the acutely sick person. Nevertheless, they only assess one aspect of pain, its intensity, and there is an assumption that the patient will be literate (MacLellan, 2006).

The most common multidimensional pain assessment tool is the McGill Pain Questionnaire (Figure 17.15). This comprehensive assessment tool contains a series of adjectives that patients can use to describe their pain. The descriptive words are divided into three classes – sensory, affective and evaluative. The questionnaire also utilises a rating scale that runs from 0 – no pain to 5 – excruciating. The assessment of pain is based on three measures: the pain rating index (PRI), which is based on the numerical values assigned to each number; the number of words selected; and the rating scale or present pain index (PPI). The McGill Pain Questionnaire also has line drawings of the human body that can facilitate the location of the pain. The McGill Pain Questionnaire is now widely used to assess chronic pain and has been shown to be very effective when measuring pain in arthritis (Grafton *et al.*, 2005).

519

Snapshot   Pain management

Graeme Jackson is a 28-year-old man with learning disabilities and complex communication needs. He lives with his Mum and Dad, who are his main carers, and his sister Jessica. Graeme attends a local day centre three times a week, but most of the time he remains at home. Graeme is often unwell. He has been admitted to hospital four times in the past year for chest infections, and it can be difficult for Graeme's parents to determine whether or not Graeme is in pain, something they both find stressful and upsetting.

Graeme's learning disabilities nurse recommends the use of a pain picture to enable them to gauge levels of pain and discomfort. Pain pictures describe displayed behaviours when Graeme is well, allowing his parents to suspect pain when his behaviour differs dramatically. Displayed behaviours could include sweating, facial expressions, body tension and vocalisation. Graeme's parents noted that when he is well he rarely sweats but when unwell or in pain he starts to sweat profusely. He is normally a happy individual who likes to smile and return the smiles of others. However, he becomes withdrawn and unwilling to engage in eye contact when in discomfort. In terms of body tension, Graeme is normally relaxed, but his parents note increased tension in his shoulders and legs when he is in pain. Graeme is a quiet and content individual, but when unwell he becomes more vocal and can scream when in pain (Moulster, 2020).

Take some time to reflect on this case and then consider the following:

1. What impact can complex communication needs have on individuals in pain?
2. What do pain pictures tell us about pain assessment?
3. What does this scenario tell you about the ethics of pain assessment?

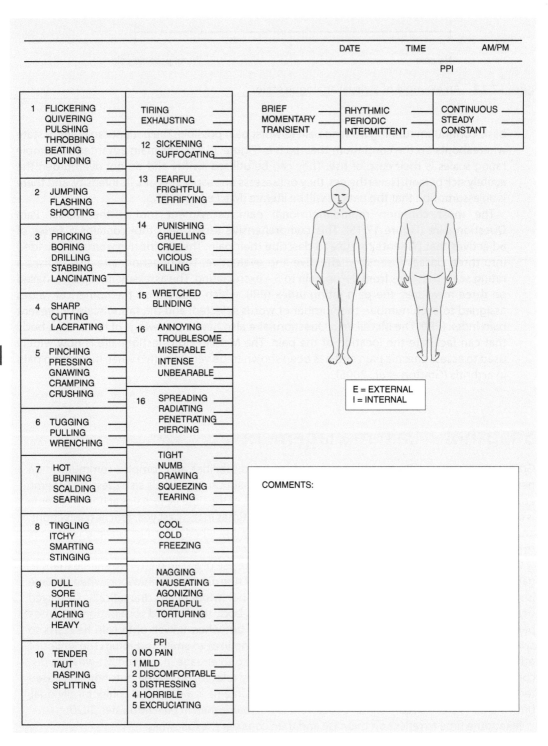

DATE TIME AM/PM

PPI

1 FLICKERING QUIVERING PULSHING THROBBING BEATING POUNDING	TIRING EXHAUSTING
2 JUMPING FLASHING SHOOTING	12 SICKENING SUFFOCATING
3 PRICKING BORING DRILLING STABBING LANCINATING	13 FEARFUL FRIGHTFUL TERRIFYING
4 SHARP CUTTING LACERATING	14 PUNISHING GRUELLING CRUEL VICIOUS KILLING
5 PINCHING PRESSING GNAWING CRAMPING CRUSHING	15 WRETCHED BLINDING
6 TUGGING PULLING WRENCHING	16 ANNOYING TROUBLESOME MISERABLE INTENSE UNBEARABLE
7 HOT BURNING SCALDING SEARING	16 SPREADING RADIATING PENETRATING PIERCING
8 TINGLING ITCHY SMARTING STINGING	TIGHT NUMB DRAWING SQUEEZING TEARING
9 DULL SORE HURTING ACHING HEAVY	COOL COLD FREEZING
10 TENDER TAUT RASPING SPLITTING	NAGGING NAUSEATING AGONIZING DREADFUL TORTURING
	PPI 0 NO PAIN 1 MILD 2 DISCOMFORTABLE 3 DISTRESSING 4 HORRIBLE 5 EXCRUCIATING

BRIEF MOMENTARY TRANSIENT	RHYTHMIC PERIODIC INTERMITTENT	CONTINUOUS STEADY CONSTANT

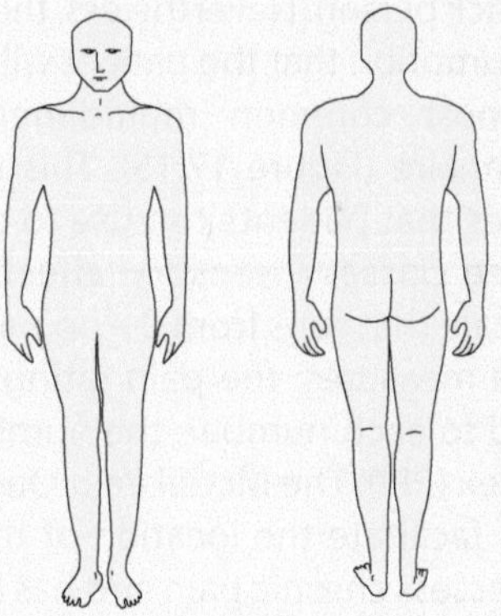

E = EXTERNAL
I = INTERNAL

COMMENTS:

Figure 17.15 The McGill Pain Questionnaire. *Source:* Melzack and Torgerson, 1971. Reproduced with permission of Wolters Kluwer Health, Inc.

Pain management

Pain management or control can be either pharmacological or non-pharmacological. Pharmacological pain management involves the administration of drugs. Drugs that are used for pain control are referred to as analgesia or analgesics. There are two main types of analgesia – opioids (or opiates) and non-opioids. As the name suggests, non-pharmacological pain management does not involve any drugs. As pain is a total experience, effective pain control is often achieved through a combination of both approaches (Ford, 2019).

Opioids

Opioid drugs are used for moderate to severe pain. They work by mimicking the body's own endogenous opiates by binding to opiate receptors in the central nervous system. Opiate receptors such as μ, κ and δ block the action of substance P when stimulated. However, unlike endogenous opiates such as endorphins, opioids are not rapidly broken down by the body. Therefore, their analgesic effects are powerful and long-lasting. The actions of opiate receptors are summarised in Table 17.4.

Table 17.4   Actions of opiate receptors.

Receptor	Physiological effects
Mu (μ)	Analgesia
	Euphoria
	Respiratory depression
	Bradycardia
	Nausea and vomiting
	Inhibition of gut motility
	Miosis
	Pruritus
	Smooth muscle spasm
	Physical dependence
Kappa (κ)	Analgesia
	Sedation
	Dysphoria
	Respiratory depression
Delta (δ)	Physical dependence analgesia
	Euphoria
	Respiratory depression
	Miosis
	Inhibition of gut motility
	Smooth muscle spasm
	Physical dependence

Red flag

Unwanted side effects of opiate analgesia

Opiate analgesia has many unwanted side effects. Nurses should continually assess for the presence of side effects, as left untreated they could be detrimental to their patient's well-being. Important side effects to look out for are:

- Respiratory depression
- Nausea and vomiting
- Constipation
- Bradycardia and hypotension
- Drowsiness.

In addition to analgesia, the stimulation of opiate receptors produces many other physiological changes (Table 17.4), which the healthcare professional needs to be aware of:

- Respiratory depression
- Constipation
- Nausea and vomiting
- Drowsiness
- Bradycardia
- Hypotension.

Opioids are controlled drugs governed by the Misuse of Drugs Act 1971 (HMSO, 1971). Opioid drugs are classified as either weak or strong. Despite their name, weak opioids are very effective analgesics. The main weak opioids are used in combination with non-opioid analgesia such as paracetamol or aspirin. Such combinations are prescription only, rather than controlled drugs (HMSO, 1968). Tables 17.5 and 17.6 summarise the main weak and strong opioids used in the NHS.

Table 17.5 Common weak opiates and their routes of delivery.

Drug	Preparations	Route
Codeine	Codeine phosphate	Oral – tablet, syrup
		Injection (controlled drug)
	Co-codamol (Paracodol®)	Oral – capsule and dispersible tablets
	Codeine phosphate 8 mg or 30 mg with 500 mg paracetamol	
	Co-codaprin®	Oral – dispersible tablets
	Codeine phosphate 8 mg with 400 mg aspirin	
Dihydrocodeine	Dihydrocodeine (DF118®)	Oral – tablet
		Injection (controlled drug)
	Co-dydramol	Oral – tablet
	Dihydrocodeine 10 mg with 500 mg paracetamol	Oral – capsule
Tramadol	Tramadol (Zydol®)	Injection
	Tramacet®	Oral – tablet
	Tramadol 37.5 mg with 325 mg paracetamol	

Table 17.6   Common strong opiates and their routes of delivery.

Drug	Examples	Route
Morphine	Morphine	Injection
		Suppository
	Oramorph®	Oral – liquid, tablet
	Sevredol®	Oral – tablet
	MST Continus®	Oral – tablet, suspension
Diamorphine	Diamorphine	Oral – tablet
		Injection
Oxycodone	Oxynorm®	Oral – tablet, liquid
		Injection
	Oxycontin®	Oral – tablet
Fentanyl	Fentanyl	Patch
		Injection
	Durogesic	Patch
	DTrans®	
Pethidine	Pethidine	Oral – tablets
		Injection
	Pamergan	Oral – tablets
	P100®	Injection

Medicines management

Patient-controlled analgesia (PCA)

PCA is a method of self-administration which is commonly used after surgery. The patient is attached to a small syringe driver that contains an opioid drug. The syringe is operated by a button, which when pressed by the patient delivers a set dosage. To protect against overdose, after each dose the syringe driver locks for a short time, and no drug can be delivered, even if the button is pressed.

   PCA has been routinely and safely used for the past 30 years. However, it is most effective when the patient is made comfortable before it is commenced. Therefore, healthcare professionals should consider pre-loading the patient with opioid analgesia prior to setting up a PCA infusion (Layzell, 2008).

Non-opioid drugs

Non-opioid analgesia is used for mild to moderate pain and is rarely effective in acute or postoperative pain. However, it can enhance the effect of opioid drugs, and when used in combination with opioids can reduce opioid use by 20–40% (MacIntyre and Schug, 2015). The most common non-opioid drug is paracetamol (acetaminophen). The precise action of paracetamol remains controversial; however, it is widely thought to suppress the production of prostaglandins. Prostaglandins are hormone-like substances that increase inflammation and also stimulate nociceptors and promote pain. Paracetamol is an effective analgesic; however, it rarely acts for longer than 4 hours and therefore may not be appropriate for prolonged pain. Despite its relative safety, paracetamol can cause liver failure even in small overdoses.

Prostaglandins are derived from arachidonic acid, which is released from damaged cells. The production of prostaglandins from arachidonic acid is accelerated by the presence of an enzyme called cyclo-oxygenase-2 (COX-2) (Figure 17.16). Non-steroidal anti-inflammatory drugs (NSAIDs) suppress the actions of COX-2 and reduce levels of prostaglandins. Many different NSAIDs are used in the UK (Box 17.1); however, the main ones are aspirin, ibuprofen, diclofenac, indomethacin and naproxen.

524

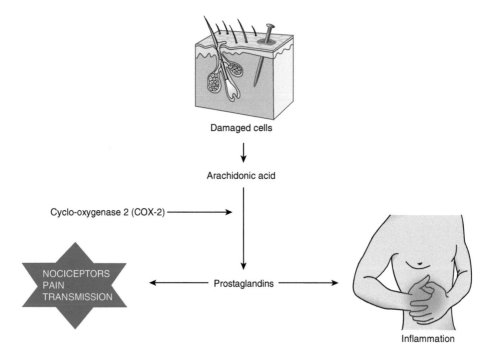

Damaged cells

Arachidonic acid

Cyclo-oxygenase 2 (COX-2) ⟶

NOCICEPTORS PAIN TRANSMISSION ⟵ Prostaglandins ⟶

Inflammation

Figure 17.16   The prostaglandin-enhancing action of cyclo-oxygenase-2 (COX-2) enhancing prostaglandin action.

Box 17.1   Common NSAIDs (trade name)

Aceclofenac (Preservex®)	Etoricoxib (Arcoxia®)	Mefenamic acid (Ponstan®)
Acemetacin (Emflex®)	Fenbufen (Fenbufen®)	Meloxican (Mobic®)
Aspirin (Caprin®)	Fenoprofen (Fenopron®)	Nabumetone (Relifex®)
Azapropazone (Rheumox®)	Flurbiprofen (Froben®)	Naproxen (Arthroxen®)
Celecoxib (Celebrex®)	Ibuprofen (Brufen®)	Piroxicam (Brexidol®)
Dexibuprofen (Seractil®)	Indometacin (Rimacid®)	Sulindac (Clinoril®)
Dexketoprofen (Keral®)	Ketoprofen (Orudis®)	Tenoxicam (Mobiflex®)
Diclofenac (Volterol®)		Tiaprofenic acid (Surgam®)
Etodolac		

Non-opioid analgesics have actions other than pain control, e.g. temperature control and prophylaxis of heart disease. Because prostaglandins promote fever as well as inflammation, NSAIDs and paracetamol may reduce core body temperature and are often used solely to reduce pyrexia. Aspirin also has antiplatelet properties. Used in small doses, it has been shown to reduce the risk of cardiovascular disease.

Medicines management

Non-steroidal anti-inflammatory drugs (NSAIDs)

NSAIDs are common and effective analgesia. They reduce inflammation by suppressing the actions of cyclo-oxygenase 2 (COX-2) and thereby reducing levels of circulating prostaglandins (hormone-like substance that promotes inflammation and increases pain sensation). In addition to the suppression of COX-2, NSAIDs can also suppress another enzyme, cyclo-oxygenase-1 (COX-1), which promotes prostaglandin production in the stomach, where it plays an important protective role by inhibiting gastric acid.

One of the most likely side effects of NSAIDs is gastric irritation and ulcers. Patients prescribed NSAIDs such as ibuprofen, diclofenac, indomethacin and naproxen should be advised to take their medication with or just after food to minimise the risk of developing gastric problems (Gilron *et al.*, 2003).

Caution is also required in patients living with asthma. NSAIDs are also associated with hypersensitive reactions in patients with asthma (Jenkins *et al.*, 2004).

525

The analgesic ladder

The World Health Organization (WHO) produced the analgesic ladder in 1986 to help combat cancer pain. However, it is now widely used to manage many different types of pain (Godfrey, 2005b). The ladder has three steps, each containing a recommended level of pharmacological treatment (Figure 17.17). If pain persists, the patient's treatment should be moved up to the next step. The goal is for the patient to be pain free at the lowest point on the ladder. Step one involves the use of non-opioid drugs, step two recommends adding a weak opioid and the final step advocates the use of strong opioids. Each step also suggests the use of an adjuvant. Adjuvants are a range of drugs that have analgesic effects, despite being normally prescribed for other conditions. Antidepressants, anticonvulsants, muscle relaxants, corticosteroids and local anaesthetics have all been shown to reduce pain when used in conjunction with opioid and non-opioid drugs.

Medicines management

Use of steroids to reduce pain

Steroids are potent anti-inflammatory agents and as such they can be effective in controlling pain caused by inflammation. Drugs such as prednisolone or dexamethasone are often used to control joint pain caused by arthritis. Steroids are also effective adjuvants if used in conjunction with analgesics.

However, steroids have many side effects, and healthcare professionals should alert their patients to the possibility that their steroid therapy could have an adverse effect on their well-being. Side effects of steroids include indigestion, heartburn, irritable mood, weight gain and difficulty in sleeping. Steroids can also weaken the immune system and render your patient susceptible to infection. Another risk is disordered blood glucose levels and the development of steroid-induced diabetes.

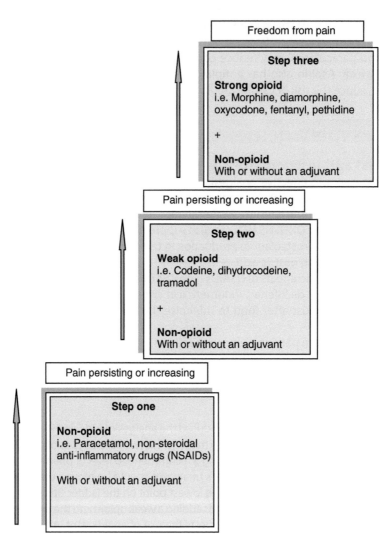

Figure 17.17   The World Health Organization analgesic ladder. *Source:* WHO, 1986. Reproduced with permission of WHO.

Non-pharmacological pain management

There are many different forms of non-pharmacological pain management interventions available in the UK:

- Cognitive behavioural therapy
- TENS
- Application of heat and cold substances
- Acupuncture
- Alexander technique
- Aromatherapy
- Massage
- Chiropractic treatment

- Hypnosis
- Homeopathy
- Meditation
- Osteopathy
- Reflexology
- Relaxation
- Shiatsu (Wigens, 2006).

There is evidence of effectiveness for only a small number of techniques, e.g. massage and cognitive behavioural therapy (Furlan *et al.*, 2015; Eccleston *et al.*, 2009). As a result, the use of non-pharmacological pain control is controversial, with many healthcare professionals being sceptical of their effectiveness (Wigens, 2006).

Snapshot   Neonatal pain

Namuna and Felix's baby daughter Blessing was born 8 weeks premature. She is thriving, and Namuna and Felix are hoping that their baby will be discharged very soon. Before she is discharged, the nurse needs to collect a sample of blood, to assess that Blessing is receiving the nutrition she needs; she also needs to remove a small dressing from the arm, which protected a cannula.

To minimise the impact of the pain caused by taking blood and removing the dressing, the nurse times the blood test to coincide with Blessing's next feed. Once blood has been taken and the dressing removed, Namuna breastfeeds Blessing. Breast feeding is an effective non-pharmacological method of reducing pain in neonates as is skin-to-skin contact or swaddling.

Take some time to reflect on this case and then consider the following:

1. Neonatal pain is difficult to diagnosis; take some time to think why that might be?
2. Babies in neonatal units are exposed to 10–15 painful procedure a day; take some time to consider what kinds of interventions could cause pain in neonates and infants?
3. Why do you think actions such as breastfeeding, skin-to-skin contact or swaddling can help reduce pain in newborn babies?

527

Physical interventions

Many non-pharmacological pain control techniques have a physiological basis. A TENS machine, for example, sends a constant stream of small electrical impulses through the skin (Figure 17.18). These impulses are thought to reduce pain in two ways. First, they may stimulate the large-diameter Aβ fibres and interrupt the pain impulse travelling along the smaller Aδ and C fibres, i.e. the same effect as rubbing a mild injury. Second, the continuous electrical stimulation may increase levels of endogenous opiates such as endorphins (Sluka and Walsh, 2003). TENS machines are a popular treatment choice for acute pain, phantom limb pain and lower back pain. However, evidence of its effectiveness remains inconclusive (Johnson *et al.*, 2015a,b).

Acupuncture is the insertion of fine needles at strategic points around the body. It too is thought to stimulate the release of endogenous opiates (Lundeberg and Stener-Victorin, 2002). Acupuncture is widely used and is accepted as an effective analgesia in many

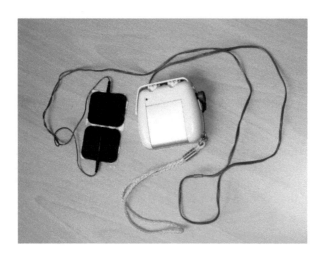

Figure 17.18   Transcutaneous electrical nerve stimulation (TENS) machine.

countries; however, there is very little evidence to suggest that it is effective. Investigations into the use of acupuncture for cancer pain, fibromyalgia and neuropathic pain suggest that it may be beneficial, but a lack of large-scale studies means it cannot be fully endorsed (Paley *et al.*, 2015; Deare *et al.*, 2013; Ju *et al.*, 2017).

The stimulation of large-diameter Aβ fibres also helps explain the therapeutic effects of pressure- and touch-based interventions such as osteopathy, reflexology and shiatsu. The most widely used touch- and pressure-based intervention is massage. Massage has been shown to be potentially effective in patients with low back pain (Furlan *et al.*, 2015). As well as sensing pressure and touch, Aβ fibres also respond to sensations of heat and cold. The therapeutic effects of mild heat and ice packs on injuries are well known. Heat can also be used to alleviate menstrual pain as well as joint and muscle strains. However, there is little evidence for the use of heat and cold substances in the clinical setting (French *et al.*, 2006).

Psychological interventions

Pain is a holistic experience, and the psychological aspects of the pain experience are an integral aspect of pain sensation. The gate control theory of pain suggests that descending pain pathways from the brain influence pain intensity. Furthermore, anxiety, stress and low mood states are significant factors that can increase pain sensation. Any non-pharmacological method that can alleviate anxiety, stress or help an individual to cope with their pain could be beneficial. It is not surprising therefore that psychological non-pharmacological pain control methods are being increasingly utilised by chronic pain sufferers (Dopson, 2010).

Psychological-based pain control interventions range from simplistic methods such as relaxation and distraction to more alternative therapies such as meditation, Alexander technique and hypnotherapy. A more intense psychological approach is cognitive behavioural therapy (CBT). CBT involves a series of structured, patient-focused sessions that aim to address the individual's psychological and emotional experience of their pain and enable them to self-manage and control their anxiety and therefore their pain. CBT should complement rather than replace traditional pharmacology-based therapies. As a pain control method for those in chronic pain, CBT has proved effective (Eccleston *et al.*, 2009).

Snapshot   lower back pain

Derek Bairstow is a 48-year-old removals operative. He has been suffering from lower back pain for the past 3 months. The intensity of the pain has increased gradually over the past couple of days, and as a result he has not been able to go to work. Although he cannot remember injuring his back, he has a very physical job working for a removals firm and believes continual muscle strain is the cause. Derek has been taking non-steroidal anti-inflammatory drugs for the pain but finds they provide little relief. The pain is such that he finds it difficult to sit comfortably or sleep. Today he has visited his GP for more advice. Derek is recently divorced, and his ex-wife and their children now live 100 miles away. He informs the GP that he has been feeling very low and has been finding it difficult to concentrate on anything and has avoided socialising with friends. The GP records a set of vital signs and asks Derek to complete a patient health questionnaire (PHQ-9) – see below. The GP reviews Derek's analgesia regime and refers him for a CT scan to rule out spinal injury.

Vital signs

The GP recorded the following vital signs and recorded the following responses to the patient health questionnaire:

Vital sign	Observation	Normal
Temperature	36.3°C	36.0–37.9°C range
Pulse	72 beats per minute	60–100 beats per minute
Respiration	13 breaths per minute	12–20 breaths per minute
Blood pressure	134/89 mmHg	100–139 mmHg (systolic) range

Patient Health Questionnaire (PHQ-9)

Over the past 2 weeks have you been bothered by any of the following problems?
I have little interest in doing things – More than half the days (2)
Feeling down, depressed, hopeless – More than half the days (2)
Trouble sleeping, staying asleep or sleeping too much – More than half the days (2)
Feeling tired or having little energy – More than half the days (2)
Poor appetite or over eating – Several days (1)
Feeling bad about yourself – or that you are a failure or have let yourself or your family down?
– Nearly every day (3)
Trouble concentrating on things, such as reading the newspaper or watching television? – More than half the days (2)
Moving or speaking so slowly that other people could have noticed?
Or the opposite – being so fidgety or restless that you have been moving around a lot more than usual? – Not at all (0)
Thoughts that you would be better off dead, or of hurting yourself in some way? – Not at all (0)
Score 14/27 – Mild Depression
Take some time to reflect on this case and then consider the following:

1. What type of pain is Derek suffering from, and how would you classify and categorise this kind of pain?
2. How do non-steroidal anti-inflammatory drugs work and what are their main side effects?
3. What further treatment options are at the GP's disposal and what advice would you provide?

Clinical investigations

Spinal computerised tomography (CT) scan

A CT scan uses X-rays and a computer to create detailed cross-sectional images of the spine. The images will provide greater depth of detail as compared to a single X-ray and will aid the discovery of spinal fractures and disc herniations.

CT scans can take between 10 and 20 minutes to complete, and the patient will be left alone and only able to communicate with staff via an intercom. For that reason, patients can often find CT scans claustrophobic and may need comfort and reassurance before the scan. In some instances, patients may require sedatives to help them cope with the stress of undergoing the scan. Healthcare professionals will need to take time to explain the procedure and answer any questions the patient may have. Clothes may need to be removed and a gown worn during the scan; care should be taken therefore to maintain privacy at all times.

In some instances, a dye is injected that highlights nerve roots on the CT images. This will provide the medical team with sensitive information on nerve lesions which could be the cause of the patient's back pain. If dyes are used, healthcare professionals should ensure that the patient is not allergic to the dye. Patient's that receive the dye will be kept in hospital for around an hour after the test to ensure there is no adverse reaction.

CT scans are not appropriate for pregnant women.

Conclusion

Pain is a personal experience. The brain plays a fundamental role in the interpretation of pain, and therefore a patient's state of mind, personality, background and culture will all shape the way in which an individual expresses or verbalises their pain. Acute pain affects the function of many body systems and left unresolved can become prolonged chronic pain. Pain control therefore is essential if homeostasis is to be maintained. There are many forms of analgesia that can be used to control pain; however, as pain is an emotional as well as physiological phenomenon, non-pharmacological methods should also be utilised, especially for the patient in chronic pain. Because pain is individualised, the selection of appropriate pharmacological and non-pharmacological pain management strategies is reliant upon a comprehensive and holistic assessment. Healthcare professionals are therefore ideally placed to provide effective care for the patient with pain.

Activities

Here are some activities and exercises to help test your learning. For the answers to these exercises, as well as further self-testing activities, visit our website at **www.wiley.com/go/fundamentalsofappliedpathophysiology/student4e**

Multiple choice questions

1. Which of the following statements is true?
   (a) Nociceptors are mainly found in the brain
   (b) Thermal stimuli includes damage caused by trauma
   (c) Ischaemia and hypoxia stimulate nociceptors and generate pain
   (d) There are three types of nociceptor: thermal, chemical and natural
2. In the ascending pain pathway, which neurons travel from the source of injury to the spinal column?
   (a) First-order neurons
   (b) Second-order neurons
   (c) Third-order neurons
   (d) Interneurons
3. Which of the following statements is correct?
   (a) C Fibres are myelinated nerve fibres
   (b) A-delta (Aδ) fibres transmit sensation faster than both c fibres and A-beta (Aβ) fibres
   (c) A-beta (Aβ) fibres are non-myelinated and transmit sensation slower than C Fibres
   (d) A-beta (Aβ) fibres transmit sensation faster than both C fibres and A-delta (Aδ) fibres
4. Which of the following best describes acute pain?
   (a) A short episode of pain of no consequence
   (b) Intense pain, with a severe sudden onset, which continues until healing begins
   (c) A syndrome and medical condition in its own right
   (d) Pain that continues after healing is complete

531

5. Which of the following statements is correct?
   (a) Superficial pain occurs due to nociceptor stimulation in the skin
   (b) Deep pain is easily located by the brain
   (c) Visceral pain emanates from bones, muscles and joints
   (d) Superficial pain can be somatic and visceral
6. Endorphins are. . ..
   (a) Neurotransmitters
   (b) Hormones
   (c) Opiate receptors
   (d) Indigenous opiates
7. Which of the following statements on pain is true?
   (a) You can teach patients to tolerate pain
   (b) The longer people have pain, the more used to it they become
   (c) Visible signs accompany pain and can be used to verify how severe it is
   (d) Pain is what they patient says it is
8. Which of the following is a non-steroidal anti-inflammatory drug?
   (a) Codeine
   (b) Pethidine
   (c) Tramadol
   (d) Ibuprofen
9. Which of the following analgesics binds with opiate receptors in the central nervous system?
   (a) Paracetamol
   (b) Morphine
   (c) Ibuprofen
   (d) Aspirin

10. Which of the following is a side effect of opiate therapies?
    (a) Respiratory depression
    (b) Constipation
    (c) Nausea and vomiting
    (d) All of the above
11. Which of the following statements describes referred pain?
    (a) Pain present in the absence of a limb
    (b) Pain created from 'pain memories'
    (c) Pain usually described as burning, tingling or electric shocks
    (d) Pain that manifests itself in one area of the body, when the source of the pain is in another area of the body
12. Which of the following conditions can lead to the development of neuropathy?
    (a) Trapped nerves
    (b) Scar tissue
    (c) Thoracotomy
    (d) All of the above
13. In the cancer pain classification, what kind of pain is caused by specific activities?
    (a) End-of-dose pain
    (b) Breakthrough pain
    (c) Incident pain
    (d) Nociceptive pain
14. Which of the following statement is correct?
    (a) Up to 90% of patients experience pain after surgery
    (b) Anxiety and apprehension prior to surgery lead to high levels of pain postoperatively
    (c) Unresolved pain leads to a complicated postsurgical recovery
    (d) All these statements are correct
15. Which of the following is a recognised effective non-pharmacological intervention for people living with chronic pain?
    (a) Reflexology
    (b) Acupuncture
    (c) Cognitive behavioural therapy
    (d) Alexander technique

Conditions

The following is a list of further conditions that are associated with pain. Take some time and write notes about each of the conditions. You may make the notes taken from textbooks or other resources (e.g. people you work with in a clinical area), or you may make the notes based on people you have cared for. If you are making notes about people you have cared for, you must ensure that you adhere to the rules of confidentiality.

Sickle cell anaemia	

Rheumatoid arthritis	
Angina	
Burns	
Chronic lower back pain	

Further resources

British Pain Society

http://www.britishpainsociety.org

This website contains publications, newsletters and information for patients, all of which can inform your care of patients with chronic pain and help you in your academic work.

Pain Concern

http://www.painconcern.org.uk

This website also hosts regular radio programmes and podcasts, which could be helpful to you in your academic work. Its discussion sites also provide insight into how individuals cope with chronic pain.

Pain Talk

http://www.pain-talk.co.uk/

This is a useful website for students studying chronic pain. Once registered, viewers can gain access to discussion forums, news, pain search engines, information on study days and conferences, and details of other useful pain websites.

NHS Choices

http://www.nhs.uk/Conditions/Back-pain

This website provides guidance to help you care for patients in pain. It gives access to advice on back pain, as well as a host of other pain conditions.

London Pain Consortium

http://www.lpc.ac.uk/html/

This website gives the latest research into pain physiology, and London Pain Consortium publications, as well as links to other pain websites and journals. This site provides an excellent resource for students studying chronic and acute pain.

Glossary of terms

Aldosterone   A hormone that increases blood pressure by increasing re-absorption of water and sodium by the kidneys.

Alexander technique   A method of teaching people how to improve their body posture and thereby avoid muscle tension.

Allodynia   Pain in response to stimuli that should not cause pain.

Amputation   Surgical removal of a limb.

Analgesic   Painkiller.

Angina   Central crushing chest pain that occurs as a result of reduced blood flow through the coronary arteries.

Antiplatelet   A substance that reduces the clotting action of platelets.

Arachidonic acid   A substance found in the cell membrane which can produce prostaglandins.

Aromatherapy   The use of odours and fragrances to alter an individual's mood.

Autonomic   Pertaining to the autonomic nervous system; associated with the maintenance of homeostasis.

Axon   The long part of a nerve cell that carries nerve impulses.

Bone metastases   Cells from a tumour that have spread to bone tissue.

Bradycardia   Having a slow heart beat (usually defined as less than 60 beats per minute).

Central nervous system   The brain and spinal cord.

Cerebral cortex   The outer surface of the brain.

Chiropractic   The manipulation and realignment of the spine.

Controlled drug   A therapeutic preparation governed by the Misuse of Drugs Act (1971).

Coronary artery   Supplies oxygenated blood to the heart.

Coronary vasoconstriction   Constriction of coronary blood vessels.

Cortisol   A hormone released by the adrenal glands, which increases resistance to stress.

Cyclo-oxygenase-2   An enzyme which speeds up the production of prostaglandins from arachidonic acid.

Deep vein thrombosis   The formation of a blood clot in the veins of the legs.

Diaphoresis   Excessive sweating.

Dorsal horn   The section of grey matter found on either side of a cross-section of the spinal cord.

Dynorphin   A neuropeptide found in the central nervous system.

Dysphoria   Low mood; opposite of euphoria.

Endorphin   A neuropeptide found in the central nervous system. Counteracts pain sensation by inhibiting substance P.

Enzyme   A protein that speeds up chemical reactions.

Epinephrine (adrenaline)   Hormone released during times of stress.

Frontal lobe   Area of the cerebrum (outer part of the brain).

Glucagon   A hormone released by the pancreas which increases blood sugar levels.

Histamine   A substance that causes constriction of smooth muscle, dilates arterioles and capillaries, and stimulates gastric juices. See serotonin.

Homeopathy   Treatment based on the principle that 'like can be cured with like'.

Hyperalgesia   Increased or heightened pain sensation.

Hypertension   Raised blood pressure.

534

Hypothalamus   A small region of the brain found in the diencephalon; important regulatory organ of the nervous and endocrine systems.

Hypoventilation   Slow and shallow breaths.

Hypoxaemia   Reduced levels of oxygen in arterial blood.

Hypoxia   Reduced levels of oxygen in the tissues.

Interneuron   Short neuron that connect nearby neurons in the brain and spinal cord.

Ischaemia   A low oxygen state in a part of the body. Usually the result of obstruction to the blood supply to tissues.

Kinin   A substances released during inflammation that causes vasodilation and increased capillary permeability; also attracts phagocytes. The primary kinin is bradykinin.

Limbic system   Part of the forebrain. Sometimes called the emotional brain, the limbic system controls feelings of emotion and behaviour.

Miosis   Contraction of the pupils.

Motor nerve   A nerve that travels from the brain and spinal cord out to an organ, muscle or gland.

Muscle atrophy   Muscle wasting.

Myelin   An electrically insulating phospholipid.

Myelinated   Covered by a protected sheath of myelin.

Neuron   A nerve cell.

Neuropeptide   A substance found in the nervous system that counteracts the effects of neurotransmitters.

Neurotransmitter   A molecule that transmits messages from one nerve to another at a junction called the synapse.

Nociceptor   A special cell that detects damage and irritants that cause pain.

Non-steroidal anti-inflammatory drug (NSAID)   A non-opioid pain killer that reduces inflammation.

Opiate   A powerful analgesic agent that stimulates opiate receptors within the central nervous system.

Opiate receptor   A receptor found in the central nervous system that is stimulated by neuropeptides and opiate drugs.

Osteopathy   The manipulation of bones and joints to diagnose and treat illness.

Patient-controlled analgesia   A method of self-administration of intravenous analgesia.

Peripheral nervous system   The nervous system outside of the central nervous system.

Prostaglandin   A complex unsaturated fatty acid produced by the mast cells and acting as a messenger substance between cells. Intensifies the actions of histamine and kinins. They cause increased vascular permeability, neutrophil chemotaxis, stimulation of smooth muscle (e.g. the uterus) and can induce pain.

Pruritus   Itchy sensation on the skin.

Pulmonary embolism   Reduced blood flow through the lungs due to a blood clot.

Pyrexia   Elevated temperature associated with fever.

Reflex arc   Nervous pathway from sensory nerve to motor nerve via the spinal cord.

Reflexology   The manipulation of various areas of the feet and hands in order to promote well-being.

Reticular formation   A network of neurons found in the central part of the brainstem.

Sensory fibre   A special nerve fibre that transmits sensations of pain, heat, cold and touch.

Serotonin   A neurotransmitter found in the central nervous system that is released from platelets in response to injury, trauma or infection. Along with other substances, such as

535

histamine, it causes temporary, rapid constriction of the smooth muscles of large blood vessel walls and dilation of the small veins (venules). This results in increased blood flow and increased vascular permeability. Associated with pain sensation.

Shiatsu   Finger pressure applied to various areas of the body in order to stimulate the internal energy of the body and thus promote healing.

Somatosensory cortex   A region of the cerebral cortex that processes feelings of touch, pain, heat, cold and muscle and joint position.

Spinothalamic tract   The sensory pathway that transmits messages of pain, temperature, touch and pressure upwards along the spinal cord.

Substance P   A neurotransmitter found in sensory nerves, spinal cord and brain; associated with the sensation of pain.

Substantia gelatinosa   A part of the spinal cord's grey matter; it is composed of large amounts of small nerve cells.

Synapse   The junction where two neurons meet or where a neuron meets tissue.

Syndrome   A collection of symptoms that characterise a specific disorder.

Tachycardia   A fast heart beat (usually defined as above 100 beats per minute).

Tachypnoea   a rapid and usually shallow respiration rate, greater than 20 breaths per minute.

Thalamus   A pair of oval masses of grey matter which account for 80% of the diencephalon area of the brain.

Thoracotomy   Incision in the chest.

Transcutaneous electrical nerve stimulation (TENS)   A method of pain control which stimulates Aβ, Aδ and C fibres with small electrical currents.

Ulceration   The erosion of skin or an internal surface.

Venous return   The volume of blood entering the right atrium.

White matter   The tissue of the spinal cord that surrounds the grey matter.

References

Alanazi, A.A. (2014). Reducing anxiety in preoperative patients: A systematic review. *British Journal of Nursing*, 23(7): 387–393.

Briggs, E. (2010). Understanding the experience and physiology of pain. *Nursing Standard*, 25(3): 35–39.

Colquhoun, L., Shephard, V. and Neil, M. (2019). Pain management in new amputees: A nursing perspective. *British Journal of Nursing*, 28(10): 638–646.

Cousins, M. and Power, I. (2003). Acute and postoperative pain. In: Melzack, R. and Wall, P.D. (eds), *Handbook of Pain Management: A Clinical Companion to Wall and Melzack's Textbook of Pain.* Edinburgh: Churchill Livingstone.

Deare, J.C., Zheng, Z., Xue, C.C.L., Ping Liu, J., Shang, J. *et al.* (2013). Acupuncture for treating fibromyalgia, *The Cochrane Database of Systematic Reviews*. DOI: 10.1002/14651858.CD007070.pub2

Dopson, L. (2010). Role of pain management programmes in chronic pain. *Nursing Standard*, 25(13): 35–40.

Eccleston, C., Williams, A. and Morley, S. (2009). Psychological therapies for the management of chronic pain (excluding headache) in adults (review). *The Cochrane Library*. Issue 2.

Ford, C. (2019). Adult pain assessment and management. *British Journal of Nursing*, 28(7): 421–423.

French, S.D., Cameron, M., Walker, B.F., Reggars, J.W. and Esterman, A.J. (2006). Superficial heat or cold for low back pain. *The Cochrane Database of Systematic Reviews*. Issue 1.

Furlan, A.D., Giraldo, M., Baskwill, A. and Irvin, E. (2015). Massage for lower back pain, *The Cochrane Database of Systematic*. DOI: 10.1002/14651858.CD001929.pub3

Gilron, I., Milne, B. and Hong, M. (2003). Cyclooxygenase-2 inhibitors in postoperative pain management. *Anaesthesiology*, 99(5): 1198–1208.

Godfrey, H. (2005a). Understanding pain Part 1: Physiology of pain. *British Journal of Nursing*, 14(16): 846–852.

Godfrey, H. (2005b). Understanding pain. Part 2: Pain management. *British Journal of Nursing*, 14(17): 904–909.

Grafton, K.V., Foster, N.E. and Wright, C.C. (2005). Test-retest reliability of the short-form McGill pain questionnaire. *Clinical Journal of Pain*, 21(1): 73–82.

Hayden, D. (2006). Pain management in palliative care. In: MacLellan, K. (ed.), *Expanding Nursing and Health Care Practice: Management of Pain*. Cheltenham: Nelson Thornes.

Her Majesty's Stationery Office (HMSO) (1968). *The Medicine's Act*. London: HMSO.

HMSO (1971). *The Misuse of Drugs Act*. London: HSMO.

Ingadottir, B. and Zoega, S. (2017). Role of patient education in postoperative pain management. *Nursing Standard*, 32(2): 50–61.

Jenkins, C., Costello, J. and Hodge, L. (2004). Systematic review of prevalence of aspirin induced asthma and its implications for clinical practice. *British Medical Journal*, 328: 434–440.

Johnson, M. (2005). Physiology of chronic pain. In: Banks, C. and Mackrodt, K. (eds), *Chronic Pain Management*. London: Whurr Publishers.

Johnson, M.I., Paley, C.A., Howe, T.E. and Sluka, K.A. (2015a). Transcutaneous electrical nerve stimulation for acute pain, *The Cochrane Database of Systematic Reviews*. DOI: 10.1002/14651858.CD006142. pub3

Johnson, M.I., Mulvey, M.R. and Bagnall, A. (2015b). Transcutaenous electrical nerve stimulation (TENS) for phantom limb and stump pain following amputation in adults. *The Cochrane Database of Systematic Reviews*, DOI:10.1002/14651858.CD007264.pub3

Ju, Z., Wang, K., Cui, J., Yao, Y., Liu, S., Zhou, J., Chen, T. and Xia, J. (2017). Acupuncture for neuropathic pain in adults. *The Cochrane Database of Systematic Reviews*. DOI: 10.1002/14651858.CD012057. pub2

Kochhar, S.C. (2002). Cancer pain. In: Warfield, C.A. and Fausett, H.J. (eds), *Manual of Pain Management*, 2nd edn. Philadelphia: Lippincott Williams & Wilkins.

Layzell, M. (2008). Current interventions and approaches to post-operative pain management. *British Journal of Nursing*, 17(7): 414–419.

Lin, L. and Wang, R. (2005). Abdominal surgery, pain and anxiety: Preoperative nursing intervention. *Journal of Advanced Nursing*, 51(3): 252–260.

Lundeberg, T. and Stener-Victorin, E. (2002). Is there a physiological basis for the use of acupuncture in pain? *International Congress Series*, 1238: 3–10.

MacIntyre, P.E. and Schug, S.A. (2015). *Acute Pain Management: A Practical Guide*, 4th edn. Boca Raton: CRC Press.

MacLellan, K. (2006). *Expanding Nursing and Health Care Practice: Management of Pain*. Cheltenham: Nelson Thornes.

Marieb, E. and Hoehn, K. (2018). *Human Anatomy and Physiology*, 11th edn. Pearson: Harlow.

McCaffery, M. (1979). *Nursing Management of the Patient with Pain*, 2nd edn. New York: J.B. Lippincott Company.

McCaffery, R., Frock, T.L. and Garguilo, H. (2003). Understanding chronic pain and the mind–body connection. *Holistic Nursing Practice*, 17(6): 281–287.

McGann, K. (2007). *Fundamental Aspects of Pain Assessment and Management*. Gateshead: Quay Books.

Melzack, R. and Torgerson, W.S. (1971). On the language of pain. *Anesthesiology*. 34(1): 50–59.

Melzack, R. and Wall, P. (1988). *The Challenge of Pain*, 2nd edn. London: Penguin.

Moulster, G. (2020). Identifying pain in people who have complex communication needs. *Nursing Times*, 116(2): 19–22.

Paley, C.A., Johnson, M.I., Tashini, O.A. and Bagnall, A. (2015). Acupuncture for cancer pain in adults, *The Cochrane Database of Systematic Reviews*. DOI: 10.1002/14651858.CD007753.pub3

Royal College of Physicians. (2020). *National Early Warning Scores (NEWS) 2*. Available at https://www.rcplondon.ac.uk/projects/outputs/national-early-warning-score-news-2 Accessed 18 June 2020.

537

Scadding, J.W. (2003). Peripheral neuropathies. In: Melzack, R. and Wall, P.D. (eds), *Handbook of Pain Management: A Clinical Companion to Wall and Melzack's Textbook of Pain*. Edinburgh: Churchill Livingstone.

Sluka, K.A. and Walsh, D. (2003). Transcutaneous electrical nerve stimulation: Basic science mechanisms and clinical effectiveness. *The Journal of Pain*, 4(3): 109–121.

Solano, J.P., Games, B. and Higginson, I.J. (2006). A comparison of symptom prevalence in far advanced cancer, AIDS, heart disease, chronic obstructive pulmonary disease (COPD) and renal disease. *Journal of Pain and Symptom Management*, 31(1): 58–69.

Theunissen, M., Madelo, L, P., Bruce, J., Gramke, H. and Marcus, M.A. (2012). Pre-operative anxiety and catastrophizing: A systematic review and meta-analysis of the association with chronic postsurgical pain. *Clinical Journal of Pain*, 28(9): 819–841.

Tortora, G.J. and Derrickson, B. (2017). *Principles of Anatomy and Physiology*, 15th edn. New York: John Wiley & Sons.

Virani, A., Green, T. and Turin, T.C. (2014). Phantom limb pain: A nursing perspective. *Nursing Standard*, 29(1): 44–50.

Wigens, L. (2006). The role of complementary and alternative therapies in pain management. In: MacLellan, K. (ed.), *Expanding Nursing and Health Care Practice: Management of Pain*. Cheltenham: Nelson Thornes.

World Health Organization (WHO) (1986). *Cancer Pain Relief*. Geneva: WHO.

World Health Organization (WHO) (2008). *National Cancer Control Programmes: Policies and Management Guidelines*, 2nd edn. Geneva: WHO.

Chapter 18

The musculoskeletal system and associated disorders

Louise Henstock[1,2]

[1]Physiotherapy Lecturer, School of Health and Society, University of Salford, Greater Manchester, UK
[2]Visiting Lecturer Cambridge University, Cambridge, UK

Contents

Introduction 540
The musculoskeletal system 541
The nervous system.......................................545
Assessing the patient with a musculoskeletal disorder..545
Disorders of the MSK system.........................547
Conclusion 559
Test your knowledge......................................559
Multiple choice questions...............................560
Conditions...562
Further resources..563
Glossary of terms..563
References..564

Key words

- Muscles
- Tendons
- Joints
- Mobility
- Independence/dependence
- Fracture
- Ligaments
- Inflammation
- Degeneration
- Osteoporosis
- Cartilage

Fundamentals of Applied Pathophysiology: An Essential Guide for Nursing and Healthcare Students, Fourth Edition. Edited by Ian Peate.
© 2021 John Wiley & Sons Ltd. Published 2021 by John Wiley & Sons Ltd.
Student companion website: www.wiley.com/go/fundamentalsofappliedpathophysiology/student4e
Instructor companion website: www.wiley.com/go/fundamentalsofappliedpathophysiology/instructor4e

- How many bones are there in the human body?
- Describe the role of osteoclasts and osteoblasts.
- Discuss a range of factors that can impinge on a person's ability to mobilise independently.
- What are the key functions of the skeleton?
- How can healthcare professionals help people become independent after sustaining a fall?

Learning outcomes

On completion of this chapter, the reader will be able to:

- Discuss the development and growth of healthy bones.

- Describe the function of the musculoskeletal system.

- Describe some of the common pathophysiological changes that may occur in the musculoskeletal system.

- Outline the care of people who have problems associated with the musculoskeletal system.

Don't forget to visit the companion website for this book
(www.wiley.com/go/fundamentalsofappliedpathophysiology/student4e)
where you can find self-assessment tests to check your progress, as well as lots of activities to practise your learning.

Introduction

The musculoskeletal (MSK) system is an organ system that provides support, stability and movement through the muscular and skeletal systems and is a crucial part of all that we do. The MSK system is required to sustain life through contraction of the diaphragm and heart muscle; to convey communication through facial expressions and body language; and to protect internal structures such as the heart and lungs.

When injury or disease affects the MSK system, it can result in the person becoming less functionally able to a greater or lesser degree. Musculoskeletal conditions are now the biggest contributor to disability worldwide, with low back pain being the single leading cause of disability globally (WHO, 2019). Unfortunately, this is predicted to rise alongside other non-communicable diseases as the global population increase (WHO, 2019).

In order to provide safe and effective care (for both the patient and the healthcare professional), we need to understand the fundamental issues related to the MSK system. This chapter provides an overview of the MSK system, and a number of common MSK-related conditions are outlined alongside their care. The healthcare professional's role is to prevent or reduce further injury, identify and reduce the risk of complications, assist in the promotion of healing, and promote and maximise independence. Healthcare professionals are now not only expected to be involved in rehabilitation, but also to ensure that every contact counts to support patients in making positive changes to their physical, mental health and well-being (NHS HEE, 2020).

The musculoskeletal system

The MSK system is also known as the locomotor system. There are 206 bones in the adult human, of various shapes and sizes; babies are born with 300 bones, but as humans age, several bones fuse to become bigger bones (Figure 18.1). A baby's bones are primarily made up of cartilage, and over time most of this cartilage turns into bone through a process called ossification. Half of the bones in the adult are in the feet and hands.

The presence of joints in the limbs (i.e. the elbow and knee joints) allows movement; if there were no joints, then there could be no movement, and the skeleton would be rigid. Cartilage, a type of firm but flexible connective tissue, provides protection for those joints that are exposed to the force that is generated during movement. Ligaments attaching bone to bone help to provide joint strength and are either incorporated into a joint capsule or

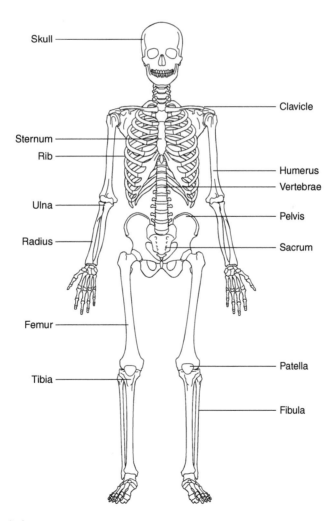

Figure 18.1   The skeleton.

they may be independent of it. Movement at the joint is achieved by contraction of muscles that pass across it.

The skeleton, the joints and skeletal muscle work together to provide basic functions that are essential to life:

- Protection for internal organs and to provide support to soft tissue
- Support – maintain an upright posture
- Blood formation – in red bone marrow, haemopoiesis
- Mineral homeostasis, storage and release of minerals as the body requires them. The bones store most of the body's calcium requirement
- Storage – fat and minerals in the yellow bone marrow
- Leverage, working with the muscles, and the bones in the upper and lower limbs pull and push, allowing for movement.

Bone structure

Bone is a collagen-based matrix with minerals laid upon it; its strength depends on both components. The mineral aspect is composed primarily of calcium, magnesium and phosphorus, and the collagen fibres help with the tension and compression the bone is subjected to. The collagen fibres and the minerals are densely packed together, resulting in a hardening of bone. Vitamin D, parathyroid hormone and calcitonin are important factors in bone mineralisation.

Bone formation is controlled by osteoblast and osteoclast activity. Osteoblasts control bone formation, and osteoclasts are responsible for bone breakdown. Bone is more than a rigid structure, and throughout life it constantly reforms and remodels itself. The way an individual moves, the amount and type of exercise taken, and an individual's diet will all influence bone structure (Figures 18.2 and 18.3).

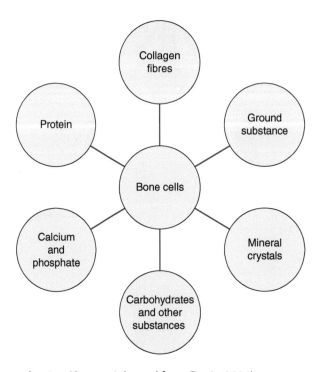

Figure 18.2   Bone production (*Source:* Adapted from Davis, 2006).

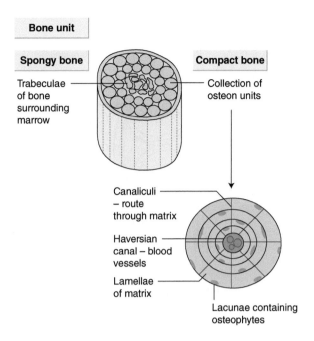

Figure 18.3   Bone structure.

The skeleton is the body's supporting framework and there are five types of bone:

1. Long, i.e. the femur
2. Short, i.e. the tarsal bones
3. Flat, i.e. the ribs
4. Irregular, i.e. the mandible
5. Sesamoid, i.e. the patella.

Joints

Where one bone meets another is a joint. There are three types of joint:

1. Those that allow free movement (i.e. diarthrosis)
2. Those that are fixed (i.e. synarthrosis)
3. Those that permit limited movement (amphiarthrosis).

Joints are classified as follows:

- Synostotic
- Cartilaginous
- Fibrous
- Synovial.

Synovial joints are the most common in the MSK system and the main ones that health-care practitioners have to assess and treat. The synovial joint allows free movement. Bony surfaces (the ends of the bones) are covered by articular cartilage and are connected by ligaments. There are different types of synovial joints including:

- Pivotal joints (i.e. the joint between the humeral radius and the ulna)
- Ball and socket joints (i.e. the hip joint)
- Hinge joints (i.e. the interphalangeal joints of the fingers).

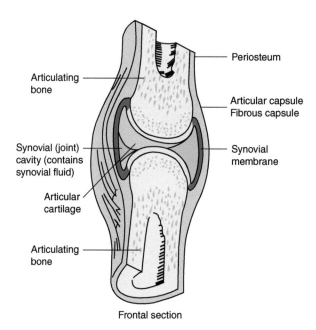

Frontal section

Figure 18.4   A synovial joint.

In synovial joints (Figure 18.4), a space exists between the bone surfaces, which allows movement of one bone against the other. Synovial fluid present in the joint provides nutrition for the articular cartilage and lubrication for the joint surfaces. Throughout life, synovial joints are subjected to normal age-related changes. These normal age-related changes can be seen in the cartilage, bone, collagen and synovial fluid. When this occurs, it may cause joint-related stiffness and pain.

Muscle

Skeletal muscle has the ability to contract and relax. A motor neuron innervates 103–3000 skeletal muscle fibres, and when contraction of the muscle occurs, the impulse that travels from the nerve to the muscle does so across the neuromuscular junction. The electrical activity causes thin actin-containing filaments to shorten, resulting in contraction of muscle. Removal of this actin-rich stimulus results in relaxation of the muscle (Figure 18.5). Electrical activity is discussed later.

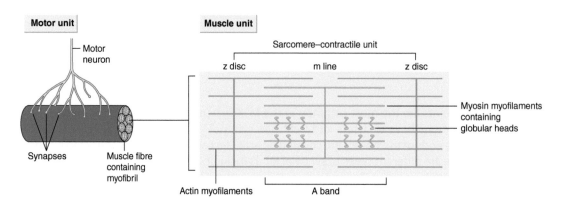

Figure 18.5   Muscle.

Muscles are often arranged in pairs associated with two or more bones and a joint. Those muscles that are associated with movement are to be found within the skeletal region where movement is caused by leverage. The pair of muscles has opposing functions: one muscle acts as the flexor (contracting and flexing) and the other as the extensor (relaxing and extending). The muscles that are attached to the bones provide the necessary force to move an object.

Body mechanics is a term used to incorporate the following coordinated efforts of the musculoskeletal and nervous systems to:

- Maintain balance
- Provide posture
- Ensure body alignment.

The muscles associated with posture are primarily the muscles of the trunk, neck and back. Working together, they provide stability and support body weight, thus allowing a sitting or standing posture to be maintained.

The nervous system

Movement and posture are both regulated by the nervous system. There is an area in the brain (the cerebral cortex) that houses the voluntary motor area. A specific area in the cerebral cortex – the precentral gyrus or motor strip – sends impulses down the motor strip to the spinal cord during voluntary movement. Muscles are stimulated after a variety of very complex neural and chemical activities take place, and movement occurs.

Movement can be impaired by a number of disorders that impede neural and chemical activity; if the muscles cannot be stimulated, movement will not occur. The concept – mobility – is complex, and there are various texts available that explain this multifaceted activity in more detail. This aspect of the chapter has merely touched on the complexities associated with mobility. In order to care for a patient with problems related to mobility, the healthcare professional needs to have a sound understanding of the many principles underpinning it.

Assessing the patient with a musculoskeletal disorder

The healthcare professional needs to be able to perform a thorough subjective and objective assessment using the biopsychosocial approach. Performing these requires excellent communication and handling skills. The competent healthcare professional will be able to identify and distinguish any psychosocial factors or any serious underlying pathologies that need referral and/or urgent attention using the Clinical Flags system (Table 18.1).

Physical examination of the patient provides much information in relation to the anatomical site. When examining the person with an MSK problem, the person undertaking the examination is generally able to make a comparison with the unaffected side of the body; usually it is advised that the unaffected side be examined first to determine what is 'normal' for the patient.

Whilst it should not necessarily be the focus of the examination, many patients will communicate that they are in pain (verbally or non-verbally). The type of pain and its distribution may give the healthcare practitioner an indication as to the type of MSK condition; a physical examination may provide information about what aspect of the anatomy has been injured.

Table 18.1   Clinical flags.

Flag	Nature	Example
Red	Sign of serious pathology	Cauda equina syndrome, severe weight loss, tumour, fracture, saddle anaesthesia, bladder and bowel disturbances, unremitting night pain, previous history of cancer
Yellow	Psychosocial issues	Unhelpful beliefs about pain, anxiety, over-dependence on passive treatments, fear avoidance, lack of job satisfaction, delayed return to work
Blue	Altered perceptions between work and health	Beliefs that work will cause injury, that there is a lack of support and acknowledgement in the workplace
Black	System or contextual obstacles	Ongoing insurance claims, legislation restricting return to work options, heavy work with minimal medication, overly solicitous family
Orange	Psychiatric	Clinical depression, personality disorder

Much can be discovered about the pain the person is experiencing by using the acronym PQRST in the subjective examination:

- **P**rovoking and **P**recipitating factors – What makes your pain worse, what makes your pain better?
- **Q**uality of pain – What does your pain feel like, how would you describe it?
- **R**adiation – Does the pain move anywhere?
- **S**everity – How much does your pain hurt right now (using an appropriate intensity scale), at its best and at its worst on a numerical rating scale of 0–10, with 0 being no pain and 10 being the worst pain you can imagine?
- **T**iming – What is the 24-hour pattern of your pain?

Table 18.2 highlights some characteristics and possible causes associated with pain in relation to the MSK system.

There are many myths, misunderstandings and unnecessary fears about pain. Most people, including some health professionals, do not have a contemporary understanding of it.

Table 18.2   Pain characteristics and possible causes associated with the MSK system.

Type of pain	Characteristics	Possible causes
Neurogenic	Sharp, stabbing, shooting, burning, pins and needles, numbness	May be neurological in nature, relating to either motor or sensory nerves
Articular	Pain that alters with movement, weight bearing and may be relieved and/or stiffens with rest, can be swollen	Likely to be associated with changes to articular structures
Phantom	Pain that is felt in a limb that is not present	Amputation, congenital limb deficiency, nerve avulsion, spinal cord injury, previous chronic pain causing altered interpretation in the brain
Inflammatory	Multiple painful joints, often symmetrical, morning stiffness but improves with exercise, swelling, erythema	May be signs of inflammation, e.g. rheumatoid arthritis
Radicular	Radiates along the upper or lower extremity along the course of a spinal nerve, pain may be in a dermatomal or myotomal pattern, reflexes may be affected	Compression, inflammation or injury to a spinal nerve root
Claudication	Cramping pain felt when walking, often relieved by rest	May mean there is an arterial insufficiency

There are two important factors we know about pain – first, the physiology of pain can be easily explained to patients and second, understanding pain physiology can change the way people think about it, decrease its threat value and improve its management. A more detailed explanation of pain is beyond the remit of this chapter; however, it is vital that the healthcare professional has an evidence-based approach and understanding and application of this to help assess and manage their patients. Chapter 17 discusses pain in more detail

When the history has been taken and a physical examination performed, in line with recommended guidelines there may be a need for further investigations, such as blood tests, X-rays and various other imaging procedures, e.g. magnetic resonance imaging (MRI) and computed tomography (CT).

Disorders of the MSK system

There are many MSK conditions, and a few of the more common pathologies will be discussed here in this chapter. MSK conditions can usually be divided into acute, sub-acute or chronic conditions, and the assessment and treatment required will reflect this. Acute conditions, particularly with soft tissue damage, can often be treated using the acronym PEACE & LOVE (Dubois and Esculier, 2019):

- **P**rotect – During the very initial stages of an injury you may need to protect the area/restrict movement (for 1 to 3 days to minimise bleeding, prevent distension of injured fibres and reduce risk of aggravating the injury) and some sort of assistive device, such as crutches or an air-cast boot may be required. Rest should be minimised (prolonged rest can compromise tissue strength and quality), and pain signals should be used to guide removal of protection and gradual reloading.
- **E**levate – Higher than the heart to promote interstitial fluid out of the tissues.
- **A**void anti-inflammatory modalities – This can impair tissue healing particularly at higher doses. Some research does question the use of ice for acute injuries – whilst it may have analgesic effects, it could disrupt the positive benefits of inflammation.
- **C**ompression – This can limit swelling and blood flow to the area and aids in venous and lymphatic drainage.
- **E**ducate – Patients should be educated on the importance of an active approach to recovery.
- **L**oad – Mechanical stress should be added, and normal activities resumed as soon as symptoms allow.
- **O**ptimism – The brain plays a huge part in recovery and psychological factors (e.g. catastrophising, depression and fear) can be barriers to recovery.
- **V**ascularisation – Cardiovascular activity should be encouraged as soon as possible to boost motivation and increase blood flow to the area.
- **E**xercise – There is strong evidence to support the use of exercise. It helps to restore mobility, strength and proprioception.

In 2018/19, MSK conditions accounted for 6.9 million lost working days in the UK (HSE, 2019). This absence from work has a huge emotional and economic impact on individuals and society. MSK conditions that last for 3 months or more can be termed chronic. These pathologies require a different treatment approach with the inclusion of psychosocial strategies. Referral to a physiotherapist for both acute and chronic MSK conditions should be arranged as they can provide expert advice on how to facilitate return to normal functioning in a safe way.

Fractures and bone healing

Many patients refer to fractures as 'broken bones': fractures are defined as a break in the continuity of bone, and this can be the result of direct or indirect trauma, underlying disease or repeated stress on a bone. Fractures that are caused by underlying disease are known as pathological fractures and those caused by repeated stress are called stress fractures.

It has already been stated that one of the unique functions of bone is its ability to constantly remodel; it is able to produce new cells and remove those cells that have died. A well-balanced diet will also aid bone healing. Calcium is a critical element in bone growth and repair; this is affected by the level of vitamin D in the body as well as renal and intestinal functioning, para-thyroid gland functioning and the ability of the adrenal glands to work effectively.

Fibroblasts (cells that take part in bone healing) originate within the connective tissue of the periosteum; therefore, the greater the damage to the periosteum, the more difficult it will be for the bone to heal (Tortora and Grabowski, 2017). There are several stages involved in the bone healing process (Table 18.3).

Whilst bone has the ability to heal by itself, this can be aided by making the broken bone immobile and restricting movement or surgical intervention, depending on the type of fracture diagnosed (see Figure 18.6 for examples of four types of fractures). There are several different classifications of fractures; listed below are some common types:

- Stress fracture (also known as hairline) – Usually affects only the outer bone.
- Transverse fracture – Breaks at a right angle to the long axis of the bone.
- Oblique fracture – Breaks in an oblique direction to the long axis of the bone.
- Spiral fracture (also known as torsion) – These can be easily confused with oblique fractures, as the break is at an oblique angle. However, rather than just being in one plane, it traverses two planes, forming a spiral shape along the bone.
- Comminuted fracture – Multiple breaks in the bone with visibly distinct fragments.
- Compression fracture – Occurs in cancellous bone, where excessive axial loading takes place.
- Greenstick fracture – In young, soft bone where the bone tends to bend and break.
- Pathological fractures – When a bone is weakened by infection, malignancy or lack of nutrition.

The aim of bone healing is to restore the normal anatomy and function of the fractured bone. Although in some circumstances, bed rest and non-weight bearing may be unavoidable, it can be counterproductive to the patient's recovery. The healthcare professional has a

Table 18.3　Osteology (*Source:* Adapted from McRae, 2016).

Time scale	Bone activity
Within the first 6 hours	As a result of the blood vessels in the bone becoming ruptured, a haematoma forms
6–48 hours	The inflammatory process begins and cytokines are released; this causes fibroblasts to migrate to the haematoma, and tissue granulation begins
2–7 days	As granulation tissue begins to form, it becomes denser and more stable, and joins with infiltrating cartilage tissue. Macrophages begin to work on the haematoma, and osteoclasts reabsorb the damaged bone
Weeks	Callus formation occurs – this is where the structure surrounding the fracture area becomes hard. This harder woven bone is eventually remodelled and becomes lamellar bone
Months	The callus, over time, becomes smaller as the bone is reconstructed

548

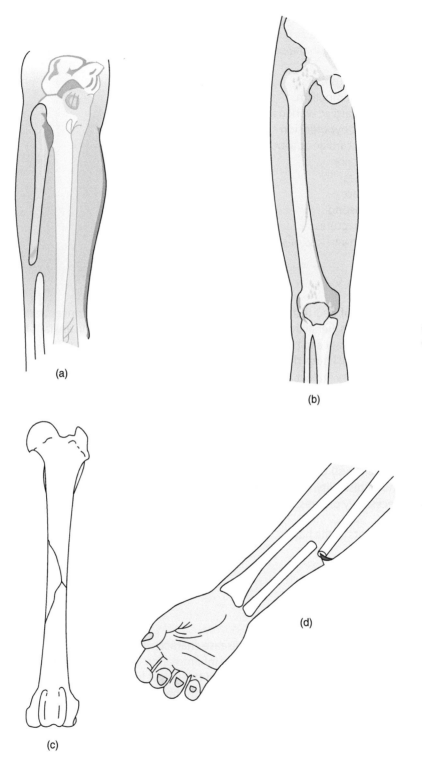

Figure 18.6 The four types of fractures: (a) simple, (b) incomplete (greenstick), (c) comminuted, (d) compound.

key role in preventing further complications that can occur and to promote mobility, normal function and exercise as far as possible, helping to encourage independence and to foster a sense of well-being in the patient. Some of the complications associated with immobility are:

- Deep vein thrombosis
- Pulmonary embolism.
- Increased cardiac workload
- Orthostatic hypotension
- Decreased cardiac output and reduced tissue perfusion
- Chest infection
- Renal stones
- Incontinence
- Muscle wasting
- Joint contractures
- Depression and loss of self-esteem

Orange flag

After several days of bed rest, a patient can experience decreased concentration, orientation and intellectual skills. Behavioural and emotional changes can result in anxiety, depression, irritability and less tolerance to pain. The healthcare professional needs to plan care that addresses not only the physical issues that are associated with bed rest and immobility but also consider those issues that may impact a person's psychological well-being.

Osteoarthritis

One of the most common disorders to affect the joints is osteoarthritis, causing potential (but not always!) pain and disability. Osteoarthritis is the single most important cause of locomotor disability. Contrary to popular belief, osteoarthritis is not caused by ageing and is not necessarily progressive. The following joints are commonly affected:

- Small joints of the hands
- Neck
- Lower back
- Big toe
- Knee
- Hip.

Osteoarthritis is a degenerative disease characterised by loss of articular cartilage, remodelling of adjacent bone and associated inflammation. The patient tends to seek help because of the pain caused by osteoarthritis and the way it interferes with their ability to function. There are known risk factors associated with the disease (CDC, 2020):

- Age 45 years and over (uncommon in younger people)
- Gender – more common in females
- Genetic predisposition
- Overweight and obesity
- Some occupations
- Previous injuries

Signs and symptoms

The patient presents with joint pain, and there is a history of joint stiffness. On examination there may be evidence of crepitus, swelling and muscle weakness and wasting; a person can become increasingly immobile – loss of function can occur. Most commonly, the patient complains of pain in the hands, cervical or lumbar spine, hips or knees.

Diagnosis

History and examination are vital. Without investigations, OA is diagnosed clinically if a person is 45 years or over *and* has activity-related joint pain *and* has either no morning joint-related stiffness or morning stiffness that lasts no longer than 30 minutes (NICE, 2014). X-ray analysis may demonstrate a reduced joint space, osteophyte formation and other abnormalities (Figure 18.7); however, it should be noted that there is very little correlation between X-ray findings and a patient's symptoms. Other investigations may be needed to exclude other causes of pain, e.g. blood tests to rule out differential diagnosis such as gout and other inflammatory arthritides, e.g. rheumatoid arthritis (NICE, 2014).

Care and management

The role of the healthcare professional is to reduce pain, increase mobility and independence and minimise progression of the disease. A core recommendation irrespective of age, co-morbidity, pain severity or disability is exercise. This should include local muscle strengthening *and* general aerobic fitness (NICE, 2014). Weight loss should also be a core treatment for those patients who are overweight or obese (NICE, 2014). Pain control can be managed by some patients with the use of paracetamol, and some patients may benefit from the use of non-steroidal anti-inflammatory drugs (NSAIDs), either orally or topically applied (NICE, 2014). Local heat or cold applied to the affected region may help to ease the pain, and transcutaneous electrical nerve stimulation (TENS) should also be considered as an adjunct to core treatments. The patient will need to be referred to a physiotherapist who can advise about exercise regimens and other adjuncts. An occupational therapist will be able to help with adaptations to the home if they are needed and a podiatrist for reviewing footwear and/or prescribing insoles. Referral to an orthopaedic surgeon may be required for joint replacement if patients experience symptoms that have a substantial impact on their quality of life.

551

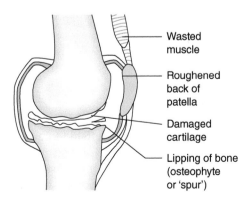

Figure 18.7   A knee joint with osteoarthritis.

Medicines management

Child-resistant packaging

The aim of child-resistant packaging is to keep little fingers out of products which could cause them harm, whilst ensuring that adults can still open and close packaging easily. Many medicines are required by law to be provided in child-proof containers, and for some people with musculo-skeletal conditions these can be impossible to open. The healthcare provider should liaise with the pharmacist to ensure the person's drugs are dispensed in a more suitable container if the person has trouble opening child-proof containers. Child-resistant closure cards can be ordered.

Osteoporosis

Osteoporotic fractures are a major cause of disability and morbidity in the elderly. The impact of fractures because of osteoporosis can have an enormous effect on the quality of a person's life. Osteoporosis is a metabolic disease resulting in loss of bone mass, particularly in postmenopausal women (NHS UK, 2019). The skeleton is affected, bone breakdown occurs faster than bone is built, and the bones become weak and break.

Osteoporosis means porous bones and is defined as a reduction in bone density, along with degenerate microarchitecture, leading to increased skeletal fragility and threat of frac-ture after minimal trauma. Everyone loses bone as they age, and the amount varies from person to person. Some people lose much more bone than others, and their bones become fragile and break more easily.

Risk factors

Everyone is at risk of developing osteoporosis as they age, but there are some factors that make some people more at risk. Risk factors associated with the development of osteoporo-sis are dependent on an interaction of multiple factors in a genetically susceptible person (NICE, 2017):

* Advancing age – risk of osteoporosis and fractures increases in women 65 years and over and men 75 years and over
* Sex hormone deficiency
* Low body mass index (BMI) – less than 18.5 kg/m^2
* Medications (current or frequent use of glucocorticosteroids)
* Chronic disease, e.g. chronic liver disease, inflammatory bowel or coeliac disease
* Previous fragility fractures
* Untreated premature menopause
* Family history of maternal hip fracture
* Immobility
* Smoking
* Excess alcohol – more than 14 units/week

Diagnosis

Diagnosis is usually made after the patient has suffered a fracture, but sometimes diagnosis of osteoporosis can be overlooked. Diagnosis can also be made by carrying out a number of investigations as well as taking an in-depth health and medical history, coupled with physi-cal examination. An X-ray cannot diagnose osteoporosis; it can, however, reveal fractures of the vertebra (and other bones) that have occurred as a result of osteoporosis. Special scans called dual-energy X-ray absorptionmetry (DXA) can be used to measure the density of the bone (bone mineral density); this can confirm diagnosis as well as quantifying the risk of fracture due to osteoporotic changes. Blood tests are required to assess a variety of bio-chemical substances, e.g.:

- Serum calcium, albumin, phosphate
- Serum creatinine
- Serum thyroid-stimulating hormone
- Alkaline phosphatase and liver transaminases.

Clinical investigations

DXA scan

A DXA scan is also known as a dual-energy X-ray absorptiometry scan and involves an advanced type of X-ray that can measure bone loss. It is the established standard for measuring bone density and helping to diagnose osteoporosis.

The patient will need to lie on their back on an X-ray table and will be required to keep very still so that images taken are not blurred. The healthcare professional may need to assist the patient prior to the investigation, during the procedure and after it has been completed. This is usually performed by a radiographer (a specialist in taking X-rays). A large scanning arm will be passed over the patient's body – this is generally the lower spine and hips; however, for some conditions, the forearm may be scanned. A narrow beam of low-dose X-ray will pass through the patient's body as the scanning arm is slowly moved. The amount of X-rays passing through the patient's body is measured, and these measurements are used to produce an image of the scanned area. This procedure normally takes around 10–30 minutes, depending upon which areas of the body are being scanned.

Test results will be in the form of two scores:

T score – This number compares the amount of bone with a young adult of the same gender with peak bone mass. Normal is a score above −1, between −1 and −2.5 is classed as osteopenia and below −2.5 is defined as osteoporotic. This figure can be used to estimate your risk of developing a fracture.

Z score – This number compares the amount of bone you have in comparison with people of the same age group, size and gender. If the score is unusually high or low, this may indicate the need for further investigations.

Care and management

Increasing awareness and encouraging activities to reduce risks is key. Pain is a predominant feature of osteoporosis – immediately when a bone fractures or in the long term in association with hip, wrist or vertebral fractures, the pain of osteoporotic fractures can be both acute and chronic. There are some over-the-counter analgesics that may help some patients, and the pharmacist may be able to provide advice; there are some patients who may, however, need stronger analgesia. Acute pain can be incapacitating, and the healthcare professional may need to engage the help of other healthcare professionals – those working in pain services – when stronger analgesics may be required, e.g. opiates.

Lifestyle advice is also a part of the care and management of the person with osteoporosis:

- Regular weight-bearing exercise
- Adequate nutrition (eating foods that are rich in calcium and vitamin D)
- Avoiding smoking
- Avoiding excessive alcohol intake.

Table 18.4 Pharmacological agents that may be used in the treatment for osteoporosis (*Source:* Adapted from Davies *et al.*, 2006).

Drug	Action
Bisphosphonates	Decreases bone loss and fracture rate
Strontium ranelate	Increases bone formation and decreases resorption of bone
Selective oestrogen receptor modulator (SERM)	Inhibit bone resorption
Hormone replacement therapy (HRT)	Postpones postmenopausal bone loss and decreases fractures

A range of pharmacological interventions can be used to improve bone mass (Table 18.4). Alternative methods of pain relief include:

- Transcutaneous electrical nerve stimulation (TENS) – Electro-analgesia using electrical signals are used to block or reduce pain impulses from getting to the brain.
- Complementary therapies, e.g. aromatherapy, homeopathy and acupuncture, may help to relieve pain, as well as increasing well-being.

Medicines management

Transcutaneous electrical nerve stimulation (TENS)

TENS is not a medication, but it is frequently used as an alternative method of pain relief for conditions such as arthritis and joint pain. A TENS machine is a small, battery-operated device that uses electrical impulses to help reduce the pain signals going to the spinal cord and brain, and this in turn may help relieve pain and muscle spasm. It is thought that TENS may also help to stimulate the production of the body's own natural painkillers – endorphins. TENS machines are often dispensed by a healthcare provider or can be bought from a pharmacy.

The machine has leads that are attached to sticky pads (either two or four pads) known as electrodes. These are placed directly on the skin and deliver electrical impulses that feel like a tingling sensation. These pads can be placed adjacent to the painful area at least 2.5 cm apart or can be placed over the spinal level pertaining to the painful site. The patient then turns on the machine and turns up the dial that controls the strength of the machine until they feel a strong but comfortable tingling sensation. TENS machines can be used whilst at work or on the move; however, they should not be used whilst driving, operating machinery or in the shower/bath. Patients must always seek medical advice before using a TENS machine as there are certain situations where they are not advised to be used such as early pregnancy, with a pacemaker or with epilepsy.

As well as the physical aspects, the healthcare professional must also consider the psychological and social aspects associated with osteoporosis. Pain can result in lack of sleep, as well as having the potential to make the patient depressed. A competent healthcare practitioner should always consider using a biopsychosocial approach to include psychological and social assessments and interventions.

Measures must be taken to reduce the risk of falls and the damage that can be caused by falls (i.e. fractures) as they are one of the biggest risk factors.

Gout

Gout, also known as crystal-induced arthritis, is an inflammatory disease (NHS UK, 2017) of the joints as the result of the deposition of crystals of the sodium salt of uric acid. The patient

554

experiences intermittent episodes of joint pain due to the uric crystals. Uric acid is the waste product formed from the breakdown of food and protein in the blood and tissues; the crystals, formed after supersaturation of the tissues, are needle like and can cause inflammation and painful swelling of the joints. There are three joints that are commonly (but not exclusively) affected:

- First metatarsophalangeal joint
- Mid-tarsal joints
- Knee.

Gout is more common in men than women, affecting men after the age of 30 years; in women it tends to occur usually after the menopause (NHS UK, 2017). There are several predisposing factors that increase the risk of contracting gout:

- Family history
- Obesity
- Excessive alcohol intake
- High purine diet (purines are found in many foods, e.g. meat, game and seafood)
- Acute infection
- Use of diuretics
- Ketosis
- Surgery
- Leukaemia
- Cytotoxic drugs
- Hypertension
- Renal failure.

Diagnosis

The person may experience intermittent episodes of acute joint pain; this is a characteristic sign, often beginning during the night, and can be brought about by trauma or another illness; it reaches a peak within a few hours. The pain may be so great that the patient is unable to tolerate the weight of bed clothes. As well as painful swollen joints, the skin over the affected area may be red and shiny, it may also peel; there may be pyrexia and fever; and the patient may have loss of appetite and malaise. More than one joint can be affected (this is termed polyarticular); particularly in the elderly person, and the joint may feel hot to touch.

Diagnosis is confirmed by in-depth history taking, examination and investigations; investigations are not carried out until the acute phase is over. Blood tests are required and may show an elevated white blood cell count and an increase in blood urate. In some instances, the fluid in the joint (the synovial fluid) may be aspirated (removed through a needle and syringe) and analysed; analysis of the synovial fluid will exclude the possibility of septic arthritis. Renal function tests may also be needed to rule out renal disease. X-rays will be unhelpful as they will usually only reveal soft tissue swelling.

Care and management

Treatment is threefold:

1. Pain management
2. Lifestyle modification
3. Lowering of urate levels.

Pain relief is a central aspect of the care and management of the person with gout. NSAIDs such as diclofenac or indomethacin may help, with the caution that such medications may cause gastrointestinal disturbances (e.g. gastric haemorrhage); if these occur, alternative medications must be given. The patient should rest, the affected limb should be elevated, and the application of an ice pack may be helpful; a bed cradle should be used to take the weight of the bed clothes off the patient's joints. The injection of steroid preparations into the joint is also effective (NHS UK, 2017).

As a health educator, the healthcare professional should encourage self-care – elevate the limb and apply ice. Lifestyle changes should also be discussed, e.g. weight loss, exercise, diet, alcohol consumption and fluid intake. If the patient is receiving aspirin (salicylate) or diuretic medications, these should be reviewed with a view to stopping them if possible.

There are some medications, e.g. allopurinol, that lower the level of uric acid. They do not control pain and once started, must be taken for a lifetime; therefore, the decision to commence this type of medication must be carefully explained to the patient using language that they understand for them to arrive at an informed decision.

Snapshot   Gout

James Willis is a 62-year-old man who presents at his GP's surgery complaining of pain and swelling over his left great toe at the metatarsal phalangeal joint. When James's foot is examined by the practice nurse (Arthur), he finds the great toe is erythematous, warm, swollen and tender to touch. James has had at least three other episodes of this type of pain, usually lasting for about 2–3 days, but he says that the pain is now worse, and he has had it for 6 days. During the examination, Nurse Arthur also notices a small rounded, subcutaneous nodule, which is tender and rubbery to the touch. The patient has a history of type 2 diabetes mellitus (controlled by diet) and of hypertension (controlled with hydrochlorothiazide). A tentative diagnosis of gout is made.

Vital signs

On admission to the ward, the following vital signs were noted and recorded:

Vital sign	Observation	Normal
Temperature	38.0°C	36.0–37.9°C range
Pulse	88 beats per minute	60–100 beats per minute
Respiration	14 breaths per minute	12–20 breaths per minute
Blood pressure	140/80 mmHg	100–139 mmHg (systolic) range
O_2 saturation	98%	94–98%
Test	Result	Normal Values
Joint fluid test	+ve urate crystals	Clear
Serum uric acid	9 mg/dL	4.0–8.5 mg/dL
Creatinine	1.1 mg/dL	0.6–1.2 mg/dL

Take some time to reflect on this case and then consider the following:

1. What information from the patient's subjective history may be required?
2. Why might joint fluid be taken from the affected joint and what might this reveal?
3. What treatment might be required in order to help Mr Willis with his condition?
4. Are there any health promotion activities the nurse might wish to discuss with Mr Willis?

NEWS 2

James Willis

Physiological parameter	3	2	1	0	1	2	3
Respiration rate				14			
Oxygen saturation %				98			
Supplemental oxygen				No			
Temperature °C					38.0		
Systolic BP mmHg				140			
Heart rate				88			
Level of consciousness				A			
Score	0	0	0	0	2	0	0
Total	2						

Low back pain

Low back pain (LBP) is the leading cause of disability globally (Maher *et al.*, 2017). The majority of LBP (>90%) is classed as non-specific LBP (nsLBP), meaning that symptoms cannot be attributed to a single pathoanatomical cause, with only 5–10% of LBP attributed to a specific pathology and <1% of LBP due to a serious pathology (Maher *et al.*, 2017). Many patients with nsLBP interpret their symptoms as tissue damage; however, it is it is widely accepted in the clinical field that this is not the case (O'Sullivan *et al.*, 2018). Pain experience is not simply an incoming message but a summary of a person's perception of how dangerous a situation is, which is also influenced by beliefs, experiences and contextual factors (O'Sullivan *et al.*, 2018). Recent evidence also highlights that clinical investigations, such as MRI and X-rays, have poor correlation with pain and disability (Brinjikji *et al.*, 2015). Interpretation of these clinical investigations, alongside diagnostic and pathological labelling, can increase patient concerns and lead to anxiety and distress (Brinjikji *et al.*, 2015).

557

Orange flag

Interpretation of clinical investigations related to nsLBP, alongside diagnostic and pathological labelling, can increase patient concerns and lead to anxiety and distress (Brinjikji *et al.*, 2015).

The biomedical approach that has been used for decades by clinicians to treat nsLBP has failed to address these issues as the prevalence and cost of nsLBP continues to rise globally (França *et al.*, 2019). There have been many conflicting and incorrect educational messages from clinicians regarding nsLBP and the vulnerability of the spine (including poor postures, lifting, pain, pathology and using passive 'fixing' treatments) have contributed to this situation (O'Sullivan *et al.*, 2018). The biopsychosocial model (BPSM) has been acknowledged to be a more effective method to reduce pain and disability in people with nsLBP.

Risk factors

- Modifiable factors – physical activity levels, cognitions and emotions, environment (socioeconomic, cultural, work, home), stress, sleep, and other comorbidities
- Non-modifiable factors – genetics, gender, life stage

Diagnosis

Acute nsLBP is usually classed as 6 weeks or less, and this type of LBP usually resolves with education on simple management and over-the-counter pain killers. An X-ray or other forms of investigation are not indicated. Patients whose nsLBP continues for longer than 6 weeks should be re-assessed, usually by a physiotherapist. X-ray is of limited benefit, and MRI is indicated if other specific causes of LBP are suspected (e.g. cauda equina, fracture, malignancy, inflammatory disorders) or within the context of a surgical referral (NICE, 2016).

Red flag

Cauda equina syndrome

This is a serious neurological condition where there is damage to the cauda equine (a bundle of spinal nerves and nerve roots from the bottom of the spinal column) and subsequent loss of function in the lumbar nerve roots. Patients may report severe back pain, bilateral pain, saddle anaesthesia or paraesthesia (pins and needles or numbness) in the groin or inner thigh region, bladder and bowel dysfunction, gait disturbances, weakness in the lower limbs and loss of sexual function. Diagnosis is initially by examination, then MRI or CT scan. Management frequently includes surgical decompression as quickly as possible to relieve the pressure on the nerve.

Care and management

Appropriate management has the potential to reduce the number of people with disabling long-term LBP and therefore reduce the personal, social and economic impacts of LBP. A healthcare professional should provide advice and education to help promote self-management of nsLBP as this is key to a successful outcome. Exercise, continuing to be active and trying to carry on with normal activities (including continuing or returning work) as much as normal should be advocated. Exercise programmes, manual therapy and acupuncture have been shown to be effective. There is no evidence that one type of exercise is more beneficial than another; it should be something the patient enjoys and will engage in. Ideally it should include aerobic activity and muscle strengthening. For those patients who have a high degree of psychological stress and disability, recommendations are to combine physical and psychological treatment programmes. These should include exercise and also cognitive behavioural approaches to manage long-term nsLBP (NICE, 2016).

Red flag

Enhancing comfort

When caring for orthopaedic/trauma patients, comfort is paramount for high-quality care and positive health outcomes. This vital element of care may be more complex for the orthopaedic/trauma patient because of the nature of their condition, injury or surgery. Musculoskeletal instability and movement may cause the patient significant pain and discomfort.

The healthcare provider should be competent in:

- Pain and comfort assessment
- Pain and comfort management (including education)
- Moving and handling.

Snapshot   Low back pain

Emma Brown is a 32-year-old primary school teacher. She lives with her husband Mike, and they have two small children aged 10 and 8 years. Emma has had LBP for 3 months which has recently got much worse. She is struggling to sleep at night due to the pain becoming so intense, despite the GP prescribing painkillers and anti-inflammatory medication. She has now been off work for 1 month and is struggling to do her personal activities of daily living (PADLs). She has an antalgic gait pattern and is feeling very depressed about the whole situation. Emma has been referred to see a physiotherapist.

There was no need for any vital signs or blood test to be taken from Emma when she visited the GP.

Take some time to reflect on this case and then consider the following:

1. What do you think the diagnosis might be? Might there be any other possible diagnoses (is there a differential diagnosis)?
2. What tests and investigations might the GP request in order to make the diagnosis?
3. How would you explain what nsLBP is to Emma?
4. What management strategies would the physiotherapist focus on?

Conclusion

Every activity of living is associated with mobility, and the degree of mobility/immobility may alter as the patient traverses the lifespan. The ability to move about freely allows us to meet our basic needs, e.g. eating, drinking and elimination, as well as being able to carry out leisure and work-related activities that will enable us to maintain our social contact and enhance our self-esteem.

Some patients may become totally dependent on others for their care; some may become transiently dependent and will then return to carrying out their activities of living in an independent manner. All body systems can be affected by the hazardous effects of immobility; the longer the patient is immobilised the greater the consequences. There are many potential complications (physical and psychosocial) associated with immobility; therefore, the healthcare professional has to assume an active role in the prevention or minimisation of the potential problems. The key elements of the healthcare professional's role are predominantly threefold – to identify, prevent and educate.

It is not possible in a chapter of this size to address in depth all concerns associated with the MSK system, and the reader is advised to read more detailed texts in order to inform clinical practice with the aim of improving their clinical skills.

Test your knowledge

- Describe the role and function of the healthcare professional in relation to the care of the person who has an MSK problem.
- Discuss the environmental, physical, psychological, politico-economic and sociocultural factors that need to be taken into account when caring for a person with an MSK problem.
- Describe the ways in which the MSK system is able to perform and fulfil several different roles.
- Provide a range of health promotion activities that would reduce the risk of OA.
- Identify the muscles of the body where it would be safe to administer an intramuscular injection. Give the reasons for your responses.

Activities

Here are some activities and exercises to help test your learning. For the answers to these exercises, as well as further self-testing activities, visit our website at **www.wiley.com/go/fundamentalsofappliedpathophysiology/student4e**

Multiple choice questions

1. What are the main functions of the skeletal system?
   (a) Protection for internal organs
   (b) Support
   (c) Blood formation
   (d) Mineral homeostasis
   (e) All of the above
2. What is the most common type of joint in the musculoskeletal system?
   (a) Synostotic
   (b) Cartilaginous
   (c) Fibrous
   (d) Synovial
   (e) Synarthrosis
3. What can be a sign of a red flag in the musculoskeletal system?
   (a) Cauda equina syndrome
   (b) Severe weight loss
   (c) Saddle anaesthesia
   (d) Bladder and bowel disturbances
   (e) All of the above
4. What is a yellow flag?
   (a) A sign of serious pathology
   (b) Psychosocial issues
   (c) Altered perceptions between work and health
   (d) System or contextual obstacles
   (e) Psychiatric issues
5. Which type of fracture usually only affects the outer bone?
   (a) Stress fracture
   (b) Transverse fracture
   (c) Oblique fracture
   (d) Comminuted fracture
   (e) Spiral fracture
6. What are some of the potential problems with immobility?
   (a) Deep vein thrombosis and pulmonary embolism
   (b) Chest infection
   (c) Muscle wasting and joint contractures
   (d) Depression and loss of self-esteem
   (e) All of the above

7. Which of the following statements about osteoarthritis is false?
   (a) The following joints are commonly affected: small joints of the hand, the neck, the lower back, the big toes, the knee and the hip
   (b) Osteoarthritis is a degenerative disease characterised by loss of articular cartilage, remodelling of adjacent bone and associated inflammation
   (c) Patients may often present with joint pain and there is a history of joint stiffness
   (d) There is always high correlation between X-ray findings and a patient's symptoms
   (e) The role of the healthcare professional is to reduce pain, increase mobility and independence and minimise progression of the disease

8. Which one of the following is NOT a risk factor for osteoporosis?
   (a) Immobility
   (b) Low body mass index (BMI) – less than 18.5 kg/m^2
   (c) Weight-bearing exercise
   (d) Smoking
   (e) Excess alcohol – more than 14 units/week

9. How long after a fracture does a callus formation normally occur?
   (a) In the first 6 hours
   (b) In 2 – 7 days
   (c) In a few weeks
   (d) In a few months
   (e) In a year

10. What is the leading cause of musculoskeletal disability globally?
    (a) Low back pain
    (b) Gout
    (c) Osteoporosis
    (d) Osteoarthritis
    (e) Fractures

11. Which of the following statements is true about non-specific low back pain?
    (a) Symptoms that can be attributed to a single pathoanatomical cause
    (b) Symptoms cannot be attributed to a single pathoanatomical cause
    (c) Symptoms that can be attributed to a serious pathology
    (d) Symptoms that cause raise red flags
    (e) Symptoms that mean there must be damage and harm to the spine

12. What can potentially make non-specific low back pain worse?
    (a) Poor/incorrect educational messages
    (b) Unnecessary investigations (e.g. using X-rays and scans)
    (c) Using catastrophising language
    (d) Using passive treatment techniques
    (e) All of the above

13. What are some of the non-modifiable risk factors in low back pain?
    (a) Gender
    (b) Physical activity levels
    (c) Stress
    (d) Sleep
    (e) Cognitions and emotions

14. Which of the following statements about cauda equina syndrome is incorrect?
   (a) This is not a serious pathology
   (b) There is damage to the bundle of nerves and nerve roots from the bottom of the spinal column
   (c) Patients may report back pain and/ or bilateral leg pains
   (d) Patients may report saddle anaesthesia or paraesthesia in the groin or inner thigh region
   (e) Patients may report bladder and bowel dysfunction
15. What percentage of low back pain is classified as non-specific low back pain?
   (a) Less than 1%
   (b) Less than 5%
   (c) Less than 50%
   (d) More than 90%
   (e) None of the above

Conditions

Below is a list of conditions that are associated with the musculoskeletal system. Take some time and write notes about each of the conditions. You may make the notes taken from textbooks or other resources (e.g. people you work with in a clinical area) or you may make the notes based on people you have cared for. If you are making notes about people you have cared for, you must ensure that you adhere to the rules of confidentiality.

Myasthenia gravis	
Sciatica	
Kyphosis	
Fibromyalgia	
Rotator cuff disorders	

Further resources

National Institute for Health and Care Excellence (NICE)

http://www.nice.org.uk/

NICE provides guidance, sets quality standards and manages a national database to improve people's health and prevent and treat ill health. There are many excellent resources on this website that can help guide and inform practice.

Arthritis Care

https://www.versusarthritis.org/about-arthritis/

Arthritis care supports people with arthritis. The website provides a range of information for people with arthritis and healthcare professionals.

Royal Osteoporosis Society

https://theros.org.uk

The Royal Osteoporosis Society is the only UK-wide charity dedicated to improving the diagnosis, prevention and treatment of osteoporosis. The website is easy to navigate and offers a wealth of useful information for people with osteoporosis and their families, and for those who care for people with osteoporosis.

Brittle Bone Society

http://www.brittlebone.org/

The Brittle Bone Society provides practical and emotional support for people affected by the rare bone condition osteogenesis imperfecta. It also provides short-term loan of specialist wheelchairs and other equipment when required. Acts as a signpost to organisations that may be able to help with queries, such as benefits and welfare issues.

American College of Rheumatology

http://www.rheumatology.org/

The American College of Rheumatology provides up-to-date information on research education and treatments for all rheumatological conditions.

Glossary of terms

Actin   A microfilament protein.

Antalgic   A posture or gait assumed so as to lessen pain.

Anticholinesterase   An agent that blocks nerve impulses by inhibiting the activity of an enzyme called cholinesterase.

Cartilage   A type of connective tissue that contains collagen and elastic fibres. This strong tough material on the bone ends helps to distribute the load within the joint; the slippery surface allows smooth movement between the bones. Cartilage can withstand both tension and compression.

Cholinesterase   An enzyme that breaks down acetylcholine to stop its action.

Claudication   Ischaemia of the muscles, causing lameness and pain during walking, particularly in the calf muscles.

Crepitus   A crinkling, cracking or grating feeling or sound in the joints.

Cytokine   A hormone-like protein that regulates the intensity and duration of immune responses.

Diplopia   A condition where a single object is perceived as two objects.

Dysarthria   A disturbance of speech and language.

Dysphagia   Difficulty in swallowing.

Effusion   A collection of fluid.

Haematoma   A localised collection of blood due to a break in the wall of a blood vessel that is often clotted.

Haemopoiesis   The formation and development of blood cells.

Immunosuppressive   Pertaining to immunosuppression – prevention or interference with the development of an immunological response.

Lesion   A wound or injury; refers to a change in the tissues.

Ligament   A tough fibrous band that holds two bones together in a joint.

Macrophage   A phagocyte produced from monocytes that engulfs and digests cellular debris, microbes and foreign matter.

Meniscectomy   The removal of the meniscus (ligament within the knee).

Opiate   A powerful analgesic agent derived from opium that stimulates opiate receptors within the central nervous system.

Ossification   The formation of bone.

Osteoblast   A cell that arises from fibroblasts; a bone-forming cell.

Osteoclasts   A cell that breaks down bone tissue and thus releases the calcium used to create bones.

Osteophyte   An overgrowth of new bone around the side of osteoarthritic joints; also known as spurs growth.

Osteoporosis   A condition characterised by reduced bone density and an increased risk of fractures.

Pathoanatomical   Of or relating to the anatomy of diseased tissues and organs (pathological anatomy).

Plasmapheresis   The removal of whole blood from the body and separation of cellular elements.

Proximal   Nearest to the trunk or point of origin.

Ptosis   Drooping of the upper eye lid.

Saddle anaesthesia   The loss or reduction of sensation around the perineum, buttocks and groin.

Septic arthritis   A pus-forming bacterial infection of a joint space.

Synapse   The junction where two neurons meet or where a neuron meets tissue.

Uric acid   The end product of the purine nucleotide (nucleoprotein) metabolism.

References

Brinjikji, W., Luetmer, P., Comstock, B. *et al.* (2015). Systematic literature review of imaging features of spinal degeneration in asymptomatic populations. *American Journal of Neuroradiology*, 36: 811–816.

CDC (2020). *Centres for Disease Control and Prevention. Arthritis: Risk Factors* https://www.cdc.gov/arthritis/basics/risk-factors.htm

Davies, R., Everitt, H. and Simon, C. (2006). *Musculoskeletal Problems.* Oxford: Oxford University Press.

Davis, G. (2006). The musculoskeletal system: Physiology, conditions and common drug therapies. *Nurse Prescribing*, 4(10): 406–411.

Dubois, B. and Esculier, J.F. (2019). Soft tissue injuries simply need PEACE & LOVE. *British Journal of Sports Medicine*, 54(2): 72–73.. https://blogs.bmj.com/bjsm/2019/04/26/soft-tissue-injuries-simply-need-peace-love/

França, A., dosSantos, V., Lordelo Filho, R., Fonseca Pires, K., *et al.* (2019). 'It's very complicated': Perspectives and beliefs of newly graduated physiotherapists about the biopsychosocial model for treating people experiencing non-specific low back pain in Brazil. *Musculoskeletal Science in Practice*, 41: 84–89.

McRae, R. (2016). *Pocketbook of Orthopaedic Trauma and Emergency Fracture Management*, 3rd edn. Edinburgh: Elsevier.

Maher, C., Underwood, M. and Buchbinder, R. (2017). Non-specific low back pain. *Lancet*, 389: 736–747.

Health and Safety Executive (HSE) (2019). *Work Related Musculoskeletal Disorder Statistics (WRMSD's) in Great Britain, 2019*. https://www.hse.gov.uk/statistics/causdis/msd.pdf

NHS Health Education England (HEE) (2020). http://www.makingeverycontactcount.co.uk/

NHS UK (2017). *National Health Service United Kingdom Choices*. https://www.nhs.uk/conditions/Gout/

NHS UK (2019). *National Health Service United Kingdom Choices*. www.nhs.uk/Conditions/Osteoporosis/Pages/Introduction

National Institute for Health and Care Excellence (NICE) (2014). *Osteoarthritis: Care and Management*. https://www.nice.org.uk/guidance/cg177

National Institute for Health and Care Excellence (NICE) (2017). *Clinical Knowledge Summaries. Osteoporosis – Prevention of Fragility Fractures*. https://cks.nice.org.uk/osteoporosis-prevention-of-fragility-fractures

National Institute for Health and Care Excellence (NICE) (2016). *Low Back Pain and Sciatica in over 16's: Assessment and Management*. www.nice.org.uk/guidance/NG59

O'Sullivan, P., Caneiro, J., O'Keeffe, M., Smith, A., Dankaerts, W., Fersum, K. and O'Sullivan, K. (2018). Cognitive functional therapy: An integrated behavioural approach for the targeted management of disabling low back pain. *Physical Therapy*, 98(5): 409–423.

Tortora, G.J. and Grabowski, S.R. (2017). *Principles of Anatomy and Physiology*, 15th edn. New Jersey: John Wiley & Sons, Inc.

World Health Organisation (WHO) (2019). https://www.who.int/news-room/fact-sheets/detail/musculoskeletal-conditions

Chapter 19

Fluid, electrolyte balance and associated disorders

Noleen P. Jones

Principal Lecturer (Ag), School of Health Studies, Gibraltar

Contents

Introduction 567
Body fluid compartments 567
Composition of body fluid..........................569
Body fluid balance 569
Disorders associated with fluid and
    electrolyte imbalance 575
Conclusion 587

Test your knowledge......................................587
Multiple choice questions............................588
Conditions..589
Further resources...590
Glossary of terms...591
References..592

Key words

- Diffusion
- Hypovolaemia
- Intracellular
- Oedema
- Electrolytes
- Hypervolaemia
- Osmosis
- Extracellular
- Interstitial fluid
- Osmotic pressure

Fundamentals of Applied Pathophysiology: An Essential Guide for Nursing and Healthcare Students, Fourth Edition. Edited by Ian Peate.
© 2021 John Wiley & Sons Ltd. Published 2021 by John Wiley & Sons Ltd.
Student companion website: www.wiley.com/go/fundamentalsofappliedpathophysiology/student4e
Instructor companion website: www.wiley.com/go/fundamentalsofappliedpathophysiology/instructor4e

- In the human body, where are the extracellular compartments?
- Where is most of the fluid volume found – in the intracellular or extracellular compartments?
- Define the function of body fluids and electrolytes.
- Define the terms hypotonic, hypertonic and isotonic solutions.
- What are the signs and symptoms of dehydration?

Learning outcomes

On completion of this section, the reader will be able to:

- Identify the fluid compartments of the body.

- List the major electrolytes of the extracellular and intracellular compartments of the body.

- Define the term *osmosis*.

- Define the term *diffusion*.

Don't forget to visit the companion website for this book (www.wiley.com/go/fundamentalsofappliedpathophysiology/student4e) **where you can find self-assessment tests to check your progress, as well as lots of activities to practise your learning.**

Introduction

Fluid and electrolytes are essential for body function and to maintain homeostasis. Fluid and electrolytes are not static in the body. There is constant movement of fluid and electrolytes between the intracellular and extracellular compartments. The movement of fluid and electrolytes ensures that the cells have a constant supply of electrolytes such as sodium, chloride, potassium, magnesium, phosphate, bicarbonate and calcium for cellular function (see Chapter 2 for a description of cellular functions). Changes in the movement of fluid and electrolytes between compartments occur as a result of disease. This chapter considers fluid and electrolyte balance and some diseases resulting from fluid and electrolyte imbalance.

Body fluid compartments

Fluid forms approximately 60% of the body weight in an adult male, 50% in an adult female and 70% in an infant (McCance *et al.*, 2019). The percentage of fluid distribution varies with age and gender. Women have less body fluid compared to men, as women have more body fat and men have more muscle mass (McCance *et al.*, 2019). Fat cells contain less water than muscle cells.

The two principal body fluid compartments are intracellular and extracellular. The intracellular compartment is the space inside a cell, and the fluid inside the cell is called intracellular fluid (ICF). The extracellular compartment is found outside the cell, and the fluid outside the cell is called extracellular fluid (ECF). However, the extracellular compartment is further divided into the interstitial compartment and the intravascular compartment (Figure 19.1). Two-thirds of body fluid is found inside the cell and one-third outside the cell. Eighty per cent of the ECF is found in the interstitial compartment and 20% in the intravascular compartment as plasma (Figure 19.2).

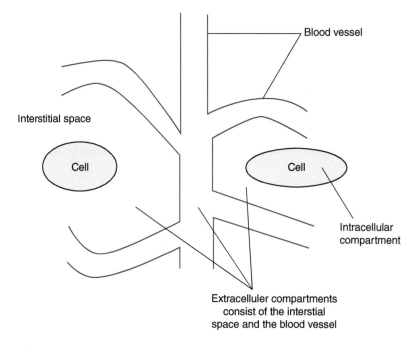

Figure 19.1　Fluid compartments.

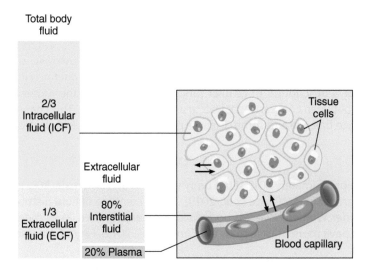

Figure 19.2　Fluid distribution.

Composition of body fluid

The body fluid is composed of water and dissolved substances such as electrolytes (sodium, potassium and chloride), gases (oxygen and carbon dioxide), nutrients, enzymes and hormones. The total body water constitutes 60% of the total body weight, and water plays an important part in cellular function. Water is essential for the body as it:

- Acts as a lubricant
- Transports nutrients, gases such as oxygen, hormones and enzymes to the cells, and waste products of metabolism, e.g. carbon dioxide, urea and uric acid, from the cells for excretion
- Helps in the regulation of body temperature
- Provides an optimum medium for the cells to function
- Provides a medium for chemical reactions
- Breaks down food particles in the digestive system.

Body fluid balance

The term *fluid balance* indicates that the body's required amount of water is present and distributed proportionally amongst the compartments. Generally, water intake equals water loss, and the body fluid remains constant. However, fluid intake varies with individuals; but the body regulates fluid volume within a narrow range. Most of the water essential for body function is obtained from drinking water, some from the food consumed and some from cellular metabolism. The kidneys play a vital role in fluid balance as water is excreted in the urine; some water is lost in respiration, skin and in faeces. See Table 19.1 for fluid intake and output.

The body regulates body fluid volume via the thirst receptors. When there is an excess of water loss through excessive sweating or by not drinking, then the body fluid balance is disrupted, which can result in dehydration. Dehydration stimulates the thirst reflex in three ways:

1. The blood osmotic pressure increases, resulting in the stimulation of the osmoreceptors of the hypothalamus.
2. Circulating blood volume decreases, which initiates the renin–angiotensin system, resulting in the stimulation of the thirst centre in the hypothalamus.
3. As a result of dehydration, the mucosal lining of the mouth is dry and the production of saliva decreases, which stimulates the thirst centre in the hypothalamus.

Osmosis

Osmosis is a process by which water moves from an area of high volume to an area of low volume through a selectively permeable membrane. The movement of water depends on

Table 19.1   Fluid intake and output.

Intake (mL)		Output (mL)	
Drinking (approx. 60%)	1400–1800	Urine (approx. 60%)	1400–1800
Water from food (approx. 30%)	700–1000	Faeces (approx. 2%)	100
Water of oxidation (approx. 10%)	300–400	Expiration (lungs approx. 28%)	600–800
		Skin (approx. 10%)	300–600
Total balance (100%)	2400–3200	Total balance 100%	2400–3200

Source: Adapted from McCance *et al.*, 2014.

Red flag

Fluid overload

Just as dehydration can be detrimental to a patient's health and well-being, so too can fluid overload. Fluid overload occurs when the circulating volume is excessive, that is, more than the heart can effectively manage. This results in heart failure, which usually causes pulmonary oedema and peripheral oedema.

Fluid overload usually presents as acute pulmonary oedema with symptoms of acute dyspnoea. Chronic fluid overload (as occurs in the context of intravascular fluid overload) usually presents with features of chronic heart failure, and the main symptoms are:

- Fatigue
- Dyspnoea
- Tachycardia
- Pitting oedema

---

the number of solutes dissolved in the solution and not on their molecular weights (Vujovic *et al.*, 2018). Therefore, the number of dissolved particles determines the concentration of the solution, which is expressed as the osmolality of the solution. The selectively permeable membrane will allow water molecules to move across, but it is not permeable to solutes such as sodium, potassium and other substances. Water accounts for the osmotic pressure in the tissues and cells of the body. Water movement between the intracellular and the extracellular compartments occurs through osmosis.

At times, the term *tonicity* is used instead of osmolality. Thus, solutions can be regarded as hypertonic, hypotonic or isotonic. The term *hypertonic solution* indicates that the solution has a high amount of solutes dissolved in it, e.g. 5% dextrose. A hypotonic solution is one that has a low concentration of solutes dissolved in it, e.g. 0.45% normal saline. An isotonic solution has the same osmolality as body fluids, e.g. 0.9% normal saline.

Electrolytes

Fluid balance is linked to electrolyte balance. Electrolytes are chemical compounds that dissociate in water to form charged particles called ions. They include potassium (K), sodium (Na), chloride (Cl), magnesium (Mg) and hydrogen phosphate (HPO_4). Electrolytes are either positively or negatively charged. Positively charged ions are called cations (e.g. Na^+ and K^+), and negatively charged ions are called anions (e.g. Cl^- and HCO_3^-). Remember that an anion and a cation will combine to form a compound; e.g. potassium (K^+) and chloride (Cl^-) will combine to form potassium chloride (KCl). The composition of electrolytes differs between the intracellular and the extracellular compartments (Figure 19.3).

Functions

Electrolytes have numerous functions in the body:

- Regulation of fluid balance
- Regulation of acid–base balance
- Essential in neuromuscular excitability
- Essential for neuronal function
- Essential for enzyme reaction.

Table 19.2 summarises the principal electrolytes and their functions.

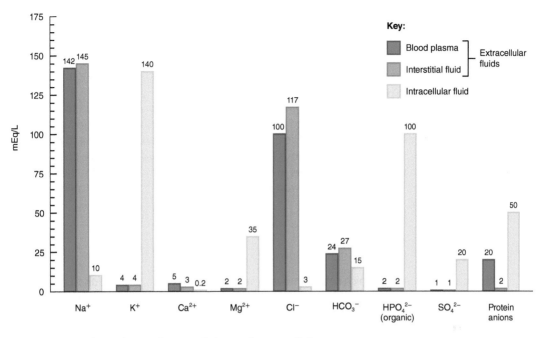

Figure 19.3 Electrolytes of intracellular and extracellular compartments.

Table 19.2 Principal electrolytes and their functions.

Electrolytes	Normal values in extracellular fluid (mmol/L)	Function	Main distribution
Sodium (Na⁺)	135–145	Important cation in generation of action potentials. Plays an important role in fluid and electrolyte balance	Main cation of the extracellular fluid
Potassium (K⁺)	3.5–5	Important cation in establishing resting membrane potential. Regulates pH balance. Maintains intracellular fluid volume	Main cation of the intracellular fluid
Calcium (Ca²⁺)	2.1–2.6	Important clotting factor. Plays a part in neurotransmitter release in neurons. Maintains muscle tone and excitability of nervous and muscle tissue	Mainly found in the extracellular fluid
Magnesium (Mg²⁺)	0.5–1.0	Helps to maintain normal nerve and muscle function; maintains regular heart rate, regulates blood glucose and blood pressure. Essential for protein synthesis	Mainly distributed in the intracellular fluid
Chloride (Cl⁻)	98–117	Maintains a balance of anions in different fluid compartments	Main anion of the extracellular fluid
Hydrocarbons (HCO₃⁻)	24–31	Main buffer of hydrogen ions in plasma. Maintains a balance between cations and anions of intracellular and extracellular fluids	Mainly distributed in the extracellular fluid
Phosphate – organic (HPO₄²⁻)	0.8–1.1	Essential for the digestion of proteins, carbohydrates and fats and absorption of calcium. Essential for bone formation	Mainly found in the intracellular fluid
Sulphate (SO₄²⁻)	0.5	Involved in detoxification of phenols, alcohols and amines	Mainly found in the intracellular fluid

Medicines management

Potassium supplement

Potassium is the main intracellular cation. Intravenous (IV) potassium must be safely and appropriately stored, prescribed and administered.

Bolus administration or rapid infusion of intravenous potassium chloride can lead to critical incidents and even death. Patients have died in hospitals after being mistakenly injected with potassium chloride instead of sodium chloride 0.9% or water for injection. In an effort to reduce the risks associated with the use of intravenous potassium chloride, guidelines have been produced nationally that describe safe practices in relation to the prescribing and administration of potassium chloride and should be followed to reduce the likelihood of a critical incident occurring due to inappropriate use.

Diffusion

Diffusion is a process by which solutes move from an area of high concentration to an area of low concentration. Diffusion is further subdivided into simple and facilitated diffusion. Liquid-soluble molecules and gases move by a process of simple diffusion through a concentration gradient (Figure 19.4). Larger molecules such as glucose and amino acids are transported across a cell membrane by a carrier protein and concentration gradient (Figure 19.5).

Hormones that regulate fluid and electrolytes

The two principal hormones that regulate fluid and electrolyte balance are antidiuretic hormone (ADH) and aldosterone (Molnar and Gair, 2015). ADH regulates fluid balance in the body. This hormone is produced in the hypothalamus by neurons called osmoreceptors and the hormone is stored by the posterior pituitary gland. Osmoreceptors are sensitive to plasma osmolality and a decrease in blood volume. The target organs for ADH are the kidneys. ADH acts on the distal convoluted tubule and the collecting ducts (see Chapter 11) and make them more permeable to water, thus increasing reabsorption of water.

Aldosterone is a steroid hormone produced by the cortex of the adrenal glands, which are situated at the top of each kidney (Figure 19.6). The adrenal gland is divided into the cortex

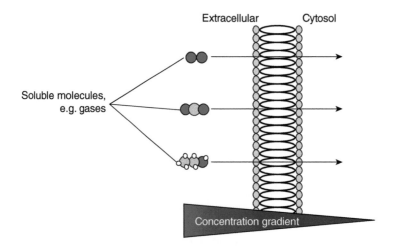

Figure 19.4   Simple diffusion.

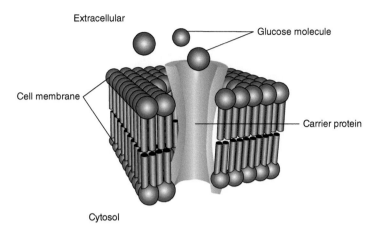

Figure 19.5   Carrier protein (facilitated diffusion).

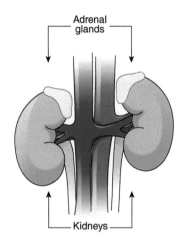

Figure 19.6   Adrenal glands.

and the medulla (Figure 19.7). Aldosterone regulates electrolyte and fluid balance by sodium and water retention.

Oedema

Oedema is the abnormal accumulation of fluid, mainly water in the body (Kumar and Clark, 2016) in the interstitial space. It is a problem of fluid distribution and does not indicate fluid excess (McCance *et al.*, 2014). The term is derived from the Greek word meaning 'swollen condition'. The accumulation of fluid may be localised as in thrombophlebitis or generalised as in heart failure, affecting all tissues. Localised oedema is normally temporary and resolves without intervention. Generalised oedema is regarded as an abnormal condition that requires treatment.

Oedema can either be pitting or non-pitting. If an indentation develops after gently pressing the swollen lower limb with a finger, this is termed pitting oedema (Wilson, 2017). The causes of oedema include:

- Heart failure
- Obesity resulting in increased fluid pressure and salt retention

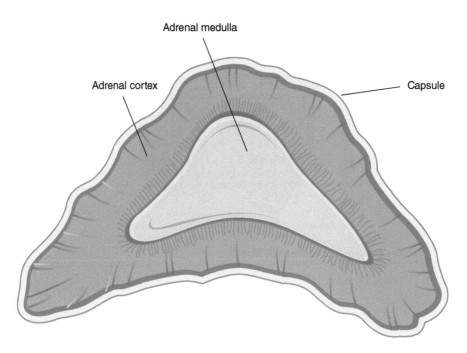

Figure 19.7   Cross-section of the adrenal gland.

- Drugs such as calcium antagonists, for example, verapamil and nifedipine, and prolonged steroid therapy
- Renal conditions such as nephrotic syndrome
- Venous stasis resulting from immobility
- Varicose veins
- Liver cirrhosis causing hypoalbuminaemia.

Pulmonary oedema

Pulmonary oedema is a condition where there is accumulation of fluid in the lungs, resulting in impaired gas (oxygen and carbon dioxide) exchange and pulmonary function. Pulmonary oedema can result from:

- Congestive heart failure
- Fluid overload as a result of renal failure
- Myocardial infarction with left ventricular failure
- Chest injury as a result of a road traffic collision
- Upper airway obstruction
- Severe chest infection.

Peripheral oedema

Peripheral oedema is a condition where there is localised soft tissue swelling as a result of fluid accumulation in the interstitial space. Fluid accumulates in parts of the body affected by gravity, e.g. the lower limbs in a mobile patient or around the sacral region in a patient who is immobile and on bed rest. Peripheral oedema can result from:

- Immobility
- Obesity

- Heart failure
- Pregnancy as a result of fluid retention and venous stasis
- Liver diseases such as cirrhosis of the liver
- Prolonged steroid therapy.

Disorders associated with fluid and electrolyte imbalance

Learning outcomes

On completion of this section, the reader will be able to:

- Describe the importance of maintaining a fluid balance chart.

- Discuss the significance of adequate hydration and the benefits of this for the health and well-being of the patient.

- Outline the management and interventions related to the patient who is nauseous and may be vomiting.

- Outline the management and interventions related to the patient who has pulmonary and/or peripheral oedema.

575

Maintaining fluid balance charts

Fluid balance occurs where the amount of fluid taken into the body equals the amount of fluid that leaves the body (Marieb and Hoehn, 2019). Maintenance of fluid balance is an important activity and is essential for optimal health. If a patient has too much fluid and there is an imbalance, health problems can result; likewise if the patient has too little fluid, this too can cause problems. There are some pathophysiological conditions that can result in fluid overloading, e.g. kidney disease and some types of heart disease; when this occurs, the person finds it difficult to rid the body of excess water and can experience oedema; i.e. there is too much fluid in the tissues of the body (care of the patient with oedema is discussed later).

For patients who are experiencing problems associated with fluid balance, the monitoring of fluid balance becomes important. The healthcare professional uses a chart called a fluid balance chart in order to monitor the patient's input and output (Figure 19.8). Sometimes these charts are known as fluid intake and output charts or intake and output flow charts. Each time the patient takes in fluids or fluids leave the body, the healthcare professional has a responsibility to record this on the fluid balance chart. The amounts are calculated at the end of a 24-hour period – usually this is from 12 midnight to 12 midnight the next night. A comparison is made between the amount of fluid taken in and the amount of fluid the patient passes out; this is the patient's fluid balance (Lister *et al.*, 2020b).

Fluid balance charts that are user-friendly should be provided, as this will help to encourage patients and their families to fill them in themselves; by doing this, independence can be promoted. There are also electronic versions of fluid balance charts. Electronic fluid balance charts enable accurate calculations of fluid balance and automated reminders to undertake assessment.

	Ward:			Date:			
Surname:				Hospital Number:			
Forename:							
Date of Birth:							

	Fluid intake			Fluid output			
Time	Oral	Intravenous	Other (specify)	Urine	Vomit	Other (specify)	
01.00							
02.00							
03.00							
04.00							
05.00							
06.00							
07.00							
08.00							
09.00							
10.00							
11.00							
12.00							
13.00							
14.00							
15.00							
16.00							
17.00							
18.00							
19.00							
20.00							
21.00							
22.00							
23.00							
24.00							
Total							

Figure 19.8　A fluid balance chart.

Orange flag

When patients are asked to complete fluid balance charts independently, this can help boost their confidence and give them a feeling of involvement in the care process. The healthcare professional must, however, ensure that the patient is able to demonstrate capacity (understand information, retain and recall when asked) concerning their fluid balance monitoring if they are to complete charts independently.

Measuring fluid balance

Intake

All of the fluid that a patient drinks and also those foods that are liquid, milk on cereals and ice cream are considered fluid intake. There are other fluids that are considered a part of fluid intake, e.g. enteral feeds and intravenous fluids. All fluid intake must be measured and documented on the patient's fluid balance chart. The healthcare professional needs to know how much various receptacles, such as cups and glasses, hold in order to chart intake effectively.

The amount of enteral feed, gastrostomy and nasogastric feeding and intravenous fluid (including blood and or blood products) being infused must also be monitored, measured and documented. There are some patients who require fluid via the subcutaneous or rectal route and the same is required here; the fluid intake must be recorded.

Output

The following are deemed fluid output, and these (just like intake) must be monitored, measured and documented on the fluid balance chart:

- Urine (in seriously ill patients with a urinary catheter *in situ*; this may need to be measured and recorded hourly)
- Vomit
- Aspirate from a nasogastric tube
- Diarrhoea
- Effluent from a stoma
- Exudate from a wound and wound drain.

There may be some instances when it is impossible to measure output accurately, e.g. where the patient has diarrhoea or a wound has excessive exudate. In these instances, the healthcare professional may need to weigh incontinence pads or dressings to determine the amount of fluid being lost via this route (Galen, 2015).

A positive fluid balance exists when the patient's intake exceeds their output, and a negative balance occurs when output exceeds intake. A record of the daily balance over several days should be carried out so that an assessment of trend can be made (Lister *et al.*, 2020b).

577

Maintaining hydration

Florence Nightingale stated that the very first requirement in a hospital is that it should do the sick no harm; this statement was made back in 1854. Having enough to eat and drink is one of the most basic of human needs (British Dietetic Association, 2019). Most people are able to maintain an adequate level of hydration – they are prompted by thirst or hunger to seek fluids or food; however, those who are ill and dependent are unable to do this and may be at risk of becoming dehydrated. Dehydration is a common fluid and electrolyte imbalance in older people (Daniels and Nicoll, 2012).

This section considers the healthcare professional's responses that are necessary to ensure that patients are adequately hydrated. It draws on previous sections of the chapter in respect of fluid and electrolyte balance. Hydration is the state of fluid balance of the body, and dehydration occurs when the state of fluid output exceeds intake. Rapid weight loss as a result of dehydration can be the consequence of a lack of fluid intake or hyponatraemia (sodium depletion) with an accompanying loss of water (Giddens, 2017).

Benefits of good hydration

Water is vital to health and should be seen as an essential nutrient. As people age, their body's needs and health concerns change as a result of an increasing susceptibility to pathophysiological disease. There are many benefits associated with good hydration. The implications of poor hydration from a pathophysiological perspective can have many ramifications, and some of these are discussed here.

Patients who are poorly hydrated have the potential to develop pressure sores (decubitus ulcers); the more an individual becomes dehydrated, the more at risk they become. Dehydration results in a reduction in padding over bony prominences. Fluid intake to correct poor hydration can increase oxygen levels with the possibility of enhancing ulcer healing. Poor outcomes of care and the person's quality of life are directly linked to dehydration.

One of the most frequent causes of chronic constipation is inadequate fluid intake. Patients who are inadequately hydrated can, by drinking more water, increase stool frequency and enhance the beneficial effects of daily dietary fibre intake (Taylor, 2015).

It is important in the prevention of urinary tract infection to ensure that the patient maintains adequate hydration. Water helps to maintain a healthy urinary tract and promotes renal function. Consumption of water at regular intervals can help by diluting bile and stimulating gallbladder emptying, which in turn has the potential to reduce and prevent gallstone formation.

In relation to heart disease, hydration reduces the risk of coronary heart disease as adequate hydration decreases blood viscosity, thereby protecting against clot formation. Extracellular volume depletion as result of dehydration is the result of a net loss of total body sodium with a reduction in intravascular volume. A well-hydrated patient will find it easier to expectorate respiratory secretions (Corroon and Hynes, 2014).

Dehydration can worsen diabetic control, and water is an essential aspect of dietary management of diabetes mellitus. In patients who have poorly controlled diabetes, there can be an increase in urinary output, and this in turn can result in dehydration; good hydration levels can slow down the development of diabetic ketoacidosis, helping to maintain healthy blood sugar levels (Effective Diabetes Education Now [EDEN], 2018).

Dehydration is a risk factor that is associated with falls in older people (Picetti et al., 2017). Dehydration can cause disorientation, dizziness, headache and tiredness, increasing the risk of fainting and falling. Adequate hydration in the older population can be part of an effective falls prevention strategy.

Failure to ensure that the patient is adequately hydrated can lead to a number of pathophysiological changes that can put the health and well-being of the individual at risk. It is therefore vital that this aspect of care is given the priority it deserves. Twenty-four hour catering can help to ensure that people can have access to hot food and drinks. People should be able to access food and drink any time, depending on their needs and preferences (Maddex, 2014; NHS England, 2014).

There may be instances where the patient requires an intravenous infusion to replace fluid loss or to hydrate them. An alternative to intravenous fluid replacement is hypodermoclysis (Galen, 2015). Hypodermoclysis involves the insertion of a small cannula (a butterfly cannula) into the subcutaneous tissues (often this is in the abdomen). Subcutaneous infusions can be carried out in the home setting if service users, relatives or carers feel confident and can be assessed by the community nurse to demonstrate safe techniques in caring for infusion and cannula sites. The cannula is secured using an occlusive type of dressing, and the prescribed infusion begins. The rate and duration of fluid to be transfused is determined by prescription, and the care and management of the patient is in accordance with local policy. It is vital that all fluids (input and output) are recorded on the fluid balance chart.

Orange flag

Maintaining normal fluid and electrolyte balance can help to prevent delirium (sudden confusion). Dehydration is a modifiable delirium risk factor. Changes in mental status begin with mild dehydration and worsen with each stage, culminating in delirium. In moderate dehydration, short-term memory loss occurs. Failure to recognise signs of dehydration predisposes older people to becoming increasingly and chronically dehydrated, which can lead to delirium.

Nausea and vomiting

There are many reasons why a person may feel nauseous and/or vomit. Most patients will experience nausea and/or vomiting during a disease process; this may be as a result of the disease pathology or the consequence of treatment. Wicker (2015) notes that post-operative nausea and vomiting is a common complication following surgery and anaesthesia. Vomiting (or emesis) according to Herlihy (2018) is and is not a stomach event. Nausea and vomiting may indicate pathophysiological changes that are occurring within the body. Both nausea and vomiting can be particularly upsetting for the patient as well as for their family; they can also impact the person's ability to perform the activities of daily living.

Nausea

Howard and Morgan (2012) describe nausea as an unpleasant sensation of imminent vomiting of the stomach contents through the mouth. The sensation produces a feeling of discomfort in the region of the stomach with a feeling of a need to vomit. Nausea can be short-lived or long-lasting. A person may experience nausea alone, with no vomiting, or they may vomit without any feeling of nausea beforehand. Some people experience nausea and then go on to vomit. Nausea, therefore, does not always lead to vomiting.

Nausea is a symptom of many conditions; it can be due to physical or psychological issues. It is not an illness, and not all of the causes are necessarily related to the stomach; e.g. patients who are receiving chemotherapy may experience nausea. Nausea can be caused by adverse drug reactions; nausea is also a common symptom of pregnancy. Usually, the presence of nausea means that there may be an underlying pathological condition occurring in the body. The following can also cause nausea:

579

- Diabetes mellitus
- Influenza
- Gastroenteritis
- Renal failure
- Adrenal insufficiency
- Peptic ulcer
- Vertigo.

Treatment of nausea will depend on its cause. Avoidance of foods in the short term may help to reduce the feelings associated with nausea. Removing or avoiding strong smells such as perfume or aftershave can also help to alleviate nausea. Some people experience nausea when they are, for example, travelling in a car, and stopping the car and sitting still can help alleviate the feelings of nausea that are caused by perceived movement and actual movement.

The healthcare professional may advise the patient to eat small meals throughout the day as opposed to three large meals, and encourage the patient to eat slowly, avoiding foods that are hard to digest. If it is the smell of food that is provoking the nausea, then foods should be eaten cold or at room temperature, avoiding the smell of cooked food or food that is cooking.

An anti-emetic (e.g. metoclopramide), a medicine that is given to prevent or stop nausea and vomiting, may also be administrated. There are also a number of mechanical aids that are used to help prevent nausea (and vomiting). These devices work by applying continuous pressure on specific acupressure points located on the wrist and can be used by children and adults.

Vomiting

Vomiting is a complex physiological activity. It can be defined as the forceful expulsion of gastric contents through the mouth and/or nose.

Excessive vomiting can have a profound effect on a person's fluid and electrolyte balance (Waugh and Grant, 2014). The vomiting centre (sometimes also known as the emetic centre) situated in the medulla oblongata of the brain is responsible for the initiation of vomiting. Both physical and psychological impulses can excite the vomiting centre, causing the patient to vomit. Some causes of excitement of the vomiting centre include:

- Fear/anxiety
- Odours
- Pain
- Unpleasant sights
- Side effects of some drugs
- Radiotherapy
- Hypercalcaemia.

The sensitivity of the vomiting centre varies in different people, and as such the healthcare professional should treat each person on an individual basis.

It is important to determine, if possible, the cause of vomiting; removal of the causative factor, if possible, should be the first line of treatment. Caring for the patient who is vomiting will include the following:

- Wash hands.
- Ask the patient if they have any tried and tested methods of dealing with vomiting, and if appropriate implement these.
- Ensure the patient is cared for in an upright (unless contraindicated) position.
- Care for the patient in the lateral position if they are unconscious and unable to protect their own airway.
- Administer prescribed anti-emetic medication.
- Ensure privacy (e.g. curtains are drawn and doors closed).
- Provide easy access to a vomit bowl and tissues (ensure a receptacle is available to dispose safely of used tissues).
- Remove the dirty vomit bowl and replace with a clean one as soon as possible.
- Offer the patient physical comfort by being with them and holding the vomit bowl or mopping their brow.
- Observe, measure, record and report vomitus.
- Provide the patient with the opportunity to use a mouthwash.
- Provide the patient with the opportunity to 'freshen up' after they have finished vomiting.
- Change and dispose any soiled clothing/bedding using local policy and procedure.
- Wash hands.
- Try to avoid strong odours such as food, perfumes and aftershaves that may induce nausea and vomiting.

If the extent of vomiting or retching has been excessive, the patient may complain of exhaustion or headache, and muscle soreness can also occur. An explanation of why the person may feel like this, as well as the administration of a prescribed analgesic, can help to provide comfort.

Excessive vomiting and anorexia as a result of this will affect a person's hydration status, leading to dehydration and loss of weight. Attention must be paid to the effects of excessive vomiting as extreme gastric secretion can lead to electrolyte imbalance and an ensuing acid–base (i.e. acidosis) discrepancy. The management of this will depend on the extent of vomiting and the patient's overall condition.

Snapshot   Dehydration

Teija Kovalainen is a 64-year-old lady who works as a clerk in a bank in the City of London. She lives at home in a flat on the 8th floor with her husband and her recently divorced daughter, Riitta. She was a fully independent lady with no significant past medical history, both her parents died about 20 years ago, her father had a myocardial infarction and her mother died as a result of cancer of the stomach.

Teija was admitted to the Emergency Department (ED). Teija's daughter Riitta heard her call for help from the bathroom and found Teija on the floor, pale and sweating. In the toilet bowl Riitta noted a foul, smelly, black-like diarrhoea as well as some blood, and she called for an ambulance. Teija was recently diagnosed with gastroenteritis and was prescribed antibiotics and an anti-emetic by her GP, and she purchased an anti-diarrhoeal medication over the counter at the pharmacy, three weeks ago. Previously Teija had been experiencing excruciating abdominal pain, she had lost some weight and was having bloody diarrhoeal stools 4–5 times a day; she was becoming increasingly tired at work, was having alternating constipation and diarrhoea, and she did not share these issues with anyone.

The paramedics assessed and transferred Mrs Kovalainen to the ED; an intravenous infusion was *in situ* with 1L NaCl in progress and 100% oxygen via a facemask. On examination she was sleepy but rousable, she looked pale and her extremities were cold. Teija reported central abdominal pain. She was feeling nauseous.

Reflect on this case study and think about the following:

1. With regards to the care of Mrs Kovalainen, what are her immediate needs?
2. What indicators may suggest that she is dehydrated and what would be the safest, most effective method of correcting her dehydration?
3. How can you help meet Mrs Kovalainen's emotional and psychological needs?

581

Medicines management

Antidiarrhoeals

Sometimes these medicines are called antimotility medicines and bulk-forming agents; they are used to treat acute diarrhoea. They include codeine phosphate, co-phenotrope and loperamide. The most commonly used antimotility medicine is loperamide (Imodium). This medication can be purchased from the local pharmacy or on prescription from a registered prescriber. Most people need to take these medicines only for a few days.

Antimotility medicines are used for the treatment of acute diarrhoea, and they work by slowing down the movement of the gut; this reduces the speed at which faecal matter passes through. As food remains in the gut for longer, this allows more water to be absorbed back into the body. This results in firmer stools passed less often.

Red flag

Antimotility medicines should not be taken by those who are under 12 years of age, if the person has blood or mucus in their faeces and a pyrexia. If there is abdominal distension, active ulcerative colitis or antibiotic-associated colitis, this type of medication should not be taken.

Clinical investigations

Colonoscopy

This type of imaging test allows the healthcare provider to visualise the inner lining of the large intestine. A thin, flexible tube, a colonoscope, is used to look at the colon.

The examination can help to determine if there is any bleeding (haemorrhage) polyps, tumours or areas of inflammation. A biopsy (a tissue sample) can be taken whilst the procedure is being performed if the examiner notices any abnormal growths.

In most cases, prior to the test, bowel preparation is usually required; however, in an emergency this may be negated. Bowel preparation is usually commenced 1 to 2 days prior to the examination, depending on local policy and procedure.

During the test, local preference may be to administer intravenous analgesia and a sedative. This helps the patient relax during the procedure, and often they remember very little about it.

The patient will be required to wear a hospital gown during the test; at all times the nurse must ensure dignity and preserve the patient's modesty. The patient will be required to lie on the left side with knees drawn up to the chest, and the nurse may need to assist the patient with this.

A thin, flexible colonoscope is slowly and gently inserted in the anus and moved gradually through the rectum and into the colon. Air will be used to inflate the colon to promote visualisation; a computer screen is connected to the colonoscope to provide images of the colon.

The patient may feel that they need to have a bowel motion or pass wind whilst the scope is in the colon, they may also feel some abdominal cramping. Encourage the patient to breathe slowly and deeply through the mouth to help to relax the abdominal muscles. The patient may be asked to change position during the test and if needed the nurse assists with this. The scope will be slowly pulled out of the anus and the anal area is cleaned with tissues. The test takes approximately 30 to 45 minutes.

Instructions are given to the patient after the test depending on what procedure was carried out, what was found and if any treatment was given. This must be documented in the patient's notes.

Red flag

There is a possibility that a colonoscope may damage the colon. This may result in bleeding, infection and perforation (rare). If any of the following occur within 48 hours after a colonoscopy, the patient should be told to consult a doctor immediately:

- Abdominal pain, in particular if this becomes gradually worse and is different or more intense from any 'usual' pains the patient may have
- Pyrexia
- Passing a lot of blood via the rectum.

NEWS 2

Teija Kovalainen

Physiological parameter	3	2	1	0	1	2	3
Respiration rate						23	
Oxygen saturation %				96			
Supplemental oxygen		Yes					
Temperature °C				36.8			
Systolic BP mmHg	90						
Heart rate					98		
Level of consciousness				A			
Score	3	2	0	0	1	2	0
Total	8						

Caring for the patient with oedema

The abnormal collection of fluid in the interstitial spaces is known as oedema (Kumar and Clark, 2016). This section provides an overview of the care required for the patient with oedema in order to maintain a safe environment and provide comfort. The causes of pulmonary and peripheral oedema have been discussed above.

Pulmonary oedema

Many patients who are diagnosed with pulmonary oedema will be acutely ill, and they (and their families) may be highly anxious and afraid. The healthcare professional must provide care that takes both the physical and psychological aspects of the condition into account for both the patient and family.

The first line of treatment should be to determine the cause of pulmonary oedema and to take steps to eliminate or reduce this; attempts should be made to reverse the specific cause(s). For example, if the cause is left-sided heart failure, then measures should be taken to improve the pumping action of the left side of the heart.

Signs and symptoms

The signs and symptoms can include some or all of the following:

- Dyspnoea/orthopnoea
- Wheeze
- Tachycardia and tachypnoea
- Hypotension
- Cardiogenic shock
- Sweating
- Pallor/cyanosis
- Nausea
- Anxiety
- Dry or productive cough (if productive pink frothy sputum).

Investigations

It is important to remember that pulmonary oedema can result in mild to severe dyspnoea; therefore, when obtaining a history from the patient in order to make a diagnosis, this must be borne in mind; questioning of the patient should be kept to an absolute minimum. The healthcare professional should ask questions that are only absolutely necessary and framed in such a way that the patient need only nod or shake their head in order to respond. After a detailed history has been undertaken from the primary source (the patient) or secondary sources (i.e. other healthcare professionals, the patient's partner, family or friends), the following investigations may be required:

- Chest X-ray
- Blood gas analysis
- Estimation of cardiac enzymes
- Liver function tests
- Estimation of urea and electrolytes
- Electrocardiograph.

The healthcare professional may be required to assist the patient prior to an investigation being performed, and they may be required to explain the procedure, both during the investigation and after the procedure (pre, peri and post procedure).

Care and management

Treatment of the specific cause of pulmonary oedema should continue, and the patient's airway must also be managed if dyspnoea becomes so severe that their life is in danger; in the acute phase, the patient may need to be resuscitated. The key aim should be to improve oxygenation, and this can be done by the administration of prescribed oxygen therapy via a facemask. As pulmonary oedema indicates that there is an abnormal collection of fluid in the interstitial spaces, it is imperative that there is strict control of fluid balance, and in some cases a urinary catheter may need to be inserted to provide close monitoring of urinary output. Here is an overview of the management of the patient with pulmonary oedema; this is not a comprehensive list, and care will be dictated by the patient's condition and response to therapeutic interventions, and as such the patient requires close monitoring and the provision of skilled care:

- Reassurance, psychological and physical support and explanations (for the patient and family) with regards to care interventions.
- Provide the patient with a nurse call bell; leave this in close proximity.
- Provide easy access to a sputum pot and tissues (ensure a receptacle is available to dispose safely of used tissues).
- Care for the patient in an upright position (unless this is contraindicated), supported by pillows.
- Administer prescribed humidified oxygen via a face mask.
- Administer prescribed medication, e.g. diuretics (i.e. furosemide) and with caution diamorphine, to alleviate anxiety, pain and distress.
- Strict monitoring of fluid balance (may include hourly urine measurements if a urinary catheter is *in situ*).
- Fluid restriction if indicated.
- Monitor, measure and report oxygen saturation, blood pressure, respiratory rate, depth and rhythm; monitoring of pulse frequency, dictated by the patient's condition.
- Assistance with all activities of daily living as appropriate.

Peripheral oedema

Whilst pulmonary oedema, as its name suggests, causes problems associated with breathing as a result of excessive fluid in the lungs, peripheral oedema presents as a collection of excessive fluid within the tissues that pools in the dependent regions, e.g. the legs, ankles, feet and sacral region (Waugh and Grant, 2014); sacral oedema tends to occur more in those patients who are bed bound. The pooling of fluid can be associated with lack of mobility, the consequence of gravitational pull, as well as the physiological factors that are related to oedema formation as described earlier.

Pitting oedema is the more serious type of oedema. The area of skin, e.g. around the ankles, when lightly pressed remains indented (a pit forms); this is a more serious type of oedema than the type that does not pit. Akbarnia *et al.* (2013) suggest that peripheral oedema does not appear or become visible until the body has retained up to 3L of fluid. If, for example, a patient retains 5.5 L of fluid, this is equivalent to 5.5 kg of weight; hence, a way of determining if the patient is retaining fluid is to record daily weight, along with meticulous fluid balance monitoring.

Snapshot   Lymphoedema

Leon Radcliffe is 72 years of age. He lives with his elderly wife, who has had a stroke, and he is her main carer; they have no children. He was diagnosed with prostate cancer and now has meta-static spread. He developed severe scrotal oedema whilst he was receiving palliative chemo-therapy. The swelling has caused him much distress, anxiety and fear. He cannot wear underpants and has to be very selective with the style of trousers he wears; he often resorts to wearing jog-ging bottoms. Because of the scrotal oedema, the pain and embarrassment, he rarely goes out, relying on neighbours to help with his shopping and odd jobs around the house.

His scrotal oedema makes standing and sitting very difficult, he finds it difficult to get com-fortable, he struggles to have a good night's sleep and there is now fluid seepage in the scro-tum. When performing his activities of living and assisting his wife with hers, he is now finding all of this a challenge as he also has metastatic spread to his bones. He is now refusing to have any more chemotherapy, and Leon has become very withdrawn. His GP has arranged for a com-munity nurse to visit and assess his needs and the needs of his wife, and a referral has been made for Mr Radcliffe to attend the lymphoedema clinic.

585

Vital signs   Physical and bloods

The following vital signs were noted and recorded:

Vital sign	Observation	Normal
Temperature	37.2 °C	36.0–37.9 °C range
Pulse	80 beats per minute (irregular)	60–100 beats per minute
Respiration	16 breaths per minute	12–20 breaths per minute
Blood pressure	170/85 mmHg	100–139 mmHg (systolic) range

A full blood count was performed.

Test	Result	Guideline normal values
White blood cells (WBC)	16×10^9/L	4 to 11×10^9/L
Neutrophils	6.8×10^9/L	2.0 to 7.5×10^9/L
Lymphocytes	3.8×10^9/L	1.3 to 4.0×10^9/L
Red blood cells (RBC)	5.0×10^9/L	4.5 to 6.5×10^9/L
Haemoglobin (Hb)	170 g/L	130–180 g/L
Platelets	320×10^9/L	150 to 440×10^9/L

Take some time to reflect on this case and then consider the following:

1. Explain the pathophysiological factors associated with the scrotal swelling.
2. What may indicate that Mr Radcliffe may have an infection?
3. It is clear Mr Radcliffe is distressed. How can the healthcare team, working in an integrated way, assist Mr Radcliffe from a psycho-social perspective?
4. What might the proposed treatment consist of to help reduce the oedema and control the pain?

Skin that has become oedematous predisposes the patient to the development of pressure sores (decubitus ulcers) and infection, particularly when the skin over the oedematous area has broken down. This risk can become more evident when healthcare professionals who handle patients with oedema have long or sharp fingernails, watches, pens, badges and scissors that can potentially catch the patient's skin and cause more trauma; hence the importance of short nails and the covering of items of equipment in the healthcare professional's pockets. It is important that the patient's fingernails are also kept short to prevent them from inadvertently causing damage to their skin. The principles of care for the patient who has peripheral oedema include the following:

- A clear explanation of the condition to the patient and, if appropriate, their family
- Assessment of skin condition in association with local policy for skin assessment
- Careful washing and patting dry (not rubbing) of the oedematous skin
- Fluid balance monitoring
- Daily weight measurement
- Administration of prescribed diuretics (e.g. furosemide)
- Elevation of oedematous ankles when sitting out of bed to aid drainage of the pooled fluid
- Assistance with those activities of daily living that the patient is unable to carry out independently.

Medicines management

Furosemide

This type of medication is known as a diuretic and is often used to reduce oedema due to heart failure, hepatic impairment or renal disease and to treat hypertension.

The drug works by inhibiting the reabsorption of sodium and chloride from the loop of Henle and distal renal tubule. It increases renal excretion of water, sodium, chloride, magnesium, potassium and calcium.

Therapeutically the medication causes diuresis and subsequent mobilisation of excess fluid (oedema, pleural effusions). It can decrease blood pressure. The drug can be administered:

- Orally
- Intramuscularly
- Intravenously.

This medication is contraindicated in:

- Those who have a hypersensitivity to the drug (and thiazides and sulphonamides)
- Hepatic coma
- Anuria (no urinary output).

It should be used cautiously in:

- Severe hepatic disease (may cause hepatic coma; concurrent use with potassium-sparing diuretics may be necessary)
- Electrolyte depletion
- Diabetes mellitus
- Hypoproteinemia
- Severe renal impairment
- In the older person, there may be an increased risk of side effects, particularly hypotension and electrolyte imbalance.

The drug should be taken as directed; recommend the patient to take missed doses as soon as possible; do not double dose.

Advise the patient to change position slowly to minimise orthostatic hypotension. Orthostatic hypotension can be exacerbated if the patient uses alcohol, exercises during hot weather or stands for long periods.

A dietician should advise regarding a diet high in potassium.

Older patients are at increased risk of falls.

Conclusion

Understanding the complex concepts and processes of fluid and electrolyte balance is vital if safe and effective care is to be provided to patients who may sometimes, as a result of fluid and electrolyte imbalance, be critically ill. The healthcare professional has a pivotal role to play when helping people who are experiencing pathophysiological changes associated with fluid and electrolyte imbalance.

This chapter has explained how the dynamics of fluid balance can have a profound effect on an individual's health and well-being. The subtle changes associated with fluid balance have to be recognised quickly by the healthcare professional in order to avert harm; this can be done in many ways, using all the senses as well as implementing the fundamentals of science.

It is not possible in a chapter of this size to address in depth all the concerns associated with fluid and electrolyte balance and the associated disorders. The reader is advised to access more detailed texts and other forms of information related to fluid and electrolytes with the key aim of providing care that is safe, effective and founded on a sound evidence base.

Test your knowledge

- List the functions of water.
- Explain how fluid and electrolytes move between compartments.
- List the major electrolytes and their functions.
- How would you encourage an older person to increase their fluid intake in order to prevent them from becoming dehydrated?
- Outline the care of a person who is feeling nauseous and vomiting.
- Describe how you would monitor a bed-bound person's fluid intake.

Activities

Here are some activities and exercises to help test your learning. For the answers to these exercises, as well as further self-testing activities, visit our website at www.wiley.com/go/fundamentalsofappliedpathophysiology/student4e

Multiple choice questions

1. Out of the average daily fluid intake of 2000–3000 mL, which of the following amounts comes from food metabolism?
   (a) 250 ml
   (b) 200 ml
   (c) 750 ml
   (d) 400 mL
2. Which of these is not a sign of fluid overload?
   (a) Tachycardia
   (b) Weight gain
   (c) Thick and sticky saliva
   (d) Oedematous skin
3. The highest potassium levels are found in:
   (a) Interstitial fluid
   (b) Intracellular fluid
   (c) Intravascular fluid
   (d) Cerebrospinal fluid
4. Extracellular fluid has a:
   (a) Higher protein content than intracellular fluid
   (b) Higher potassium content that intracellular fluid
   (c) Higher sodium content than intracellular fluid
   (d) Higher nutrient content than intracellular fluid
5. Which of the given statements best describes osmosis?
   (a) The movement of particles through a semi-permeable membrane from low concentrations to high concentration
   (b) The movement of particles through a permeable membrane from a high concentration to a low concentration
   (c) The movement of particles through a semipermeable membrane from a high concentration to a low concentration
   (d) The movement of particles through a permeable membrane from a low concentration to a high concentration
6. Renin is released by the:
   (a) Stomach
   (b) Liver
   (c) Kidney
   (d) Heart
7. Antidiuretic hormone (ADH):
   (a) Increases plasma osmolality
   (b) Is secreted by the anterior pituitary
   (c) Increases water reabsorption in the kidneys
   (d) Causes the production of a large volume of urine

8. Under normal conditions, most water loss from the body is through the:
   (a) Skin
   (b) Kidneys
   (c) Lungs
   (d) Sweat
9. Which of the options given is a sign of water conservation by the body?
   (a) Diarrhoea
   (b) Perspiration
   (c) Decreased water intake
   (d) Decreased urine volume
10. An acceptable pH for blood plasma is
    (a) 7.00
    (b) 7.25
    (c) 7.40
    (d) 7.55
11. Blood osmotic pressure increases:
    (a) Stimulation of the osmoreceptors of the hypothalamus
    (b) An increase in the production of saliva
    (c) A reversal of the renin-angiotensin-aldosterone feedback system
    (d) Equalisation of intracellular and extracellular membrane selectivity
12. On which part of the renal tubule does ADH work?
    (a) The proximal tubule
    (b) The glomerulus
    (c) The collecting duct
    (d) The loop of Henle
13. Furosemide promotes the excretion of all of the followings, except:
    (a) Sodium
    (b) Uric acid
    (c) Potassium
    (d) Magnesium
14. The functions of calcium do not include:
    (a) Nerve conduction
    (b) Clotting aid
    (c) Buffer of hydrogen ions
    (d) Maintenance of muscle tone
15. What amount of extracellular fluid is found in the intravascular compartment?
    (a) 30%
    (b) 40%
    (c) 15%
    (d) 20%

Conditions

The following is a list of conditions that are associated with fluid and electrolyte balance. Take some time and write notes about each of the conditions. You may develop the notes from textbooks or other resources (e.g. people you work with in a clinical area), or you may make the notes based on people you have cared for. If you are making notes about people you have cared for, you must ensure that you adhere to the rules of confidentiality.

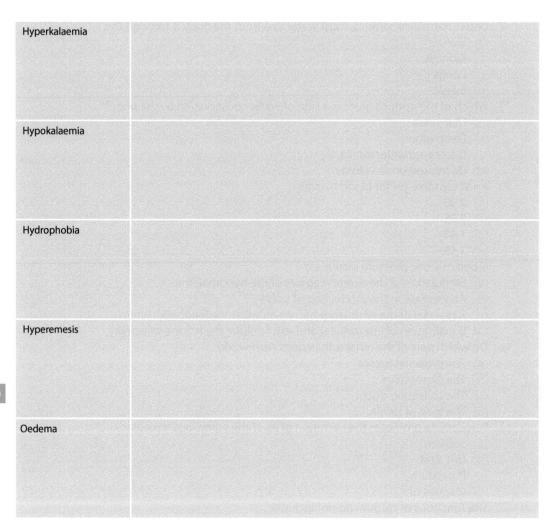

Hyperkalaemia	
Hypokalaemia	
Hydrophobia	
Hyperemesis	
Oedema	

Further resources

Scottish Intercollegiate Guidelines Network (SIGN)

http://www.sign.ac.uk/index.html

SIGN develops evidence-based clinical practice guidelines for the NHS in Scotland. SIGN guidelines are selected from a systematic review of the scientific literature and are designed to accelerate the translation of new knowledge into action.

National Institute for Health and Care Excellence (NICE)

http://www.nice.org.uk/

NICE provides guidance, sets quality standards and manages a national database to improve people's health and prevent and treat ill health. There are many excellent resources on this website that can help guide and inform practice.

Lymphoedema Support Network

http://www.lymphoedema.org/

The Lymphoedema Support Network is the only national patient-led organisation offering information and support to people with this condition and has a unique understanding of the patients' experience. It provides a high standard of information as well as promoting self-help.

Water UK

http://www.water.org.uk/

This website includes a section called Water for Health, and it describes The Water for Health initiative that was launched to guide and inform health professionals and health authorities, to stimulate interest and research in hydration, and to help move water up the public health agenda. This is a user-friendly, helpful site.

Public Health England

https://www.gov.uk/government/organisations/public-health-england

Public Health England (PHE) aims to protect and improve the nation's health and well-being and to reduce health inequalities. PHE is responsible for making the public healthier, supporting the public so they can protect and improve their own health, protecting the nation's health, sharing information and expertise and researching, collecting and analysing data to improve our understanding of health.

Age UK

http://www.ageuk.org.uk/

This national website is packed with information for the general public and healthcare professionals concerning the older population. It includes a section called professional resources; this contains links to (amongst other things) policy and research.

Glossary of terms

Amine   Organic compound that contains nitrogen.

Anion   Negatively charged ion.

Anti-emetic   A drug that reduces nausea and vomiting.

Anuria   Failure of the kidneys to produce urine

Cation   Positively charged ion.

Dehydration   Excessive fluid loss from the body.

Detoxification   Removal of toxic substances from the body.

Electrolyte   A chemical element or compound that includes sodium, potassium, calcium, chloride and bicarbonate.

Extracellular   Outside the cell.

Hypertonic   Solution that has large amounts of solutes dissolved in it.

Hypodermoclysis   Insertion of a small cannula into the subcutaneous tissues.

Hypotonic   A solution that has a low concentration of solutes.

Interstitial space   Space between cells.

Intracellular   Inside the cell.

Isotonic   A solution that has the same osmolality as the body fluids.

Metabolism   The collective name for all the physical and chemical processes occurring within a cell/living organism, but often referring only to reactions involving enzymes.

Nausea   An unpleasant sensation that produces a feeling of discomfort in the region of the stomach with a feeling of a need to vomit.

Oedema   The abnormal accumulation of fluid in the interstitial spaces. It may be localised (following an injury resulting in swelling) or it may be generalised (as in heart failure).

Oliguria   The production of abnormally small amounts of urine.

Osmolality   Osmotic concentration of a solution.

Osmosis   The passive movement of water through a selectively permeable membrane from an area of high concentration of a chemical to an area of low concentration.

Osmotic pressure   The pressure that must be exerted on a solution to prevent the passage of water into it across a semipermeable membrane from a region of higher concentration of solute to a region of lower concentration of solute.

Plasma   Fluid component of the blood.

Stoma   Any opening; a mouth. Usually used to refer to a surgically created opening.

Tonicity   Another term for osmolality.

Vomiting   A disagreeable experience that occurs when the stomach contents are reflexly expelled through the mouth or nose.

References

Akbarnia, H., Vo, V. and Chan, S. (2013). " I'm Swollen":Evaluation of Peripheral Edema in the Emergency Department. *Emergency Medicine Reports*, 34(2): 13.

British Dietetic Association (2019). *The Importance of Hydration*. https://www.bda.uk.com/resource/the-importance-of-hydration.html (Accessed 29/06/2020).

Corroon, A.M. and Hynes, G. (2014). Nursing care of conditions related to the respiratory system. In: Brady, A.M., McCabe, C. and McCann, M. (eds), *Fundamentals of Medical–Surgical Nursing. A Systems Approach*. Oxford. *Wiley, Chapter* 12, pp. 176–209.

Daniels, R. and Nicoll, L. (2012). *Contemporary Medical-Surgical Nursing*. New York: Delmar.

Effective Diabetes Education Now (EDEN) (2018). *Sick Day Rules: Type 1 Diabetes*. Available from: https://static1.squarespace.com/static/5a6439bab7411c94f2ebe216/t/5dcd223fc05f010766bd0bf6/1573724736814/Sick_Day_Rules_Infographic_V2.pdf. (Accessed 29/06/2020).

Galen, G.T. (2015). Underpad weight to estimate urine output in adult patients with urinary incontinence. *Journal of Geriatrics Cardiology*, 12: 189–190.

Giddens, J.F. (2017). *Concepts for Nursing Practice*, 2nd edn. Missouri: Elsevier.

Herlihy, B. (2018). *The Human Body in Health and Illness*, 6th edn. Missouri: Elsevier.

Howard, J. and Morgan, A. (2012). The patient with acute gastrointestinal problems. In: Peate, I. and Dutton, H. (eds), *Acute Nursing Care. Recognising and Responding to Medical Emergencies*. Harlow: *Pearson, Chapter* 10, pp. 240–261.

Kumar, P. and Clark, M. (2016). *Clinical Medicine*, 9th edn. Edinburgh: Elsevier.

Lister, S., Hofland, J and Grafton, H. (2020a). Medicines optimization. The Royal Marsden Manual of Clinical Procedures, 10th edn. Chapter 15.

Lister, S., Hofland, J and Grafton, H. (2020b) Nutrition, Fluid Balance and Blood Transfusion. The Royal Marsden Manual of Clinical Procedures, 10th edn. Chapter 7.

Maddex, S. (2014) Assessing and meeting fluid and nutritional needs. In: Baillie, L. (ed.), *Developing Practical Nursing Skills*, 4th edn. Chapter 10, pp. 453–506.

Marieb, E.N. and Hoehn, K. (2019). *Human Anatomy and Physiology*, 11th edn. Boston: Pearson.

McCance, K.L., Huether, S.E., Brashers, V.L. and Rote, N.S. (2019). *Pathophysiology: The Biologic Basis for Disease in Adults and Children*, 8th edn. St Louis: Mosby.

Molnar, C. and Gair, J. (2015). *Concepts of Biology: 1st Canadian Edition*. Victoria, B.C.: BC campus.

NHS England (2014). *Five Year Forward Plan*. Available at: https://www.england.nhs.uk/wp-content/uploads/2014/10/5yfv-web.pdf. (Accessed 29/06/2020).

Picetti, D., Foster, S., Pangle, A.K., Schrader, A., George, M., Wei, J.Y. et al. (2017). Hydration health literacy in the elderly. *Nutrition and Healthy Aging*, 4(3): 227–237.

Taylor, C.R. (2015). *Fundamentals of Nursing: The Art and Science of Fundamental Nursing Care*. Philadelphia: Wolters Kluwer.

Vujovic, P., Chirillo, M. and Silverthorn, D.U. (2018). Learning (by) osmosis: An approach to teaching osmolarity and tonicity. *Advances in Physiology Education*. 42(4): 626–635.

Waugh, A. and Grant, A. (2018). *Ross and Wilson Anatomy and Physiology in Health and Illness*, 13th edn. Edinburgh: Elsevier.

Wicker, P. (2015). *Perioperative Practice at a Glance*. Oxford: Wiley.

Wilson, S.F. (2017). *Perfusion*. In: Giddens, J.F. (ed.), *Concepts for Nursing Practice*. Missouri: Elsevier, pp. 148–160.

Chapter 20

The skin and associated disorders

Melanie Stephens

Senior Lecturer in Adult Nursing and Head of Interprofessional Education, School of Health and Society, University of Salford, Manchester, UK

Contents

Introduction 594
The anatomy and physiology of the skin...596
Disorders of the skin...603
Conclusion 618
Test your knowledge..618

Multiple choice questions..............................618
Further resources..620
Glossary of terms..621
References..621

Key words

- Dermis
- Dermatology
- Health promotion
- Psychological
- Epidermis
- Self-esteem
- Chemotherapy
- Integumentary system
- Cancer
- Radiotherapy
- Stigma

Fundamentals of Applied Pathophysiology: An Essential Guide for Nursing and Healthcare Students, Fourth Edition. Edited by Ian Peate.
© 2021 John Wiley & Sons Ltd. Published 2021 by John Wiley & Sons Ltd.
Student companion website: www.wiley.com/go/fundamentalsofappliedpathophysiology/student4e
Instructor companion website: www.wiley.com/go/fundamentalsofappliedpathophysiology/instructor4e

- Name the layers of the skin.
- List the appendages of the skin.
- What is the role of the skin in health?
- Describe the aesthetic properties of the skin.
- How can a healthcare professional help in the prevention of skin cancer?

Learning outcomes

On completion of this section, the reader will be able to:

- Describe the anatomy and physiology of the skin.

- Outline the numerous functions of the skin.

- Discuss the appendages of the skin.

- Detail the care and management of some skin conditions.

- Consider the role of the healthcare and social care professional as health and care educator.

Don't forget to visit the companion website for this book
(www.wiley.com/go/fundamentalsofappliedpathophysiology/student4e)
where you can find self-assessment tests to check your progress, as well as
lots of activities to practise your learning.

Introduction

Skin diseases affect a significant proportion of the population and can seriously impact a person's health and well-being. They can affect how a person undertakes their activities of daily living as well as how they interact with others and how others interact with them. Each time a healthcare and social care professional interacts with those they care for, they are observing the patient's skin as they undertake care activities; it is essential therefore that they have an understanding of the function of the skin so as to recognise problems that can occur. There are several areas of practice where the healthcare professional will come into contact with those who experience skin problems, and they are ideally placed to offer these people support with respect to some of these conditions.

Some skin conditions have the potential to cause stigma, such as eczema and psoriasis; the healthcare and social care professional, as advocate, can correct any misunderstanding concerning contagion and help to improve the individual's social well-being. Often, appearance and image are associated with success and achievement, and the blemish-free fair-skinned individual represented in the media (in many Western societies) is the image to which many strive; however, this is not always possible for those with skin conditions nor necessary in modern society. Society places much emphasis on physical appearance, and for those who have skin problems, this can become increasingly challenging. People with skin problems may experience difficulties in other aspects of their lives, e.g. from a sexual relationship perspective, and also concerning issues associated self-esteem and self-concept – altered body image can have a profound effect on the individual, their partner and their family.

Red flag

A study by the National Psoriasis Foundation found that nearly a third of people with psoriasis and psoriatic arthritis reported that their disease interferes with their love lives. Even though psoriasis is not contagious, the appearance of the skin rash can have a negative impact on intimacy.

Patients may report feeling ostracised, stigmatised and isolated. It is unusual for skin diseases to kill; however, the psychological morbidity they cause is huge and often largely unrecognised or ignored by healthcare and social care professionals. Every disease brings with it a psychological as well as a physical burden, but the visual nature of skin diseases means that people with skin disease are more susceptible to embarrassment and as a result of this, loss of self-esteem. The impact of skin disease on quality of life is well documented (Balieva et al., 2017).

Weller (2014) notes that skin disease is not only a cosmetic nuisance, emphasising that it can have a profound impact on a person's life. Weller (2014) considers the five 'Ds' often associated with dermatology:

595

- **D**isfigurement
- **D**iscomfort
- **D**isability
- **D**epression
- **D**eath.

Balieva et al., (2017) and Page (2006) summarise some of the problems that patients with skin conditions may experience (Table 20.1).

Dermatology is the study of the skin and its diseases; dermatologists are specialist practitioners who diagnose and treat diseases of the skin, nails and hair. The healthcare and social care professional can help enhance the quality of life for the person who has a skin problem.

This chapter introduces the reader to the structure and function of the skin. The skin (including its appendages), the only visible and largest organ of the body, is also known as the integumentary system. An overview of the anatomy and physiology of the skin is provided; the function of the skin is also discussed, and a number of skin conditions are considered along with the management of a patient with a skin disorder. A brief discussion is also provided of the skin appendages – hair follicles, eccrine and apocrine glands and nails. This chapter considers preventative strategies that the healthcare and social care professional may wish to introduce to prevent conditions such as skin cancer.

Table 20.1   Problems that patients with skin conditions may experience.

Emotional problems	Low self-esteem
	Feeling unclean
	Problems with relationships
	Feeling stared at
	Being regarded as infectious or contagious
	Anxiety and depression
Clothing restrictions	Avoiding wearing short sleeves
	Avoiding the wearing of dark clothing due to skin shedding
	Avoiding the wearing of summer clothing which exposes the skin
	Clothing can become stained or ruined when using greasy, oily skin preparations
Social restrictions	Skin becomes itchy in hot places where people congregate
	Avoiding swimming or sports facilities
	Avoiding communal changing rooms
	Avoiding participating in activities in classroom if hands affected
	Impaired mobility due to surface area of skin affected, leakage of exudate or topical agents, malodour, slippage of dressings, pain and lack of equipment
Financial implications	Routine prescriptions are expensive but essential
	No allowances are made to replace clothing or bedding
	No allowances are made for fuel bills due to extra laundering and bathing

Source: Adapted from Page, 2006; Zaidi and Lanigan, 2010; Balieva *et al.*, 2017.

596

The anatomy and physiology of the skin

The skin in humans (as in most other mammals) consists of two layers: the outer layer – the epidermis – and an underlying layer made of fibrous tissue – the dermis. Below the dermis is subcutaneous fat. At a cellular level, the skin is composed of a number of types of cells; these cells and their functioning are essential to maintaining health and the promotion of well-being (Figure 20.1).

The skin is estimated to weigh between 2.5 and 4 kg in an adult and is thickest at the palms and soles (about 1 mm thick) and at the eyelids it is at its thinnest (about 0.1 mm thick). There are over 1 million nerve endings in the skin, and it covers a surface area of 2 m². The skin performs a number of vital functions:

- Protects from harmful external factors (e.g. microbes, ultraviolet light and chemicals)
- Maintenance of internal homeostasis (a balanced internal environment)
- Acts as a shock absorber
- Provides thermoregulation
- Insulation
- Sensation

- Provides lubrication
- Protection and grip
- Calorie reserve
- Synthesises vitamin D
- Body odour
- Psychosocial.

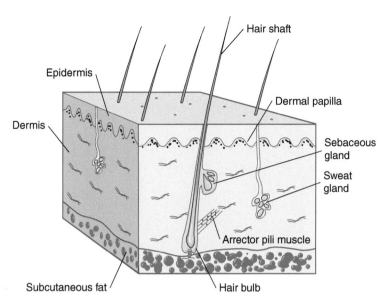

Figure 20.1 The structure of the skin.

The epidermis

The outer layer of the skin is the epidermis and is composed mainly of keratinocytes (approximately 95% of cells), including other specialised cells, e.g. melanocytes, Langerhans cells and Merkel cells. Table 20.2 outlines the functions of these cells.

The epidermis is made up of stratified epithelium; it has no blood vessels. The cellular nourishment (including oxygenation) and removal of waste products occurs through diffusion from the vascular network in the superficial dermis.

The key functions of the epidermis are to provide a physical and biological barrier to the environment – the penetration of irritants is prevented by the epidermis, as is the loss of water, and the management of internal homeostasis. There are three key features associated with the layers of the epidermis:

1. Division and migration of epidermal cells to the skin surface on a regular basis
2. Keratinisation of the epidermal cells
3. Rubbing away of the epidermal cells (desquamation).

Table 20.2 The functions of melanocytes, Langerhans and Merkel cells.

Cells	Functions
Melanocytes	These cells are located in the basal layer of the epidermis. The melanocytes produce the pigment melanin; melanin is found in the eyes, hair and skin. Melanin is responsible for providing protection and the absorption of ultraviolet rays. Melanin is the primary determinant of human skin colour
Langerhans cells	Langerhans cells are a part of the body's immune system; they activate the immune response and in particular the T-helper cells. They play an important role in contact allergies
Merkel cells	These cells are found in small numbers in the basal layer. They play a role in sensation, are associated with sensory nerve endings and are found in specific areas such as the palms, soles and genitalia. Their exact function is unclear

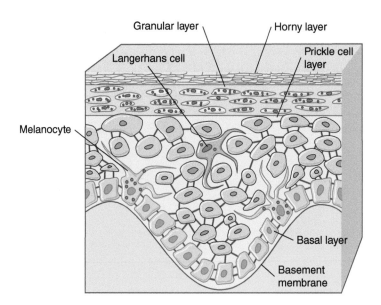

Figure 20.2   The layers of the epidermis.

The layers of the epidermis are shown in Figure 20.2. The basal layer (also called the stratum basale) is located close to the cells that are nearest to the dermis at the dermo-epidermal junction; it is at this point that cell division occurs. Cells migrate upwards from the dermoepidermal junction, and over a period of approximately 12–18 days, they keratinise prior to being shed.

The next layer is the prickle cell layer (stratum spinosum), and this protects against shearing forces or trauma to the skin; the cells in this layer move upwards above the basal layer.

Fine granules are formed from within the granular layer (stratum granulosum). These granules are the precursor of keratin, which will eventually replace the cytoplasm of the cells.The clear cell layer (stratum lucidium) is only present in areas where the skin is thick, e.g. the soles and palms. The cells in this layer have large amounts of keratin; they are flattened and closely packed. When injury or trauma occurs, the production of these cells is increased, and calluses or corns are formed.

The horny layer (stratum corneum) is the uppermost part of the epidermis and is made up of thin, flat and non-nucleated cells. These are dead cells and are shed from the skin.

The dermis

The dermis is chiefly composed of a network of connective tissue (mostly collagen) underlying the epidermis of the skin, which acts as the anchor joining the dermis and epidermis (Figure 20.3). The connective tissue gives strength and elasticity, as well as providing a supportive meshwork for the specialised structures throughout the dermis. This layer of the skin is much thicker than the epidermis; the key function is to support and sustain the epidermis. The dermis provides a protective pad for the deeper structures, protecting them from trauma, and it also nourishes the epidermis and has a vital role to play in wound healing.

The dermis has a number of specialised cells, e.g. mast cells and fibroblasts, as well as:

- Blood vessels
- Lymphatics
- Nerves
- Sweat glands.

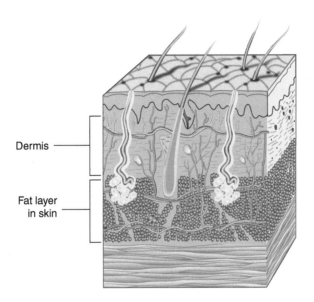

Figure 20.3   The structure of the dermis.

Just as the epidermis has layers, so too does the dermis; the dermis has two layers. The first layer, the superficial papillary dermis, is predominantly made up of loose connective tissue that contains blood vessels in the form of capillaries; elastic fibres and collagen are also components. The depth of the superficial papillary dermis depends on age and anatomical location.

The second layer is called the reticular dermis. This layer is thicker than the superficial papillary dermis; a dense connective tissue and larger blood vessels are interlaced with elastic fibres (providing flexibility), and thick bundles of collagen are present. There are also mast cells and fibroblasts as well as nerve endings and lymphatic vessels. These structures are surrounded by a viscous gel that bathes the structures, allowing nutrients, hormones and waste products to pass through the dermis. The viscous gel helps to provide bulk, allowing the dermis to act as a buffer.

Blood supply

Thermoregulation is largely controlled by a complex network of blood vessels within the dermis. Lying close to the epidermal border is the superficial plexus, which is made up of a number of interconnecting arterioles; these vessels wrap themselves around the structures in the dermis, and through this interconnecting network, oxygen and nutrients are supplied to the cells. At the border with the subcutaneous layer (the dermis) is the deep plexus. These vessels, when compared to those in the superficial plexus, are more substantial; they connect vertically to the superficial plexus.

Lymph vessels

The lymph vessels play an important role in draining excess tissue fluid and plasma proteins from the dermis; this results in internal homeostasis – ensuring the correct volume and composition of tissue fluids. Lymph also searches for foreign matter such as bacteria and antigenic substances.

Nerves

Free sensory nerve endings (the Merkel cells) are found in the basal layer of the epidermis and the dermis, and they detect pain, irritation and temperature. The skin is supplied with around 1 million nerve fibres; sensory perception is an important protective mechanism of these cells. Specialist receptors responding to pressure and vibration (Pacinian corpuscles) and touch/sensitivity (Meissner's corpuscles) are also found in the dermis. Autonomic nerves supply the blood vessels and sweat glands and the arrector pili muscles.

Red flag

Because nerves are essential to all that we do, nerve pain and damage can seriously affect a person's quality of life. Sensory nerve damage may produce the following symptoms:

- Pain
- Sensitivity
- Numbness
- Tingling or prickling
- Burning
- Problems with positional awareness.

In people with sensory nerve damage, the healthcare and social care professional must ensure that those people are safe and protected from harm.

The subcutis

The subcutis is a subcutaneous layer that lies below the dermis. This layer, composed chiefly of fat (adipose tissue), provides the skin with support and acts as a shock absorber (Figure 20.3). The subcutis is also responsible for insulating the body and storage of nutrients; it is interlaced with blood vessels and nerves.

The appendages

There are three important components of the skin known as the appendages of the epidermis:

1. The sweat glands
2. Hair follicles and sebaceous glands
3. Nails.

Sweat glands

Sweat glands are coiled tubes of epithelial tissue; they open out to pores on the skin surface (Figure 20.4). Each gland has its own nerve and blood supply. The glands secrete a slightly acidic fluid containing water and salts (excess excretory products). Keratin maintains its suppleness because of the action of sweat. There are two types of sweat glands: eccrine and apocrine. The production of secretions by the eccrine glands in response to, for example, heat or fear, is controlled by the sympathetic nervous system. These glands are found all over the body; however, they are more numerous at some sites, e.g. the forehead, axillae, soles and palms.

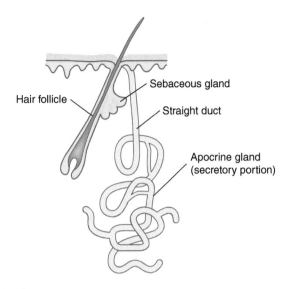

Figure 20.4   Sweat gland.

The apocrine glands are also coiled; they are not as numerous as the eccrine glands and are found in more localised sites – the pubic and axillary regions, the nipples and perineum – they are not functional until the person reaches puberty; it is understood that they secrete pheromones released into the external environment. A viscous material is excreted that causes body odour when acted upon by the surface bacteria.

Hair follicles and sebaceous glands

Hair is found on all surfaces of the body apart from the palms, soles and lips; its amount, distribution, colour and texture vary depending on its location, and the sex, age and ethnic group of the individual. It contributes to an individual's unique appearance. Hair colour is determined by the melanocytes that are within the hair bulb, and hair growth is influenced by genetic and hormonal factors.

Hair is a keratin structure of the epidermis; each hair is a thread of keratin and is formed from cells at the base of a single follicle. It has several functions:

- Sexual
- Social
- Thermoregulation
- Protection.

The key role of hair is to prevent heat loss. The whole skin surface is provided with hair follicles; each pore is an opening to a follicle, and they are situated deep in the dermis. Attached to each gland is a small collection of smooth muscles known as the arrector pili; these muscles contract and become erect in response to cold, fear and emotion. The contraction of the muscle can be seen on the skin in the form of 'goose bumps'. When heat leaves the body through the skin, it becomes trapped in the air between the hairs.

The hair follicles are accompanied by sebaceous glands, and sebum (a liquid substance) is secreted by these glands, moisturising the skin as well as ensuring that the skin and hair are waterproof. Sebum is a slightly acidic substance that has antibacterial properties, protecting the skin form infection (Stephens, 2014). The distribution of the sebaceous glands varies;

they are most prominent on the scalp, face, upper torso and anogenital region, and during puberty these glands are at their most active – sebum production is influenced by sex hormone levels. Figure 20.5 demonstrates what is known as a pilosebaceous unit; the pilosebaceous unit is composed of the follicle, the hair shaft and the sebaceous gland.

Red flag

Alopecia is the general medical term for hair loss. There are many types of hair loss with different symptoms and causes. Loss of hair (for whatever reason) for some people can result in emotional issues, and hair loss can be difficult to come to terms with.

The hair on a person's head can be a defining part of their identity. If a person starts to lose their hair, they may feel that they are losing a part of their identity; this can affect self-confidence, and sometimes this can lead to depression.

Speaking with a practice nurse or GP might help if the person is finding it difficult to deal with hair loss. The person may also benefit from joining a support group or speaking to other people in the same situation – for example, through online forums.

Nails

The final appendage is the nails; these are also made of keratin, and they have a tough texture because the keratin is formed in concentrated amounts; they can be described as horn-like. Nails have no nerve endings. They act as protectors; fingernails and toenails provide some protection to the digits. Nails also make it easier to grab or grasp things, acting as a counterforce to the fingertips which have many nerve endings to allow an individual to receive a substantial amount of information about the objects that we touch.

The rate of nail growth varies; on average, nails grow at a rate of 0.1 cm per day (1 cm per 100 days). Fingernails require 4–6 months to regrow completely; toenails take longer to grow, between 12 and 18 months to regrow completely. The rate of growth depends upon factors such as the age of the person, the time of year, the amount of exercise undertaken and hereditary factors (Woodard, 2014). Nail growth can be impeded by trauma and

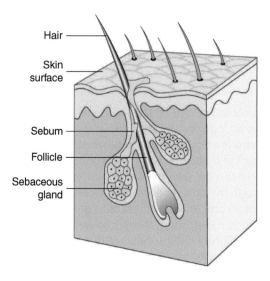

Figure 20.5 The pilosebaceous unit.

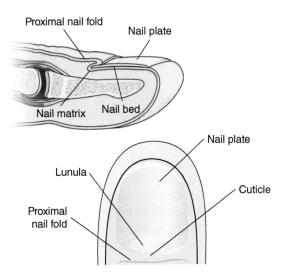

Proximal nail fold

Nail plate

Nail matrix   Nail bed

Nail plate

Lunula

Cuticle

Proximal
nail fold

Figure 20.6 The structure of the nail.

inflammation; changes in the integrity of the nails can be the result of injury or infection and in some instances is evidence of systemic diseases, e.g. chronic cardiopulmonary disease (College of Podiatry, 2019). Figure 20.6 demonstrates the structure of the nail.

Disorders of the skin

Learning outcomes

On completion of this section the reader will be able to:

- Describe some of the pathophysiological changes that may occur to the skin.

- Highlight the role and function of the healthcare professional when caring for those who may suffer with a skin condition.

A picture is worth a thousand words is an often used saying; this saying is particularly true when caring for those people with skin, hair and nail disorders. It is important that you understand what some of the most common skin lesions look like. The reader may benefit from consulting a colour skin atlas to enhance their skills of observation (Wolff *et al.*, 2017) or the latest literature from British Association of Dermatologists (2020) for common skin manifestations of COVID-19. When discussing skin conditions, the term lesion describes a small area of disease, whereas a rash or eruption describes a widespread area of skin.

Many skin lesions can be diagnosed on sight; however, there is still the need to adopt a systematic approach to diagnosis, and this will entail a detailed health and medical history as well as a physical examination. To confirm diagnosis, other investigations may also be needed. Weller *et al.* (2015) and Chowdhury *et al.* (2013) provide details of what a full history should entail (Box 20.1). The healthcare professional needs to use effective and sensitive communication skills to help reveal the diagnosis and also the person's description and understanding of the disorder, as well as their perception and the perceptions of others of living with it.

Box 20.1   Some components of the history are as follows

- Any known allergies.
- Onset, initial site continuous or intermittent, how long.
- Associated symptoms such as itch, burning, redness, oozing, scaling, blisters.
- Actions that might make the condition worse, e.g. exposure to heat or cold, any stress including activities.
- Family history, e.g. genetic predisposition, anyone at work/school with a similar condition.
- Associated systemic symptoms, e.g. asthma.
- Current prescribed medications, including any medications that are being applied to the skin as well as any oral preparations. How often are they taken and their effect.
- Current over-the-counter medications, including any medications that are being applied to the skin as well as any oral preparations. How often are they taken and their effect.
- Social history, including details about occupation, hobbies, amount of exercise, housing, smoking, alcohol intake, recent travel and use of recreational drugs.
- Impact of the disorder on them as an individual, their self-esteem, self-image, ability to manage on a daily basis and any coping mechanisms used.
- Impact of the disorder on others they live or work with.

Adapted from Morris-Jones (2014), Weller *et al.* (2015) and Chowdhury *et al.* (2013).

Table 20.3   Some intrinsic and extrinsic factors that can predispose a person to skin disease.

Extrinsic	Intrinsic
Extremes of heat	Genetic/hereditary factors
Allergens	Internal disease
Chemicals	Medications
Irritants	Infections
Trauma	Psychological factors
Friction	
Infections	
Sunshine	
Sun lamps	

Source: Adapted from Weller *et al.*, 2015

Wolff *et al.* (2017) report that the type, frequency and prevalence of skin disorders is closely associated with and depends on an individual's social, economic, geographical and cultural circumstances. There are a number of factors that can predispose a person to skin disorders; both extrinsic and intrinsic (Table 20.3).

Skin disorders can be minor or life-threatening, with people sometimes seeking their own remedies to some of the problems they encounter. There are, however, a number of conditions that require more intensive interventions; these interventions can take place in the patient's own home, in the primary care setting or there may be a need for the person to be admitted to hospital.

Skin cancer

Sunlight is the main cause of skin cancer, and the incidence of this cancer has increased steadily over the years (Chang *et al.*, 2014). In the UK, skin cancer is the fifth most common form of cancer (Cancer Research UK, 2017). There are three forms of skin cancer:

1. Malignant melanoma
2. Basal cell carcinoma (BCC)
3. Squamous cell carcinoma (SCC).

Malignant melanoma

This is the most dangerous form of skin cancer, and it accounts for 10% of all cases of skin cancer (Wolff *et al.*, 2017). The cells of the body that become cancerous in malignant melanoma are the melanocytes. Melanoma usually develops in a naevus (also known as a mole); it can metastasise rapidly via the circulatory and lymphatic systems.

This type of skin cancer spreads rapidly, and because of the speed with which it spreads, it is the most dangerous type. These cancers are more common in young people and are closely related to sunburn and overexposure (Foss and Farine, 2007).

Risk factors:

- Exposure to sun
- Use of sunbeds
- Being female (evidence to suggest that hormones play a part if risk is inconclusive)
- Age
- Presence of moles
- Being fair-skinned
- History of sunburn, having been sunburned at least once, and risk rises if this occurred as a child
- Geographical factors (where the person was born)
- Family history.

605

There is one key risk factor for melanoma, i.e. sun or sunbeds (ultraviolet light). There are, however, some people who are more at risk than others. More women than men get melanoma; it is the fifth most common cancer in women. The disease is rare in those who are aged under 14 years; after age 15 years, the incidence steadily rises, and the highest incidence is in those aged 85 years and over. Risk increases the more moles a person has.

Those who are fair-skinned are more at risk than those who are dark-skinned; however, dark-skinned people can and do get malignant melanoma. Skin cancers in skin of Black, Asian and minority ethnic people, including melanoma, often present at an advanced stage or atypically with a poorer prognosis than skin cancer in lighter-skinned populations (Kailas et al., 2016).

Those who are fair and have a tendency to freckle in the sun are more at risk as are those who do not tan at all; these people are usually those who peel before getting a tan. People with melanoma are twice as likely to have been badly sunburned at least once in their lives; sunburn as a child is even more damaging than sunburn as an adult, because during childhood the skin is at its most vulnerable. Risk is also associated with geography and where the person was born. Those who are fair-skinned and were born in a hot country, e.g. Australia, have an increased risk of melanoma for life, in contrast to those who went to live there as a teenager or those with similar skin colour who live in cooler climates. The skin would have been exposed to the effects of the sun whilst the person was young, when the skin was at its most delicate. A family history, i.e. a family member who has had melanoma, places a person at risk.

Signs and symptoms

There are a number of warning signs that may indicate malignant melanoma (Page, 2006; Stephens, 2014):

- New or existing moles getting bigger
- Changes in the shape of a mole; if there is a change in the edge of the mole, it becomes irregular in shape around the edges
- Changes in the colour of a mole – it gets darker or becomes patchy or multi-shaded
- A mole becomes itchy or painful
- A mole starts to bleed or becomes crusty
- Any surrounding or underlying inflammation.

Diagnosis

A patient's history as well as full physical examination is required. The healthcare professional should examine and observe the whole of the body. Hutchinson's freckle (also known as lentigo maligna) is a premalignant melanoma condition (Weller *et al.*, 2015). Hutchinson's freckle can be seen on the face or other areas of the body that are exposed to the sun; in some patients, the condition will have been slowly enlarging for a number of years.

Dermatoscopy may be performed in order to examine the lesion. This is a painless test that has the ability to magnify the area up to ten times.

The only method used to confirm diagnosis of a malignant melanoma is to take a biopsy of the lesion and subject it to histological testing (histology). Usually, the specimen is obtained under a local anaesthetic, but this will depend on the part of the body where the lesion is. The lesion is measured and usually photographed in order to make comparisons at a later stage.

Urgent referral must be made if the lesion is suspected to be cancerous. A seven-point scale is advocated by the National Institute for Health and Care Excellence (NICE, 2016) to help make the decision to refer to a specialist (Table 20.4). Within the scale, there are three major features and four minor ones. Two points are given for any of the major features and one for the minor features; if the mole (the lesion) scores three points or above, then urgent

Table 20.4   Assessing changes in moles (lesions).

Characteristic	Points
Change in size*	2
Change in colour (e.g. getting darker, becoming patchy or multi-shaded)*	2
Change in shape*	2
7 mm or more across in any direction	1
Inflammation	1
Oozing or bleeding	1
Change in sensation (e.g. itching or pain)	1

* Major feature.
Source: Adapted from NICE, 2016

referral is required. However, NICE (2016) suggests that if there is any cause for concern, regardless of the score, then the person should be referred to a specialist.

Care and management

Precancerous moles can be treated by excision under local anaesthetic; early malignant melanomas can also be treated in this way. The longer a suspicious mole is left, the more difficult it can be to treat and the poorer the prognosis. If the mole is removed, the patient will have sutures in place and they will need to stay *in situ* for up to a week; the patient returns to the centre where the lesion was removed and usually receives the results of the histology. If the histology reveals that the lesion was non-cancerous, then no further treatment is needed; however, if there is evidence of cancerous cells, more tests will be required.

One of the proposed tests will determine how deep the melanoma is – this is called staging. The deeper the cancerous cells, the more likely it is that the cancer has spread within the body (American Joint Committee on Cancer, 2018; Thompson *et al.*, 2005). The following tests may also be required:

- Blood tests
- Chest X-ray
- Ultrasound scan
- Bone scan
- CT scan.

Wide local excisions may be required, depending on the individual's unique circumstances, e.g. how much of the mole (lesion) was left behind and how deep the melanoma has grown into the tissues. In some circumstances, if a large area of skin has been excised, this may require skin grafting.

Lymph node removal, if there is lymph involvement, may be needed, and treatment can also include chemotherapy; another type of treatment that may be offered is interferon or immunotherapy treatment. Chemotherapy and interferon/immunotherapy (biological therapy) are also known as adjuvant treatment. These treatments may be given intravenously, topically, or directly into the melanoma (intralesional therapy) or affected arm or leg (isolated limb infusion). Radiotherapy, the use of high-energy radiation, to kill cancer cells can also be used; again, this will depend on the individual needs and circumstances. Laser treatment using carbon dioxide laser is also an available treatment. Sharpe (2006) suggests that there is no improvement regarding survival when adjuvant therapy is used; however, disease-free intervals may be prolonged.

Often patients are anxious and concerned about the results of tests and the decisions they will have to make. The healthcare professional has a duty to provide the patient with physical and psychological support before, during and after all interventions; this will include providing information in a manner that the patient understands and is able to assimilate, so that they can make an informed decision.

Regular follow-up is needed, and the frequency at which this is required will depends on the individual circumstances. The aim of follow-up is to see how the patient is coping and to determine if they need any further physical or psychological support, if there is recurrence around the scar, if there is any spread to the lymph nodes or other parts of the body or if there are any new melanomas.

Basal cell carcinoma and squamous cell carcinoma

BCC is a skin cancer of the epidermis. BCC is slow to develop and commonly occurs on the face. SCC occurs to the outermost layers of the skin. Often it appears as a scaly or crusty

607

patch of skin bigger than 1 cm (but it may be smaller); it does not heal. Both these types of cancer are called non-melanoma skin cancers and are the most common type of cancer in the UK (NICE, 2016). Usually, they appear on body parts that are exposed:

- Face
- Neck
- Ears
- Forearms
- Fingers
- Hands.

These types of skin cancer are more common in the older population (NICE, 2010). Prognosis for those with this type of cancer is very good.

The main treatment for BCC and SCC is surgery (NICE, 2010). The type of surgery is classed as minor surgery and involves the use of a local anaesthetic to remove the cancer. Radiotherapy may be used to treat large areas of skin cancer or if the cancer is in a difficult place to operate on or if the patient is unable, due to ill health or incapacity, to have surgery performed safely (Sharpe, 2006). Chemotherapy is another option, but for BCC and SCC this is rarely used. Creams that contain chemotherapeutic medications may, however, be used, particularly when the cancer is limited to the top layer of the skin.

In all cases of skin cancer, malignant or non-malignant, and for all patients, the healthcare and social care professional should be prepared to provide health promotion advice. Healthcare and social care professionals in any situation can encourage regular checking of the skin; they are ideally placed to provide information concerning skin self-examination. Effective treatment depends on early detection of skin cancer and a prompt diagnosis (NICE, 2016).

Health promotion advice – skin cancer

When the opportunity arises, the healthcare and social care professional should be proactive in providing health promotion advice concerning the damaging effects of the sun and the avoidance of skin cancer to those who may need it, e.g. those working outdoors and younger members of the population.

Not everyone's skin offers the same protection in the sun, and because of this, it is important to know about skin types (Table 20.5). Those with skin types I–IV need to take most care in the sun, particularly those who have skin types I and II. Those who have skin types V and

Table 20.5   Skin types.

Type	Characteristics
Type I	Pale skin, burns very easily and tans rarely. Generally these people have light-coloured or red hair and freckles
Type II	These people usually burn but may gradually tan. Often they have light hair, blue or brown eyes. Some may have dark hair but still have fair skin
Type III	Generally tan quite easily, but with long exposure to the sun burn. Usually, they have dark hair with brown or green eyes
Type IV	Tan very easily, but with long exposure to the sun will burn. Often they have olive skin, brown eyes and dark hair
Type V	Naturally brown skin with dark hair and brown eyes. These people burn only with prolonged exposure to the sun, and their skin further darkens easily
Type VI	Have black skin with dark brown eyes and black hair. These people burn only with extreme exposure to the sun, and their skin further darkens easily

Source: Adapted from British Association of Dermatologists, 2016

Box 20.2   Some points related to sun protection

- Select a waterproof sunscreen, one with an adequate sun protection factor (SPF). An SPF of 15 multiplies the period of time it takes to burn by 15. An SPF of at least 15 should be used by everyone. Those who have paler skin should use a higher SPF rating. The sunscreen should screen out both ultraviolet A (UVA) and ultraviolet B (UVB) rays. A lip balm with a high SPF should also be applied to the lips.
- The sunscreen should be rubbed in well and applied approximately 15–30 minutes before going out into the sun. Every 2 hours throughout the day the sunscreen should be reapplied and also after swimming.
- Avoid excessive exposure to the sun. Light-coloured loose-fitting clothing should be worn as this will help the person feel cooler. Garments should be closely woven as lightweight clothing provides little protection to UV light which will pass through it. A wide-brimmed hat protects the head and neck.
- The sun should be avoided between 1100 hours and 1500 hours, particularly in those countries that are close to the equator.
- Sunglasses should be worn as prolonged exposure can cause damage to the lens of the eye, resulting in an opaqueness (cataract). Sunglasses that conform to British standards are advocated.
- The skin's sensitivity is increased when cosmetics are worn in the sun; therefore they should be avoided.
- UV light can be reflected by water, snow and buildings; therefore, it is important to apply sunscreen when sitting in the shade. Cloud is no barrier to UV light, and it is still possible to burn on a cloudy day as UV light can penetrate cloud.

Adapted from Foss and Farine (2007)

VI generally only need to protect their skin when the sun is particularly strong or they go out in the sun for a long period of time. Box 20.2 provides some advice the healthcare professional can give to patients concerning sun protection. Skin cancer is a significant and increasing health problem for the nation; prevention according to Sharpe (2006) is a long-term issue and will require major attitude and behavioural changes of the population.

Legislation is now in force to protect people aged under 18 years from the harmful effects of sunbeds (ultraviolet tanning equipment). The Sunbeds (Regulation) Act 2010, which is enforced by local councils, requires sunbed operators to ensure that no person under the age of 18 uses a sunbed on their premises.

There is much evidence to suggest that sunbeds can lead to malignant melanoma. The International Agency for Research on Cancer (IARC, 2007), an expert body that examines the evidence on causes of cancer, have re-classified sunbeds as a Group 1 carcinogen. This classification is the highest cancer risk category and is reserved for things where the evidence is strongest. IARC has demonstrated that, on average, people who start using sunbeds under the age of 35 years increase their risk of malignant melanoma by 75%.

Eczema

According to Weller *et al.* (2015), the word *eczema* comes from the Greek word meaning 'boiling', associated with the tiny vesicles (bubbles) that are often seen in the early, acute stages of the disorder. The terms eczema and dermatitis are used interchangeably; they can be described as acute or chronic, and the severity can vary. The condition can affect all age groups. There is no specific diagnostic test for eczema, and the diagnosis is based on clinical assessment (Weller *et al.*, 2015). With the correct treatment, the inflammation can be reduced; however, there is currently no cure for eczema.

As with most skin conditions that are visible, eczema can have a profound effect on an individual's self-esteem. The patient may also experience disturbed sleep as a result of the clinical manifestations. For younger patients, there may be a significant impact on their behaviour and development as a result of disturbed sleep, lowered self-esteem and social isolation (ostracism). Frequent visits to the doctor, the need to apply messy topical applications and the use of special clothing can add to the burden of the disease. Eczema can have a profound effect not only on the patient but also on their family.

The pathophysiology of atopic eczema is a complex interaction of susceptible genes, environmental triggers, defects in the skin barrier and immunological responses (McCann and Huether, 2014). Raised serum immunoglobulin E (IgE) levels are seen in atopic eczema, but the exact role of IgE in the disease is unclear (Flohr *et al.*, 2004).

Wolff *et al.* (2017) describe the characteristics of both acute and chronic eczema. Acute eczema is characterised by:

- Pruritus
- Erythema
- Vesiculation.

  and chronic eczema by:

- Pruritus
- Xerosis
- Lichenification
- Hyperkeratosis
- Fissure formation (rare).

In darker-pigmented skin, erythema is inapparent and is replaced by patches of darkened skin colour. Inflammation results in the release of inflammatory mediators that increase melanogenesis by the melanocytes, resulting in post-inflammatory hyperpigmentation (Myers, 2015).

Endogenous eczema

Atopic eczema

This condition is described as a chronic relapsing inflammatory skin condition; the patient tends to scratch and itch at a red rash that is often found in skin creases, such as the elbows and behind the knees. Black people are more prone to developing small bumps on the torso, arms and legs. This is called papular eczema, and it may resemble permanent goosebumps. These bumps can develop around hair follicles, which is called follicular accentuation. Weller *et al.* (2015) and Schofield (2013) note that other features include:

- Crusting
- Scaling
- Cracking
- Swelling of the skin.

The cause of atopic eczema is unknown. The condition is also associated with other diseases such as hay fever and asthma. Adults make up nearly one-third of community cases of atopic eczema.

Pathophysiological changes are the result of complex interactions between:

- The skin barrier
- Genetic responses
- Environmental issues
- Pharmacological factors
- Immunological causes.

Microscopically, atopic eczema appears as excessive fluid between the cells in the epidermis (this is known as spongiosis); when the condition worsens, the fluid erupts into the epidermis and forms vesicles – small collections of fluid, and vesiculation occurs. In atopic eczema, a hypersensitivity response occurs in reaction to an antigen and antibody effect; however, Wolff *et al.* (2017) suggest that the antigen–antibody response is still not fully understood. A genetic predisposition and a combination of allergic and non-allergic factors appear to be influencing features.

Discoid eczema

Also called nummular eczema, the aetiology of this type of eczema is unknown. It appears to peak twice a year in autumn and winter (Wolff *et al.*, 2017) and is more common in middle-aged and older people; it usually lasts for only a few weeks. Characteristically, the disease appears as coin-shaped plaques with small papules and vesicles on an erythematous base. In darker skin, the plaques appear darker in pigmentation and are more commonly found on the lower legs.

Seborrhoeic eczema

The main areas affected are the hairy areas of the body, and the patient may complain of itching and have a red scaly rash. In darker-skinned patients, this scaling can have a flower-like shape (petaloid seborrheic dermatitis). Discolouration of the skin with lightening or darkening of affected areas may also occur. The disease is more common in men and may be associated with patients who are immunosuppressed, e.g. those with human immunodeficiency virus (HIV). This type of eczema can become complicated as a result of fungal infection.

Varicose eczema

This type of eczema commonly affects the lower limbs and can occur with or in the presence of varicose ulcer. The aetiology is associated with chronic venous stasis; often the area involved becomes red and itchy. On darker skin, it tends to look dark brown, purple or grey and can be more difficult to see, and the patient may also have varicose veins and oedema (Gawkrodger, 2016).

Diagnosis

It has already been stated that diagnosis is made on clinical examination; referral to a dermatologist may be required. Other diagnostic tests include:

- Blood tests
- Patch test
- Allergy tests.

Exogenous eczema

In industrial settings, exogenous eczema is common (Mitchell and Kennedy, 2006). It is usual for this type of eczema to erupt at the point of contact, and the way in which the patient presents will depend on the irritant. The immune system overreacts to a substance that would otherwise be harmless.

There are many irritants that can cause allergic contact dermatitis, e.g. the wearing of earrings or jewellery that contains nickel may cause allergic contact dermatitis, and hypersensitivity will occur; perfumes and cosmetics can also cause contact dermatitis. Dermatitis may be triggered by the wearing of disposable gloves; if this is the case, the user should be advised to use hypoallergenic, commercially supplied, disposable gloves. In such cases, the person may have to consider a change in occupation. Occupations that are considered high risk include:

- Hairdressing
- Catering
- Health and social care
- Printing
- Engineering
- Agriculture
- Horticulture
- Construction
- Cleaning
- Medicines management.

Latex gloves

Natural Rubber Latex (NRL) is found in a number of products used in health and social care, such as non-sterile examination gloves and surgical gloves. It is also used in a range of medical devices.

As the use of such products has increased, particularly of single-use latex gloves in infection control, NRL allergy and sensitisation has been identified as a problem:

- Powdered latex gloves should therefore not be used in the workplace.
- Staff with latex allergy, latex sensitivity or latex-induced asthma should use non-latex gloves.
- Staff who are latex allergic/sensitised should take latex avoidance measures; their symptoms will reduce or disappear.
- In employees who have latex-induced asthma or rhinitis, the use of powder-free, low-protein gloves by colleagues reduces symptoms and indices of severity in the affected employee to a similar degree as the use of non-latex gloves by colleagues.
- There is a lack of published primary research comparing occupational interventions for those sensitised to latex (without symptoms), with those with clinical latex allergy.

Health and Safety Executive (2019)

Care and management

The care and management of the various types of eczema are similar. In atopic eczema, one of the main complications is infection (bacterial and fungal) as a result of a break in the skin. When the skin is infected, it contains pustules that are green or yellow in colour, with large blisters; the patient may feel unwell and have an elevated temperature. The role of the healthcare professional is to prevent infection in this instance, and this can be done by educating the patient in how the infection may be caused and spread by scratching.

The healthcare and social care professional should explore with the patient what it is that causes or makes the eczema worse; the answers to these questions can provide information that will lead to the testing of the patient for certain things with a patch test. If an allergen or irritant is identified, then this should, if possible, be avoided. The following outlines the general approach to the management of atopic eczema; however, it should be noted that approaches to care should be tailored to meet individual needs:

- Remove, if possible, the irritant or allergen that causes the antibody–antigen reaction.
- Offer support to the patient and their family to empower, educate and motivate. The overall aim should be to raise self-esteem and self-awareness and as such to prevent stigma.
- If the eczema, for example, is varicose eczema, then the patient may be advised to wear support hosiery or if appropriate and possible, surgical intervention may be required.
- Creams, ointments and oils can be used to act as emollients to reduce the drying and itching effects of the disease.
- Aqueous cream may be used as a substitute for soap. Soaps can have the effect of further drying the skin. Perfumed products should be avoided.
- If infection occurs, then antibiotics or antifungal medication may need to be prescribed. These medications are often given systematically but may be applied topically.
- In some instances, topical steroid preparations can be used to reduce inflammation, but these should be used with caution and should not be used for longer than is necessary.
- Topical preparations containing both antibiotics and steroids are available, but again these should only be used for the short-term.
- Antihistamines may be prescribed.

Examples of other issues that will need to be considered are the following:

- Encourage rest as it may be difficult for some people to get proper sleep.
- Dietary advice may be needed if the allergen is a food product; a multidisciplinary approach is advocated with referral to a dietician.
- Complementary therapies may help some people. Complementary therapies are not a substitute for conventional medicine; however, the healthcare and social care professional must respect the person's wishes.
- At all times when applying medications, wear gloves not only to combat the risk of cross-infection but also to avoid absorbing the person's medicines.

Case study

Martin Halpin, a 25-year-old retail assistant in a large (do-it-yourself) DIY store, is at his GP surgery seeing the practice nurse. He is shortly to be interviewed for a promotion. Martin has had eczema for over 10 years; this comes and goes but is particularly bad during periods of stress. The eczema is usually symmetrical and his skin itches uncontrollably, and this can affect his ability to sleep. Mr Halpin has used steroid cream prescribed by his doctor; this has helped with the itching, but it was less effective when the situation became severe and the itching became worse. Mr Halpin is also an asthmatic, and he uses an inhaler when his breathing troubles him; this is often caused by dust, and flares up during the winter.

Currently he is experiencing itching at his elbow and in the elbow crease, and behind the knees. He feels very tired and is hot and irritable. Red thick areas with erythema located at the back of knees and elbows are present on examination.

Vital signs   Physical

The following vital signs were noted and recorded:

Vital sign	Observation	Normal
Temperature	36.8°C	36.0–37.9°C range
Pulse	80 beats per minute	60–100 beats per minute
Respiration	12 breaths per minute	12–20 breaths per minute
Blood pressure	130/60 mmHg	100–139 mmHg (systolic) range

No blood was taken during this consultation.
Reflect on this case and then consider the following:

1. What are the factors that might cause a flare-up of eczema?
2. Are there any ways in which you can help promote comfort?
3. How might you help Mr Halpin with this condition?
4. Are there any complications that may arise? What are they?

Clinical investigations

Patch testing
Patch testing can be useful in helping to determine if a person is allergic to a specific substance. Small amounts of different substances are placed on the skin under an adhesive coating. The specialist nurse or doctor will then check for a skin reaction under the patches. Patch testing may help to identify the exact cause of an allergy, but it can only test for allergic contact dermatitis. It cannot diagnose other types of allergy, for example, food allergy or urticaria.

On day one of testing, tiny amounts of up to 25 or more substances are applied as small patches to the skin, usually on the upper aspect of the back, fixed on with non-allergic tape.

The person returns to the department two days after, and the patches are removed. The skin is examined to determine if there is a reaction to any of the substances used.

After another two days, a further examination of the skin is undertaken in case the patient has a delayed reaction to any substance.

If the patient has had a reaction to any of the substances, the specialist nurse or doctor will be able to tell them what it is and what materials contain that substance, and the patient is given advice on how to avoid that substance. Avoiding the substance can help to prevent any further flare-ups of the rash.

The patient should be advised to keep the area of skin being tested dry until the final skin examination, usually four days after the patches are put on the skin. The person should avoid activities that cause them to sweat a lot whilst patch testing is in progress.

Sunlight and other sources of ultraviolet (UV) light should be kept off the skin whilst the test is underway.

Psoriasis
There are several forms of psoriasis; this skin disorder is a non-infectious, inflammatory disorder that can appear as purple patches with grey scales on black skin. The patches can also appear as a dark brown colour. Generally, psoriasis patches appear more purple or brown on darker skin. However, for black people with lighter skin, these patches may look like those

that appear on white skin: red, raised demarcation of skin patches with silvery whitish scales (Stephens, 2014); the condition can vary from mild to severe. The aetiology is unknown.

The patient may also experience an itch. If itching occurs, the scales are easily shed. It occurs most frequently on the back, elbows, knees and scalp. This skin condition has the potential to cause the patient to feel ashamed and dirty.

Pathophysiologically, the cells of the basal layers of the epidermis reproduce, and the more rapid upward progression of these cells through the epidermis results in an incomplete maturation of the upper layer (Weller et al., 2015); there is an overproduction of skin cells. Sometimes psoriasis is associated with arthritis, and this is called psoriatic arthropathy. The rash associated with psoriasis can occur when the patient is experiencing an episode of arthritis.

There is often a familial history associated with this condition; Page (2006) points out that there are other precipitating/aggravating factors:

- Infection (streptococcal throat infection)
- Some medications, e.g. antimalarials, antidepressants, beta blockers
- Sunlight (can help or hinder)
- Hormones – psoriasis can get better or worse during pregnancy or menstruation
- Psychological stress, e.g. bereavement, divorce or sitting examinations
- Trauma, e.g. burns, the site of an injury or a surgical scar.

The diagnosis of psoriasis is made on clinical presentation (Chowdhury et al., 2013). Skin biopsy, skin swab, throat swab and blood tests as well as clinical examination will be required to confirm diagnosis (Page, 2006). Treatment will include psychological support for the patient and the family.

A range of topical therapies is available to manage psoriasis. The healthcare professional has a role to play in motivating and encouraging the patient to apply the therapies meticulously, adhering to the treatment regimen. The following is a list of some of the topical therapies. It must be noted that whatever treatment is chosen is not a cure for the disease, and no single treatment will suit everyone; individual assessment is required:

- Emollients with the aim of lubricating the skin and easing scaling, as well as providing patient comfort.
- Coal tar ointments – These preparations have an antipruritic and anti-inflammatory effect (they may stain clothing).
- Dithranol – this is used to suppress cell proliferation.
- Vitamin D analogues such as calcipotriol, tacalcitol and calcitriol; these are used, amongst other things, to inhibit cell proliferation.
- Phototherapy can be used to inhibit cell division in some forms of psoriasis.
- Methotrexate – This is often used in the treatment of cancer; it causes inhibition of cell division.
- Retinoids – These influence the activity of the epidermis.
- Topical steroids – Used only for a short period.

Red flag

Bath additive emollients will coat the bath, and this will make it greasy and slippery. People should be advised to use a mat and/or grab rails in order to reduce the risk of slipping. Anybody else who may use the bath after additive emollients have been used should be warned that it will be very slippery.

Case study   Mark Gonzales

Mark, a 20-year-old university student, arrived at the emergency department with severe second- and third-degree burns from a fire in the university halls of residence. He was rescued from his burning room. He had fallen asleep at night when a candle he lit fell and started a fire. By the time the fire brigade arrived, and rescued him, he had suffered severe burns and was unconscious. He was transport to the emergency department with oxygen mask applied and an intravenous infusion *in situ*.

In the resuscitation room, his burns were evaluated, and he was found to have primarily second-degree burns over the upper half of his posterior chest and his whole right arm including his hand. Oxygen therapy was maintained, a further two large-bore cannulae were inserted, and he was given intravenous lactated Ringer's solution. A urinary catheter was inserted. His vital signs were recorded, and he was now responding, complaining of severe pain and asking what happened. His oxygen saturation was 96% on 100% oxygen.

Vital signs   Physical and bloods

The following vital signs were noted and recorded:

Vital sign	Observation	Normal
Temperature	38.1°C	36.0–37.9°C range
Pulse	120 beats per minute	60–100 beats per minute
Respiration	10 breaths per minute	12–20 breaths per minute
Blood pressure	106/55 mmHg	100–139 mmHg (systolic) range

A full blood count was performed.

Test	Result	Guideline normal values
White blood cells (WBC)	8×10^9/L	4 to 11×10^9/L
Neutrophils	7.2×10^9/L	2.0 to 7.5×10^9/L
Lymphocytes	3.2×10^9/L	1.3 to 4.0×10^9/L
Red blood cells (RBC)	6.4×10^9/L	4.5 to 6.5×10^9/L
Haemoglobin (Hb)	155 g/L	130–180 g/L
Platelets	390×10^9/L	150 to 440×10^9/L

Take some time to reflect on this case and then consider the following:

1. How can infection be controlled in those people who experience burns?
2. How will you manage Mr Gonzales's pain?
3. What activities of living will Mr Gonzales require assistance with?

News

Mark Gonzales

Physiological parameter	3	2	1	0	1	2	3
Respiration rate			10				
Oxygen saturation %				96			
Supplemental oxygen		Yes					
Temperature °C			38.1				
Systolic BP mmHg			106				
Heart rate		120					
Level of consciousness				A			
Score		4	3	0	0	0	0
Total	7						

Skin manifestations of COVID-19

Since the outbreak of the Covid 19 pandemic in Wuhan, China, dermatologists from across the globe have been reporting on lesions and rashes commonly associated with the corona virus. Five major patterns were identified by researchers (Galván Casas *et al.*, 2020).

1. Acral areas of erythema-oedema with some vesicles or pustules (pseudo-chilblain) of young patients. Asymmetrical small itchy lesions with red or purple spots caused by bleeding under the skin.
2. Other vesicular eruptions in middle-aged patients, which present as small blisters on the limbs and trunk, that may be filled with blood and become larger and spread out.
3. Urticarial lesions presenting as very itchy pink or white raised areas of skin resembling nettle rash, spread across the body, and occasionally seen on the palms of hands.
4. Other maculopapules that are described as small, flat, and raised red bumps, distributed around hair follicles, similar to pityriasis rosea with blood spots.
5. Livedo or necrosis due to impaired circulation of the skin a blotchy red or blue appearance with a net-like pattern emerges. This skin manifestation is associated with older patients who have severe Covid 19 infection.

Skin lightening products

Skin lightening or bleaching creams include the aesthetic use of an assortment of products broadly available in the Middle East, Asia and South America. These products are illegal and can include the use of the following products to lighten the skin:

- Mercury and caustic agents.
- Hydroquinone-based compounds and corticosteroids.

The side effects and risks can include periorbital hyperpigmentation, skin infections, including cellulitis, scabies, and impetigo. Long-term use can lead to steroid-induced acne, skin atrophy, hypercortisolism and adrenal insufficiency.

Conclusion

The skin, also called the integumentary system, is the largest organ in the body and has several important functions. This chapter has provided an overview of the skin and has discussed a number of pathological changes that can result in disease or illness. Some of the more common skin conditions have been discussed with an emphasis on skin cancer. The reader is advised to consult other texts to fully appreciate the scope and potential the healthcare professional has in helping people with skin conditions; this chapter has merely touched on the topic. The healthcare professional has a vital role to play in assisting the individual with problems associated with the skin; however, this can only be achieved with insight and understanding.

As well as the physiological disturbances resulting in problems of skin, there are also important psychological ramifications that must be given much consideration. The healthcare professional has a role to play in empowering and motivating the patient in order to adhere to prescribed treatment regimens that can often be messy and potentially damage clothing and bedding. Many patients with skin conditions and their families voice concerns about social isolation and ostracism; education and explanation may help to reduce these feelings; the healthcare professional is ideally placed to do this, acting as a key resource.

Test your knowledge

- What is the rule of Nines?
- Outline the advice to be given to a person concerning latex allergy.
- Describe the pathophysiological changes that occur in a grade 2 pressure sore.
- Discuss the role of the healthcare professional in offering psychosocial support to a person with a disfiguring skin condition.
- Discuss the first-aid needed for a toddler who has sustained a burn to the finger.

Activities

Here are some activities and exercises to help test your learning. For the answers to these exercises, as well as further self-testing activities, visit our website at **www.wiley.com/go/fundamentalsofappliedpathophysiology/student4e**

Multiple choice questions

1. What are the five D's that Weller associates with the profound effect dermatological conditions have on a person's quality of life:
   (a) **D**isfigurement, **D**istress, **D**isability, **D**epression, **D**eath.
   (b) **D**eformity, **D**iscomfort, **D**isability, **D**epression, **D**eath.
   (c) **D**isfigurement, **D**iscomfort, **D**isability, **D**espair, **D**eath.
   (d) **D**isfigurement, **D**iscomfort, **D**isability, **D**epression, **D**read.
2. Who are dermatologists?
   (a) Nurses who diagnose and treat diseases of the skin.
   (b) Specialist practitioners who diagnose and treat diseases of the skin, nails, and hair.
   (c) Healthcare practitioners who diagnose and treat diseases of the skin.
   (d) Specialist practitioners who diagnose and treat diseases of the skin.

3. What is the estimated weight of the skin?
    (a) 2.5 and 4 kg
    (b) 2 and 4 kg
    (c) 2.8 and 4 kg
    (d) 2.6 and 3.9 kg
4. How many functions does the skin have?
    (a) 4.
    (b) 5.
    (c) 9.
    (d) 11.
5. Where are melanocytes found?
    (a) Epidermis
    (b) Dermis
    (c) Subcutaneous layer
    (d) Peritoneum
6. What are the functions of hair?
    (a) Sexual, social, thermoregulation, protection.
    (b) Protection, thermoregulation.
    (c) Protection, touch and thermoregulation.
    (d) Protection, touch, social.
7. Which cells are a part of the body's immune system?
    (a) Langerhans cells
    (b) Melanocytes
    (c) Merkel cells
    (d) Keratinocytes
8. What do sebaceous glands produce?
    (a) Sebum
    (b) Melanocytes
    (c) Sex hormones
    (d) Langerhans cells
9. Which layer of the epidermis is nearest to the dermo-epidermal junction?
    (a) Stratum basale
    (b) Stratum spinosum
    (c) Stratum granulosum
    (d) Stratum lucidium
    (e) Stratum corneum
10. What does the dermis mainly consist of?
    (a) Collagen
    (b) Blood vessels
    (c) Nerve cells
    (d) Lymphatics
11. What is the main cause of skin cancer?
    (a) Genetics
    (b) Diet
    (c) Obesity
    (d) Sunlight
12. SPF is an abbreviation of:
    (a) Sun protection factor
    (b) Sun prevention factor
    (c) Sun protection freedom
    (d) Sun prevention factor

13. Acute eczema is characterised by:
- (a) Pruritus, erythema and vesiculation.
- (b) Pruritus, erythema and lichenification
- (c) Pruritus, erythema and xerosis
- (d) Pruritus, erythema and hyperkeratosis

14. Which contagious skin condition causes sores and blisters?
- (a) Psoriasis
- (b) Eczema
- (c) Melanoma
- (d) Impetigo

15. How many major patterns were identified by researchers of COVID-19 skin manifestation?
- (a) 4
- (b) 5
- (c) 6
- (d) 3

Further resources

Alopecia UK
https://www.alopecia.org.uk/

This is a national charity that provides information, offers advice and support to people with alopecia. The charity has support groups and online forums where people can talk to others who are experiencing hair loss.

Alopecia UK aims to improve the lives of those affected by alopecia. They will provide impartial information, advice and support to help people feel less isolated and raise awareness to the general public and healthcare professionals about alopecia and its psychological impact. The charity supports medical and psychological researchers who aim to find effective treatments

British Association of Dermatologists
https://www.bad.org.uk/#

This website provides information sheets about skin diseases, as well as general information about the skin, current issues in skin disease, and changes to dermatology services in the UK and those areas experiencing problems with providing access to care for their patient population.

Brown Skin Matters
https://www.brownskinmatters.com/

This website provides pictures of skin disorders and how they present on Black, Asian and minority ethic skin.

Changing Faces
https://www.changingfaces.org.uk/

Changing Faces is the leading UK charity that supports and represents people who have disfigurements to the face, hand or body from any cause. Changing Faces helps people to face the challenges of living with a disfigurement and equips them with the appropriate tools to build self-confidence and self-esteem. Its work involves providing support for children, young people, adults and their families, working with schools and employers to ensure a culture of inclusion and with healthcare and social care professionals to provide better psychological care for people with disfigurement, and campaigning for better policies and practices that are inclusive of people with disfigurements and for social change by working with the media, government and opinion leaders

The Psoriasis Association
https://www.psoriasis-association.org.uk/

The Psoriasis Association is the leading national membership organisation for people affected by psoriasis – patients, families, carers and healthcare professionals. This site provides easy to understand information concerning psoriasis, as well as offering information concerning research related to the condition.

UK National Eczema Society

https://eczema.org/

The National Eczema Society has two key aims: first, to provide people with independent and practical advice about treating and managing eczema; second, to raise awareness of the needs of those with eczema amongst healthcare professionals, teachers and the government. A very useful, practical site.

Glossary of terms

Adjuvant   An agent that modifies the effects of another agent.
Antibiotic   A drug used to kill bacteria.
Antifungal   A drug used to treat fungal infections.
Chemotherapy   The use of chemical substances to treat diseases, primarily to treat cancer.
Dermatitis   Inflammation of the skin.
Dermatoscope   A magnifier with a light allowing illumination of the lesion.
Erythema   A superficial redness of the skin.
Extrinsic   Originates externally.
Fissure   A groove or tear.
Histology   The study of a tissue's microscopic anatomy.
Hyperkeratosis   Excess keratins are produced resulting in thickening of the skin.
Integumentary   The external covering of the body – the skin.
Intrinsic   Originates internally.
Keratin   A tough insoluble protein.
Keratinise   To convert into keratin.
Lichenification   Thickening of the skin as a result of chronic scratching.
Naevus   A pigmented lesion of the skin.
Pheromone   A chemical that triggers an innate behavioural response in another.
Prognosis   A prediction about how a person's disease will progress.
Pruritus   Itchy sensation on the skin.
Radiotherapy   The medical use of radiation to treat cancer.
Relapsing (relapse)   When the person is again affected by a condition that has occurred in the past.
Sebum   An oily substance made of fat and the debris of fat-producing cells.
Suture   Stitch.
Topical   A medication applied to the body surface.
Vesiculation   Collection of fluid in the skin.
Viscous   Relating to the thickness of a fluid.
Xerosis   Dry skin.

621

References

Balieva, F., Kupfer, J., Lien, L., Gieler, U., Finlay, A.Y. *et al.* (2017). The burden of common skin diseases assessed with the EQ5D™: A European multicentre study in 13 countries. *British Journal of Dermatology*, 176(5): 1170–1178.

British Association of Dermatologists (2020). *Five Common Skin Manifestations of COVID-19 Identified*. Retrieved from https://www.skinhealthinfo.org.uk/five-common-skin-manifestations-of-covid-19-identified/ 15th May 2020.

British Association of Dermatologists (2016). *Skindex*. Retrieved from https://www.bad.org.uk/shared/get-file.ashx?id=3910&itemtype=document 15th May 2020.

Cancer Research UK (2017). *Cancer Incidence for Common Cancers. Retrieved from https://www. cancerresearchuk.org/health-professional/cancer-statistics/incidence/common-cancers-compared 15th May 2020.*

Chang, C., Murzaku, E.C., Penn, L., Abbasi, N.R., Davis, P.D. *et al.* (2014). More skin, more sun, more tan, more melanoma. *American journal of public health*, 104(11), e92–e99. https://doi.org/10.2105/ AJPH.2014.302185.

Chowdhury, M.M.U., Katugampola, R.P. and Finlay. A.Y. (2013). *Dermatology at a Glance*. Oxford: Wiley.

College of Podiatry (2019). *Nail Surgery Guidelines.* Retrieved from file:///C:/Users/steph/AppData/ Local/Packages/Microsoft.MicrosoftEdge_8wekyb3d8bbwe/TempState/Downloads/ NailSurgery%20with%20name%20changes%20(1).pdf

Flohr, C., Johansson, S.G., Wahlgren, C.F. and Williams, H. (2004). How atopic is atopic dermatitis? *Journal of Allergy and Clinical Immunology*, 114(1): 150–158.

Foss, M. and Farine, T. (2007). *Science in Nursing and Health Care*, 2nd edn. Harlow: Pearson.

Galván Casas, C., Català, A., Carretero Hernández, G., Rodríguez-Jiménez, P., Fernández Nieto, D. *et al.* (2020). Classification of the cutaneous manifestations of COVID-19: A rapid prospective nationwide consensus study in Spain with 375 cases. *British Journal of Dermatology*, 183(1): 71–77.

Gawkrodger, D.J. (2016). *Dermatology: An Illustrated Colour Text*, 6th edn. Amsterdam: Elsevier.

Gershenwald, J.E. and Scolyer, R.A. (2018). Melanoma Staging: American Joint Committee on Cancer (AJCC) 8th edition and beyond. *Annals of Surgical Oncology*, 25, 2105–2110 https://doi.org/10.1245/ s10434-018-6513-7.

Health and Safety Executive (2019). *Latex Allergies in Health and Social Care*. Retrieved from https:// www.hse.gov.uk/healthservices/latex/ 15th May 2020.

International Agency for Research on Cancer (IARC) (2007). The association of use of sunbeds with cutaneous malignant melanoma and other skin cancers: A systematic review. *International Journal of Cancer*, 120(11): 116–122.

Jackson-Richards, D. and Pandya, A.G. (Eds.) (2014). *Dermatology Atlas for Skin of Color* (eds.). Springer-Verlag: Berlin Heidelberg.

Kailas, A., Solomon, J.A., Mostow, E.N., Rigel, D.S., Kittles, R. and Taylor, S.C. (2016). Gaps in the under-standing and treatment of skin cancer in people of color. *Journal American Academy of Dermatology*, 74: 1020–1021. DOI: 10.1016/j.jadd.2015.11.028.

McCann, S.A. and Huether, S.E. (2014). Structure, function, and disorders of the integument. In: McCance, K.L., Heuther, S.E., Brashers, V.L. and Rote, N.S. (eds), *Pathophysiology. The Biologic Basis for Disease in Adults and Children*, 7th edn. St Louis: Elsevier, pp. 1616–1667.

Mitchell, T. and Kennedy, C. (2006). *Common Skin Disorders*. Edinburgh: Churchill Livingstone.

Myers, J. (2015). Challenges of identifying eczema in darkly pigmented skin. *Nursing Children and Young People*, 27: 24–28. DOI: 10.7748/ncyp.27.6.24.e571

Morris-Jones, R. (2014). Introduction. In: *ABC of Dermatology*, 6th edn. Oxford: Wiley, pp. 1–10.

National Institute for Health and Care Excellence (NICE) (2016). *Skin Cancers – Recognition and Referral*. Retrieved from https://cks.nice.org.uk/skin-cancers-recognition-and-referral#!scenario 15th May 2020.

National Institute for Health and Care Excellence (NICE) (2010). *Improving Outcomes for People with Skin Tumours Including Melanoma (update). The Management of Low-Risk Basal Cell Carcinomas in the Community. Retrieved from* https://www.nice.org.uk/guidance/csg8/resources/improving-outcomes-for-people-with-skin-tumours-including-melanoma-2010-partial-update-pdf-773380189

Page, B.E. (2006). Skin disorders. In: Alexander, M.F., Fawcett, J.N. and Runciman, P.J. (eds), *Nursing Practice, Hospital and Home: The Adult*, 3rd edn. Edinburgh: Churchill Livingstone, pp. 525–552.

Sharpe, G. (2006). Skin cancer: Prevalence, prevention and treatment. *Clinical Medicine*, 6: 333–334.

Stephens, M. (2014). *The Principles of Skin Integrity*. In: Peate, I., Nair, M. and Wild, K. (eds), *Nursing Practice Knowledge and Care*. Oxford: Wiley, pp. 355–382.

Thompson, J.F., Scolyer, R.A. and Kefford, R.A. (2005). Cutaneous melanoma. *Lancet*, 365: 687–701.

Weller, R.B. (2014). *Skin Disease in Perspective – Clinical Dermatology*, 5th edn. Oxford: Wiley.

Weller, R.B., Hunter, J.A. and Mann, W.M. (2015). *Clinical Dermatology*, 5th edn. Oxford: Blackwell Scientific.

Woodard, I. (2014). *Assessment of Integumentary Function*. In: Hinkle, J.L. and Cheever, K.H. (eds), *Brunner and Suddarth's Textbook of Medical-Surgical Nursing*, 13th edn. Philadelphia: Lippincott, pp. 1752–1766.

Wolff, K., Johnson, R.A. and Saavedra, A.P. (2017). *Fitzpatrick's Color Atlas and Synopsis of Clinical Dermatology*, 8th edn. New York: McGraw-Hill.

Zaidi, Z. and Lanigan, S.W. (2010). *Dermatology in Clinical Practice*. London: Springer-Verlag.

Chapter 21

The ear, nose and throat, and eyes, and associated disorders

Carl Clare

Senior Lecturer, Department of Adult Nursing and Primary Care, School of Health and Social Work
University of Hertfordshire, Hatfield, Hertfordshire, UK

Contents

Introduction 624
Physiology of the ear, nose and throat.......624
Conclusion 646
Multiple choice questions.............................647

Conditions...648
Further resources...649
Glossary of terms...649
References...651

Key words

- Pinna
- Tympanic membrane
- Eustachian tube
- Cochlea
- Septum
- Turbinates
- Epiglottis
- Larynx
- Iris
- Retina
- Sclera
- Humour

Fundamentals of Applied Pathophysiology: An Essential Guide for Nursing and Healthcare Students, Fourth Edition. Edited by Ian Peate.
© 2021 John Wiley & Sons Ltd. Published 2021 by John Wiley & Sons Ltd.
Student companion website: www.wiley.com/go/fundamentalsofappliedpathophysiology/student4e
Instructor companion website: www.wiley.com/go/fundamentalsofappliedpathophysiology/instructor4e

Test your prior knowledge

- Which part of the ear contains the sensory organ for balance?
- Which structure is completely removed from the throat during a laryngectomy?
- Which part of the eye is affected by a cataract?
- How many sections is the ear divided into?

Learning outcomes

On completion of this section, the reader will be able to:

- Describe the functions of each of the three sections of the ear.

- Explain the functions of the nose in respiration.

- Describe the functions of the true vocal cords and the false vocal cords.

- Describe the roles of the two types of photoreceptors of the eye.

Don't forget to visit the companion website for this book
(www.wiley.com/go/fundamentalsofappliedpathophysiology/student4e)
where you can find self-assessment tests to check your progress, as well as lots of activities to practise your learning.

Introduction

Disorders of the structures of the head and neck range from the relatively minor to some of the most challenging you may be asked to care for. The special senses of the ear, nose and eye are something that are often taken for granted, but conditions that affect these senses can profoundly influence the daily activities of a person. The aim of this chapter is to introduce the reader to the physiology and associated disorders of the special senses and, in line with the speciality of ear, nose and throat (ENT) care, the physiology and disorders of the throat will also be reviewed.

Physiology of the ear, nose and throat

Ear

The ear is divided into three sections (Figure 21.1):

1. External
2. Middle
3. Inner.

Each of these three sections is integral to the process of hearing and the inner ear is also essential to the maintenance of the sense of balance.

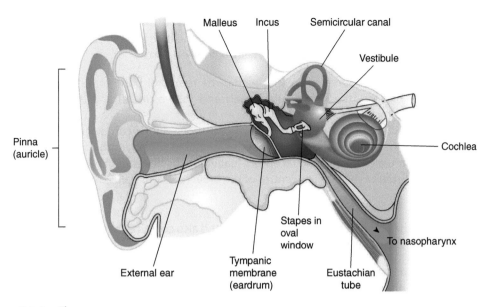

Figure 21.1   The ear.

External ear

The external ear consists of the pinna, the external ear canal and the tympanic membrane:

- Pinna – A skin-covered flap of elastic cartilage shaped somewhat like the end of a horn and surrounding the end of the external auditory canal.
- External ear canal – A slightly 'S'-shaped tube lined with skin, fine hairs, sebaceous (oil) glands and ceruminous (wax) glands. The purpose of the oils and the wax is to lubricate the ear canal, kill bacteria and, in conjunction with the hairs, keep the canal free of debris (Lewis *et al.*, 2016).
- Tympanic membrane – Composed of epithelial cells, connective tissue and mucous membrane. It acts as a partition between the external and middle ears and is responsible for the transmission of sound from the external to the middle ear.

Middle ear

The middle ear is an air space lined with a mucous membrane; it is connected to the naso-pharynx by the eustachian tube, thus allowing for the equalisation of air pressure between the middle ear and the throat (and therefore atmospheric air). This equalisation of pressure ensures free movement of the tympanic membrane in response to sound waves conducted along the external ear canal.

Within the middle ear are three bones (the ossicles or ossicular chain):

1. Hammer (malleus)
2. Anvil (incus)
3. Stirrup (stapes).

These interlink and are connected with the tympanic membrane. Vibrations of the tympanic membrane are conducted along the bones to the oval window; these vibrations are then transmitted via the oval window into the fluid of the inner ear. Movement in this fluid leads to stimulation of the hearing receptors.

Inner ear

The inner ear is also known as the labyrinth due to the complicated series of canals it contains. The inner ear is composed of two main, fluid-filled parts:

1. Bony labyrinth – A series of cavities within the temporal bone that contains the main organs of balance (the semicircular canals and the vestibule) and the main organ of hearing (the cochlea).
2. Membranous labyrinth – A series of sacs and tubes that is contained within the bony labyrinth. Movement of the fluid within the membranous labyrinth contained within the cochlea stimulates the hearing receptors, leading to the generation of nerve impulses that are transmitted to the hearing centres of the brain (Hall and Hall, 2020).

Nose

The nose is the first part of the respiratory tract and also contains the receptors for the sense of smell. The functions of the nose are threefold:

1. Warming, moistening and filtering inhaled air
2. Detecting olfactory stimuli
3. Resonance chamber that modifies the quality of speech.

The nose can be divided into external and internal sections:

- External nose – A framework of bone and cartilage covered by muscle and skin and lined with a mucous membrane. This framework is attached to the frontal and maxillary bones of the skull. The external nose is divided by the septum into two airways (nares or nostrils) of roughly equal size, which form part of the framework of bone and cartilage.
- Internal nose – A large chamber lined with ciliated mucous membrane and containing coarse hairs that filter out large particles from inhaled air. Finer particles that enter the nose become trapped in the sticky mucus created by the membrane and are then transported to the nasopharynx by the ciliary system. The internal nose is divided into two by a continuation of the septum. Each side contains three shelves formed by projections of bone known as the turbinates (Figure 21.2); these increase the surface area that inhaled air must pass over (Hall and Hall, 2020). The internal nose has an extremely rich vascular

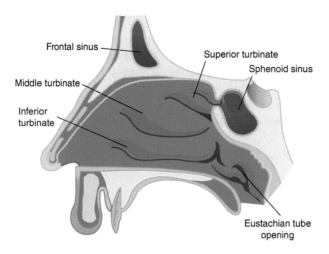

Figure 21.2   The nose.

supply, which in conjunction with the turbinates, maximises the humidification and warming of the air passing through. The internal nose also contains openings (ostia) from the sinus cavities (contained within the bones of the skull).

Throat

The throat consists of the oropharynx and the hypopharynx (Figure 21.3).

Oropharynx

Tonsils

The tonsils are five collections of lymphatic nodules mostly located in a ring around the junction of the oral cavity and the oropharynx:

- Two palatine tonsils located at the back of the oral cavity
- Two lingual tonsils located at the base of the tongue
- A single pharyngeal tonsil (adenoid) located at the junction of the nasal cavity and the nasopharynx.

The role of the tonsils is to participate in the fight against inhaled or ingested foreign substances.

Hypopharynx

Larynx

The larynx is a short tube that connects the lower hypopharynx with the trachea. It is composed of a mucous membrane covering several pieces of cartilage including:

- Thyroid cartilage (Adam's apple)
- Epiglottis – a large piece of cartilage that covers the opening of the glottis during swallowing, thus protecting the airway

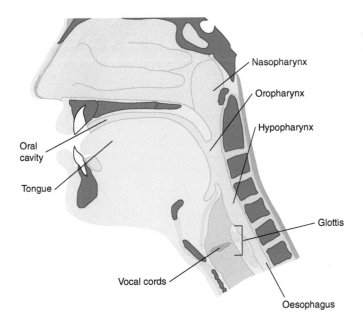

Figure 21.3   The throat.

- Cricoid cartilage – a ring of cartilage that forms the inferior wall of the larynx and connects to the first cartilage ring of the trachea.

The mucous membrane of the larynx is formed to create two pairs of folds:

1. Ventricular folds (false vocal cords) – When they are brought together, they enable the holding of the breath against the pressure in the thoracic cavity, such as when lifting a heavy object.
2. Vocal cords (folds; true vocal cords) – Situated below the ventricular folds, the vocal cords are fundamental to the generation of speech. Sound is generated by the vibration of these cords, but the mouth, nasal cavity and nasal sinuses are also required to create recognisable speech.

Physiology of the eye

The eyeball (globe) is made up of three layers (Figure 21.4):

1. A tough outer layer – fibrous tunic
2. A middle layer – vascular tunic
3. The retina – sensory tunic.

Fibrous tunic

The fibrous tunic is composed of the cornea and the sclera, and contains no blood vessels. The cornea is a curved, transparent coat which helps focus light onto the retina. The sclera (the 'white' of the eye) covers the entire eyeball, except where the cornea is present; it gives

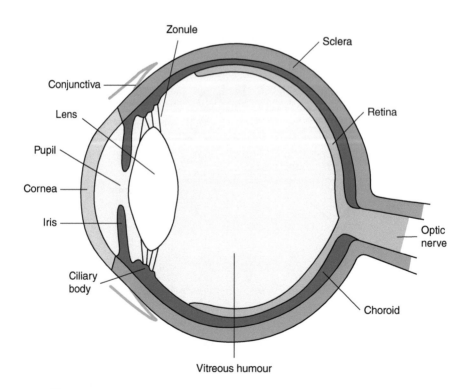

Figure 21.4   The eye.

shape and protection to the eyeball. The anterior sclera (but not the cornea) is covered by the conjunctiva, which produces a lubricating mucus that prevents the eye from drying out (Marieb and Hoehn, 2018).

Vascular tunic

The vascular tunic (uvea) is composed of the iris, the ciliary body and the choroid:

- Choroid – A highly vascular membrane; its blood vessels supply nutrition to all the tunics of the eye (Marieb and Hoehn, 2018).
- Ciliary body – At the front of the eye, the choroid becomes the ciliary body – a thickened ring of smooth muscle that circles the lens and has an important role in controlling the shape of the lens. The choroid is connected to the lens by a suspensory ligament (zonule).
- Iris – Coloured part of the eye lying between the cornea and the lens; it contains a hole (the pupil) through which light can enter the eye. The size of the pupil is controlled by the contraction and relaxation of two separate layers of muscle fibres contained within the iris.

Sensory tunic

The retina has two layers; however, only the neural layer is directly involved with vision (Marieb and Hoehn, 2018). Within this neural layer are the photoreceptors:

- Rods for peripheral and dim light vision
- Cones for bright light and colour vision.

629

Impulses generated as a result of stimulation of these photoreceptors are transmitted to the visual cortex via the optic nerve.

Internal structure

Internally, the eye is divided into two chambers by a barrier formed by the lens and the zonule:

1. Anterior segment – In front of the lens and zonule. This chamber is filled with aqueous humour, which is constantly formed and drained. Aqueous humour provides the lens and the cornea with nutrients and oxygen.
2. Posterior segment – Filled with a gel-like substance called vitreous humour. The thick vitreous humour supports the back of the lens, holds the retina against the choroid and contributes to intraocular pressure, thus helping to maintain the shape of the eye.

Lens

The lens is the main apparatus for focusing light onto the retina. The thickness of the lens is varied by the contraction and relaxation of the ciliary muscles, depending on whether the eye is focusing on near or far objects.

Movement of the eye

Movement of the eye is controlled by the extrinsic eye muscles; neuromuscular coordination ensures the simultaneous movement of both eyes (Lewis et al., 2016).

Disorders of the ear, nose and throat and eye

Learning outcomes

On completion of this section, the reader will be able to:

- Describe the care of a patient following ear surgery.

- Describe the care of a patient following nasal surgery.

- Explain the difference between a tracheostomy and a laryngectomy.

- Discuss the two types of glaucoma.

Disorders of the ear, nose and throat

Ear

Ear wax

Impaction of ear wax in the external ear canal is a common complaint often related to a patient's attempts to remove ear wax with fingers or cotton buds. Impaction of ear wax reduces the ability of sound to travel the length of the external ear canal and the responsiveness of the tympanic membrane to sound waves, leading to a temporary reduction in the ability to hear. This is especially common in older patients, who have a tendency to produce more, and drier wax.

One method for the removal of ear wax is the syringing of the external ear canal, often preceded by the use of a cerumenolytic (a substance that actively helps to break down wax) or a wax softener (Schwartz *et al.*, 2017), though commercially available ear drops have not been proven to be any better than saline or tap water (Aaron *et al.*, 2018).

Otitis externa

This is diffuse inflammation of the external ear canal, often associated with regular swimming ('swimmer's ear'). The condition is characterised by pain, itching and a discharge from the ear canal (Wiegand *et al.*, 2019). The discharge is usually watery at the beginning but becomes purulent as the condition progresses.

The spread of infection can lead to pyrexia and systemic symptoms such as malaise. The infection is usually caused by a mixture of microorganisms, and swabs should be sent for microbiological culture and sensitivity.

The care of this condition includes:

- Careful removal of any debris from the external ear canal.
- The administration of topical antibiotics and a steroid preparation (Wiegand *et al.*, 2019).
- If the infection has become systemic (entered the bloodstream) or extensive, the patient may require oral antibiotics, analgesia and bed rest.
- The patient should be discouraged from scratching the affected ear and advised to prevent water from entering the ear canal.

Tympanic membrane rupture

Rupture of the tympanic membrane due to improper ear syringing technique, blows to the side of the head or blast injuries are often self-healing as long as infection is not present.

Patients should be advised to avoid:

- The entry of water into the ear
- Introducing foreign objects such as cotton buds.

Persistent deafness may indicate damage or displacement of the ossicular chain and may require surgical intervention.

Otitis media

Acute otitis media is a condition that is often associated with upper respiratory tract infections and sinusitis (Schilder *et al.*, 2016). The infection tracks up into the middle ear via the eustachian tube, leading to infection and the collection of pus. The infection and the pressure resulting from the collection of pus may lead to a range of potential symptoms including (Schilder *et al.*, 2016):

- Pain
- Pyrexia
- Malaise
- Headache
- Nausea and vomiting
- Tinnitus
- Reduction in hearing.

Treatment includes:

- Antibiotics
- Pain relief
- Antipyretics
- Nasal decongestants may reduce inflammation of the eustachian tube and allow drainage of the middle ear into the nasopharynx though this is unproven (Roditi *et al.*, 2019)
- Application of warmth to the affected ear in order to reduce pain
- Avoiding entry of water into the ear canal.

631

Untreated or repeated episodes of acute otitis media may lead to chronic infection of the middle ear, which may eventually spread to the mastoid process of the temporal bone of the skull (mastoiditis) (Laulajainen-Hongisto *et al.*, 2016). Tympanic membrane rupture is common, and destruction of the bones of the ossicular chain is also possible. Symptoms include:

- Purulent discharge
- Pain – may be associated with redness and swelling of the bone behind the pinna (mastoid process)
- Pyrexia
- Hearing loss
- Nausea and vomiting
- Vertigo.

Treatment for the chronic complications of otitis media is usually surgical and depends on the structures that are affected:

- Myringoplasty – repair of the tympanic membrane, often using grafted tissue
- Ossiculoplasty – reconstruction of the ossicular chain

- Tympanoplasty – myringoplasty and ossiculoplasty performed at the same time
- Mastoidectomy – removal of infected tissue from the middle ear and mastoid bone; often performed with a tympanoplasty.

The care of patients following surgery of the ear is detailed in Box 21.1.

Otosclerosis

Otosclerosis is the formation of new bone around the footplate of the stapes. It is often hereditary (Batson and Rizzolo, 2017) and is associated with a gradual deterioration in hearing. The treatment is surgical (e.g. stapedectomy or stapedotomy) and involves the removal of part of the stapes and insertion of a prosthesis (Batson and Rizzolo, 2017).

Ménière's disease

Ménière's disease is a disorder of the inner ear characterised by episodes of:

- Vertigo
- Nausea and vomiting
- Tinnitus
- Varying hearing loss
- Aural fullness (a feeling of 'stuffiness' in the ear)
- 'Drop attacks' – a feeling of being pulled to the ground; alternatively some patients feel as though they are whirling through space.

Box 21.1 Care of the patient following ear surgery

- Recovery period – Position the patient flat on the opposite side to the operation side with no pillows.
- Advise the patient to avoid sudden movements of the head.
- Administer analgesia as prescribed.
- Pillows are introduced for comfort when the patient feels able to tolerate them; most patients are able to tolerate sitting up after 24 hours.
- Following operations on the inner ear, observe for signs of neurological damage (neurological observations at least 4 hourly for the first 24 hours).
- Facial nerve damage may occur at the time of the operation or subsequently due to inflammation or oedema. The patient should be asked to show their teeth or smile to assess for facial palsy.
- Patient should avoid coughing, sneezing and blowing their nose, or straining during bowel movements for 7–10 days as this will lead to an increased pressure in the ear via the eustachian tube. If coughing or sneezing is unavoidable, then the patient is advised to keep the mouth open to reduce the pressure on the middle ear (Lewis et al., 2016). Laxatives may be provided to avoid straining during bowel movements.
- Most patients can be discharged after 2–3 days, but should be advised to avoid water entry into the ear, crowded places (where respiratory infections may be contracted) and changes in air pressure (such as flying or high altitudes) until advised by the surgeon (Lewis et al., 2016).

The duration of an episode may be hours or days. The care of a patient experiencing an acute episode of Ménière's disease includes:

- Reassurance and counselling
- A quiet, darkened, environment
- Comfortable position (often semi-recumbent)
- Avoidance of sudden head movements
- Fluorescent and flickering lights, and watching television should be avoided as they can exacerbate symptoms
- Vomit bowls should be provided
- All drugs should be administered parenterally
- The bedside call bell should be put in the patient's reach and the patient advised to not mobilise without assistance.

Treatment of the disease requires lifestyle changes and long-term medication (e.g. diuretics or steroids). Patients who experience a reduced quality of life (frequent incapacitating attacks and/or loss of employment) or who are resistant to other treatments may require surgery (Sood *et al.*, 2014).

Snapshot Antiepileptic drugs and vertigo

Victoria is a 24-year-old lady with learning disabilities; recently she has been reporting recurrent bouts of dizziness, slowly increasing in length and intensity. Examination of the ear for obvious signs of infection revealed no signs, and blood tests showed no abnormal results (low sodium levels can be a cause of vertigo). Her blood pressure is stable on lying and standing, ruling out orthostatic hypotension. On review of Victoria's medication history, it is noted that she is taking phenytoin and the dose was increased two months ago. It is known that phenytoin is associated with vertigo, especially at higher doses (Behere *et al.*, 2019). Victoria's medication was changed to one of the newer anti-epileptics with a much lower side effect profile (Palleria *et al.*, 2017), and the vertigo stopped.

633

Clinical investigation

Tilt table testing

In cases of vertigo where the diagnosis is uncertain, it is important to rule out cardiovascular causes (Cheshire and Goldstein, 2019). This can be done by having the patient lie down for a few minutes, recording the blood pressure and then have them stand up and retaking the blood pressure. However, in younger people with vertigo, this can often be inconclusive, and the patient may be referred for tilt table testing. For a tilt table test, the patient is strapped to a bed (table) with their feet against a foot board. The patient is laid flat for 5–20 minutes, and continuous ECG monitoring and repeated blood pressure measurements are taken. After the defined period of time, the patient is raised through 90° and kept there for 20–45 minutes. Vertigo that is due to cardiovascular causes will show in the ECG tracing or blood pressure response.

Nose

Epistaxis (nose bleed)

Epistaxis is often associated with trauma to the nose or upper respiratory tract infections. Control is achieved by applying pressure to the upper part of the nose by pinching it between the finger and the thumb whilst the patient sits with their head tilted forward to avoid blood draining into the throat and being swallowed. Nasal packing may be required, and in some cases this may be modified by the use of a Foley catheter or postnasal pack to provide a firm base against which to pack the nose (Tikka, 2016). Further care for difficult-to-control bleeds may include:

- Frequent observations (blood pressure and pulse half-hourly)
- Assessment of blood loss and blood transfusion if hypovolaemia is suspected
- Cold compresses applied to the nose and back of the neck to reduce blood flow to the nose
- Antihypertensive drugs for hypertensive patients
- Cauterisation with silver nitrate stick or electrocautery
- Surgical ligation of blood vessels may be used in cases that are resistant to other treatment (Tikka, 2016).

Snapshot   Child with recurrent epistaxis

Samuel is a 9-year-old boy presenting to the emergency department via his GP with an epistaxis that is not responding to standard treatment (pressure to the nasal bridge). Except for the continued bleeding, Samuel is otherwise well with vital signs within normal range. On questioning the parents, it is clear that Samuel has a three-year history of recurrent epistaxis in the winter, suggesting a bacterial cause from recurrent infection. They deny any coagulation disorders in Samuel or his family. The paediatric registrar feels that the epistaxis is manageable with local anaesthetic and silver nitrate. The affected nostril was sprayed with lidocaine and phenylephrine spray to anaesthetise the area and vasoconstrict the local blood vessels. Silver nitrate was applied to the bleeding area whilst Samuel was reassured by his mother (application of silver nitrate is unpleasant and can be painful). Samuel was discharged with a prescription for a neomycin cream (topical antibiotic) to apply to the nostril twice a day as colonisation with *Staphylococcus aureus* is common in children with recurrent epistaxis (Yaneza and Amiraraghi, 2018).

634

Medicines management

Silver nitrate sticks degrade over time and must be kept in an airtight and light-proof container. If there is no response to the silver nitrate, it may be worth trying a new stick in case the previous one has degraded.

Red flag

Cauterising the nasal septum
When using cautery for a septal bleed, only one side of the nasal septum should be cauterised to prevent perforation of the nasal septum.

Deviated nasal septum
This is a condition that may be congenital or acquired (due to trauma); the patient may present with nasal obstruction. Treatment is normally surgical:

- Submucous resection (SMR) – removal and resection of the parts of the septum causing the deviation
- Septoplasty – septum is completely freed, and the removal of areas around its margin may allow it to be repositioned in the midline.

The care of patients following surgery of the nose is detailed in Box 21.2.

Nasal polyps

These are soft fleshy swellings inside the nose and are the end product of prolonged oedema of the nasal mucosa caused by prolonged infection or allergy. The patient may present with nasal obstruction, nasal discharge and headaches. The treatment for severe cases is the surgical removal of the polypi (ethmoidectomy) and treatment of the underlying cause (DeMarcantonio and Han, 2011), although some cases may be managed medically.

Sinusitis

Following a viral infection of the nose, the natural resistance of the mucosa is reduced, and a secondary bacterial infection occurs, which rapidly spreads into the sinuses. The swelling of the mucosa may close off the ostia of the sinuses; thus, the infected mucus is unable to escape. The symptoms include:

- Pain
- Nasal obstruction
- Malaise
- Pyrexia
- Localised tenderness.

If untreated, there is the possibility of complications such as:

- Spread of infection to the eyes
- Intracranial infection or abscess formation
- Osteomyelitis (infection of the bone).

635

Box 21.2 Care of the patient following nasal surgery

- In the immediate post-operative period, patients will normally have a nasal pack in place. This is removed 24–48 hours after the operation.
- Monitoring of the patient's airway is essential in the immediate post-operative period due to the risk of blood or nasal packing entering the respiratory tract.
- When the patient is fully conscious, their head should be raised above the level of the heart, and they should be encouraged to sleep with at least three pillows. This reduces bleeding and swelling. Ice packs may also be used to reduce swelling if allowed by the surgeon.
- Administer analgesia and antibiotics as prescribed.
- Patient should avoid sneezing, blowing their nose and straining during bowel movements for 10–14 days as this may lead to bleeding. If sneezing is unavoidable, then the patient is advised to keep the mouth open to reduce the pressure on the nose. Laxatives may be provided to avoid straining during bowel movements.
- After the removal of nasal packs, steam inhalations or a saline spray will help to keep the nasal mucosa moist and loosen any crusts.

The treatment of sinusitis includes:

- Nasal decongestants to reduce the mucosal swelling and allow drainage
- Antibiotics
- Pain relief
- Saline lavage to relieve symptoms (Rosenfeld *et al.*, 2015)
- Abscesses require surgical intervention.

The care of patients includes:

- A warm, well-ventilated environment
- Fluid intake of at least 3 L a day
- Good oral hygiene
- Use of a humidifier
- Bed rest may be required for 24–48 hours
- Whilst recovering, the patient should avoid extremes of temperature, crowded environments and smoking.

Throat

Tonsillitis and quinsy

Tonsillitis is a condition characterised by inflammation of the tonsils, leading to the patient presenting with:

- Bilateral sore throat
- Dysphagia
- Pyrexia
- Malaise.

Treatment is usually:

- Antibiotics
- Encourage a fluid intake of 1–3 L per day
- Pain relief
- Good oral hygiene
- Recurrent bouts of tonsillitis may require surgical removal of the tonsils (tonsillectomy).

A peritonsillar abscess (quinsy) may develop, and patients may present with:

- An inflamed tonsil with swelling due to the collection of pus
- Worsening dysphagia often with an associated inability to swallow saliva
- Worsening pain on one side of the throat
- Trismus – an inability to open the mouth due to spasm of the jaw muscles.

This is considered a much more serious condition and is managed by needle aspiration (with antibiotic cover), surgical incision and drainage, or quinsy tonsillectomy (Galioto, 2017).

Tracheostomy

Tracheotomy is the surgical procedure of making an incision in the anterior tracheal wall for the purpose of creating an airway; a tracheostomy is the opening (stoma) that is created by the tracheotomy. Tracheostomies are created for several reasons:

- Relief of upper airways obstruction
- Protection of the lungs from the aspiration of food or regurgitation of the stomach contents

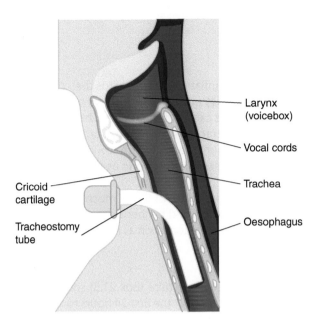

Larynx
(voicebox)

Vocal cords

Cricoid
cartilage

Trachea

Tracheostomy
tube

Oesophagus

Figure 21.5 Temporary tracheostomy.

- Respiratory insufficiency
- Long-term ventilation
- Following a laryngectomy.

Most tracheostomies are temporary, and a plastic or metal tube is inserted into the stoma to maintain the patency of the airway (Figure 21.5). Following a laryngectomy, the trachea is brought to the surface of the neck and a permanent stoma is formed.

Potential complications following tracheostomy include:

- Tube dislodgement – avoided by correctly securing the tube with tapes and sutures
- Tube obstruction – due to the build-up of secretions or the formation of a mucous plug, which is then coughed into the tube
- Surgical emphysema – the escape of air into the soft tissue of the neck, characterised by a 'crackling' sensation when palpated
- Pneumonia
- Tracheo-oesophageal fistula – created by excessive or prolonged inflation of a cuffed tracheostomy tube leading to necrosis of the tracheal wall and the development of a hole (fistula) between the trachea and the oesophagus; the fistula allows the entry of food and fluids into the lungs.

Early identification and intervention is crucial, with up to 50% of airway-related deaths post tracheostomy being due to tube displacement (Patton, 2019).

The care of a patient following the creation of a tracheostomy includes the following:

- Position the patient upright to reduce oedema formation.
- Frequent observations – Blood pressure, pulse, respirations and oxygen saturations should be noted every 15 minutes for the first 2 hours, then reducing to half-hourly for 2 hours and then hourly for 24 hours.

Box 21.3   Cuffed and uncuffed tracheostomy tubes

Cuffed tracheostomy tubes have an inflatable cuff towards their distal end; this is used to create an airtight seal in the trachea. They are generally used in patients who require a tracheostomy for ventilation (e.g. in intensive care) or for patients who are at risk of aspirating food or body fluids (e.g. immediately post-tracheostomy formation, there is a risk of bleeding from the operative site). Cuffed tracheostomy tubes have a low-pressure cuff, and therefore there is no requirement to deflate the cuff regularly so long as the pressure is checked with a pressure gauge.

Uncuffed tracheostomy tubes (as in Figure 21.5) are much more common. However, in the acute setting it is recommended that a cuffed tracheostomy tube of the correct size is kept by the bedside for use in an emergency situation (such as resuscitation).

- A low-pressure cuffed tracheostomy tube (Box 21.3) should be placed in the operating theatre and should be left inflated for the first 24 hours to reduce the chance of bleeding. To reduce the chance of pressure necrosis, the cuff pressure should be checked every 4 hours (NCEPOD, 2014). The correct cuff pressure is maintained by the use of a pressure gauge.
- Suctioning – This is dependent on patient requirements (patients will produce secretions at different rates), but indications include audible secretions, cyanosis, alterations in arterial blood gas results and reduced breath sounds (Patton, 2019). The type and quantity of the suctioned mucus should be monitored and recorded.
- Humidification – As the air entering the patient's lungs is no longer warmed and humidified by the upper airway, the provision of humidification is essential to prevent the formation of crusts which may block the tracheostomy tube (Mitchell *et al.*, 2013).
- Dressings should be kept clean and dry as wet dressings encourage the growth of bacteria and may lead to wound infections or, if inhaled, respiratory infections (Feber, 2006). However, a recent meta-analysis has suggested that moist dressings may be beneficial for wound care (Yiu *et al.*, 2019).

638

Red flag

Tracheostomy tube changes

The first tracheostomy tube change should be performed by a clinician experienced in tracheostomy care. All tracheostomy changes must involve two people, one of whom is experienced in tracheostomy care (Mitchell *et al.*, 2013).

Longer-term care of the patient with a tracheostomy is geared towards enabling the patient to perform their own care (including tube care, tube changes, suctioning and dressing changes).

Laryngectomy

Laryngectomy is the removal of the entire structure of the larynx (Figure 21.6) and is the treatment for advanced laryngeal cancer where partial laryngectomy is not possible (NICE, 2018).

Snapshot   Laryngectomy

John Derwent is a 47-year-old man who is being cared for on the ward having undergone a laryngectomy for cancer. He currently has a tracheostomy tube in place and is beginning to mobilise around the ward, though at present he is sat on the edge of the bed in a 'tripod position'. He is frequently visited by his wife and 13-year-old daughter, although his daughter does not seem keen to stay at the bedside and is often to be found in the day room whilst her mother stays at her father's bedside. Mr Derwent was a police officer and will not be returning to work as he has been advised to retire on health grounds. He is depressed and anxious about the future, but finds it hard to communicate and thus he can become quite frustrated.

On careful questioning, Mr Derwent reports that he feels that it is harder to breathe. On examination it was found that his tracheal tube has become encrusted with dried secretions. The inner tube was removed and changed for a new one easing airflow and improving Mr Derwent's ability to breathe. The need for humidification was reinforced to Mr Derwent as it appears that he does not like being attached to a 'pipe' as it upsets his daughter to see it. Nursing staff were also reminded that the inner tube of Mr Derwent's tracheostomy should be cleaned every two hours for the first 48 hours and every four hours after that.

Vital signs

The following vital signs were noted and recorded:

Vital sign	Observation	Normal
Temperature	37.0°C	36.0–37.9°C range
Pulse	82 beats per minute	60–100 beats per minute
Respiration	24 breaths per minute	12–20 breaths per minute
Blood pressure	155/90 mmHg	100–139 mmHg (systolic) range
O_2 saturation	92%	94%–98%

Take time to reflect on this case study and then consider the following:

1. What are Mr Derwent's immediate care needs on a daily basis?
2. What should be done to prepare Mr Derwent for his eventual discharge?
3. It is too early for Mr Derwent to begin using artificial speech, so what can be done to help him communicate in the short term?
4. Mr Derwent and his family have psychological needs. What are these and how could the family be aided in overcoming and adapting to the new situation?

During a laryngectomy, the trachea is brought to the surface of the neck and a permanent tracheostomy is formed through which the patient breathes; therefore, there is no connection between the mouth, nose and lungs. Immediately postoperatively, the stoma will be protected by a tracheostomy tube, and the care of the patient is similar to that of a patient with a temporary tracheostomy. The greater trauma to the trachea raises the risk of bleeding and oedema formation, and it is therefore common practice for oxygen saturations to be monitored with pulse oximetry continuously for 24 hours and then overnight for 2–3 days. Once the risk of bleeding and oedema formation has reduced, about 5–10 days

NEWS2

John Derwent

Physiological parameter	3	2	1	0	1	2	3
Respiration rate						24	
Oxygen saturation %		92					
Supplemental oxygen				No			
Temperature °C				37.0			
Systolic BP mmHg				155			
Heart rate				82			
Level of consciousness				A			
Score	0	2	0	0		2	0
Total	4						

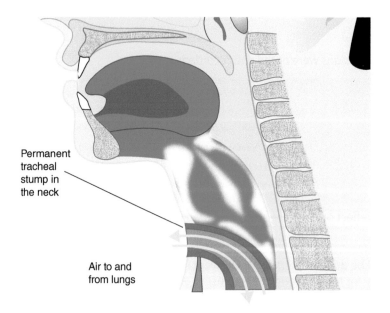

Permanent
tracheal
stump in
the neck

Air to and
from lungs

Figure 21.6   Laryngectomy.

postoperatively, the tracheostomy tube is removed and replaced with a silicone stoma button or stud to prevent the closure of the stoma as scar tissue forms (Feber, 2006). Patients are normally discharged 14 days postoperatively.The loss of the normal humidification and warming mechanisms of the mouth and nose will lead to the drying of the mucous lining of the lower respiratory tract and a significant increase in water loss via exhaled air. This leads to changes in respiratory mechanisms and a significantly increased risk of respiratory infections (Jackson *et al.*, 2019). The loss of moisture will lead to the creation of thick secretions and crust formation, which may completely block the stoma and thus threaten life. Humidification is essential for a laryngectomy patient, and once the patient is discharged, they must use a passive heat and moisture exchanger (HME) worn over the stoma; these are usually made of foam that traps the heat and moisture in expired air, which are then transferred into the inspired air.

The loss of the patient's voice following laryngectomy can have significant psychological effects, and several communication methods are available (Ruddy *et al.*, 2016):

- Voice prostheses (speaking valve) – A valve placed between the trachea and the oesophagus which diverts expired air into the oesophagus when the tracheostomy is manually blocked; thus, air passes into the mouth.
- Electrolarynx – A battery-powered device held against the mouth that creates speech with the use of sound waves.
- Artificial larynx – Similar to an electrolarynx except that the device is held to the neck rather than the mouth.
- Oesophageal speech – This involves the patient swallowing air, trapping it in the oesophagus and releasing it to create sound.

It is important that laryngectomy patients wear a medical alert bracelet identifying them as a 'neck breather' in the event of an emergency situation.

Laryngectomy is a procedure with lifelong implications; it leaves patients with lifelong disfigurement, disability and complex care needs (Bickford *et al.*, 2019). The need for social support, for instance, via laryngectomee clubs, helps patients to adjust to their new situation. A list of clubs can be found at https://www.laryngectomy.org.uk/.

Red flag

Hypoxia in laryngectomy patients
In the event of a hypoxic event in a patient who has undergone a laryngectomy, it is important that any airway management/ventilation is performed via the stoma (not the mouth) as normal airway patency no longer exists. However, in tracheostomy patients, the upper airway may be patent.

If specialist equipment is not immediately available, then oxygen can be delivered via a standard facemask turned sideways and held against the stoma.

If you are unsure if the patient has a tracheostomy or a laryngectomy, then it is advised that you apply oxygen to both the mouth and the stoma until expert staff arrive.

Orange flag

Anxiety
Patient anxiety before and after laryngectomy is very high. Patients will react in a variety of ways to anxiety, and it is important for the healthcare professional to remain calm and understanding. Whilst anxiety will reduce following the teaching and mastery of self-care, it will never completely resolve (Almonacid *et al.*, 2016). The levels of anxiety must also be viewed in the light of alterations of body image

Disorders of the eye
Cataracts
A cataract is opacity within the lens and has several causes (Liu *et al.*, 2017):

- Congenital
- Age related – occurring in patients over the age of 60 years

- Traumatic – penetrating or blunt trauma
- Toxic – radiation therapy or drugs such as topical steroids
- Secondary – to diseases of the eye or systemic disease such as diabetes mellitus.

Patients may report:

- Decrease in vision
- 'Misty vision'
- Abnormal colour perception
- Glare – dazzling by bright lights due to abnormal light refraction.

The treatment of cataracts is surgical and requires the removal of the diseased lens and replacement with a prosthetic lens (Liu *et al.*, 2017). The procedure is normally carried out under local anaesthetic, and the patient is given sedation. Postoperatively, the patient can be discharged the same day (Zhuang *et al.*, 2019). Post-operative self-care advice may include:

- Administration of antibiotic and steroid eye drops as prescribed
- Covering the eye with an eye patch and protective shield for 24 hours, then only at night
- Avoiding situations that increase intraocular pressure (stooping, coughing or lifting)
- A reduction in visual acuity in the immediate post-operative period is not unusual – it may take up to 2 weeks for vision to improve
- Once full healing has occurred (approximately 6–8 weeks), a prescription for glasses will be required as the prosthetic lens is not able to correct for near vision (e.g. reading).

Macular degeneration

Snapshot　Visual hallucinations and macular degeneration

Joyce Kirkpatrick is a 72-year-old widow who has been diagnosed with mild dementia, but otherwise she is fit and active. Recently, she has noticed that her eyesight is deteriorating, and she finds that she is unable to focus on objects that are in front of her and has to turn her head in order to 'catch them in the corner of my eye'. Joyce's family have been concerned as she is reporting 'being followed in the street' and people in her house. A recent visit to the optician led to a referral to the ophthalmologist at the local hospital. Amongst the tests performed, Mrs Kirkpatrick underwent fluorescein angiography. The ophthalmologist informed Mrs Kirkpatrick that she has macular degeneration in both eyes. The left eye has mostly dry macular degeneration, but the right eye has both wet and dry macular degeneration. The ophthalmologist has advised Joyce that there is little that can be done for the left eye at present, but she can help prevent the condition from worsening. The ophthalmologist has also advised Mrs Kirkpatrick that a treatment is available for the wet macular degeneration which involves injecting a drug into the eye, but it is still quite new and expensive so permission to use the treatment will need to be sought from the local health authority. Unfortunately, visual hallucinations are common in older people with visual problems (Gordon, 2016), and there is no treatment that can be offered except reassurance and reorientation.

Take some time to reflect on this case and then consider the following:

1. What is the treatment the ophthalmologist is referring to for the treatment of the wet macular degeneration?
2. What can Mrs Kirkpatrick do to help prevent her macular degeneration from worsening?
3. What support groups are available to help Mrs Kirkpatrick with her condition?
4. Mrs Kirkpatrick lives alone and would like to continue living in her house. What changes to the home could be made to maintain her safety and independence?

Fluorescein angiography

Otherwise known as fundus fluorescein angiography, this test involves the injection of dye into the veins via a peripheral cannula. The dye rapidly spreads throughout the circulation, and photographs are then taken of the back of the eye using a specialised camera which is filtered to record only yellow-green light from the fluorescence. This gives a detailed picture of the blood vessels. This test is especially useful in diagnosing wet macular degeneration.

The test takes about 10–15 minutes, and patients are asked to remain in the department for 30 minutes afterwards and may not drive for 2 hours afterwards.

Side effects of the test are usually rare and include transient nausea, itching skin or a rash. Very rarely the patient may have an anaphylactic reaction to the dye, and this is dealt with according to standard hospital guidelines.

A new, non-invasive, procedure called optical coherence tomography (OCT) angiography is becoming increasingly common. Using no dye, the potential side effects of anaphylaxis and itching are removed, and no intravenous access is required (Mitchell *et al.*, 2018).

643

Macular degeneration is characterised by a gradual loss of central vision, but peripheral vision is maintained. There are two types of macular degeneration:

1. Dry macular degeneration – Associated with small, round, white yellow areas (drusens) in the macula. There is no treatment available, but progression is slow and thus sight loss is limited. Some lifestyle changes can be made to help reduce the deterioration and possible progression to wet macular degeneration, e.g. protecting the eyes from UV light, eating a healthy diet rich in antioxidants and stopping smoking.
2. Wet macular degeneration (neurovascular) – Caused by the development of abnormal blood vessels below the retina. All patients with wet macular degeneration will have had dry macular degeneration first. Current treatments are controversial and include dietary changes to include high levels of vitamins C and E, beta-carotene and zinc (Mukhtar and Ambati, 2019). A small number of patients may be suitable for photodynamic therapy (PDT) (Mitchell *et al.*, 2019), which involves the injection of a dye into the blood vessels; subsequent excitation of the dye by a 'cold' laser (which does not damage the retina) coagulates the targeted blood vessels. Increasingly, drug therapies (antivascular endothelial growth factor) are being developed and are becoming more common in clinical use (Mitchell *et al.*, 2019).

Glaucoma

Glaucoma is a term relating to a series of disorders characterised by (Davis *et al.*, 2016):

- Increased intraocular pressure (IOP)
- Optic nerve atrophy
- Loss of peripheral vision – 'tunnel vision'.

Loss of vision is related to a loss of balance in the generation and reabsorption of aqueous humour; the subsequent rise in IOP damages the head of the optic nerve.
Treatment is dependent on the particular type of glaucoma (Conlon *et al.*, 2017):

- Open angle glaucoma – The mechanisms for the drainage of aqueous humour become blocked. The onset is subtle and without symptoms until the patient finally notices the loss of peripheral vision, by which time the visual loss is usually large (Weinreb *et al.*, 2014). Primary treatment is the reduction of IOP with eye drops. Laser treatment is effective in the short term, but surgery remains the main option for treatment.
- Acute closed angle glaucoma – The lens bulges forward and restricts aqueous humour drainage. The onset is rapid and the patient may report:
  - Headaches
  - Nausea and vomiting
  - Eye pain
  - Blurred vision.

Medicines management

Some of the medications used for reducing IOP can cause systematic problems. This is especially true of beta blockers, which can be problematic for people with asthma, COPD or heart rhythm disturbances.

If the patient blinks rapidly after the instillation of eye drops, the medication can be drained from the eye into the throat and then absorbed into the systemic circulation

When there is a need to prevent eye drops from entering the systemic circulation, the patient can be advised to either keep the eyelid shut for two minutes or to put pressure near the inside corner of the eye for two minutes with a finger (this is known as punctal occlusion). Either method reduces the drainage of the tears and reduces the amount of medication being drained away before it has been absorbed by the eye.

Acute closed angle glaucoma is an ocular emergency and requires immediate medical attention. The patient will require laser iridotomy (creation of a hole in the iris) as a matter of urgency.
Care includes:

- Caring for the patient in a quiet, darkened, environment
- Providing vomit bowls, tissues and mouth washes as required
- Administering analgesia as prescribed
- Cold compresses to the forehead to reduce pain
- Administering of prescribed drugs, including an intravenous infusion of mannitol, anti-emetics and eye drops
- Reassurance and explanation.

Orange flag

Glaucoma and depression

Depression is a common but underdiagnosed co-morbidity found alongside glaucoma. Whilst an obvious mechanism is related to the loss of vision and the loss of role and independence leading to depression, there are some theories related to the reduced absorption of light leading to a reduction in the synthesis of melatonin and thus causing sleep disturbance and depression (Jeong *et al.*, 2016).

Retinal detachment

Retinal detachment is the detachment of the neural layer from the rest of the retina. Patients may experience:

- Flashing lights
- Floaters – small dark particles in the vision caused by small haemorrhages
- Loss of vision – related to the area of detachment.

Treatment is with surgery:

- Laser therapy or photocoagulation is used to seal tears or holes in the retina and prevent the further accumulation of subretinal fluid, which would otherwise make the detachment worse.
- Plombage (scleral buckling) – A small square of material is sutured onto the sclera over the site of the hole, thus pushing the retinal layers back together.
- Encirclement – A silicone band is placed around the eyeball. This is used where there is a large area of detachment or multiple holes.
- Vitrectomy (Pars plana vitrectomy) – Removal of the vitreous humour, allowing the surgeon better access to the tear. Cryotherapy or laser therapy is then used to heal the break. The vitreous is then replaced with gas or fluid to splint the retina in place. Post-operative positioning is vital to ensure that the gas or fluid remains in the correct place. If a gas is used, then the patient must not fly until given permission by a doctor as changes in pressure can cause increased IOP. The most commonly used gas is air, but other gases are used (such as perfluoropropane). The gas will remain in place for 2–12 weeks and will be gradually replaced by vitreous humour over that time. If fluid (such as silicone based oil) is used, then this will need to be removed at a later date.
- Pneumatic retinopexy – Injecting a gas into the vitreous humour. The gas expands in place, pushing the retina back in place. The break is treated with cryotherapy before the gas is injected or laser therapy after the retina has flattened in place.

Subretinal fluid is drained during all these procedures to allow the separated layers to come into contact again.

Patient care includes:

- Bed rest to prevent further detachment occurring before and after surgery.
- The patient may be required to rest in a position that causes the detachment to lie against the underlying layers and also encourage the subretinal fluid to be reabsorbed.
- Analgesia – Patients will experience eye pain after surgery.
- Eye care – The eyelids and conjunctiva are usually swollen after surgery.

645

Medicines management

Other than air, the most commonly used gases in vitrectomy and pneumatic retinopexy can interact with nitrous oxide (used as pain relief in childbirth and for pain relief in emergency situations). It is important that midwives and any emergency healthcare practitioners are informed of the gas in the eye so that they avoid the use of nitrous oxide. If the patient requires a general anaesthetic, it is important that the anaesthetist is informed.

Retinopathy

The leading cause of retinopathy in the UK is diabetes mellitus (Khan *et al.*, 2017). It can be divided into two types:

1. Non-proliferative retinopathy – Aneurysms of the capillaries of the eyes, retinal haemorrhages and hardened exudates of lipids.
2. Proliferative retinopathy – The retina has become ischaemic, and in response there is a development of new blood vessels in the eye; however, new blood vessels are fragile and have a tendency to bleed. These blood vessels also grow into the vitreous humour. Eventually, fibrous bands develop which pull on the retina and cause retinal detachment.

Treatment of retinopathy includes:

- Control of cholesterol levels.
- Advice on diet and glycaemic control.
- Laser therapy to the retina – Dead retinal tissue does not encourage new blood vessel formation. Therefore, a laser beam is used to create multiple small areas of dead retinal tissue (scotomas), which will not have an effect on vision but will reduce the growth of new blood vessels.
- Vitrectomy – Removal of the vitreous humour; this removes blood vessels and haemorrhages. Vitreous humour is not naturally replaced by the body; however, replacement with aqueous humour will occur.

646

Conclusion

Disorders of the senses can lead to the loss of the ability to maintain the activities of daily living and may even threaten life. When faced with these possibilities, the patient will often be anxious and frightened. In this situation, being cared for by a professional with knowledge of both the condition and the care required will help the patient to overcome these feelings. This chapter has introduced the reader to the physiology of the eye, ear, nose and throat and some of the conditions associated with these structures. Knowledge of the physiology and the associated conditions of these structures enables the healthcare professional to deliver care that is safe and effective. Whilst this chapter cannot hope to cover all the conditions associated with the special senses and the throat, it gives the reader a firm base from which to deliver competent and knowledgeable care and to develop their knowledge in these fascinating areas.

Activities

Here are some activities and exercises to help test your learning. For the answers to these exercises, as well as further self-testing activities, visit our website at
www.wiley.com/go/fundamentalsofappliedpathophysiology/student4e

Multiple choice questions

1. The tympanic membrane is composed of a variety of tissues including:
   (a) Epithelial cells
   (b) Connective tissues
   (c) Mucous membrane
   (d) All of the above
2. The main organ of hearing is:
   (a) The semicircular canals
   (b) The oval window
   (c) The cochlea
   (d) The eustachian tube
3. How many turbinates are contained within each side of the internal nose?
   (a) 1
   (b) 2
   (c) 3
   (d) 4
4. The tonsils are made of how many collections of lymphatic nodules?
   (a) 3
   (b) 4
   (c) 5
   (d) 6
5. The lubricating mucus that prevents the eye from drying out is produced by:
   (a) The sclera
   (b) The conjunctiva
   (c) The cornea
   (d) The zonule
6. Nutrition is supplied to the tunics of the eye by:
   (a) The choroid
   (b) The ciliary body
   (c) The retina
   (d) The vitreous humour
7. A cerumenolytic is:
   (a) A type of antibiotic
   (b) A steroid type of medication
   (c) A substance that breaks down wax
   (d) A substance that coats the ear canal
8. When treating otitis media, nasal decongestants are useful because
   (a) They reduce the inflammation in the eustachian tube
   (b) They reduce the production of the mucus
   (c) The infection is mostly based in the nose
   (d) They reduce pain
9. The treatment to cure otosclerosis is:
   (a) Steroid medications
   (b) Antibiotics
   (c) Surgery
   (d) All of the above

10. Immediately following ear surgery, the patient should be placed:
    (a) Feet down
    (b) Head down
    (c) Flat
    (d) Head up
11. Nasal polyps are caused by:
    (a) Cancer
    (b) Trauma
    (c) Infection
    (d) Oedema
12. The most common cause of death in patients with a tracheostomy is:
    (a) Surgical emphysema
    (b) Infection
    (c) Tube displacement
    (d) A fistula
13. Optical coherence tomography (OCT) is a replacement for which test?
    (a) Fluorescein angiography
    (b) Retinal photography
    (c) Snellen test
    (d) Tonometry
14. Plombage is
    (a) Suturing material over a retinal hole
    (b) Removal of vitreous humour
    (c) Placing a rubber band around the eyeball
    (d) Injecting gas into the vitreous humour
15. In macular degeneration, which vision is lost?
    (a) Peripheral
    (b) Colour
    (c) Central
    (d) All vision

Conditions

The following is a list of conditions that are associated with the ear, nose, throat and eyes. Take some time and write notes about each of the conditions. You may make the notes taken from textbooks or other resources (e.g. people you work with in a clinical area), or you may make the notes based on people you have cared for. If you are making notes about people you have cared, for you must ensure that you adhere to the rules of confidentiality.

Nasal polyps	
Stridor	

Ménière's disease	
Cataracts	
Eye infections	

Further resources

National Tracheostomy Safety Project

http://www.tracheostomy.org.uk/e-learning
This is a free multimedia course on the care of the patient with a tracheostomy.

Royal National Institute of Blind People

www.rnib.org.uk
This website is of interest to all health professionals. There is information on how to help patients with
poor vision in any setting, resource pages on various conditions (some produced in conjunction
with the Royal College of Ophthalmologists) and patient stories to help you understand the real
impact of sight loss.

The National Association of Laryngectomee Clubs

www.laryngectomy.org.uk
This site has a useful glossary of terms related to laryngectomy and a wide range of leaflets for professionals and patients.

The Royal College of Ophthalmologists

www.rcophth.ac.uk
This website has a large electronic library both for professionals and the public. You will find many
eye-related disorders explained here as well as information on eye health.

Sign Station

www.signstation.org
This is an interactive website that helps you to understand British Sign Language (BSL). It is free to
register and registered users can access the BSL dictionary, view video scenarios on dealing with
deaf people and take a free online course to learn the basics of BSL.

Glossary of terms

Aneurysm   A localised dilatation of the wall of a blood vessel, usually the aorta or the arteries
at the base of the brain.

Anticholinergic   A drug that blocks the action of acetylcholine and thus inhibits the transmission or effect of parasympathetic nerve action.

Anti-emetic   A drug that reduces nausea and vomiting.

Antihistamine   A drug that inhibits the effect of histamines.

Antipyretic   A drug that can reduce high temperatures (e.g. paracetamol, aspirin, ibuprofen).

Aspiration   Inhalation of a foreign body (such as food).

Atrophy   Wasting away; a diminution in the size of a cell, tissue or organ.

Aural   Related to the ear.

Cannula   A flexible tube containing a stiff, pointed trocar. Once inserted into the body, the trocar is removed, allowing fluid to pass along the cannula.

Cartilage   A type of connective tissue that contains collagen and elastic fibres. This strong tough material on the bone ends helps to distribute the load within the joint; the slippery surface allows smooth movement between the bones. Cartilage can withstand both tension and compression.

Cauterisation   Coagulation of tissues by heat or caustic substances.

Cilia   Small, hair-like processes on the outer surface of some cells; used to propel liquids.

Coagulation   The process of transforming a liquid into a solid (especially blood) or the hardening of tissue by physical means.

Congenital   Present at birth, rather than acquired during life.

Connective tissue   A primary tissue characterised by cells separated by a matrix; supports and binds other body tissue.

Distal   Away from the beginning.

Dysphagia   Difficulty in swallowing.

Epithelial cell   A cell that covers the internal and external organs of the body.

Exudate   Escaping fluid that spills from a space; contains cellular debris and pus.

Facial palsy   Paralysis of some or all of the muscles of the face.

Fistula   An abnormal passage from an internal organ to the surface of the skin or between two organs.

Foley catheter   A rubber catheter with an inflatable balloon tip.

Glycaemic control   The control of blood sugar levels.

Haemorrhage   Bleeding.

Hereditary   Transmitted from parent to child.

Humidification   Increasing the water content of inhaled air.

Hypertension   Raised blood pressure.

Hypovolaemia   Low levels of fluid in the circulation.

Intracranial   Within the skull.

Intraocular pressure   Pressure within the eye.

Ischaemia   A low oxygen state in a part of the body. Usually the result of obstruction to the blood supply to tissues.

Laxative   A drug that promotes evacuation of the bowel.

Ligation   Tying off a blood vessel to stop or prevent bleeding.

Lipid   An energy-rich organic compound that is soluble in organic substances such as alcohol and benzene.

Lymph node   Part of the lymphatic system; it contains many white cells to destroy bacteria that are trapped within the lymph node.

Malaise   A feeling of body weakness.

Mucosa   Mucous membrane.

Mucous membrane   Thin sheet of tissue lining a part of the body that secretes mucus. Cover all the passageways leading into or out of the body (e.g. the mouth, nose, bronchi, urethra).

Mucus   The secretions of mucous membranes.

Necrosis   Tissue death.

Needle aspiration   The removal of fluid by a fine needle.

Neurological   Pertaining to the nervous system.

Olfactory   Pertaining to the sense of smell.

Opacity   Referring to the opaque quality of a substance.

Opaque   Does not allow the passage of light.

Palpation   Using the fingers or hands to examine by touch.

Pneumonia   A condition characterised by acute inflammation of the lungs.

Polyp (plural polypi)   Abnormal growth of tissue projecting from a mucous membrane.

Postnasal pack   Packing the upper nasopharynx with gauze or sponge to prevent the flow of blood into the nasopharynx. Also provides a firm base against which to pack the nasal cavity if required.

Pressure necrosis   Tissue death caused by prolonged or excessive pressure.

Prosthesis   An artificial replacement for a missing part of the body.

Pulse oximetry   Non-invasive measurement of the oxygen content of the blood (SpO_2).

Purulent   Producing or containing pus.

Pus   A thick green or cream fluid found at the site of a bacterial infection. It consists of millions of dead white blood cells of the immune system as well as dead bacteria.

Pyrexia   Elevated temperature associated with fever.

Regurgitation   The return of swallowed food to the mouth.

Respiratory insufficiency   Inability to breathe due to weakness of the muscles of respiration.

Sac   A pouch.

651

Secondary bacterial infection   A bacterial infection following viral infection.

Sedation   State of calm or sleepiness brought about by drugs.

Semi-recumbent   Reclining position.

Stoma   Any opening; a mouth. Usually used to refer to a surgically created opening.

Suture   Stitch.

Syringing   The procedure of introducing a fluid into a cavity to flush out debris or foreign bodies.

Tinnitus   Ringing noise in the ear.

Trocar   A sharp pointed rod that fits inside a tube (cannula).

Vertigo   Dizziness.

Visual acuity   Detailed central vision.

References

Aaron, K., Cooper, T.E., Warner, L. and Burton, M.J. (2018). Ear drops for the removal of ear wax. *Cochrane Database of Systematic Reviews*, (7).

Almonacid, C.I.F., Ramos, A.J. and Rodríguez-Borrego, M.A. (2016). Level of anxiety versus self-care in the preoperative and postoperative periods of total laryngectomy patients. *Revista latino-americana de enfermagem*, 24.

Batson, L. and Rizzolo, D. (2017). Otosclerosis: An update on diagnosis and treatment. *Journal of the American Academy of PAs*, 30(2): 17–22.

Behere, P.B., Das, A. and Behere, A.P. (2019). Antiepileptics. In *Clinical Psychopharmacology*. Springer, Singapore, pp. 117–130.

Bickford, J., Coveney, J., Baker, J. and Hersh, D. (2019). Validating the changes to self-identity after total laryngectomy. *Cancer Nursing*, 42(4): 314–322.

Cheshire, W.P. and Goldstein, D.S. (2019). Autonomic uprising: The tilt table test in autonomic medicine. *Clinical Autonomic Research*, 29(2): 215–230.

Conlon, R., Saheb, H. and Ahmed, I.I.K. (2017). Glaucoma treatment trends: A review. *Canadian Journal of Ophthalmology*, 52(1): 114–124.

Davis, B. M., Crawley, L., Pahlitzsch, M., Javaid, F. and Cordeiro, M.F. (2016). Glaucoma: the retina and beyond. *Acta Neuropathologica*, 132(6): 807–826.

Demarcantonio, M.A. and Han, J.K. (2011). Nasal polyps: Pathogenesis and treatment implications. *Otolaryngologic Clinics of North America.* 44(3): 685–695.

Feber, T. (2006). Tracheostomy care for community nurses: Basic principles. *British Journal of Community Nursing.* 11(5): 186–193.

Galioto, N.J. (2017). Peritonsillar abscess. *American Family Physician*, 95(8): 501–506.

Gordon, K.D. (2016). Prevalence of visual hallucinations in a national low vision client population. *Canadian Journal of Ophthalmology*, 51(1): 3–6.

Hall, J. and Hall, M. (2020). *Guyton and Hall Textbook of Medical Physiology*, 14th edn. Philadelphia: Elsevier Saunders.

Jackson, C., Grigg, C., Green, M. and Grigg, R. (2019). Care of laryngectomy stomas in general practice. *Australian Journal of General Practice,* 48(6): 373.

Jeong, A.R., Kim, C.Y., Kang, M.H. and Kim, N.R. (2016). Psychological aspects of glaucoma. *The Journal of Nervous and Mental Disease*, 204(3): 217–220.

Khan, A., Petropoulos, I. N., Ponirakis, G. and Malik, R.A. (2017). Visual complications in diabetes mellitus: Beyond retinopathy. *Diabetic Medicine*, 34(4): 478–484.

Laulajainen-Hongisto, A., Jero, J., Markkola, A., Saat, R. and Aarnisalo, A.A. (2016). Severe acute otitis media and acute mastoiditis in adults. *Journal of International Advanced Otology*, 12(3): 224–230.

Lewis, S.L., Bucher, L. Heitkemper, M.M., Harding M.M. and Kwong, J. (2016). *Medical – Surgical Nursing: Assessment and Management of Clinical Problems*, 10th edn. St Louis: Mosby Elsevier.

Liu, Y.C., Wilkins, M., Kim, T., Malyugin, B. and Mehta, J.S. (2017). Cataracts. *The Lancet*, 390(10094): 600–612.

Marieb, E.N. and Hoehn, K. (2018). *Human Anatomy and Physiology*, 11th edn. San Francisco: Pearson Benjamin Cummings.

Mitchell, R.B., Hussey, H.M., Setzen, G., Jacobs, I.N., Nussenbaum, B. *et al.* (2013). Clinical consensus statement tracheostomy care. *Otolaryngology – Head and Neck Surgery*, 148(1): 6–20.

Mitchell, P., Liew, G., Gopinath, B. and Wong, T.Y. (2018). Age-related macular degeneration. *The Lancet*, 392(10153): 1147–1159.

Mukhtar, S. and Ambati, B.K. (2019). The value of nutritional supplements in treating Age-Related Macular Degeneration: A review of the literature. *International Ophthalmology*, 1–9.

National Confidential Enquiry into Patient Outcome and Death (NCEPOD). (2014). *On the Right Trach? A Review of the Care Received by Patients Who Underwent a Tracheostomy*. London: NCEPOD

National Institute for Health and Care Excellence (NICE) (2018). *NG:36 Cancer of the Upper Aerodigestive Tract: Assessment and Management in People #aged 16 and Over*. London: NICE.

Palleria, C., Cozza, G., Khengar, R., Libri, V. and De Sarro, G. (2017). Safety profile of the newest antiepileptic drugs: a curated literature review. *Current Pharmaceutical Design*, 23(37): 5606–5624.

Patton, J. (2019). Tracheostomy care. *British Journal of Nursing*, 28(16): 1060–1062.

Roditi, R.E., Caradonna, D.S. and Shin, J.J. (2019). The proposed usage of intranasal steroids and antihistamines for otitis media with effusion. *Current Allergy and Asthma Reports*, 19(10): 47.

Rosenfeld, R.M., Piccirillo, J.F., Chandrasekhar, S.S., Brook, I., Kumar, K.A. *et al.* (2015). Clinical practice guideline (update) adult sinusitis. *Otolaryngology – Head and Neck Surgery.* 152(Suppl. 2): S1–S39.

Ruddy, B. H., Lewis, V. and Sapienza, C. (2016). *Rehabilitation of the laryngectomized individual: alaryngeal communication options. Cases in Head and Neck Cancer: A Multidisciplinary Approach*, 219.

Schilder, A.G., Chonmaitree, T., Cripps, A.W., Rosenfeld, R.M., Casselbrant, M.L. *et al.* (2016). Otitis media. *Nature Reviews Disease Primers*, 2(1): 1–18.

Schwartz, S.R., Magit, A.E., Rosenfeld, R.M., Ballachanda, B.B., Hackell, J.M. *et al.* (2017). Clinical practice guideline (update): earwax (cerumen impaction). *Otolaryngology–Head and Neck Surgery*, 156(1_Suppl): S1–S29.

Sood, A.J., Lambert, P.R., Nguyen, S.A. and Meyer, T.A. (2014). Endolymphatic sac surgery for Meniere's disease: A systematic review and meta-analysis. *Otology & Neurotology*, 35(6): 1033–1045.

Tikka, T. (2016). The aetiology and management of epistaxis. *Otolaryngology Online Journal*. Available from: http://www.alliedacademies.org/articles/the-aetiology-and-management-of-epistaxis.html) Accessed 10th June 2020.

Wiegand, S., Berner, R., Schneider, A., Lundershausen, E. and Dietz, A. (2019). Otitis Externa: Investigation and evidence-based treatment. *Deutsches Ärzteblatt International*, 116(13): 224.

Weinreb, R.N., Aung, T. and Medeiros, F.A. (2014). The pathophysiology and treatment of glaucoma: A review. *JAMA*, 311(18): 1901–1911.

Yaneza, M.M. and Amiraraghi, N. (2018). Epistaxis. *Surgery (Oxford)*, 36(10): 543–552.

Yue, M., Lei, M., Liu, Y. and Gui, N. (2019). The application of moist dressings in wound care for tracheostomy patients: A meta-analysis. *Journal of Clinical Nursing*, 28(15–16): 2724–2731.

Zhuang, M., Fan, W., Xie, P., Yuan, S.T., Liu, Q.H. and Zhao, C. (2019). Evaluation of the safety and quality of day-case cataract surgery based on 4151 cases. *International Journal of Ophthalmology*, 12(2): 291.

Appendix A

Reference values in venous serum (adults)

Analysis	Reference range	
	SI units	Non-SI units
Albumin	36–47 g/L	3.6–4.7 g/100 mL
Alkaline phosphatase	40–125 U/L	–
Amylase	<100 U/L	–
Bilirubin (total)	2–17 μmol/L	0.12–1.0 mg/100 mL
Calcium	2.12–2.62 mmol/L	4.24–5.24 mEq/L or 8.50–10.50 mg/100 mL
Chloride	95–107 mmol/L	95–107 mEq/L
Cholesterol (total)	<5.5 mmol/L	–
HDL-cholesterol		
Male	0.5–1.6 mmol/L	19–62 mg/100 mL
Female	0.6–1.9 mmol/L	23–74 mg/100 mL
Copper	13–24 μmol/L	83–153 μg/100 mL
Creatine kinase (total)		
Male	30–200 U/L	–
Female	30–150 U/L	–
Creatinine	55–120 μmol/L	0.62–1.36 mg/100 mL
Ferritin		
Male	17–300 μg/L	17–300 ng/mL
Female	14–150 μg/L	14–150 ng/mL
Glucose (fasting)	3.6–5.8 mmol/L	65–104 mg/100 mL
Glycated haemoglobin (HbA$_1$)	5.0–6.5%	–
Immunoglobulin A	0.5–4.0 g/L	50–400 mg/100 mL
Immunoglobulin G	5.0–13.0 g/L	500–1300 mg/100 mL
Immunoglobulin M		

Fundamentals of Applied Pathophysiology: An Essential Guide for Nursing and Healthcare Students, Fourth Edition. Edited by Ian Peate.
© 2021 John Wiley & Sons Ltd. Published 2021 by John Wiley & Sons Ltd.
Student companion website: www.wiley.com/go/fundamentalsofappliedpathophysiology/student4e
Instructor companion website: www.wiley.com/go/fundamentalsofappliedpathophysiology/instructor4e

Analysis	Reference range	
	SI units	Non-SI units
Male	0.3–2.2 g/L	30–220 mg/100 mL
Female	0.4–2.5 g/L	40–250 mg/100 mL
Iron		
Male	14–32 µmol/L	78–178 µg/100 mL
Female	10–28 µmol/L	56–156 µg/100 mL
Magnesium	0.75–1.0 mmol/L	1.5–2.0 mEq/L or 1.82–2.43 mg/100 mL
Osmolality	280–290 mmol/kg	280–290 mOsm/L
Phosphate (fasting)	0.8–1.4 mmol/L	2.48–4.34 mg/100 mL
Potassium (plasma)	3.3–4.7 mmol/L	3.3–4.7 mEq/L
Potassium (serum)	3.6–5.1 mmol/L	3.6–5.1 mEq/L
Protein (total)	60–80 g/L	6–8 g/100 mL
Sodium	132–144 mmol/L	132–144 mEq/L
Total CO_2	24–30 mmol/L	24–30 mEq/L
Transferrin	2.0–4.0 g/L	0.2–0.4 g/100 mL
Triglycerides (fasting)	0.6–1.7 mmol/L	53–150 mg/100 mL
Urate		
Male	0.12–0.42 mmol/L	2.0–7.0 mg/100 mL
Female	0.12–0.36 mmol/L	2.0–6.0 mg/100 mL
Urea	2.5–6.6 mmol/L	15–40 mg/100 mL
Zinc	11–22 µmol/L	72–144 µg/100 mL
Haematological values		
Bleeding time (Ivy)	Less than 8 min	–
Body fluid (total)	50% (obese) to 70% (lean) of body weight	–
Intracellular	30–40% of body weight	–
Extracellular	20–30% of body weight	–
Blood volume		
Male	75 ± 10 mL/kg	–
Female	70 ± 10 mL/kg	–
Coagulation screen		
Prothrombin time	8.0–10.5 s	–
Activated partial thromboplastin time	26–37 s	–
Erythrocyte sedimentation rate[a]		
Adult male	0–10 mm/h	–
Adult female	3–15 mm/h	–
Fibrinogen	1.5–4.0 g/L	0.15–0.4 g/100 mL
Folate		

(Continued)

Analysis	Reference range	
	SI units	Non-SI units
Serum	1.5–20.6 µg/L	1.5–20.6 ng/mL
Red cell	95–570 µg/L	95–570 ng/mL
Haemoglobin		
Male	130–180 g/L	13–18 g/100 mL
Female	115–165 g/L	11.5–16.5 g/100 mL
Leucocytes (adults)	$4.0–11.0 \times 10^9$/L	$4.0–11.0 \times 10^3$/mm³
Differential white cell count		
Neutrophil granulocytes	$2.0–7.5 \times 10^9$/L	$2.0–7.5 \times 10^3$/mm³
Lymphocytes	$1.5–4.0 \times 10^9$/L	$1.5–4.0 \times 10^3$/mm³
Monocytes	$0.2–0.8 \times 10^9$/L	$0.2–0.8 \times 10^3$/mm³
Eosinophil granulocytes	$0.04–0.4 \times 10^9$/L	$0.04–0.4 \times 10^3$/mm³
Basophil granulocytes	$0.01–0.1 \times 10^9$/L	$0.01–0.1 \times 10^3$/mm³
Packed cell volume (PCV) or haematocrit		
Male	0.40–0.54	–
Female	0.37–0.47	–
Platelets	$150–350 \times 10^9$/L	$150–350 \times 10^3$/mm³
Red cell count		
Male	$4.5–6.5 \times 10^{12}$/L	$4.5–6.5 \times 10^6$/mm³
Female	$3.8–5.8 \times 10^{12}$/L	$3.8–5.8 \times 10^6$/mm³
Red cell lifespan (mean)	120 days	–
Red cell lifespan T½ (^{51}Cr)	25–35 days	–
Reticulocytes (adults)	$25–85 \times 10^9$/L	$25–85 \times 10^3$/mm³
Vitamin B_{12}	130–770 pg/mL	–

[a] Higher values in older patients are not necessarily abnormal.

Index

Note: Page numbers are in *italics* for illustrations/figures and **bold** for tables

A

allodynia, 534
abducens nerve, **157**
A-beta fibres, 504, **504**
ablation, 497. *See also* endometrial
    ablation
ABO blood groups, *263,* 263–264
absorption, 395
ACE inhibitors, *see* angiotensin-
    converting enzyme inhibitors
acetylcholine, 182
acidaemia, 460
acid–base balance, 255, 296, 570
acid phosphatase, 491
acid reflux, 380–381
acinar cells, 439
acquired immunity, 125
actin, 262, 563
active immunity, 125
active transport, 25, 45
acupuncture, 511, 526
acute closed angle glaucoma, 648
acute eczema, 610
acute kidney injury, 305–309
    care and management, 308
    case study, 309
    investigations, 307
    pathophysiology, 305–306, **306**
    pharmacological interventions, 308
    signs and symptoms, 307
    staging, 307–308, **308**
acute lymphoblastic leukaemia (ALL),
        79–83, 279
    bone marrow biopsy, *81*
    case study, 79–81
    causes, 82
    neutropenia, 82
    prognosis, 83
    treatment, 83
    vital signs, 80
acute myeloid leukaemia (AML), 279
acute pancreatitis, 388–390
    gallstones, 389–390

care and management, 389
pathophysiology, 388
signs and symptoms, 389
acute pyelonephritis, 301–303
    care and management, 302
    investigations, 302
    pharmacological interventions, 303
    signs and symptoms, 302
Adam's apple, 627
Addison's disease, 447–450, *448*
    thyroid function tests in
        undiagnosed, 451
Addison's Disease Self-Help Group,
        459
A-delta fibres, 504, **504,** 511
adenohypophysis, *433*
adenoma, 460
adenopathy, 91
adenosine diphosphate (ADP), 25,
        46, 249
adenosine triphosphate (ATP), 25, 46,
        288, 460
adipose tissue, 40
adjuvant, 624
adrenal crisis, 450
adrenal glands
    anatomy, *436*
    cortex, 436, *436,* 437–439
    disorders, 447–452
    insufficiency, 448–452. *See also*
        adrenal insufficiency
    medulla, *436,* 436–437
    physiology, 436–439
adrenal insufficiency, 448–452
    adrenal crisis, 450
    case study, 450–452
    Cushing's disease, *447,* 447–448
    primary, 448, *448*
    secondary, 448, *448*
    signs and symptoms, 449
    treatment, 449–450
    types, 448, *448*
adrenalitis, 460

adrenocorticotropic hormone (ACTH),
        434, 437, 451
aerobic, 150
aerobic respiration, 47
aetiology, 213
Age UK, 591
agglutination, 288
agranulocytes, 260
albumin, 255
alcohol consumption, 409
    cancer, 71
    folate deficiency, 269
aldosterone, 437, *438,* 534, 572
Alexander technique, 526, 534
alkaloid, 91
allele, 91
allergen, 125
allergy, 125
allodynia, 513
Alopecia UK, 617
alteplase, 169
alveolar sac, 213
Alzheimer's disease (AD), 173–175
    care and management, 173
    non-pharmacological
        management, 174
    pathophysiology, 173–174
    pharmacological management, 174
    stages, **174**
amantadine (Symmetrel), in
        Parkinson's disease, 172
amenorrhoea, 478–481
    care and management, 479
    diagnosis, 479
    vital signs, 480–481
American College of Rheumatology,
        563
amiloride (Midamar), 232
amine, 591
amino acid, 460
amino acids, 46, 402
amitriptyline (Elavil), in multiple
        sclerosis, 176

Fundamentals of Applied Pathophysiology: An Essential Guide for Nursing and Healthcare Students, Fourth Edition. Edited by Ian Peate.
© 2021 John Wiley & Sons Ltd. Published 2021 by John Wiley & Sons Ltd.
Student companion website: www.wiley.com/go/fundamentalsofappliedpathophysiology/student4e
Instructor companion website: www.wiley.com/go/fundamentalsofappliedpathophysiology/instructor4e

amphiarthrosis, 543
amputation, 534
amrinone, for shock, **146**
amyotrophic lateral sclerosis, 356
anaemia, 91, 265–277, 356
    aplastic, 271–273
    haemolytic, 274–275
    iron deficiency, 266–269
    macrocytic, 269–271
    microcytic, 266
    normocytic, 271
    sickle cell, 275–277
anaerobic, 150
anaerobic metabolism, 206, 213
anaerobic respiration, 47
analgesic, 534
analgesic ladder, 525–526
anaphase, 29, *29*, 31
anaphylactic shock (anaphylaxis),
       136–137, 151, 264
    causes, **137, 140**
    signs and symptoms, 136–137
    stages, *137*
anastomosis, 395
anatomical planes, 5, *5*
anatomical regions, 6
    of head and neck, **6**
    of lower limbs (leg), **7**
    of trunk, **6**
    of upper limbs, **7**
anatomy
    anatomical planes, 5, *5*
    anatomical regions, 6, **6, 7**
    body cavities, 6–7, *8*
    body map, 2–3, *3*, **4,** *4*
    cell, 21–22
aneurysm, 233–236, 249, 649
    aetiology, 233
    care and management, 234–235
    case study, 235–236
    classification, 233
    Dacron graft, *234*
    dissecting, 233, *233*
    fusiform, 233, *233*
    investigations, 234
    pharmacological treatment, 235
    saccular, 233, *233*
    symptoms, 234
    vital signs, 235–236
angina, 207–210, 534
    blockage in coronary arteries, 207,
       208
    care and management, 209
    investigations, 207
    non-pharmacological treatment,
       209
    pathophysiology, 207–209
    pharmacological treatment, 209
    signs and symptoms, 209

    stable, 208
    types, 208
    unstable, 208
    variant, 208
angiogenesis, 91
angiogenic growth factor, 91
angiotensin-converting enzyme (ACE)
       inhibitors, 204
angular cheilitis, 395
anion, 591
anorexia, 91
antalgic, 563
anterior, 319
anterior segment, eye, 629
anthropometry, 423
antibiotic, 91, 624
antibodies, 125, 151, 288
    functions of, 117
antibody, 91
anticholinergic, 649
anticholinesterase, 563
antidiarrhoeals, 581
antidiuretic hormone (ADH), 214,
       434, 572
anti-emetic, 579, 591, 650
antifungal, 624
antifungal therapy, 107
antigens, 91, 125, 151, 263, 288
antihistamine, 650
antihypertensives, 169
antimotility medicines, 581
antiplatelet, 534
antipyretic, 356, 650
anti-rheumatoid drugs, 110–111
anuria, 151, 319, 591
anus, *363*
aorta, 188, *208*, 249, 356
    ascending, *189*
    chemoreceptors in, 143
    elastic recoil, *221*
    functions, **190**
aortic arch, *187, 189*
aplastic anaemia (AA), 271–273
    aetiology, 271
    blood transfusion, 273
    care and management, 272–273
    pathophysiology, 272
    pharmacological treatment, 273
    symptoms, 272
apoptosis, 66, *67*, 91, 125
appendages, 600
appendix, *363*
aqueous humour, 629
arachidonic acid, 524, 534
areolar tissue, 40
aromatherapy, 534
arrhythmia, 460
arterial insufficiency, 237–239
    aspirin, 239

    care and management, 238–239
    pain control, 238
    pathophysiology, 237
    pharmacological treatment, 239
    signs and symptoms, 237
    versus venous insufficiency, **238**
arteries, 214, *220*, 221–222, 249
    atheroma build-up, *227*
    elastic, 221
    insufficiency, *see* arterial
       insufficiency
    muscular, 222
    structure, *220*
arteriogram, 226
arterioles, 43, 222, 249
arteriosclerosis, 225–229, 249. *See also*
       atherosclerosis
Arthritis Care, 563
artificial larynx, 641
asbestos, risk of cancer, 72
ascites, 214
aspiration, 650
aspirin, 169, 307, 524
    in arterial insufficiency, 239
asthma, 338–342
    care and management, 340–341
    case study, 342
    pathophysiology, 339, *339*
Asthma UK, 356
asymptomatic, 125, 460, 497
atelectasis, 356
atherosclerosis, 214, 225–229, 233
    aetiology, 225–226
    arteriogram, 226
    care and management, 228
    effects, **228**
    investigations, 226
    pathophysiology, 227–228
    pharmacological treatment,
       228–229
    signs and symptoms, 228
atheroma build-up, in artery, *227*
atheromatous plaque, 213
atopic eczema, 610–611
atria, 188, 214
atrioventricular (AV) bundle, *191*
atrioventricular (AV) node, *191*, 192
atrioventricular valves, 188, *189*, 214
atrophy, 460, 497, 650
atropine, for shock, **146**
aural, 650
aural fullness, 632
autoimmune, 460
autoimmune diseases, 117
autoimmunity, 117, 125
autonomic nervous system (ANS),
       160–161, 534
AVERT, 124
axon, 534

B

bacillus, 356
baclofen, in multiple sclerosis, 176
bacteraemia, 151
bacteria, 103–104, *104*, 125
  bacilli, 104, *104*
  cocci, 104, *104*
  reproduction, 104, *105*
  shapes, 103, *104*
bactericidal, 125
barium meal, 395
baroreceptor, 249
Bartholin's glands, 468, 497
basal cell carcinoma, 91
basal cell carcinoma (BCC), 607–608
basal ganglia, 156
basophils, 261
b-cell lymphocytes, 125
benign, 91, 460, 497
benign prostate, 490–493
  care and management, 491–492
  diagnosis, 490–491
  PSA testing, 493
  sexual health history language, 492
  TURP and sexual function, 493
  TURP procedure, 492
beta-blockers, for angina, 210
bicuspid valve, 188, *189*, 214
bifurcation, 319
bile, 288, *375*, 395
bile duct, *374*
bilirubin, 288
The Biology Project, 124
Biomedical Central, 287
biotin, **406**
biphosphonates, for osteoporosis, **554**
blast cell, 91
blood
  clotted, *254*
  composition, 254, 255
  diseases, 264–284
  formed elements, 257–261
  functions, 255
  glucose levels, 401
  groups, 263–264, 288
  overview, 253
  plasma, 253, 255
  platelets, 261
  properties, 254–255
  protection, 255
  red blood cells, 257–259
  regulation, 255
  transportation, 255
  white blood cells, 259–261
blood-brain barrier, 159, 182
blood cells, 115–118
  leucocytes, 115
  mediator cells, 116
  phagocytic cells, 115–116, *116*

blood clotting, 57, 261–262, **262**
blood pressure, 224, 249
  factors affects, 224
  regulation, 224
blood supply, 599
blood vessels
  ACE inhibitor effects, 204
  arteries, *220*, 221–222
  blood flow, *219*
  blood pressure, 224
  capillaries, *220, 222*, 222–223
  diseases, 224–245
  haemorrhagic stroke, 169
  kidney, *294*
  liver, 373
  overview, 218
  parasympathetic effects, **161**
  structure, 219–223, *220*
  sympathetic effects, **161**
  veins, *220*, 223, *223*
  venules, *220*, 223
B lymphocytes, 261, 288
BMC Cancer, 93
body cavities, 6–7, *8*
body fluid, 569
body map, 2–3, *3*, **4**, *4*
body mass index (BMI), 411, 417, 423
body mechanics, 545
bolus, *368*
bone, 541
  production, 541, *541*
  structure, 542–543, *543*
  types of, 543
bone healing, 548–550
bone marrow, 125
bone marrow biopsy, *81*
bone metastases, 534
botulism, 356
Bowman's capsule, 293, *295*
brachytherapy, 497
bradycardia, 534
bradykinin, 151
brain, 155–159
  blood supply to, 158
  brainstem, *156*, 157–158
  cerebellum, 156, *156*
  cerebrum, 155–156, *156*
  damage to, **169**
  diencephalon, *156*, 157
  parts, *156*
  trauma, 163
breast, *86*
breast cancer
  causes, 86
  signs and symptoms, *86*, 86–87
British and Irish Hypertension Society, 249
British Association of Dermatologists, 617

British Cancer Journal, 93
British Heart Foundation, 213, 249
British Liver Trust, 394
British Lung Foundation, 356
British Medical Journal, 423
British Nutrition Foundation Task Force, 414
British Pain Society, 533
British Society for Allergy and Clinical Immunology, 151
British Society of Gastroenterology, 395
British Thoracic Society, 355–356
Brittle Bone Society, 563
bronchiectasis, 348
bronchospasm, 214
Brown Skin Matters, 617
buffer, 423
bundle branches, *191*, 192
bundle of His, *191*, 192
BUPA, 213

C

cachexia, 91
caecum, *363*
calcium, **407**
calculus, 319
calf-muscle pump, *240*
calories, 401
calprotectin, 385, 395
calyces, 319
cancer, 91
  acute lymphoblastic leukaemia, 79–83
  alcohol and risk of, 71
  biology, 66–69
  breast, 85–88
  causes, 69–73
  clinical model, 68, *69*
  colon, 78
  definition, 65
  development, 68, *68*
  diet and risk of, 71
  drug therapy, 75–76
  environmental factors, 70–73
  environmental pollution, 72
  genes, role of, 69–70
  gene therapy, 77
  hormonal therapy, 77
  hormones and risk of, 72
  immunotherapy, 76
  lung, 83–85
  molecular biology model, 68, *68*
  occupational exposure, 72
  overview, 65–66
  pain, 514–517, **515**
  photodynamic therapy, 77
  prevention, 77–78

cancer (cont'd)
  radiation exposure, 70–71
  radiation therapy, 76
  sexual and reproductive behaviour, 71
  signs and symptoms, 74, 74–75
  sites, 74
  smoking and risk of, 71
  staging, 73–74
  surgical therapy, 76–77
  treatment, 75–77
  viruses and, 73
cancerous cell, 67
Cancer Research UK, 93
Cancer Symptoms, 93
Candida albicans, 376
candidiasis, 376
Cannon, Walter, 50
cannula, 650
capillaries, 220, 222, 222–223, 249
captopril, for heart failure, 204
carbamazepine (Tegretol), in epilepsy, 179
carbohydrates, 46, 400–401, 423
carcinogen, 91, 356
carcinogenesis, 66
cardia, 369
cardiac accelerator nerves, 192, 192–193
cardiac muscle, 41, 188
cardiac output, 142
cardiogenic shock, 134, **140,** 205–207
  aetiology, 205
  causative factors, **140**
  cycle of, 206
  investigations, 205
  pathophysiology, 205–206
  pharmacological treatment, 207
  signs and symptoms, 206
cardiovascular (CV) centre, 192
cardiovascular system, 131
Caring for people with a learning
      disability. Resources from the
      Royal College of Nursing, 497
carotid arteries, 158
  endarterectomy, 169
carotid artery, 356
carrier/transport protein, 46
cartilage, 40, 356, 563, 650
catalysts, 46
cataracts, 641–642
cation, 591
cauda equina syndrome, 558
cauterisation, 650
cauterising the nasal septum, 634
cell(s)
  anaerobic metabolism, 206
  anatomy, 21–22
  apoptosis, 66, 67
  cancerous, 67

characteristics, 20–21
clotted, 253, 254
differentiation, 91
division, 91
immune system, 111
mediator, 116
microscopic, 98
neuroglia-supporting, 42
nucleus, 21, 21, 27–28
organelles, 22, 32–35, 47
phagocytic, 43, 115–116
precancerous, 67
structure, 21
tissues, 36–43
types of, 35
cell cycle, 30, 30–31
cell-mediated immunity, 125
cell membrane, 22–27, 47
  anatomy, 22–23, 23
  degree of permeability, 24–25
  functions, 22–23, 24
  transport across, 23–27
cell stability, 51–52
cell theory, 20
central cyanosis, 356
central nervous system (CNS), 155,
      155–161, 156, 534
  cerebrospinal fluid, 159
  meninges, 159
  spinal cord, 159, 160
centrioles, 35
cerebellum, 156, 156, 158
cerebral arterial circle, 158
cerebral cortex, 156, 534
cerebrospinal fluid (CSF), 159, 356
cerebrovascular accident, 167, 183
cerebrum, 155–156, **156,** 156, 158
cerumenolytic, use of, 630
cervix, 469, 470
C fibres, 504, **504,** 511
Changing Faces, 617
cheeks, 364, 364
chemical barriers, 114–115
chemical compensatory mechanisms, 143
chemical digestion, 363, 370
chemical reaction, 46
chemical stimuli, 503
chemoreceptor, 249, 356
chemotherapy, 624
child resistant packaging, 552
chiropractic, 534
chlamydiae, 108
cholecystokinin (CCK), 374, 403
cholesterol, 404
cholesterol reducing drugs, 169
cholinesterase, 563
chordae tendineae, 189
choroid plexus, 183, 628, 629
chromatids, 29, 46

chromosomes, 27, 28, 46
chronic bronchitis, 344–345
chronic eczema, 610
chronic kidney disease, 309–313
  aetiology, 310
  care and management, 311
  case study, 312
  investigations, 310
  pathophysiology, 311
  pharmacological interventions, 312
  signs and symptoms, 310
  staging, **311**
  vital signs, 312–313
chronic lymphoblastic leukaemia
      (CLL), 279
chronic myeloid leukaemia (CML), 279
chronic obstructive pulmonary
      disease, 342–343
  breathlessness, 346
  care and management, 345
  case study, 346
  oxygen therapy, 346
  vital signs, 346–347
chronic pancreatitis, 391
  care and management, 389
  medicines management, 389
  pathophysiology, 391
  signs and symptoms, 391
chronic pyelonephritis, 303–304
  aetiology, 304
  care and management, 304, 305
  investigations, 304
  signs and symptoms, 304, 305
chyme, 370, 374, 395
cilia, 35, 356, 497, 650
  as mechanical barrier, 114
ciliary body, 628, 629
ciprofloxacin, 303
circle of Willis, 158, 158
cisternae, 32
CJD, see Creutzfeldt-Jakob Disease
claudication, 563
clitoris, 468, 497
clotting cascade, 249
coagulation, 262, 288, 650
cocci, 104, 104
coccobacilli, 104, 104
codeine, **522**
coenzyme, 288, 424
cognitive behavioural therapy (CBT), 526
cold therapy, 528
collagen, 214
  fibres, 39, 249
colon, 363, 371
colonoscopy, 582
colorectal cancer, 91
columnar epithelium, simple, 37, 38
commensal, 125

comminuted fracture, 548
complement, 125
compression fracture, 548
computerised tomography (CT) scan, 530
concentration gradient, 25, 46
concordance, 460
cones, 629
congenital, 650
congestive heart failure, 199–205
conjunctiva, 628, 629
connective tissue, 39–41, 288, 650
    characteristics, 39
    dense, 40
    functions, 39
    loose, 40
    reticular, 41
consciousness, level of, 60
contaminated intermediate, 101, 125
controlled drug, 534
control of breathing, 330, 330, **331,** 331
cornea, 628, 628
coronary arteries
    blockage, 207, 208
    function, **190**
coronary artery, 534
coronary ligament, 374
coronary vasoconstriction, 534
coronary veins, **190**
coronavirus disease 2019 (COVID-19), 126
cor pulmonale, 356
corpus callosum, 156
corticotropin, 434
corticotropin-releasing hormone (CRH), 434
cortisol, 437, 439, 534
cranial nerves, **157**
C-reactive protein (CRP), 126
crepitus, 563
crescendo angina, 208
Creutzfeldt-Jakob disease (CJD), 106, 126
cricoid cartilage, 628
Crohn's and Colitis UK, 395
Crohn's disease, 384–388
    care and management, 385
    pathophysiology, 384
    pharmacological intervention, 385–386
    psychological support, 385
    signs and symptoms, 384
    surgical intervention, 386
crystal-induced arthritis, 554
cuboidal epithelial tissue, 37
Cushing's disease, 447, 447–448
cyanosis, 203, 208
cyclo-oxygenase-2, 534
cystic medial degeneration, 233

cystitis, 126, 304–305
cystoscope, 497
cystoscopy, 315
cytokine, 563
cytokines, 126
cytoplasm, 21, 22, 27, 46, 92
cytoskeleton, 34
cytotoxic drugs
    aplastic anaemia, 271–272
    cancer, 75
cytotoxicity, 92
cytotoxic T lymphocytes, 67, 92

D
Dacron graft
    abdominal aortic aneurysm, 234
    peripheral vascular disease, 238
daughter cell, 92
death rates, 65
debridement, 460
deep pain, 509
deep vein thrombosis (DVT), 243–245, 534
    aetiology, 243
    care and management, 245
    clot formation, 244
    formation, 243
    pathophysiology, 243–244
    pharmacological treatment, 245
    platelet plug formation, 244
    signs and symptoms, 245
degranulation, 126
dehydration, 577–578, 581, 591
dementia, 173, 183
demyelination, 175, 183
deoxyribonucleic acid (DNA), 46
    functions, 28
Department of Health (DH), 124, 423
Department of Health and Social Care (DHSC), 213, 249
dermatitis, 611, 624
dermatoscope, 624
descending pain pathways, 506–507
determinants of health, 14–15, 15
detoxification, 591
diabetes insipidus, 442
diabetes mellitus (diabetes), 118
    foot ulcers, 456
    mobilising the patient, 455
    signs and symptoms, 452–453
    type 1 diabetes, 454
    type 2 diabetes, 453, 454–455
Diabetes UK, 459
diabetic foot ulcers, 456
diamorphine, **523**
diapedesis, 260
diaphoresis, 534
diaphragm, 187
diarthrosis, 543
diazepam, in multiple sclerosis, 176

diencephalon, 156, 157
diffusion, 46, 356
    facilitated, 25, 46
    process, 25
digestion, 363, 395
    accessory organs, 373–375
    chemical, 370
    disorders, 376–391
    protein, 370
    swallowing, 368
digital rectal examination (DRE), 491
dihydrocodeine, **522**
dilate, 126
diplobacilli, 104
diplococci, 104, 104
diplopia, 563
disaccharides, 400
discoid eczema, 611
distal, 650
distributive shock, 134, 134–135
    case study, 135–136
    clinical investigation, 136
    vital signs, 135–136
diuresis, 319
diuretics, 460
    heart failure, 204
    hypertension, 232
diverticulum, 497
dobutamine, for shock, **146**
docusate sodium (Colace), 269
donepezil (Aricept), in Alzheimer's disease, 174
dopamine, 183
    in Parkinson's disease, 172
    for shock, **146**
dorsal, 497
dorsal horn (spinal cord), 505, 505, 534
drop attacks, 632
dual energy X-ray absorptiometry (DXA) scan, 553
duct, 395
ductal carcinoma, 86
duodenal ulcers, 377
duodenum, 363, 369, 370–371, 371, 374, 374
dynorphins, 507, 534
dysarthria, 563
dysmenorrhoea
    care and management, 477
    diagnosis, 477
    NSAIDs, 478
    oral contraceptive, 477–478
    pathophysiology, 476–477
    risk factors, 476
    types of, 475, **476**
dyspareunia, 497
dyspepsia, 395
dysphagia, 424, 563, 650
dysphonia, 92
dysphoria, 534

dyspnoea, 92, 151, 214
dysuria, 319

E

ear, 624–626, *625*
  disorders of, 630–633
  external, 625
  inner, 626
  middle, 625
ear surgery, and care, 632
ear wax, 630
eclampsia, 460
ectocervix, 470
eczema, 609–610
  acute, 609–610
  care and management, 612–613
  case study, 613–614
  chronic, 610
  endogenous, 610–611
  exogenous, 611–613
effectors, 52, 53
effusion, 563
elastic arteries, 221
elastic cartilage, 357
elastic fibres, 39
electroencephalogram (EEG), 178
electrolarynx, 641
electrolytes, 460, 570–571, **571,**
  571, 591
emotional brain, *see* limbic
  system
emphysema, 344, *345*
encephalins, 507
encirclement, in retinal detachment,
  645
endocardium, 187, *188*, 214
endocrine glands, 38, 395, 429, 460
  physiology, 433–440
  receptors, 431
endocrine-releasing organs, 429–430
The Endocrine Society, 459
EndocrineSurgeon.co.uk, 459
endocrine system, 429–430
  disorders, 440–456
  physiology, 433–440
  response to stress, *439*
endocytosis, 21, 23, *24*, 46, 126
endogenous, 126
endogenous infection, 98
endogenous opiate, 507
endometrial ablation, **484**
endoplasmic reticulum, *21*, 32–33
  agranular, *32*, 33
  anatomy, *32*, 32–33
  granular, *32*, 33
endorphins, 507, 534
endothelium, 249
enteral nutrition, 419, 424
enteric fevers, 126

enzymes, 46, 126, 357, 395, 534
eosinophils, 261
epicardium, 187, *188*
epiglottis, *368*, 627
epilepsy, 176–179
  care and management, 178
  non-pharmacological
    management, 179
  pathophysiology, 177
  pharmacological management, 179
  psychosocial impact of, 178
epinephrine (adrenaline), 534
  for shock, **146**
epistaxis, 288, 633–634
epithelial cell, 650
epithelial tissue, *36*, 36–38, *38*
epitopes, 126
eructation, 395
erythema, 249, 610, 624
erythroblasts, 258
erythrocytes, *see* red blood cells
erythropoietin, 259, 288, 319
Escherichia coli (E. coli), 98
estimated glomerular filtration rate
  (eGFR), 310
eukaryotic cell, 46
euphoria, 460
excretion, 319
exocrine glands, 38, 395, 460
exocytosis, 25, 46
exogenous, 126
  infection, 98
exophthalmos, 460
expectorate, 357
external intercostal muscle, 357
external respiration, 327–329, *329*, 357
extracellular, 424, 591
extracellular fluid (ECF), 46, 249, 568
extracellular matrix, 46
extrinsic, 624
extrinsic asthma, 357
exudate, 357, 650
eye
  case study, 642–643
  disorders of, 641–646
  physiology of, 628, *628*

F

facial nerve, **157**
facial palsy, 650
facilitated diffusion, 25, 46
fallopian tubes, 470
false vocal cords, 628
fatty acids, 402–403, 424
feedback
  negative, 53–54, *55*
  positive, 54–57, *56*
female breasts, 472, *472*
femur, *240*

fibres, 39, 46
fibrin, 357
fibrinogen, 256
fibroblast cells, 46, 249, 548
fibroid, 497
fibrosis, 319, 357
fibrous, 357, 395
fibrous tunic, 628–629
fibula, *240*
filtration, 25, 319
finger clubbing, 357
fissure, 624
fistula, 395, 424, 650
flagella, *21*, 35
fluid and electrolytes, 567
  balance, 569–575
  clinical investigations, 582–583
  compartments, 567–568, *568*
  composition of, 569
  dehydration, 581
  intake and output, **569**
  lymphoedema, 585
  overload, 570
  vital signs, 585–586
fluid balance chart, 575–576, *576*
  disorders associated, 575
fluid balance monitoring, 142
fluke, 126
fluorescein angiography, 643
fluoxetine, in multiple sclerosis, 176
folate deficiency, 269–270
Foley catheter, 634, 650
folic acid (folate), 273, **407**
follicle-stimulating hormone (FSH),
  434, 471
fomites, 101
Food Allergy and Anaphylaxis
  Network (FAAN), 151
food groups, *408*
foramen magnum, 158, 183
fossa ovalis, *189*
fractures, 548–550
  and bone healing, 548–550
  classifications, 548, *549*
  immobility, complications with, 550
  pathological, 548
  stress, 548
free fatty acids, 403
free T$_4$, 460
frontal lobe, 534
fundus, *369*, 395
fungi, 106, *107*, 126
furosemide, 584, 586–587

G

galantamine (Reminyl), in Alzheimer's
  disease, 174
gallbladder, *363*, 374, *374*
gametes, fusion of, 32

gastrectomy, 288, 424
gastric bypass surgery, *416*
gastric gland, *369*
gastrin, 370
gastrointestinal system, 362, *363*.
        See also digestion
    function, 362–363
    length, 363
    salivary glands, 366–367
    structure, *363*
    upper, 364–373
gastro-oesophageal reflux disease
        (GORD), 381
gastroscopy, 395
general malaise, 92
genetic material, 46
germline cell, 92
gland, 460
glandular epithelium, 38–39
Glasgow Coma Scale (GCS), 164,
        165, 182
glaucoma, 644–645
    acute closed angle, 644
    open angle, 644
globulins, 256
glomerulus, 319
glossopharyngeal nerve, **157**
glucagon, 424, 439–440, 534
glucocorticoids, 437
gluconeogenesis, 401, 424
glucose, 25, 46
glycaemic control, 650
glycaemic index (GI) and control,
        401–402
glyceryl trinitrate (GTN), for angina,
        210
glycogen, 395, 401, 424, 460
glycogenolysis, 401, 424
glycoprotein, 47
goblet cell, 47, 357
goitre, 460
golgi apparatus, *21,* 33
gonadotropins, 434
gout, 554–557
    care and management, 555–556
    diagnosis, 555
    predisposing factors, 555
granulocytes, 260
granzyme, 67
gray, 92
greater omentum, *371*
greenstick fracture, 548
grey matter, 156
ground substance, 47
growth hormone-inhibiting hormone
        (GHIH), 434
growth hormone-releasing hormone
        (GHRH), 434
gut helminths, *see* helminths
Guts UK, 395

H
haem, 257
haematocrit, 288
haematoma, 564
haematuria, 319
haemoglobin (Hb), 92, 257–258, *258,*
        288, 357
    defects, 274
haemoglobinopathies, 274
haemolysis, 259, *260*
haemolytic anaemia, 274–275
    aetiology, 274
    care and management, 274–275
    pathophysiology, 274
    signs and symptoms, 274
haemolytic–uremic syndrome (HUS),
        281
haemopoiesis, 564
haemoptysis, 92, 357
haemorrhage, 650
haemorrhagic stroke, 169
haemostasis, 261–262, **262,** 288
    coagulation, 262
    platelet aggregation, 262
    vasoconstriction, 262
hair follicles, 601–603
head injury, management of, 166
Health concerns (web site), 287
heart
    apex of, *187*
    base of, *187*
    blood flow, 190
    cardiac muscle, *188*
    chambers, 188, *189*
    chest pain and hypertension, 193
    conducting system, 190–192
    diseases, 193–210
    failure, *see* heart failure
    location, 186, *187*
    output to, *192*
    structure, 187–190
    12-lead ECG, 195
    valves, 188, *189*
    vessels, 188, *189*
heart failure (HF), 199–205
    ACE inhibitors, 204
    aetiology, 201
    care and management, 203–204
    case study, 200
    echocardiography, 202
    investigations, 201
    left, 199, 202
    non-pharmacological treatment,
        204
    pathophysiology, 201
    pharmacological treatment, 204
    right, 199, 202
    signs and symptoms of, 203
    vital signs, 200–201
heat therapy, 528

heavy menstrual bleeding (HMB), 480
    care and management, 482–484
    contraceptive implant, 482
    diagnosis, 481–482
helminths, 108–109, 126
hepatic artery, 373
hepatic duct, *374*
hepatic portal vein, 373
hepatic vein, 373
hepatopancreatic ampulla, *374*
hepatosplenomegaly, 92
herd immunity, 126
hereditary, 650
hilus, 319
histamine, 151, 534
histology, 624
histoplasmosis, 126
HIV tutorial (University of Utah), 125
homeopathy, 534
homeostasis, 151, 288, 460
    components for, 52
    overview, 50–51
    stable psychological condition, 52
    systems and, **58–59**
    vital signs and, 57–60
homeostatic cycle, 51–52, *52*
hormone replacement therapy (HRT),
        for osteoporosis, **554**
hormones, 430–433, 460
    adrenocorticotropic, 434
    amino acid-based, 431
    antidiuretic, 214
    circulating, *430*
    compensatory mechanisms,
        141–143
    definition, 47
    glucocorticoid, 437
    growth, 433
    hypothalamus, 433–434, **434**
    local, *430*
    parathyroid, 436
    pituitary gland, 433–434, **434**
    position, *431*
    receptors, *430,* 431
    regulation, 431
    release, *430,* 432
    response, 432
    target cells, 429
    thyroid, *435,* 435–436
    thyrotropin-releasing, 434
    transport, *430*
HPV, *see* human papillomavirus
HPV vaccines, 79
human papillomavirus (HPV),
        71, 78
human physiology, 8
humidification, 650
humoral immunity, 126
hydration, 577
hydrocele, 489–490

hydrochloric acid, 370
hydronephrosis, 498
hydrostatic pressure, 357
hydroureter, 498
hyperalgesia, 513, 534
hypercalcaemia and cardiac
        arrhythmias, 447
hypercapnia, 357
hyperglycaemia, 453, 460
hyperkalaemia, 319, 460
hyperkeratosis, 610, 624
hyperparathyroidism, 446
hypersecretion, 460
hypersensitivity reaction, 151
hypertension, 229–233, 249, 357, 460,
        534, 650
    aetiology, 230
    diuretics, 232
    FAST test, 230
    investigations, 230
    isolated systolic, 231
    malignant, 231
    non-pharmacological treatment,
        231–232
    pathophysiology, 230–231
    pharmacological treatment, 232
    primary, 230–231
    secondary, 231
    symptoms, 230
    types, 230
hyperthermic, 460
hyperthyroidism, 443–444
    long-term effects, 444
    signs and symptoms, 443–444
    thyroid storm, 445
    treatment, 444
hypertonic, 591
hyperventilation, 151
hyphae, 106, 127
hypnotherapy, 528
hypodermoclysis, 578, 591
hypoglycaemia, 460
hyponatraemia, 319, 460
hypoparathyroidism, 446
hypoperfusion, 151
hypopharynx, *627*, 627–628
hypopituitarism, 441–442
    causes, 441, *441*
    signs and symptoms, 442
    treatment, 442
hypoproteinaemia, 357
hyposecretion, 460
hypotension, 357, 460
hypothalamus, 157, 535
    hormones, **434**
    physiology, 433–440
hypothermic, 460
hypothyroidism, 444–446
    causes, 444
    elderly patients, 445

myxoedemic coma, 446
    signs and symptoms, 445
    thyroxine replacement therapy, 445
    treatment, 445
hypotonic, 591
hypoventilation, 535
hypovolaemia, 461, 650
hypovolaemic shock, 133–134
    causative factors, **140**
    clinical presentation, **141**
hypoxaemia, 357, 535
hypoxia, 141, 151, 357, 535
hysterectomy, **484**
hysterosalpingogram, 498

I

ibuprofen, 307
idiopathic thrombocytopenic purpura
        (ITP), 281
IgA, 116–117
IgD, 116–117
IgE, 116–117
IgG, 116–117
IgM, 116–117
ileocaecal valve, *371*
The Ileostomy and Internal Pouch
        Support Group, 395
ileum, *363, 371*, 372
imipramine (Tofranil), in multiple
        sclerosis, 176
immune system, 97, 111–118
    blood cells, 115–118
    cells, 111
    immune surveillance, 67
    immunity, 113–115. *See also*
        immunity
    innate, 114–116
    lymphatic system, 111–113, *112*
    malfunctioning, 117
    organs, 111
    proteins, 111
immunity, 114–115, 288
    herd, 126
    non-specific, 114–116
    specific, 116
    types, 113
immunodeficiencies, 117, 127
immunoglobulins, 127, 151, 288
immunoglobulin tests, 116–117
immunology, 111
immunosuppressant drugs, 110–111
immunosuppressive, 564
infection, 97
    aerosol transmission, 99
    airborne transmission, 99
    case study, 102–103
    contact transmission, 100
    contaminated intermediates, 101
    droplet spread, 98–99

endogenous, 98
exogenous, 98
faecal-oral route, 101
of host cells, 105
inoculation, 100–101
peripheral intravenous cannula,
        133
person-to-person transmission, 100
soil, 100
spreading/transmission, 98–103
vector transmission, 101
vital signs, 102
waterborne transmission, 99
inferior vena cava, *189*, **190,** *208*, 214,
        219
inflammation, 118–120, 127
    blood test to detect, 120
    causes, 120
    effects, 120
    process, 118, *119*
    symptoms and signs, 119
inflammatory bowel disease, 383, 395
    Crohn's disease, 384–388
    investigations for, 384–385
    ulcerative colitis, 383–384
inflammatory breast carcinoma, 86
infundibulum, *433*
inhaler technique, 342–343
inoculation, 100–101
inorganic substance, 47
inotrope, 461
insulin, 439–440
    resistance, 461
integral plasma membrane proteins,
        22
integumentary, 624
intercostal nerve, 357
intermediate filaments, 34
intermittent claudication, 235
internal carotid artery, *158*
internal intercostal muscle, 357
internal respiration, 357
interstitial fluid, 151
interstitial space, 214, 591
intestine, 396
intracellular, 424, 591
intracellular fluid (ICF), 568
intracellular space, 214
intracranial, 650
intracranial pressure (ICP), increased,
        163–165
    care and management, 164
    cerebrovascular accident, 167
    effects, 164
    head injury, management of,
        166–168
    signs and symptoms, 163
    vital signs, 167
intraocular pressure (IOP), 644, 650
intravenous pyelogram (IVP), 315

intravenous urogram (IVU), 315
intrinsic, 624
    asthma, 357
    factor, 288
intubation, 357
involuntary, 319
ionising radiation, 70, 71
ions, 23, 47, 461
iris, *628, 629*
iron, **407**
iron deficiency anaemia, 266–269
    aetiology, 266
    bone marrow sample, 267
    care and management, 268
    investigations, 266–267
    pathophysiology, 267–268
    pharmacological treatment,
        268–269
    signs and symptoms, 268
iron supplements, 269
ischaemia, 151, 498, 535, 650
ischaemic heart disease, 461
ischaemic stroke, 169
islets of Langerhans, 439
isoproterenol, for shock, **146**
isotonic, 591

J

jejunum, *363, 371, 372, 374*
joints, 543–544, *544*
Journal of Kidney Care, 319
Journal of Renal Care, 319

K

keratin, 597, 600–602, 624
keratinise, 624
ketone, 424
ketosis, 461
kidney, 292–298, 320
    acute kidney injury, 305–309
    blood supply, 296
    chronic kidney disease, 309–313
    composition of urine, 297–298
    external structure, 292, *293*
    functions, 296
    internal structure, 292–293, *294*
    nephrons, 293–296, *295*
    urine formation, 296–297
kinin, 43, 535
Kinin System, 127
kwashiorkor, 424
kyphosis, 357

L

labia majora, 498
labia minora, 498
lactic acid, 214
laparoscopy, 498
laparotomy, 498

large intestine, 372–373, *373,* 396
    anatomy, 372, *373*
    functions, 372
    length, 372
laryngectomy, 637, 638–641, *640*
    case study, 639–640
    and hypoxia, 641
    loss of patient's voice after, 641
laryngopharynx, *368*
larynx, *324,* 324–325, 627–628
laxatives, 650
    in multiple sclerosis, 176
left heart failure (LHF), 199, 202
    backward effects, 203
    forward effects, 203
Legionnaire's disease, 99, 127
lens, 629
leptospirosis, 99, 127
lesion, 564
leucocytes, *see* white blood cells
leukaemia, 276, 278–281
    aetiology, 279
    care and management, 280
    case study, 278
    non-pharmacological treatment,
        280–281
    pathophysiology, 279–280
    pharmacological treatment,
        280–281
    symptoms, 280
    types, 279
    vital signs, 278
leukocytosis, 127
levodopa, in Parkinson's disease, 172
lichenification, 610, 624
ligament, 564
ligamentum atreriosum, *189*
ligation, 650
limbic system, 506, *506,* 509, 535
lingual frenulum, *367*
lipids, 47, 402–404, 424, 650
    absorbed, 403
    solubility in, 25
lipodermatosclerosis, 241, *242*
lipoprotein, 424
lipoproteins, 403, *404*
lips, 364, *364*
liver, *363,* 373–374
    anatomy, *374*
    blood vessels, 373
    functions, 373–374
    lobes, *374*
lobular carcinoma, 86
London Pain Consortium, 533
low back pain (LBP), 529, 557–559
    care and management, 558
    diagnosis, 558
    risk factors, 557
lower respiratory tract, 325–327, *326,
    327*

lumen, 249, 498
    artery, *220*
    vein, *220*
lung (pulmonary) function test,
        347–348
lungs
    cancer, 71, 78, 83–85, 349
    epithelial tissue, 37
    location, *187*
    sympathetic/parasympathetic
        effects, **161**
    types, 85
luteinising hormone (LH), 434, 471
lymph
    node, 92, 113, *113,* 357, 650
    vessels, 599
lymphoblast, 92
lymphocytes, 261, 357
lymphoedema, 585
Lymphoedema Support Network, 590
lymphoid tissue, 113
lymph vessel, 357
lysosomes, *21,* 23, 33, 47
lysosyme, 47, 288

M
MacMillan Cancer Support, 356
macrocytic anaemia, 269–271
    aetiology, 269
    care and management, 271
    folate deficiency, 269–270
    vitamin B$_{12}$ deficiency, 270–271
macronutrients, 400–405, 424
    carbohydrates, 400–401
    glycaemic index (GI) and control,
        401–402
    lipids, 402–404
    proteins, 402
macrophages, 127, 250, 261, 357, 564
macular degeneration, 642–643
    case study, 642
    dry, 643
    fundus fluorescein angiography,
        643
    wet, 643
magnesium, **407**
Magnetic resonance angiography
        (MRA), 307
magnetic resonance imaging (MRI)
        scan, 171
malaise, 630, 650
male reproductive tract, 484–486, *485*
    benign prostate, 490–493
    disorders, 486–487
    genitalia, 484–486
    malignant prostate, 490–493
    testicular torsion, 487
    vital signs, 487
malignant, 92, 461, 498

malignant melanoma, 605–607
  care and management, 607
  changes in moles, **606**
  diagnosis, 606–607
  risk factors, 605–606
  signs and symptoms, 606
malnutrition, 411–419
  aetiology, 417
  assessment, 418–419
  care and management, 417–418
  complications, 416
  screening tools, 417
  signs and symptoms, 417
Malnutrition Universal Screening Tool
    (MUST), 413
marasmus, 424
Marfan's syndrome, 233
massage, 528
mast cell, 357
mast cell degranulation, 43
mastication, 396
mastoidectomy, 632
mastoiditis, 631
McGill Pain Questionnaire, 519, *520*
mechanical barriers, 114
mechanical digestion, 363, 370
mechanical stimuli, 502
mechanoceptors, 503
mediastinum, 214
mediator cells, 116
medulla oblongata, 158, 214, 358
megakaryocyte, 92
meiosis, 31–32, 47
  fusion of gametes, 32
  stages, **31,** 31–32
melanoma, 92
memantine (Ebixa), in Alzheimer's
    disease, 174
menarche, 92
Ménière's disease, 632–633
meninges, 159
meniscectomy, 564
menorrhagia, drugs for treatment,
    483–484
Men's Health Forum, 496
menstrual cycle, *471,* 471–472
  case study, 473
  clinical investigation, 474–475
  female breasts, 472
  menstrual disorders, 472
  vital signs, 473–474
mesencephalon, 157
mesenchyme, 288
mesentery, *371*
metabolism, 47, 591
metabolite, 47
metaphase, 29, *29,* 31
metastasise, 75, 92
metoclopromide, 579
microcytic anaemia, 266

microfilaments, *21,* 34
micronutrients, 405–409, 424
  minerals, 405, **407**
  vitamins, 405, **406–407**
microorganisms, 97–98, 127
  bacteria, 103–104, *104,* 125
  chlamydiae, 108
  fungi, 106, *107,* 126
  helminths, 108–109
  mycoplasmas, 108
  protozoa, 106
  rickettsiae, 107
  types of, **103,** 103–111
  viruses, 104–106, *105*
Microscopy, Culture and Sensitivity
    test, 103
microtubules, 34
micturition, 320
midbrain, 157
middle cerebral artery, *158*
milk teeth, 365, *365*
mineralocorticoids, 437
minerals, 405, **407**
miosis, 535
mitochondria, *21,* 34, 288
mitosis, 28–31, 47
  anaphase, 29, *29*
  metaphase, 29, *29*
  prophase, 28–29, *29*
  stages, 28–29
  telophase, 30, *30*
mitral valve, 214
modality, 53
mole, 605
molecule, 214, 288
monocytes, 261
monosaccharides, 400
mons pubis, 498
morphine, **523**
motor nerve, 535
mucosa, *369,* 650
mucosal membranes, 127
  as physical barrier, 114
mucous membrane, 650
mucus, 370, 651
multiple sclerosis (MS), 175–76
  care and management, 176
  pathophysiology, 175
  pharmacological management, 176
  signs and symptoms, 176
muscle, *544,* 544–545
  atrophy, 535
  cardiac, 41
  skeletal, 41
  smooth, 41
  tissue, 41
muscular arteries, 222
muscular dystrophy, 358
muscularis, *369*
musculoskeletal system, *541,* 541–545

  bone, 542–543, *543*
  case study, 556
  clinical investigations, 553
  disorders of, 547–559
  joints, 543–544, *544*
  muscle, *544,* 544–545
  nervous system, 545
  vital signs, 557
mutagen, 92
mutation, 92
Mycoplasma genitaleum, 108
Mycoplasma hominis, 108
Mycoplasma pneumoniae, 108
mycoplasmas, 108
myelin, 535
myelinated, 535
  nerve axons, 156
mylohyoid muscle, *367*
myocardial infarction (MI), 196–199,
    197, 214
  aetiology, 196
  care and management, 197–198
  investigations, 196
  non-pharmacological treatment,
    198
  pathophysiology, 196–197
  pharmacological treatment, 198
  signs and symptoms, 197
  sublingual glycerine trinitrate, 199
myocardium, 187, *188,* 214
myomectomy, **484**
myosin, 262
myringoplasty, 631
myxoedemic coma, 446

N

naevus, 605, 624
nails, *602,* 602–603, *603*
nasal packing, 634
nasal polyps, 635
nasal septum, deviated, 634–635
nasal surgery, and care, 635
nasogastric (NG) tube feeding, 419
nasojejunal (NJ) tube feeding, 419
nasopharynx, *368*
The National Association of
    Laryngectomee Clubs, 649
National Early Warning Score (NEWS),
    214
National Heart, Lung and Blood
    Institute, 287
National Institute for Health and Care
    Excellence (NICE), 17, 164,
    182, 213, 248, 249, 287, 319,
    355, 423, 496, 563, 590
National Institute for Health and Care
    Excellence (NICE) – Obesity,
    423
National Resource for Infection
    Control (NRIC), 124

National Tracheostomy Safety Project, 649
Natriuretic Peptide Test (NT-proBNP), 215
natural killer cells, 127
Natural Rubber Latex (NRL), 612
nausea, 579, 591
necrosis, 651
needle aspiration, 651
negative feedback, 53–54
neonatal pain, 527
neoplasm, 92
nephrons, 293–296, 295, 320
  with capillaries, 297
  produces dilute urine, 295
nerve cell, 35
nervous system, 154
  autonomic, 160–161, 545
  central, 155–156, 155–161
  disorders, see nervous system disorders
  parasympathetic, 161, 161
  peripheral, 155, 155, 155–161, 183
  somatic, 159
  structure, 42, 155–161
  sympathetic, 161, 161, 183
nervous system disorders, 161–179
  Alzheimer's disease, 173–175
  brain trauma, 163
  dementia, 173
  epilepsy, 176–179
  intracranial pressure, raised, 163–165
  multiple sclerosis, 175–176
  Parkinson's disease, 171–173
  road traffic collision, 162
  seizures, 176–179
  status epilepticus, 177–178
  stroke (cerebrovascular accident), 168–171
  traumatic brain injury, 163
  vital signs, 162, 166
nervous tissue, 41–42
neural compensatory mechanisms, 141
neurogenic (vasogenic) shock, 140
  causative factors, 140
  clinical presentation, 141
neuroglia-supporting cells, 42, 47
neurohypophysis, 433
neurological, 651
neuron, 503–504, 535
neuropathic pain, 513
neuropathy, 461
neuropeptide, 535
neurotransmitter, 535
neutropaenia, 127
neutropenia, 82
neutrophils, 127, 260, 358
NHS Choices, 213, 533

NHS Clinical Knowledge Summaries, 150
niacin, 406
NICE, see National Institute for Health and Care Excellence
nociceptive-specific (NS) neurons, 505
nociceptors, 502–503, 535
nocturia, 320
non-invasive positive pressure ventilation (NIPPV), 358
non-opioid analgesia, for pain management, 523–525
non-steroidal anti-inflammatory drugs (NSAIDs), 524, 525, 535
norepinephrine, 183
  for shock, 146
normocytic anaemia, 271
  nose, 626, 626–627
nose bleed, see epistaxis
nuclear membrane, 47
nucleolus, 47
nucleoplasm, 27, 47
nucleosome, 47
nucleotide sequence, 92
nucleus, 21, 21, 27–28, 35, 105, 288
nulliparous, 92, 498
nummular eczema, see discoid eczema
Nursing and Midwifery Council Code, 268
nursing/medical dictionary
  hints and tips for using, 15–16, 16
nutrient, 424
nutrition, 400–420
  disorders, 410–420
  enteral, 419
  parenteral, 420
  requirements, 408
  during shock, 145
Nutrition Facts, 423

O
obesity, 411–415, 424
  aetiology, 412–413
  assessment tools, 413
  BMI assessment, 413
  care and management, 414
  case study, 415–416
  complications, 412
  nutritional status, 413
  orlistat, 414–415
  pharmacological intervention, 414
  signs and symptoms, 413
  surgery, 415–416, 416
obligate intracellular parasites, 127
oblique fracture, 548
O blood group, 263
obstructive lung disorders, 337–338
obstructive shock, 134
  causative factors, 140

oculomotor nerve, 157
oedema, 127, 358, 573–575, 591
  care and management, 583–587
  causes, 573–574
  definition, 573
  generalised, 573
  localised, 573
  peripheral, 574–575, 584–586
  pitting, 573
  pulmonary, 574, 583–584
oesophageal speech, 641
oesophageal sphincter, 369
oesophagus, 363, 367, 368–369, 396
olfactory, 651
  nerve, 157
oliguria, 215, 320, 396, 591
oncogene, 92
oncogenic viruses, 69–73, 92
opacity, 651
opaque, 651
open angle glaucoma, 644
opiate, 535, 564
  endogenous, 507
  receptor, 507, 521, 521, 535
opioids, for pain management, 521, 521–523
opportunistic screening, 461
opsonisation, 127
optic nerve, 157
oral candidiasis, 376
oral cavity, 363–366, 396
  cheeks, 364, 364
  lips, 364, 364
  palates, 364, 365
  teeth, 365–366, 365–366
  tongue, 364, 365
oral contraceptives, and cancer risk, 72–73
oral hygiene, 376
oral hypoglycaemic, 461
organelles, 22, 32–35, 47, 289, 424
  centrioles, 35
  cilia, 35
  cytoskeleton, 34
  endoplasmic reticulum, 32, 32–33
  flagella, 35
  Golgi apparatus, 33
  lysosomes, 33
  mitochondria, 34
  peroxisomes, 33–34
orlistat, for obesity, 414–415
oropharynx, 368, 627, 627
orthopnoea, 203, 215
os, 498
osmolality, 591
osmolarity, 320
osmosis, 26, 47, 289, 461, 569–570, 591
  and movement of solute, 26
  process, 25

osmotic pressure, 47, 358, 591
ossiculoplasty, 631
ossification, 564
osteoarthritis, 550–552, *551*
    care and management, 551
    diagnosis, 551
    joints affected, 550
    risk factors, 550
    signs and symptoms, 551
osteoblast, 564
osteoclasts, 461, 564
osteology, **548**
osteopathy, 528, 535
osteophyte, 564
osteoporosis, 461, 552–554, 564
    care and management, 553–554
    diagnosis, 552–553
    risk factors, 552
otitis externa, 630
otitis media, 631–632
otosclerosis, 632
ovulation, 92
oxidation, 250
oxidative phosphorylation, 47
Oxybutynin (Ditropan), in multiple
        sclerosis, 176
oxycodone, **523**
oxygen saturation, 60
oxygen therapy, 142, 145
oxytocin, 434

P
pacemaker, 215
Paget's disease, 250
pain, 501
    acute, 507
    ascending pathway, *503*, 503–505
    assessment, 517–520
    cancer, 514–517, **515**
    chronic, 508
    classification, 507–509
    deep, 509
    descending pathways, 506–507
    effects of, **514**
    experience, 509
    gate control theory, *510*, 510–511
    impulses, 504
    management, 511–512, 519–530
    neonatal, 527
    pathophysiology, 511–512
    phantom limb, 511–512
    physiology of, *502*, 502–507
    superficial, 509
    theories, 510–511
    visceral, 509
Pain Concern, 533
pain rating index (PRI), 519
Pain Talk, 533
pain threshold, 509
palates, *364*, 365, *368*, 396

palpation, 651
palpitations, 461
pancreas, *363, 374*, 375
    disorders, 452–456
    endocrine function, 375
    exocrine function, 375
    hyperglycaemia, 453
    physiology, 439–440
    type 1 diabetes, 454
    type 2 diabetes, 453, 454–455
pancreatitis, 388–391, 396
    acute, 388–390
    chronic, 391
papilloedema, 250
paracetamol, 524
paralytic ileus, 396
paraphimosis, 489
parasite, 127
parasthaesia, 461
parasympathetic nervous system
        (PNS), 161, **161,** 183, 192–193,
        215
parathyroid glands
    disorders, 446
    hyperparathyroidism, 446
    hypoparathyroidism, 446
    physiology, 436
parathyroid hormone (PTH), 436
parenchyma, 320
parenteral nutrition, 396, 420
Parkinson's disease (PD), 171–173
    care and management, 173
    non-pharmacological
        management, 173
    pathophysiology, 172
    pharmacological management, 172
parotid gland, *363, 367*
passive immunisation, 127
passive transport, 25, 47
patch testing, 614
pathoanatomical, 564
pathogen, 127, 289
pathological fractures, 548
pathophysiology, 13–14
    objectives of, 14
    terms and definitions, **13**
patient-controlled analgesia (PCA),
        523, 535
peak expiratory flow rate, 358
pelvic inflammatory disease (PID), 127
pelvis, 466–467, *467*
    female external genitalia, 467–468,
        468
pepsinogen, 370
peptic ulcer, 377–383, *378*
    care and management, 380
    case study, 380–381
    clinical investigation, 379–380
    complications, 379
    GORD, 381

investigations, 379
    medicines management, 382–383
    obesity management, 382
    pathophysiology, 378–379
    pharmacological interventions, 380
    risk factors, 377–378
    signs and symptoms, 379
    sites, *378*
    vital signs, 381
percutaneous endoscopic
        gastrostomy (PEG), 419
pericardial cavity, *188*
pericardium, 187, *188,* 215
peripheral artery disease, 461
peripheral intravenous cannula (PVC),
        133
peripheral nervous system (PNS), 155,
        155, 159, 183, 535
peripheral oedema, 574–575, 584–586
peripheral plasma membrane
        proteins, 22
peripheral vascular disease (PVD),
        236–237
    aetiology, 237
    Dacron graft, *238*
    Doppler ultrasound, 237
    investigations, 237
peripheral vascular resistance, 151
peristalsis, *42,* 396, 498
peritoneum, 396
peritonsillar abscess, 636
permanent teeth, 365–366, *366*
pernicious anaemia (PA), 270
peroxisomes, 33–34
pethidine, **523**
phagocytic cells, 43, 115–116, 120,
        289
phagocytosis, 22, 48, *116,* 127
phantom limb pain, 511–512
pharynx, *363,* 367, *368,* 396
phenytoin (dilantin), in epilepsy, 179
pheromones, 468, 601, 624
phimosis, 488
phospholipids, *404*
phosphorus, **407**
photocoagulation, 645
photodynamic therapy (PDT), 643
photoreceptors, 629
phrenic nerve, 358
physical barriers, 114
physiological parameters, 60
pinocytosis, 22, 48
pitting oedema, 573
Pituitary Foundation, 459
pituitary glands, *158,* 433–440
    diabetes insipidus, 442
    disorders, 441–442
    hormones, **434**
    hypopituitarism, *441,* 441–442
    physiology, 433–434

plasma, 253, 255, 289, 592
  anti-A antibody, *263*
  anti-B antibody, *263*
  electrolytes, 256
  gases, 256
  nutrients of metabolism, 257
  proteins, 256
  waste products of metabolism, 257
  water, 255
plasma membrane, *21*
plasma membrane proteins (PMPs), 22
  integral, 22
  peripheral, 22
plasmapheresis, 564
plasma protein systems, 43
platelets, 261, 289
  aggregation, 262
pleural disorders, 350–352, *351*
  care and management, 352
  signs and symptoms, **351**
plombage (scleral buckling), 645
pneumatic retinopexy, 645
pneumonia, 334–337, 651
  aetiology, 334–335
  care and management, 335–336
  case study, 336
  chest x-ray, 337
  investigations, 335, **335**
  signs and symptoms, 335
podiatrist, 461
poliomyelitis, 358
polycythaemia, 358
polymodal nociceptors, 503
polyp (plural polypi), 651
polypeptide, 289
polysaccharides, 400
pons, 158, *158*, 358
porphyrins, 92
posterior, 320
  segment, eye, 629
postnasal pack, 651
postural hypotension, 461
potassium, **407**
  sparing agents, 232
  transport, 27
precancerous cell, 67, 92
prepuce, 498
present pain index (PPI), 519
pressure necrosis, 651
primary cancer, 92
prions, 105–106, 127
proctitis, 396
prognosis, 92, 624
prokaryotic cell, 48
prolactin, 498
prolactin-inhibiting hormone, 434
prolactinoma, 498
prophase, 28–29, *29*, 31
prostaglandins, 127, 396, 498, 524, 535
Prostate Cancer UK, 497

prostate-specific antigen (PSA), 491
prosthesis, 651
protective isolation, 115
proteins, 402, 424
  immune system, 111
  plasma membrane, 22
proteinuria, 320
proto-oncogene, 92
protoplasm, 48, *105*
protozoa, 106, 127
proximal, 564
pruritus, 535, 610, 624
PSA testing, 493
pseudostratified ciliated columnar
    epithelium, 358
psoriasis, 614–617
  case study, 616–617
The Psoriasis Association, 617
psychological-based pain, 528
psychological impact of isolation, 334
ptosis, 564
ptyalin, 396
Public Health England, 125, 591
puerperal fever, 127
pulmonary artery, **190**, 215
pulmonary circulation, 215
pulmonary embolism, 535
pulmonary oedema, 215, 574
pulmonary rehabilitation, 349–350
pulmonary trunk, *187*
pulmonary veins, **190**, 215
pulmonary ventilation, 327, *328*, 358
pulse oximetry, 358, 651
pulse rate, 60
pulsus paradoxus, 358
Pumping marvellous, 213
pupil, *628*, 629
Purkinje fibres, 190, *191*, 192
purulent, 651
pus, 128, 651
pyelonephritis, 128, 301–304
  acute, 301–303
  care and management, 302
  chronic, 303–304
  investigations, 302
  pharmacological interventions, 303
  signs and symptoms, 302
pyloric region, 396
pylorus, *369*, *371*
pyrexia, 320, 358, 535, 631, 651
pyridoxine, **406**
pyuria, 320

Q
quinsy, 636

R
radiation therapy, 92
radiotherapy, 624

rasagiline, in Parkinson's disease, 172
receptor-mediated endocytosis, 48
receptors, 52, 53
receptor sites, 22, 48
rectum, *363*
red blood cells, 257–259, 357
  destruction of, 259
  formation, *258*, 258–259
  haemoglobin, 257–258, *258*
  haemolysis, 259, *260*
  haemolytic anaemia, 274–275
  respiratory gases, transport of, 259
  sickled, 275
referred pain, 511–512, *513*
reflex arc, 506, *507*, 535
reflexology, 528, 535
regurgitation, 651
relapsing (relapse), 624
renal artery, 320
The Renal Association, 319
renal calculi, *314*, 314–316
  aetiology, 314
  care and management, 316
  investigations, 314
  pharmacological interventions, 316
  signs and symptoms, 315
renal cortex, 320
renal medulla, 320
renal pelvis, 320
renal pyramid, 320
renal system, 291–300, *292*
  disorders, 300–316
  kidneys, 292–298
  ureter, *298*, 298–299
  urethra, 299–300, *300*
  urinary bladder, 299, *299*
renal vein, 320
renin, 320
renin-angiotensin-aldosterone system,
    438
renin angiotensin mechanism, *143*
reproductive health, 465–466
reservoir of infection, 128
respiration rate, 60
respiratory acidosis, 358
Respiratory Education UK, 356
respiratory insufficiency, 651
respiratory system
  anatomy, 324–331
  disorders of, 331–352
  physiology, 324–331
restrictive disorders, 348–349
Resuscitation Council (UK), 150
reticular activating system, 157
reticular connective tissue, 41
reticular fibres, 39
reticular formation, 535
retina, *628*, 629
retinal detachment, 645
retinopathy, 646

rhesus factor (Rh), 264
rheumatoid arthritis, 117
ribosomal ribonucleic acid
        (rRNA), 48
ribosome, *21*, 48
rickettsiae, 107
right heart failure (RHF), 199, 202
rivastigmine tartrate (Exelon), in
        Alzheimer's disease, 174
rods, 629
The Royal College of
        Ophthalmologists, 649
Royal College of Physicians, 182
Royal National Institute of Blind
        People, 649
Royal Osteoporosis Society, 563
rugae of mucosa, *369*

S
sac, 651
saddle anaesthesia, 564
salbutamol, 128
saliva
    composition, 366
    functions, 367
salivary glands, *363*, 366–367, *367*
SBAR Communication tool, 60, **60**
schistosomiasis, 99, 128
Schwann cell, 183
sclera, *628*, 629
scoliosis, 358
Scottish Intercollegiate Guidelines
        Network (SIGN), 17, 590
sebaceous glands, 601–603
seborrhoeic eczema, 611
sebum, 601, 625
secondary bacterial infection, 651
sedation, 651
seizures, 176–179
    care and management, 178
    classification, **177**
selective oestrogen receptor
        modulator (SERM), for
        osteoporosis, **554**
selective permeability, 23, 48
selegiline (Eldepryl), in Parkinson's
        disease, 172
selenium, **407**
semilunar valves, 188, *189*, 215
semi-recumbent, 651
sensory fibre, 535
sensory tunic, 629
sepsis, 137–138
    case study, 137–138
    red flags, **139**
    risk factors for, 139
Sepsis Six care bundle, **146**
septic arthritis, 564
septic shock, 138–139, **140**
    causative factors, **140**

clinical presentation, **141**
septoplasty, 635
septum, 187, 215
serosa, *369*
serotonin, 128, 504, 535–536
set point, 53
Sexual Advice Association, 497
sexual health history language, 492
shiatsu, 527, 536
shock
    anaphylactic (anaphylaxis), 136–137
    cardiogenic, 134, 205–207
    care of patient, 144–146
    case study, 132–133
    causative factors, **140**
    clinical presentation, **141, 144**
    compensatory (non-progressive)
        stage, 141–143, **144**
    distributive, *134,* 134–135
    hypovolaemic, 133–134
    irreversible (refractory) stage,
        143–144, **144**
    neurogenic, 140
    oxygen therapy, 142
    pathophysiology, 140–141
    pharmacological management,
        146, **146**
    physiological changes, **144**
    physiological parameters, 133
    progressive (decompensated)
        stage, 143, **144**
    septic, 138–139
    stages, 141–146
    types, 131–140, **140**
    vital signs, 132
sickle cell anaemia, 275–277
    care and management, 276
    case study, 277
    pain management, 276
    pathophysiology, 275
    symptoms, 276
    vital signs, 277
SIGN: Health Improvement Scotland,
        182
Sign Station, 649
silver nitrate sticks, 634
simple epithelial tissues, 37, *37*
simvastatin, 169
sinoatrial (SA) node, 190, *191*, 192, 215
sinusitis, 635–636
skeletal muscle, 41
skin
    anatomy, 596–603
    appendages, 600
    blood supply, 599
    cancer, 605–609
    case study, 613
    clinical investigations, 614
    dermis, 598–599, *599*
    disorders of, 603–617

eczema, 610–611
epidermis, 597–598, *598*
    lightening products, 617
    manifestations of COVID-19, 617
    physical barrier, 114
    physiology, 596
    problems, **596**
    sensory nerve, 600
    structure, *597*
    subcutis, 600
    sweat glands, 600–601, *601*
    types, **608**
slough, 498
small intestine, 370–372, 396
    duodenum, 370–371, *371*
    functions, 370
    Ileum, *371*, 372
    jejunum, *371*, 372
    length, 370
    mesentery, *371*
smooth muscle, *35*, 41
sodium, **407**
sodium pump, 45
sodium valporate (Epilim), in epilepsy,
        179
solute, 48, 92
solvent, 92
somatic cell, 93
somatic nervous system, 159
somatosensory cortex, 536
source isolation, 115
specific gravity, 320
spherocytosis, 274
sphincter, 320
spinal accessory nerve, **157**
spinal cord, 159, *160*
spinal nerves, 159, *160*
spinothalamic tract, 505, *505*, 536
spiral bacteria, 104, *104*
spiral fracture, 548
spirochetes, 104, *104*
spirometry, 358
spironolactone (Aldactone), 232
spleen, 93, 112, 113
spongiform encephalopathy, acute,
        105–106
squamous cell carcinoma (SCC), 93,
        607–608
squamous epithelium, 37
stable angina, 208
staphylococci, 104, *104*
Staphylococcus aureus, 140
statins, for atherosclerosis, 229
status epilepticus, 177–178
sternum (breastbone), 267
steroids, for cancer, 77
stoma, 592, 651
stomach, *363*, 368–370, *371*, 396
    anatomy, 368, *369*
    layers, *369*

lumen of, *369*
stratified cuboidal epithelial tissue, 38
stratified epithelium, 37, *37*
stratified squamous epithelial tissue, 37, *37*
streptobacilli, 104
streptococci, 104
Streptococcus pyrogenes, 140
stress fracture, 548
stroke (cerebrovascular accident), 168–171
  care and management, 170–171
  factors, 168
  haemorrhagic, 169
  ischaemic, 169
  non-pharmacological management, 169–170
  pathophysiology, 168–169
  pharmacological treatment, 169
  signs and symptoms, **169**
  transient ischaemic attack, 169
Stroke Association, 182
strontium ranelate, for osteoporosis, **554**
subcutis, 600
sublingual gland, *367*
sublingual glyceryl trinitrate, 199
submandibular area, 128
submandibular duct, *367*
submandibular gland, *363, 367*
submucosa, *369*
submucous resection (SMR), 635
substance P, 504, 506, 536
substantia gelatinosa (SG) cells, 511, 536
substantia nigra, 183
sulphur, **407**
superficial pain, 509
superior vena cava, *187,* **190**, *191, 208, 215, 219*
surgical emphysema, 358, 637
Surviving Sepsis Campaign Guidelines, 145
suture, 625, 651
swallowing, *368*
sweat glands, 600–601, *601*
swimmer's ear, 630
sympathetic nerve, 192–193, 215
sympathetic nervous system, 161, **161,** 183
symptomatic, 128
synapse, 536, 564
synarthrosis, 543
syndrome, 536
synovial joints, 543–544, *544*
synthesis, 424
syringing, 651
systemic circulation, 215, 358
systemic lupus erythematous (SLE), 109
systolic blood pressure, 60

T
tachycardia, 358, 461, 536
tachypnoea, 536
T cell lymphocyte, 128
tears, as mechanical barrier, 114
teeth, 365–366, *365–366*
  milk, 365, *365*
telophase, 30, *30*
terminal cancer, 93
terminology, 8–10, **9,** *9,* **11–13**
tetany, 461
thalamus, 157, 536
thermal stimuli, 502
The UK Sepsis Trust Professional Resources, 150
thiamine, **406**
thoracotomy, 536
thorax, 358
throat, *627,* 627–628
  disorders of, 636–641
  hypopharynx, *627,* 627–628
  oropharynx, *627, 627*
thrombin, 262
thrombocytopenia, 93, 281–284
  aetiology, 281
  care and management, 282
  case study, 283
  non-pharmacological treatment, 282–283
  pathophysiology, 281
  pharmacological treatment, 282–283
  signs and symptoms, 282
  vital signs, 283–284
thrombolytic agents, 169
thromboplastin, 262
thromboplastinogenase, 262
thrombotic thrombocytopenic purpura (TTP), 281
thromboxane, 250
thymus gland, 128
thyroid gland
  disorders, 442–447
  hormones, *435,* 435–436
  hypothyroidism, 443–446
  negative feedback control, *435*
  physiology, 435–436
thyroiditis, 461
thyroid nodule, 461
thyroid-releasing hormone (TRH), *435,* 436
thyroid-stimulating hormone (TSH), 434–436, *435*
thyroid storm, 445
thyrotropin, 434
thyrotropin-releasing hormone (TRH), 434
thyroxine replacement therapy, 445
tibia, *240*

tinnitus, 631, 651
tissues, 36–43
  areolar, 40
  connective, 39–41
  epithelial, 36–38
  glandular epithelium, 38–39
  inflammatory response, 43
  injury, 43, 120
  lymphoid, 113
  muscle, 41
  nervous, 41–42
  perfusion, 206, 215
  repair, 42–43
  types, 36
T lymphocytes, 261
tongue, *364, 365, 367*
tonicity, 592
tonsillitis, 636
tonsils, 627
topical, 625
toxic shock syndrome (TSS), 140, 151
trabeculae carneae, *189*
tracheo-oesophageal fistula, 637
tracheostomy, 358, 636–638, *637*
  care after, 637–638
  complications, 637
  cuffed tracheostomy tubes, 638
  purpose of, 636–637
  temporary, 637, *637*
  uncuffed tracheostomy tubes, 638
tramadol, **522**
transcutaneous electrical nerve stimulation (TENS), 527, 536, 554
transient ischaemic attack (TIA), 169
transitional epithelium, 38
transmembrane ion gradient, 48
transmission (T) cells, 511
transport of gases, 358
  and internal respiration, 330
transport proteins, 25
transrectal ultrasound (TRUS), 491
transverse fracture, 548
trauma and shock factsheet, 150
traumatic brain injury, 163
triamterene (Dyrenium), 232
tricarboxylic acid cycle, 48
tricuspid valve, 188, *189,* 215
trigeminal nerve, **157**
triglycerides, *404,* 424
trocar, 498, 651
trochlear nerve, **157**
trypanosomiasis, 128
tryptase test, 136
T score, DXA scan, 553
tuberculosis, 333–334
  pharmacological therapy, 334
tubulin, 34
tumour, 93
tumour suppressor gene, 93

tunica externa, *220, 250*
tunica interna, *220*
tunica intima, 250
tunica media, *220, 250*
tunnel vision, 644
TURP procedure, 492
tympanic membrane rupture, 630–631
tympanoplasty, 632
type A antigen, 263
type A blood group, 263
type B antigen, 263
type B blood group, 263

U
UK National Eczema Society, 617
ulceration, 536
ulcerative colitis, 383–384
    case study, 386–387
    pathophysiology, 383
    signs and symptoms, 384
    surgical intervention, 386–388
ultraviolet radiation, 70–71
undernutrition, 424
unilateral, 498
unstable angina, 208
upper respiratory tract, *324,* 324–325
ureter, *298,* 298–299, 320
urethra, 299–300, 320
urgency, 320
uric acid, 564
urinary bladder, 299, *371*
urine
    composition of, 297–298, **298**
    formation, 296–297
urobilinogen, 289
uterine artery embolisation (UAE), **484**
uterus, 469, *469*
uvula, *368*

V
vaccine, 93
vagus nerves, **157,** 192–193
variant angina, 208
variant CJD (vCJD), 106
varicose eczema, 611
varicose veins, 239–242

care and management, 241–242
    complications, 241, *242*
    signs and symptoms, 241
vascular permeability, 128
vascular tissue, 41
vascular tunic (uvea), 629
vasoconstriction, 151, 215, 250, 262
vasodilatation, 151, 250
vasopressin, 434
vectors, 93, 105, 128
veins, *220, 223, 223,* 250
    leg susceptible to varicosity, *241*
    lumen, *220*
    structure, *220*
    varicose, 239–242, *240*
venous eczema, 241, *242*
venous insufficiency, 239–242
    versus arterial insufficiency, **238**
venous return, 536
venous ulcer, *242*
ventricles, 183, 188, *189, 191,* 215
ventricular folds, 628
venules, *220, 223,* 250
verbal rating scale, 518, *518*
Verity, 497
vertigo, 632, 651
vesicles, 48
vesiculation, 610, 625
vestibulocochlear nerve, **157**
vibrios, 104, *104*
villi, *372*
viruses, 104–106, *105,* 128
    infection of host cells, 105
    oncogenic, 69–73, 92
    prions, 105–106
    replication, *105*
    unconventional slow, 105–106
visceral pain, 509
viscous, 625
visual acuity, 642, 651
visual analogue scale, 519, *519*
vitamin B$_{12}$ deficiency, 270–271
vitamins, 405, **406–407,** 424
vitrectomy, 646
vitreous humour, 629
vCJD, *see* variant CJD
vocal cords, *627,* 628
voice prostheses, 641

voluntary, 320
vomiting, 579–580, 592

W
waste products
    cell membrane and, 22
    liver, 373
    by micro-organisms, 98
    nephrons, 293–296, *295*
    plasma, 257
water, 577–578
    balance, 569
    body fluid, 569
    osmotic pressure, 569
    in plasma, 255
    total body water, 569
water-soluble vitamins, **406**
Water UK, 591
wax softener, 630
weight gain, 410
white blood cells, 115, 259–261, 289
white coat syndrome, 138
white matter, 156, 536
wide dynamic range (WDR) neurons, 505
Women's Health Forum Royal College of Nursing, 497
World Health Organisation (WHO), 423, *526*
    analgesic ladder, *526*
wound healing, *119*

X
xerosis, 610, 625

Y
yeasts, 106

Z
zinc, **407**
zona fasciculata, 437
zona glomerulosa, 437
zona reticularis, 437
zonule, *628,* 629
Z score, DXA scan, 553
zygomatic arch, *367*
zygotes, 32